THE ENCYCLOPEDIA OF

ASTHMA AND RESPIRATORY DISORDERS

THE ENCYCLOPEDIA OF

ASTHMA AND RESPIRATORY DISORDERS

Tova Navarra, B.A., R.N.

Foreword by
Charles K. Dadzie, M.D., F.A.A.P., F.C.C.P., Director of
Pediatric Pulmonology and Critical Care Medicine,
Jersey Shore Medical Center, Meridian Health System;
Clinical Assistant Professor, Pediatrics, U.M.D.N.J.,
Robert Wood Johnson Medical School

☑®
Facts On File, Inc.

The Encyclopedia of Asthma and Respiratory Disorders

Facts On File, Inc.
132 West 31st Street
New York NY 10001

Library of Congress Cataloging-in-Publication Data

The encyclopedia of asthma and respiratory disorders / Tova Navarra ; foreword by Charles K. Dadzie
p. cm.
Includes bibliographical references and index.
ISBN 0-8160-4467-8
1. Respiratory organs—Diseases—Encyclopedias. 2. Asthma—Encyclopedias. I. Title.
RC732 .N37 2002
616.2'38'003—dc21   2002002445

Text and cover design by Cathy Rincon

Printed in the United States of America

VB FOF 10 9 8 7 6 5 4 3 2 1

This book is printed on acid-free paper.

To Vincent Paul Fleming, my first grandchild,
whose every breath reinforces and imbues my life
with all manner of inspiration.

CONTENTS

FOREWORD

Asthma is a very common problem worldwide with incidence in the United States on the rise, especially among children.

I remember a 12-year-old patient of mine some years ago whose pulmonary status was that of severe obstruction. I first saw him when he was in the intensive care unit, but he refused to come for continuous care. He took his medications at home. He was a tough kid—one of the toughest I'd ever encountered—and he was angry and did not accept that he had life-threatening asthma. I warned his parents, and I sat down with him to tell him with proper treatment he could be like any other kid. He said, "I'm not like any other kid, and I won't go to the emergency room." Unwilling to seek preventive measures, the boy died. A preventable death.

Another patient of mine, about nine years old, thought he had only mild asthma. I'll never forget him, because he wanted to go to a slumber party with his friends, much to the dismay of his mother, who was accused of being overprotective. He needed treatment episodically, and his mother agreed to let him go to the party as long as he took his inhaler with him, which he did. The group then went to a recreational facility similar to Great Adventure, where the boy must have felt sick but was hiding it because he didn't want to have to leave the party. He collapsed. By the time people got him to the ER, he was brain dead. Again, preventable.

A somewhat happier story involves a 13-year-old girl I was treating with continuous nebulization for frequent asthma attacks. She kept a pet guinea pig in her bedroom. Sometimes she even let the guinea pig on the bed. When I did a radioallergosorbent test (RAST) on her, I found her to be a Class 6 for allergy to guinea pigs! I believed she should get rid of the pet, but it's very hard to tell a kid to do that. So she takes Serevent and other medications that help ward off asthma attacks.

Parents of children who have been diagnosed with asthma, as well as those parents who have been questioning the validity of giving their children drugs to control asthma, will find this book extremely informative and useful. This book will help in understanding some of the basic concepts and definitions of asthma that have boggled their minds for a while.

Tova Navarra has a knack for making complex concepts and definitions easy to comprehend. This quality is easily appreciated in perusing her previous publications *The Encyclopedia of Allergies*, Second Edition and *The Encyclopedia of Vitamins, Minerals and Supplements*. She has written this book, *The Encyclopedia of Asthma and Respiratory Disorders*, with both professional and lay public in mind because they can all benefit from reading it. No one with interest in asthma should be without this book. Tova Navarra, an erudite clinical professional, has done it again!

—Charles K. Dadzie, M.D., F.A.A.P., F.C.C.P.,
Director of Pediatric Pulmonology and Critical
Care Medicine, Jersey Shore Medical Center,
Meridian Health System; Clinical Assistant
Professor, Pediatrics, U.M.D.N.J.,
Robert Wood Johnson Medical School

PREFACE

Breath is life, and breathing disorders threaten life.

Lung disease is the third leading cause of death in America. Over the last decade, the death rate from lung disease has been growing faster than the death rate from almost any other leading killer.

Approximately 30 million people in the United States suffer from some form of chronic breathing disorder, which generates a cost of $85 billion in health care a year. It is important to realize that 5 percent of all adults and 10 percent of children in the United States suffer from asthma, according to the American Medical Association. Asthma is the most common diagnosis among children's diseases, and it seems to be on the rise because of increased air pollution and, possibly, increased stress factors. More than 5,000 people die from asthma each year, a good portion of them children and blacks.

In addition to asthma, other enemies of breath are still lurking among millions of people all over the world. Tuberculosis has made a comeback with resistant strains of the *Mycobacterium*. Lung cancer and emphysema haven't ceased to haunt persistent smokers as well as strike nonsmokers for some known and some unknown reasons. Influenza, bronchitis, and pneumonia continue to loom large every winter, particularly for infants, the infirm, and the elderly. In 1918, a flu epidemic killed 548,000 people in the United States and 20 million worldwide. Today, flu and pneumonia combined are the sixth leading cause of death in America, which warrants many physicians' urging their patients to get a "flu and/or pneu" shot each year well before the difficult cold weather is able to stress the human system a bit more than warmer temperatures do. It seems, too, that when hay fever lets up, the common cold rushes in.

The "heat" is on to protect our respiratory systems in an age that claims to be more aware and knowledgeable about prevention, but, unfortunately, prevention remains the most elusive of common medical and hygienic practices. Organizations such as the American Lung Association and others seek to answer as many questions as they can as a way to educate the general population, sponsor research toward cures and treatments, and keep tabs on the trends and statistics related to respiratory disorders, lest we become complacent and thereby vulnerable to whatever new or old strain of microorganism may be waiting in the wings.

This book's "reason to breathe" is to promote prevention and add comprehensively and accessibly to the literature on diseases that affect our airways, which more often than not we take for granted.

—Tova Navarra, B.A., R.N.

ACKNOWLEDGMENTS

Whenever I face the daunting task of writing a book that must be scientific, accurate, comprehensive, and accessible, I realize the importance of those who encourage me and provide valuable assistance. For their generous help with this volume, I heartily thank my daughter and journalist/lyricist, Yolanda Fleming, the late Myron A. Lipkowitz, R.P., M.D., my former coauthor, and Martin Corbo, who provided important reference materials. I offer a very special thank-you to Jim Reme. Many thanks to Dr. Charles Dadzie for praising my work so highly and adding his distinguished name to this book. In addition, Facts On File's James Chambers and his staff are excellent, diligent editors with whom I am honored to work, and my agent Faith Hamlin deserves high praise for making a "perfect match." Thanks also go to Frederic C. Pachman, director of the medical library at Monmouth Medical Center in Long Branch, New Jersey. I am also infinitely grateful to Victor Zak, Paul Boyd, Bunny Schuler, Mona Wichman, Dorothy Fox, Johnny and Mitzi Navarra, Guy, Amanda, and Wesley Fleming, Jacquie, Tony, and Matthew Munoz, Lilo Meany, Sallie and Stan Tillman, Jordan Stinemeyer, Trista Clayton, Richard Conley, Dr. Andrea Campbell, and Betty Sorrentino, who lighten and brighten my days, do me endless favors, and tolerate a lot of whining.

Finally, I feel moved to acknowledge a CD entitled *One Single Breath*, produced in 2000 by my daughter and son-in-law (Yolanda and Guy Fleming) as I began to write this book. The music is meditative and nothing short of awe-inspiring.

The group itself, called One Single Breath, hopes to promote and raise money through its music for a charitable organization that focuses on asthma and breathing disorders.

INTRODUCTION

Losing my breath again, never wanted to,
what am I to do, can't help it.

—from "Falling in Love Again,"
the signature song in the film *The Blue Angel*

Inspiration.

From the Latin *inspirare*, to breathe in, we inherit a word that has dual meaning. First and foremost, it gives verbal acknowledgment to the most fundamental of all human activities: to take in the air our bodies crave in order to live. It tops the medical list of priorities commonly known as "ABC," a mnemonic for assessing the status of emergency patients' airway, breathing, and circulation.

Breathing ranks supreme in religious teachings as well. In *The Upanishads: Breath of the Eternal*, part of the oldest Hindu scriptures, it is written: "O Prana, lord of creation, thou movest in the womb, and art born again. To thee, who, as breath, dwellest in the body, all creatures bring offerings." *Pranayama* refers to yoga exercises during which one concentrates intensely on breathing patterns.

The Incan word for God is expressed as "ha" in a forceful puff of air without the need for any more than a whisper-like sound—as much a reverence for the Greater Power as for the very ability to breathe. The exchange of oxygen for the exhaled carbon dioxide, then, goes far beyond the human requirement for the preferred gas, as author Dannion Brinkley put it, to symbiotic breathing described as "in for me, out for the universe." He pointed even more emphatically to the significance of breathing by conducting an exercise in which people were instructed to breathe in rhythm with each other. If nothing else, the exercise induced a keener awareness of taking in and letting out that all-important air, and brought to mind the 1974 pop song performed by the Hollies whose refrain ends with the line, "All I need is the air that I breathe and to love you."

Inspiration also means, perhaps more literally than we think, having ideas, decisions, or other concepts "breathed" into our minds from "nowhere," usually toward a creative goal. "Breathtaking" is often the adjective that applies well to the panoramas of the Rocky Mountains, Michelangelo's *David*, and other wondrous accomplishments.

To be deprived of breath seems the ultimate enemy.

Impaired breathing of any sort, frequently explained within the categories of various respiratory disorders, may be as symbolic as it is physical and is employed heavily as an artistic motif. In emergency medicine, one relates immediately to the choking victim's hand at his throat—an image instinctively meant to alarm others—indicating that he can't breathe. Similarly in literature and other arts, the plight of society's victims may well be intensified by a respiratory disorder. Mildred in Somerset Maugham's *Of Human Bondage* and Thomas Mann's protagonist in *The Magic Mountain* suffered from tuberculosis. The leading female characters of the 1937 film *Camille*, Kathryn Hulme's *The Nun's Story*, and Puccini's opera *La Boheme* also had TB. In the television series

I, Claudius, the demented Caligula solved his intolerance of a young boy's chronic cough by having him beheaded.

On the lighter side, the hapless Adelaide in Broadway's *Guys and Dolls* sneezed endlessly and worried about catching "la grippe" because her fiance, Nathan Detroit, kept eluding a wedding day. One may speculate whether the character called Wheezer in *The Little Rascals* had asthma or some breathing or allergy problem. In one episode, he suffers a coughing fit when he is near ducks. Many a dark-humored line in television sitcoms refers to an asthmatic child's missing inhaler. Monmouth University photographer Jim Reme remembers his Little League coaching days during which one of his players had asthma. Before each game, the boy would give Jim custody of his inhaler and forget to retrieve it afterward. Late into the night, Jim would receive a call from the boy's mother asking for the inhaler's safe return.

Real-life stories offer as much drama and impact as fictional ones. In December 1988, artist Linda Troeller exhibited 20 photocollages entitled *TB-AIDS Diary* at the City Without Walls Gallery in Newark, New Jersey. The images drew biting parallels between the disease that attacked her mother and countless others in the 1930s and the disease of the 1980s that initially burst into the male homosexual community. In both cases, the artist said, the diseases are deadly and infectious, and the victims have been stigmatized by people around them out of ignorance and fear. Dr. Richard Conviser, then health policy analyst of the State Department of Health in Trenton, New Jersey, praised Troeller's exhibit, which won the PhotoMetro portfolio award in 1987 and other recognitions.

On the everyday scene, one woman recounted to a group of friends that after she had legally parked in a spot designated for those with handicapped symbols on their cars and walked to a store, a man confronted her and said angrily, "You don't look handicapped to me!"

"Sir," she replied, "I have a breathing disorder."

Asthma—the disorder synonymous with a chronic delicacy of constitution and the bane of famous individuals including French novelist Marcel Proust—beleaguers one of William Golding's protagonists in *Lord of the Flies.* In the book's first chapter, Piggy, as he is called, admitted his physical ineptitude to the robust leader, a boy named Ralph:

> "'My auntie told me not to run,' he explained, 'on account of my asthma.'
> 'Ass-mar?'
> 'That's right. Can't catch me breath. I was the only boy in our school what had asthma,' said the fat boy with a touch of pride. 'And I've been wearing specs since I was three.'"

The impact of asthma is clear, particularly for children who are set apart by it. Representative Nita M. Lowey of New York referred to the number of children suffering from asthma as "nothing short of a crisis," following news reports in May 2000 that about 130,000 children in New York City are afflicted and that asthma is the leading cause of absenteeism from school. The recent film *As Good as It Gets,* which earned actors Jack Nicholson and Helen Hunt Academy Awards, focuses on a woman's son who has severe asthma, and because she has limited resources and keeps taking him to the emergency room for treatment, the child receives no continuous medical care or follow-up until the protagonist appears and offers to pay for the doctors. This is not unlike situations that actually happen, and, unfortunately, all too often.

On a larger scale in real life, as historian Paul Boyd wrote, there is the "well-documented phenomenon called 'the toxic ghetto.' The term reflects the fact that where there's a dirty manufacturing plant, a smokestack industry, a landfill or a dump looking for a site, disproportionately, the selection falls on poor neighborhoods. The result is that bad-ecology illnesses are poverty illnesses in toxic ghettos, probably with asthma as one of the top outcomes."

The Centers for Disease Control and Prevention (CDC) reported in a 1998 survey that black children were 31 percent more likely than white children to have had an episode of asthma or an asthma attack during the previous year. Lara Akinbami, of the CDC's National Center for Health Statistics, said, "In 1998, 68 out of 1,000 black children had asthma versus only 52 out of 1,000 white children. Black children are much more likely to be hospitalized or die from asthma." So the racial gap expands for young people with a chronic respiratory disease.

In addition, more inner-city children fall victim to asthma triggered by cockroach and mouse allergens than by cats, dogs, and house-dust mites, according to a federally funded report. Researchers at Johns Hopkins University found that in eight urban areas studied, 95 percent of the tested homes harbored mouse allergens, and 18 percent of the children who live in them are allergic to mice and tend to have severe asthma. In 1996, information from the National Cooperative Inner-City Asthma Study conducted in Baltimore, Washington, the Bronx and Brooklyn in New York City, St. Louis, Chicago, Cleveland, and Detroit brought forth the discovery that, of the 1,528 children ages 4 to 9 in the study, all had asthma and lived in communities in which 30 percent or more household incomes dipped below the 1990 poverty level. Hence, "inner-city asthma" has become a bona fide diagnosis attributable to insects, rodents, and the rank of the underprivileged.

Urban areas in which there is a significant amount of industry—and the bad air that accompanies it—thunder into the picture as well. The *New York Times* reported on February 28, 2001, that the U.S. Supreme Court unanimously decided "in setting national air quality standards, the Environmental Protection Agency must consider only the requirements of public health and safety and may not engage in the cost-benefit analysis that a coalition of industry groups sought to import into the (Clean Air Act) statute. . . . The decision today dealt with new standards for two pollutants—ground-level ozone, which causes smog, and fine airborne particles, commonly known as soot—that the Environmental Protection Agency issued in 1997." At last, facing the grim toll taken by asthma, bronchitis, and other respiratory disorders caused and/or aggravated by air pollution, the federal government has rejected an industry attack in one of the most important environmental rulings in years.

The *Asthma in America: Executive Summary,* conducted by Schulman, Ronca & Bucuvalas, a national research firm specializing in health issues, took the asthma connection a few steps further into the realm of what might be called the "secondary smoke" of the condition: "Nearly half of the American public (48 percent) have had asthma themselves, or in their household, or in their immediate family. Another three out of 10 (29 percent) know friends, coworkers, or someone else personally who has asthma. Hence, nearly four out of five Americans (77 percent) are affected."

It stands to reason that if the person next to you, familiar or unfamiliar, suddenly starts gasping for air, your psyche will be moved. "'I didn't want to wake up this morning,' said Northwestern coach Randy Walker, still fighting back tears and trying to control his emotions yesterday afternoon. . . ." in the *Asbury Park Press*'s August 5, 2001, story about a college football player. "The breathing problems that forced Rashidi Wheeler out of a conditioning drill didn't seem to be any different from the 30 other asthma attacks he'd had while playing football the past three years. But the Northwestern safety was never able to catch his breath Friday afternoon and later died. Bronchial asthma was the preliminary cause of death, the Cook County coroner's office ruled yesterday."

Boyd also points out that asthma has been dubbed "The Breath Robber You Can Stop." Numerous self-help books for adults and children with asthma pepper the shelves, including *Go Blow Your Nose, Robert!* by Nancy Sander, president of the Allergy and Asthma Network/Mothers of Asthmatics, Inc., based in Fairfax, Virginia. In addition, the pervasive disorder prompted a movement called "asthma-friendliness" in schools, and asthma camps provide a tremendous service for children who may not otherwise be able to enjoy summer outdoor sports and activities.

Modern literature and scientific advances stand as the fine result of an entire time-line of effort and study so people can "breathe easier," as the saying goes. As early as the second century A.D., Aretaeus of Cappadocia described "bronchial asthma," a term widely used for hundreds of years. In 1565, Leonardo Botallo described an asthma-like condition he called the "Rose Cold." J. B. van Helmont in 1607 wrote of "spasmodic attacks of difficult breathing" with symptom-free periods between attacks. In 1713, Ramazzini recognized a hypersensitivity-pneumonitis-like lung disease in grain workers. The English physician John Bostock in 1819 was one of the first to describe multiple cases suggestive of hay fever, which was called "Bostock's summer catarrh." Eleven years later John Elliotson noted a patient's observation that pollen might be responsible for his symptoms.

In 1890 Robert Koch discovered and extracted the tubercle bacillus, *Mycobacterium tuberculosis,* that causes tuberculosis. A worldwide malady transmitted by the inhalation of minute droplets from the cough or sneeze of an infected person, tuberculosis is still one of the chief causes of death in Third World countries. Even animals, such as cattle and other domestic animals, are susceptible to certain forms of TB. During the early 20th century, poor hygienic standards and periods of war and catastrophe resulted in high death rates from tuberculosis, but the drugs rifampin, isoniazid, para-aminosalicylic acid, and streptomycin eventually came about to fight it. Before the drugs were developed, sanatoriums operated to foster good nutrition, hygiene, fresh air, and exercise for the prevention and treatment of the disease.

Potions falling under the moniker of folk medicine had their day, too. Until 1905 when coca leaf extracts were eliminated from Coca-Cola's original formula, which contained "a little something to put color in your cheeks," as Dr. Sigmund Freud put it, heroin was a popular over-the-counter cough suppressant. No doubt it was so effective that some patients saw to it they never coughed again.

Recently, tuberculosis made a gruesome comeback in Japan, particularly in the elderly who had at one time been exposed to the infection but did not previously exhibit symptoms. A New York City television newscast of February 11, 2001, reported that Japanese officials were embarrassed that a disease for which there has been effective early detection and treatment for decades re-exploded among the frailest of their population.

Tuberculosis has also presented as a complication in AIDS patients, in which the victim's immune system cannot effectively ward off the invader, and in emigrants from certain countries who arrive in the United States with the infection, who do not understand contagion, and may refuse to comply with hospital treatment that seems to them like a punishing incarceration.

Professionals as well shared in some of the misunderstandings that unwittingly allow disease to flourish. After Dr. Alexander Fleming of St. Mary's Hospital Medical School in London brought forth penicillin in 1928, it languished unused for nearly 10 years. By 1943, people had to pay $20 per 100,000-unit dose of the drug that proved effective against pneumonia and a host of other diseases. About 30 years passed after Austrian chemist Paul Gelmo discovered the white crystalline sulfanilamide in 1908, derivatives of which were eventually recognized as enemies of *Staphylococcus* and *Streptococcus* infections, pneumonia, meningitis, dysentery, and leprosy.

The history of pathology always includes an evolution of sorts, for as one "devil" is recognized and perhaps conquered, another appears. In the late 19th century, Henry Salter concluded a correlation between asthma and hay fever and animal exposure. Sir Henry Dale discovered histamine in 1910 while working on rye poisoning by ergot. He noted the shock-like drop in blood pressure histamine caused by its effect on smooth muscle. Three years later, W. P. Dunbar reproduced the symptoms of hay fever using pollen extracts. Also in the 1900s Charles F. Cole established a test for histamines, and in the 1920s, Kern, Cooke, and Storm van Leeuwen demonstrated that many asthmatics had positive skin-test reactions to house dust. Storm van Leeuwen also removed asthma patients from their homes to demonstrate that changing one's environment could improve asthma.

Medical studies progressed. In 1942, the French produced the first antihistamine safe for human use—phenbenzamine (Antergan), closely followed by pyrilamine maleate (Neo-Antergan). In the United States, researchers developed diphenhydramine (Benadryl) and tripelennamine (Pyribenzamine). In 1950 corticosteroids were first used to treat asthma. The history of medicine continued to make stride after stride in the effort to treat or eradicate both major and minor infections and to understand the body's immune system and why it suffered repeated attacks of determined microorganisms.

Enter the "super bug" of the 21st century. "Shortly after the introduction of penicillin-G in the 1940s, it was recognized that certain strains of staphylococci have a potent enzyme called ß-lactamase which inactivates penicillin," writes

Jacqueline Fuccello-Breuer, R.N., in the February 5, 2001, issue of the New York-New Jersey *Nursing Spectrum.* "In patients with such staphylococcal infections, penicillin-G has no therapeutic effect. Since then some organisms have not only developed resistance to one antibiotic, but have developed resistance to many. Pharmaceutical companies in the 1970s and into the late 1980s developed newer and stronger antimicrobial agents—three generations of cephalosporins and the fluoroquinolones. These antibiotics were considered sophisticated enough to control bacterial infections; and drug development efforts were redirected to cardiovascular, metabolic, and psychoactive drugs."

Fuccello-Breuer goes on to describe the toll of "super bugs" as a major new health problem and how we've set the stage for their success: "Ninety-five percent of physicians in office practice issue one or more prescriptions to a patient diagnosed with the 'common cold.' Similarly, a hospital study revealed that there was no evidence of infection in as many as 70 percent of patients who received antimicrobial therapy."

In the category of "super bugs" also stands the problem of vermin- and insect-related incidences of asthma, particularly in New York City, where the respiratory environment is compromised. In the article "Asthma: A Public Health Partnership Tackles a Neighborhood Terror" (*Columbia University Magazine,* Winter 2001), author Dodi Schultz says the Columbia Center for Children's Environmental Health (CCCEH) was established in 1998 "with the far-reaching mission of preventing environmentally related disease in children. It receives support from the National Institute of Environmental Health Sciences (NIEHS), the Environmental Protection Agency (EPA), and several foundations. Its 'patients' are the children of northern Manhattan and the South Bronx. Its special areas of concern are three: low birthweights coupled with impaired growth and development; unusually high, and inexplicably rising, local rates of childhood cancer; and—the primary child-health concern as perceived by both researchers and residents themselves, based on community surveys—the devastating impact of asthma. Asthma levels in the Columbia study area are startling: In the South Bronx, 17 percent of all children—two of every dozen kids—are asthmatic."

The study expects to involve 600 African-American and Latino women and their children through prenatal clinics. CCCEH director Frederica Perera said this is a pioneering study to examine prenatal and perinatal influences on the children's medical status through analysis of the home environment, and blood and other body-substance analysis. Reported exposure to tobacco smoke, for example, may be assessed through cotinine levels (cotinine in the urine is considered a biomarker for exposure to nicotine).

The study also plans to include environmental factors such as pollutants—ozone, oxides of sulfur and nitrogen, particulates (ash and soot), etc.—because they affect the quality of breathable air. "Particulate matter—known in the trade simply as PM—broadly includes all small airborne solids, ranging in size from visible smokestack effluent to the tiniest microscopic bits," according to Schultz. "It's the latter category that worries pulmonary specialists and public-health researchers, in particular those particles known as $PM_{2.5}$; that designation denotes those with a diameter of 2.5 microns or less. Larger particles, as irritating as they are, are relatively harmless, since they're trapped, coughed up, or blown out of the nose. The smaller particles, though, easily penetrate the bronchial tubes and even the lung's small passageways. Researchers have repeatedly found these particulates statistically associated with markedly higher risks of disease and death." Diesel and other exhaust fumes from vehicles are another concern to be addressed by the Columbia study, along with dust mites, cockroaches, pets, and other aspects of what has been dubbed "the toxic home."

The leading investigator on the CCCEH asthma project is Jean Ford, M.D., chief of pulmonary medicine at Harlem Hospital. He also heads the Harlem Asthma Research Team (HART), which operates (in affiliation with Columbia) under a grant from the National Institutes of Health. Ford is also a member of the National Heart, Lung, and Blood Institute's expert panel on asthma management, and sits on the board of West Harlem Environmental Action (WE ACT), an activist group dedicated to environmental justice.

While New York City, with the highest asthma mortality rates in the country, combats asthma and respiratory disorders, the diseases exist all over the globe. Schultz goes on to report that "scientists are more and more inclined to believe that, while who you are (family, race) may play a part, what you do and where you live may play far more significant roles. Speculations have postulated roles for factors ranging from day care and too many (or too few) childhood infections to junk food and use of computers. But we are, after all, talking about the lungs. The most significant factor of all may be the air you breathe, both indoors and out. The ethnic groups with the highest incidence are chiefly city dwellers. Even within broad ethnic groups, noted differences—again, particularly in acute-attack data—may be suggestive. Asthma mortality rates, for example, are markedly higher among Hispanics from the Caribbean; the rate among Puerto Ricans is approximately four and one half times that of Mexican Americans."

New drugs are being investigated to help fight all the entities that terrorize the respiratory system, but risk is always at hand in well-meaning research. A June 15, 2001, article in The *New York Times* reports that a 24-year-old healthy volunteer in a Johns Hopkins University breathing study died June 2 after inhaling hexamethonium, a drug used to determine how the lung protects the airways from narrowing, which plays a crucial role in asthma. The drug had been used in several studies of lung physiology at leading academic medical centers without any unexpected ill effects, said Johns Hopkins, but volunteer Ellen Roche died from progressive lung and kidney failure brought on by hexamethonium inhalation. The day after the chemical was administered to her, Ms. Roche developed a cough, fever, runny nose, and fatigue. Before her death, the article says, "a CAT scan revealed that her lungs had the appearance of ground glass, indicating severe damage, and two days later she was put on a ventilator." The study has been suspended, and the case is now under federal investigation.

One may conclude that breathing, which ought to be easy, is all too frequently impaired either voluntarily or involuntarily. Alexander Lowen, M.D., said, "Most people are poor breathers. Their breathing is shallow, and they have a tendency to hold their breath in any situation of stress. Even in such simple stress situations as driving a car, typing a letter, or waiting for an interview, people tend to limit their breathing. The result is an increase of their tension."

Furthermore, Paul Bragg said, "Shallow breathers poison themselves," and Hans Weller, M.D., said, "Nearly every physical problem is accompanied by a disturbance of breathing. But which comes first?" Andrew Weil, M.D., agrees that "improper breathing is a common cause of ill health."

According to the teachings of Tibetan mystics, "mastery over breath conquers all passion, anger and carnal desires, acquires serenity, prepares the mind for meditation and awakens spiritual energy." Thich Nhat Hanh adds, "Without full awareness of breathing, there can be no development of meditative stability and understanding."

Given that we take between 17,000 and 20,000 breaths each day, it seems reasonable to believe that breathing truly does create a bridge between body and spirit. We all are breathing beings. It is our responsibility to honor and respect each breath and the intriguing physical system that facilitates it.

ENTRIES A–Z

acapnia The absence of carbon dioxide. From the Greek word *akapnos,* meaning smokeless, acapnia indicates a level of carbon dioxide lower than the normal amount found in blood and bodily tissues, such as the level resulting from voluntary over-breathing or hyperventilation. Symptoms of acapnia include depressed respiration, giddiness, paresthesia, cramps, involuntary contractions of the fingers and, on occasion, seizures.

Accolate The trade name for the drug zafirlukast, which is used to treat bronchoconstriction.
  See also ZAFIRLUKAST.

acidosis, respiratory An excess of acidity in body fluids. Also known as hypercapnic acidosis, respiratory acidosis may be the result of diabetes, renal disease, or an excessive loss of bicarbonate (or alkalinity). The body requires an acid-base balance for optimal functioning. Therefore, when the hydrogen ion concentration increases, the pH decreases and causes an imbalance, or acidosis. Carbon dioxide acidosis is another form of excessive acidity caused by carbon dioxide retention, particularly as a result of drowning or a situation in which there is decreased respiration.

acquired immune deficiency syndrome (AIDS), respiratory complications of See AIDS.

active immunity Protection from disease via the body's production of antibodies in response to a foreign, potentially pathogenic, organism. In the fifth century B.C., Greek physicians observed that persons who had recovered from the plague were immune to subsequent attacks of the plague. This acquired natural, or "active," immunity results when B cells and T cells of the immune system are "programmed" at the time of first exposure to an invading microorganism. In response to a foreign antigen, B cells and T cells manufacture antibodies that remember and attack the invader if it is encountered in the future. Mounting an immune response depends on one's inherited disposition to do so to a particular antigen.

  Vaccinations (immunizations), as well as invading infections, can stimulate acquired active immunity. This immunity then prevents a manifestation of a particular disease, or, in the event immunity develops in response to having an active disease, or from contracting the disease again. Active immunity differs from passive immunity in that preformed antibodies injected into the body allow a more immediate protection. The advantage of active immunity is its longer lasting, perhaps lifelong, protection. A disadvantage is the delay between administration of a vaccine and its effectiveness.

  Active immunity is the basis for the immunizations known as "baby shots" because infants are usually immunized shortly after birth against a variety of diseases. Vaccines contain killed, modified, or parts of microorganisms in sufficient amounts to trigger an antibody response without causing the actual disease. In rare cases, a subclinical infection, a weakened manifestation of a disease, is produced by the vaccine. Some live-virus vaccines have been sufficiently diluted to render them safe for immunization. The medical breakthrough of genetic engineering has allowed the manufacture of safer vaccines.

  The duration of immunity depends on the type of antigen, quantity encountered, and its means of entering the body, but active immunity generally lasts from many months to a lifetime. Active immunity requires an inductive (latent) period between immunization and the development of protective antibodies. This process could take from several days to several months and may require "booster" doses of the vaccine. Some immunizations that produce active immunity are tetanus, diphtheria, pertussis, poliomyelitis, measles, mumps, Rubella or German measles, *Haemophilus influenzae* type b, viral influenza (flu), pneumonia, and hepatitis vaccines. These immunizations are given according to a schedule recommended by the Centers for Disease Control and Prevention.

See also ALLERGY SHOTS; INFLUENZA; IMMUNITY, PASSIVE; AND VACCINE.

acupressure Similar to acupuncture, a technique involving use of the fingers to press on the appropriate body meridians to unblock stagnant energy at painful sites.

See also ACUPUNCTURE.

acupuncture An ancient Chinese technique for reducing pain and/or promoting restoration which calls for the insertion of extremely fine needles into the skin over points related to other parts and functions of the body. A point near the wrist, for example, is associated with respiration. Acupuncture is said to be effective in treating sinusitis, asthma, pains and addictions (including depression), and many other digestive, nervous, musculoskeletal, and respiratory conditions. Traditional Chinese medicine refers to the qi or chi (pronounced chee), the life force or a flow of healthy energy along specific channels or meridians.

Disease is thought to be caused by the blockage in one or more of these meridians, and the goal of acupuncture is to relieve the blockages at any of the 14 major "acupuncture points" or meridians. Each meridian contains numerous points and serves as a site for the insertion of the needles. Studies suggest that acupuncture stimulates the release of the body's natural, opiate-like substances called endorphins. Endorphins act as painkillers, sometimes as effective as morphine or anesthesia, and are thought also to contribute to the feeling of well-being.

In an article in the National Auxiliary Publication Service (NAPS) (from the American Society for Information Science), Bryan Frank, M.D., president of the American Academy of Medical Acupuncture (AAMA), said, "Treating allergies with medical acupuncture stimulates the immune system to help the body more efficiently heal itself, diminishing the frequency and severity of allergic reactions." A medical acupuncture session includes an extensive medical history and physical examination, possibly a prescription for medication, and the stimulation of points on the body that correspond to the symptoms experienced by each individual patient, which "customizes" the treatment. The AAMA encourages allergy sufferers to consider acupuncture treatments in conjunction with allopathic treatments. The AAMA's patient referral service may be accessed by calling (800) 521-2262 or visiting www.medicalacupuncture.org.

acute mountain sickness See ALTITUDE SICKNESS; PULMONARY EDEMA.

addiction A physical and often psychological dependence on a substance such as a narcotic, alcohol, or tobacco that affects the central nervous system. Repeated use and abuse of these substances may lead to substantial debilitation of one's health and well-being, and increased dependence may lead to overdose and death. When an addict does not get the substance his body craves or when use of the substance is discontinued, withdrawal symptoms (also known as delirium tremens, or DTs) occur. Individuals who smoke, for example, develop a dependence on nicotine, which frequently leads to mouth, throat, lung, and other serious illnesses. Treatments abound for addictions of all types and include behavior modification, in which an individual is counseled psychologically as well as weaned off a particular substance by using increments of smaller and smaller doses until the dependence is gone.

See also LUNG CANCER; SMOKING, PASSIVE; SMOKE POISONING.

adenoids Lymphatic tissue, the same as the pharyngeal tonsils, named from the Greek word for "glandular." This tissue forms lymph fluid that contains nutrients and lymphocytes (white blood cells that help form antibodies), which fight infections by attacking pathogenic bacteria. Lymph is found throughout the body.

The adenoids located on the wall of the nasopharyngeal area, often become overactive and swollen, resulting in nasal stuffiness. They can be removed by surgical adenoidectomy, or, when removed with the tonsils, a tonsillectomy, known as a "T and A" procedure. This is not routinely recommended as it was years ago, probably because it may be more advantageous to keep organs serving the immune system intact and also to avoid the risks of anesthesia.

See also ADENOTONSILLECTOMY.

adenotonsillectomy   A surgical procedure in which the tonsils and adenoids are removed.

See also ADENOIDS.

adult respiratory distress syndrome (ARDS)   A lung disease that causes difficulty in breathing, rapid breathing, rapid heartbeat, excessive sweating, pink, frothy sputum, rhonchi, and changes in the level of consciousness. Affecting approximately 150,000 people each year, with a statistic that half of these will die despite treatment, ARDS is attributed to abnormal permeability of either the pulmonary capillaries or the alveolar epithelium. Most patients diagnosed with ARDS have suffered a severe infection, trauma, or other illness, and the disease often strikes young patients who were previously healthy. Treatment includes assisted ventilation, the administration of oxygen, antibiotics effective against the infecting microorganism, tests for continuous positive airway pressure and positive end-respiratory pressure, adequate nutrition (parenteral [injected] nutrition if required), prevention of side effects of the patient's immobility, and emotional support for anxiety of both the patient and his family.

adverse drug reactions   Hypersensitivity to medication that causes various symptoms, ranging from unpleasant to life-threatening, and may preclude a medication's use as treatment. New medical guidelines have been established on drug hypersensitivity by a national task force of allergists/ immunologists and were published in the American College of Allergy, Asthma and Immunology's (ACAAI) December 1999 *Annals of Allergy, Asthma and Immunology*. The guidelines, titled "Disease Management of Drug Hypersensitivity: A Practice Parameter," are one of a series that includes asthma, allergy diagnostic testing, immunodeficiency, rhinitis, atopic dermatitis, anaphylaxis, immunotherapy, insect stings, and sinusitis. They are designed to help prevent medical errors.

Risk factors for drug hypersensitivity include the chemical properties and molecular weight of a drug; dosage; route of administration; duration of treatment; repetitive exposure to the drug; concurrent illnesses; and a patient's age, gender, atopy, and genetics. The new guidelines include components for clinical evaluation and diagnosis of drug hypersensitivity, including history, physical examination, and clinical tests. Parameters stipulate that prevention of allergic reactions may be accomplished by attention to:

1. A careful history to determine host risk factors;
2. Avoidance of cross-reactive drugs;
3. Use of predictive skin tests when available;
4. Proper and prudent prescribing of drugs (especially antibiotics) frequently associated with adverse reactions, and
5. Use of oral medication in preference to parenteral (injected) drugs when possible.

aeration   The process of exchanging carbon dioxide for oxygen in the blood of the lungs. Aeration also refers to "airing" something out and to putting gases into a fluid.

aeroallergens   Substances that, when transported through the air, are capable of causing an allergic reaction when inhaled by an allergic individual. Airborne allergens include pollen grains, fungal spores, and the so-called inhalant allergens such as house dust (which is actually a mixture of many allergens), dead dust mite bodies and pellets of their fecal waste, human and animal danders, and flakes of dead skin. Animal proteins from saliva and urine become aeroallergens as they are absorbed into the environment. Cooking odors of highly allergenic foods and allergenic industrial chemicals behave in a similar manner.

Most airborne allergens range in size from 2 to 60 microns (1 micron = 1/25,000 inch), but some are even smaller. Finer aerosolized particles may pass into the distant terminal bronchioles, but ragweed-sized pollen grains do not usually reach that far.

Since most pollens do not reach the areas where bronchoconstriction is greatest, it is thought that reflex mechanisms occur when the allergen comes in contact with mucosal surfaces within its reach in the upper air passages. For some reason so far undiscovered, this triggers a spasm of the bronchial tubes and an asthma attack.

aerobic   The characteristic of an organism or microorganism able to thrive in the presence of oxygen. Aerobic exercise, therefore, means physical activity that specifically uses and metabolizes oxygen to produce energy (as opposed to anaerobic exercise, which does not require inspired oxygen for energy and is limited to short bursts of strenuous activity; an anaerobe is a microorganism that can thrive in an oxygen-free atmosphere). Aerobic training fosters aerobic conditioning, generally with exercise three to five times a week for 20 to 30 minutes per session and at a level intense enough to produce a heart rate of 220 minus the age of the individual. Aerobic training is typically incorporated into cardiac and other rehabilitation programs.

AeroBid   The trade name (also Nasalide) for the corticosteroid drug flunisolide, which is used to treat rhinitis, allergies, and nasal polyps. In metered doses obtained via nasal spray, flunisolide suppresses the migration of polymorphonuclear leukocytes. Contraindications include administering the drug to children younger than six years and to anyone with hypersensitivity to flunisolide. Precautions include nonasthmatic bronchial disease, bacterial, viral, or fungal infections of the mouth, throat, and/or lungs, respiratory tuberculosis, any untreated infection, pregnancy, and glaucoma. Flunisolide is available as a nasal solution of 25 micrograms (Nasalide) or 250 micrograms (AeroBid).

aeropathy   A disorder or condition caused by a significant change in atmospheric pressure.

See also CAISSON DISEASE; EDEMA, PULMONARY.

aerophobia   Morbid fear of fresh air or a draft.

aerosol   A solution administered in the form of a mist from a spray bottle or can. Aerosol therapy refers to the inhalation of beneficial aerosolized solutions, such as corticosteroids or mucolytic agents, by patients with asthma, bronchitis, emphysema, and other respiratory disorders. Aerosol devices include pressurized canisters called metered-dose inhalers, hand-held nebulizers, machine-powered jet or ultrasonic nebulizers, or dry powder inhalers. There are several types of aerosol nasal sprays. Aerosols are also used in the cosmetic and other industries.

See also INHALATION THERAPY.

aerotherapy   The treatment of disease by using air, particularly changes in composition and density of air, such as a decompression chamber and hyperbaric oxygen.

See also HYPERBARIC OXYGEN THERAPY.

aerothorax   See PNEUMOTHORAX.

agonist   A drug that mimics the body's own regulatory function. An agonist binds to a cell's receptors and stimulates the receptors' function. There are at least two different receptor systems, alpha and beta. Alpha-adrenergic receptors are associated primarily with excitatory functions, such as the constriction of smooth muscle in blood vessels, bronchi, and the urinary bladder. They also cause relaxation of smooth muscle in the intestines. Stimulation of these receptors may raise blood pressure and increase heart rate. Beta-adrenergic stimulation primarily affects the airways or air passages by allowing smooth-muscle relaxation. There are $beta_1$ and $beta_2$ receptors and drugs that have very broad actions affecting both $beta_1$ and $beta_2$

receptors. More selective drugs react primarily or only with the beta$_2$ receptors. These medicines have fewer side effects and are the most frequently prescribed for the treatment of asthma.

AIDS   A life-threatening disease caused by the human immunodeficiency virus (HIV) and characterized by a breakdown of the body's immune defenses. The disease was first recognized in 1981 in a group of homosexual males in California, who were diagnosed as having a rare form of pneumonia, *Pneumocystis carinii,* seen only in immunosuppressed individuals. Then a rare cancer, Kaposi's sarcoma, which affects the skin and other parts of the body, was reported in alarming numbers in this same population.

In 1984, French and American scientists identified HIV as the virus responsible for AIDS. Persons at the highest risk appear to be homosexual or bisexual men and their partners, intravenous drug abusers, patients who received blood transfusions from unscreened donors (before adequate screening was available), and children of infected women. Heterosexuals are becoming increasingly infected, although heterosexuality itself still poses a somewhat lower risk. AIDS is not present in all patients who are infected with HIV. One to 5 percent of people who have a positive blood test for HIV but have no symptoms may eventually develop AIDS. Less than 1 percent of those infected with HIV appear to be immune to developing AIDS, and the virus and antibodies to it disappear spontaneously.

Once the diagnosis has been confirmed, it is considered a fatal illness. Death usually results from an opportunistic infection such as *P. carinii* (a protozoan one-celled organism) or tuberculosis. Opportunistic infections are caused by commonplace organisms that do not usually trouble people whose immune systems are healthy, but take advantage of the opportunity provided by an immunosuppressed, or debilitated, person. Some individuals infected with HIV may remain well. In others, minor illness suggestive of infectious mononucleosis may occur between three weeks and three months following exposure to HIV. Symptoms including fever, sore throat, malaise,

muscle and joint aches, swollen glands, fatigue, weight loss, diarrhea, rash, and thrombocytopenia (decreased blood platelet count) appear suddenly and last about two weeks. These symptoms persist in many individuals, and up to 25 percent of those with this persistent condition, known as AIDS-related complex or ARC, may progress to AIDS within one year. Those with AIDS may have one or more of a variety of disorders, including anomalies of the nervous system; severe and unusual infections, such as *P. carinii* pneumonia, fungal, tuberculosis, herpes simplex, and zoster (shingles), and oral yeast infections (thrush); cancerous tumors, such as Kaposi's sarcoma, non-Hodgkin's lymphoma, or primary lymphoma of the brain.

A positive HIV-antibody test result in a person with signs and symptoms of an opportunistic infection or tumor characteristic of the disease must be confirmed by the Western blot blood test. A negative test result may occur in someone recently exposed to HIV. If that person is at high risk for developing AIDS, a repeat test should be performed in six months or sooner. AIDS is a contagious disease. Any person infected with the HIV can transmit the infection, even if that person does not have AIDS or ARC. It is spread by sexual contact, by direct contact of the HIV with the bloodstream from re-use of contaminated needles or accidental needle-sticks, and from mother to her unborn child through the placenta. Adequate screening at blood banks has made the blood supply for transfusions in the United States virtually free of HIV. The transmission of this disease requires intimate contact, such as sexual intercourse, in which an exchange of infected body fluids takes place. Researchers currently believe that HIV is not transmitted through casual or social contact.

There is no cure for HIV infection or AIDS, and mutant strains of HIV have already emerged. However, attempts to develop a vaccine are under way. Various antiviral agents, such as zidovudine (Retrovir), formerly called azidothymidine, or AZT, appear to inhibit the progression of the disease. There are serious side effects from these drugs, including anemia, granulocytopenia, dizziness, and severe headache. It is often difficult to differentiate between adverse drug reactions and effects of the illness. Antibiotics and antifungals have been known to be effective against some of the opportunistic infections. Chemotherapy with interferon has shown promise in early studies, and radiation is used against Kaposi's sarcoma and other malignancies. The 1990 Behavioral Risk Factor Surveillance System, or BRFSS, a government-sponsored study, assessed public awareness of HIV/AIDS. In random telephone interviews, 81,556 adults in 44 states and the District of Columbia were surveyed. Results are listed in the table below.

Have you heard of the AIDS virus HIV?	83.0%	Yes
Are you aware that drugs can lengthen life of persons with HIV?	46.6%	Yes
Are you aware that infected individuals can look normal?	67.7%	Yes
Do you think that persons giving blood can get AIDS?	72.2%	No
Do you think that AIDS can be transmitted by insect bites?	83.9%	No

Source: *Journal of the American Medical Association*, 1992.

air A mixture of gases consisting of approximately 78 percent nitrogen and 21 percent oxygen, water vapor, carbon dioxide, and traces of ammonia, argon, helium, neon, krypton, xenon, and other gases. *Clean air* is odorless, tasteless, invisible, and surrounds the entire Earth. *Alveolar air* refers to air in the alveoli, or air sacs, of the lungs. *Complemental air* refers to the volume of air available over and above the air taken in by the deepest possible inspiration. This is also known as the inspiratory reserve (supplemental) volume. The amount of air remaining in the lungs after one exhales fully is called *residual air*. After a normal, full exhalation, approximately 1,600 cubic centimeters of air are available in an adult. This is known as the expiratory reserve volume. In an adult male, an average of 500 cubic centimeters of air flows in and out with each normal respiration, and that volume is called *tidal air*. Air that fills the structures of the respiratory system's passageways but is not available for exchange of gases with the blood is called *dead space air*.

When a lung collapses with the thorax (chest cavity) open, the small amount of air trapped in the alveoli is referred to as *minimal air*.

air bronchogram sign In pulmonary edema and pneumonia, a radiograph or X ray of the lung that shows a bronchus filled with air as it passes through an area of increased anatomic density. A diagnostic technique, bronchography is accomplished by instilling a radiopaque substance into the trachea or bronchial tree so the lung may be viewed by X ray.

air conditioning The use of a ventilation device that controls air temperature and humidity, particularly to lower the temperature and humidity during the warm seasons. Air conditioning may prove beneficial to individuals with respiratory disorders because cool air is easier to breathe and may help shrink swollen membranes of the airways. On the other hand, there are dangers that certain infectious lung diseases may be spread by contaminated spray water from commercial air-conditioning systems. Actinomycetes are one cause of hypersensitivity pneumonitis, an allergic disease. Legionnaire's disease is an infectious pneumonia also spread by contaminated water in cooling systems. Air-filtration systems, such as the high-efficiency particulate air (HEPA) filters, are available to keep the air clean and free of contaminants. They also may actually worsen exposure to allergens by lifting them into the air where they can be inhaled, so it is best to seek the advice of a physician or other health care professional when air purification is considered.

air curtain A method of directing air currents around a patient in order to divert air that might otherwise irritate or contaminate the patient with dust-borne allergens and other undesirable microorganisms.

air flow, laminar A system of filtered air flow in areas such as operating theaters, nurseries, bacteriology work areas, and places designated for food preparation. The system helps prevent bacterial contamination of the air and collects chemical fumes that may be harmful.

air hunger A common term for shortness of breath or dyspnea (difficulty breathing), especially rapid, labored breathing.

air pollution Any contamination of the air we breathe, including industrial waste, fumes and exhaust from vehicles, and the spraying of pesticides, insecticides, or other noxious substances. Air pollution is also known as smog.

air quality The degree of purity or pollution in the atmosphere in which we breathe. According to the American Lung Association, its new report, *State of the Air: 2000,* provides easy-to-understand summaries of the quality of the air based on concrete data and sound science. Cities and counties are assigned grades "A" through "F" based on how often the air quality exceeds the "unhealthful" categories of the U.S. Environmental Protection Agency's Air Quality Index. The report confirms that air pollution remains a major threat to Americans and contributes substantially to the nation's ill-health burden. The report also says more than 132 million Americans live in areas that received an "F"—approximately 72 percent of the nation's population who live in counties where there are ozone monitors. Of the 678 counties examined, nearly half (333) received an "F." Furthermore, in "F"-rated areas, there are an estimated 16 million Americans older than 65, more than 7 million people with asthma (5 million adults and 2 million children), 29 million children younger than 14, and 7 million adults with chronic bronchitis.

According to the report, "while emissions of some air pollutants have generally gone down and the nation's overall air quality has improved over the past 30 years, much of that progress has been in eliminating obvious pollution and sources, bans on open burning, for example. Many of the pollutants that are literally invisible, such as ozone, have been reduced far less, and as understanding of the health effects of air pollution has advanced, it has become clear that much of the nation still faces major air pollution problems. *State of the Air* is the first annual 'report card' on America's air quality. It focuses on the most widespread air pollutant, ozone, sometimes called smog . . . among the most dangerous of the common air pollutants. . . . Many major metropolitan areas in the United States are plagued by high levels of ozone. As of 1998, almost 100 million Americans still lived in areas classified as not meeting the earlier one-hour national ozone standard."

The American Lung Association has also declared May "Clean Air Month," which will involve national and local events designed to emphasize the link between environmental conditions and respiratory wellness: "The quality of the air we breathe, both indoors and out, has a great impact on lung health. Fragile lung tissue is easily damaged by pollutants in the air, resulting in increased risk of asthma and allergies, chronic bronchitis, lung cancer and other respiratory diseases." (May 28, 2000)

See also OZONE.

air travel (related to impaired pulmonary function) Individuals with pulmonary impairment may require supplemental oxygen (appropriate to their respiratory system's functional capacity) when traveling by airplane, and those with blocked sinuses or eustachian tubes may be advised not to fly until the disorder has been resolved. Anyone with an infectious disease that can be transmitted to others by the airborne route is advised not to fly.

air vesicle An alveolus of the lung.

See also ALVEOLUS.

airways Passageways allowing air from the atmosphere to reach the lungs, beginning at the nostrils and mouth, and gradually branching into bronchi and bronchioles. They end at the alveolar sacs in the lungs, where oxygen is absorbed into the bloodstream.

During an asthma attack, the airways narrow or become obstructed by either constriction or mucous plugs. At first, muscles in the walls of the bronchioles constrict or go into spasm, called bronchospasm. If this is not relieved immediately, spontaneously, or with medication, blood vessels in the airway dilate and fluid leaks into the tissues. Resulting swelling (edema) further narrows the airway. This is followed by an inflammatory response and secretion of mucus, restricting airflow even more.

Wheezing may not be heard until there is at least a 50 percent narrowing of the airways. However, in extremely severe obstruction, there may be no audible wheezing. This can be misleading in a life-threatening situation. In an emergency room or doctor's office, the degree of narrowing of the airways can be measured by a spirometer or a peak flow meter. Inexpensive peak flow meters are available so patients can measure their peak flow at home, school, or work. Peak flow meters also aid physicians in making treatment decisions.

See also PEAK FLOW METER; SPIROMETER.

albuterol (Gen-Salbutamol, Novosalmol, Proventil, Proventil HFA, Proventil Repetabs, Salbutamol, Ventodisk, Ventolin, Ventolin Rotacaps, Volmax) A fast-acting bronchodilating drug used to open constricted airways in the treatment of asthma and in the prevention of exercise-induced asthma, bronchospasm, and the prevention of premature labor. It is in investigational use for hyperkalemia in dialysis patients. Albuterol is contraindicated for patients with severe cardiac disease and hypersensitivity to sympathomimetics. The most widely used of the beta-agonist drugs, its use is rarely limited by minor tremors or palpitations. Possible other side effects include headache, dizziness, restlessness, hallucinations, flushing, irritability, dry or irritated nose and throat, heartburn, nausea, vomiting, muscle cramps, hypotension, and paradoxic bronchospasm. Albuterol also interacts with other aerosol bronchodilators, tricyclic antidepressants, MAO inhibitor antidepressants, and other adrenergics, increasing their action. Other beta-blockers may inhibit the action of albuterol. The therapeutic response is absence of wheezing and difficulty breathing, and improved airway exchange and arterial blood gases (ABGs).

Albuterol is available as an aerosolized metered-dose inhaler (MDI), as a solution for use with an aerosol nebulizer, or as a tablet or syrup for oral use. For children or other persons who lack the coordination to use an MDI, the product Ventolin is available in a dried powder form dispensed in Rotacaps and inhaled by using a device known as a Rotahaler.

alcohol A chemical used as a solvent, an antiseptic, an astringent, and a component in intoxicating beverages, alcohol is also a common ingredient in cough syrups. It is thought to be a depressant to the cough center of the brain and may have some muscle-relaxing effect on the bronchial tubes. Two common adverse effects of alcohol (ethanol) are sedation and drying of the mucous membranes of the upper respiratory tract. Alcoholism may eventually result in respiratory arrest and death.

alkalosis, respiratory Excessive alkalinity (as opposed to acidity) in the body's fluids because of an acid-base imbalance, either an increase in alkalines or decrease in acid. Altitude alkalosis is caused by decreased oxygen in the air at high altitudes, which then causes respiratory alkalosis. Symptoms include numbness and tingling, carpopedal spasm, tetany, lightheadedness, and paresthesias. Respiratory alkalosis may also be the result of anxiety, fever, hyperventilation due to hypoxia (lack of oxygen), salicylate intoxication, exercise, and excessive assist, such as in the use of a respirator, to breathing. Initial treatment for hyperventilation includes having the person calm down by breathing into a paper bag, thus rebreathing carbon dioxide. Also, the patient may find some relief by breathing with one nostril closed off and the mouth closed. Other treatments depend upon the severity of the patient's symptoms and his or her medical history, including cardiac and neurologic status, vital signs, and arterial blood gases.

allergen A particle, substance, or other agent that causes hypersensitivity in certain individuals who come in contact with it.

See also AEROALLERGENS.

allergic rhinitis (pollinosis, hay fever) An inflammatory condition of the nasal passages, adjoining sinuses, ears, and/or throat that occurs when an allergic person inhales an allergen to which he or she is sensitive. Allergic rhinitis is an immune response that does not occur in a normal or nonallergic individual. Allergic rhinitis may occur periodically (seasonally) or continuously (perennially).

Cause

During the allergic reaction of hay fever, mast cells in the lining of the nose rupture when exposed to an allergen in a susceptible person. The mast cells release chemicals, called mediators, that are responsible for allergic symptoms.

Hay fever is an English name given because of symptoms caused by exposure to grass allergens coinciding with the bailing of hay. It usually refers to seasonal allergies, occurring with exposure to the airborne (windblown) pollens of trees, grasses, ragweed, and other weeds and outdoor mold spores. A person may suffer the symptoms during spring, fall, or both seasons.

Perennial, or year-round, allergic rhinitis is usually due to exposure to indoor allergens called "inhalants." Cats, dogs, rodents, house-dust mites, and indoor molds are examples of perennial allergens.

Allergic rhinitis is often confused with colds, sinus infections, nasal polyps or other nasal obstructions, and nonallergic, vasomotor rhinitis. Vasomotor rhinitis is nasal congestion that cannot be attributed to another cause, such as allergy. A deviated septum, an abnormality of the cartilage separating the nostrils, is a frequent cause of stuffy noses and can occur in allergic as well as nonallergic individuals. Rarely, more serious conditions such as tumors or nonhealing granulomas may exist. These conditions should be considered in patients who fail to respond promptly to treatment and who have blood-stained nasal mucus.

Overuse or abuse of over-the-counter nasal sprays can result in a common and troublesome disorder called rhinitis medicamentosus (rhinitis means an inflamed nose; medicamentosus means caused by medication). This condition is often confused with allergy and may occur in both allergic and nonallergic individuals.

Signs and Symptoms

These vary in severity from person to person. Symptoms include pruritus (itching), sneezing, rhinorrhea (runny and watery discharge from the nose), postnasal drip, and congestion of the nose, ears, and sinuses. A general state of fatigue and malaise (a feeling of being "unwell") may exist during allergy attacks. Loss of smell or taste occurs in severe cases.

Persons with hay fever frequently suffer from allergic conjunctivitis (itchy, watery, and red eyes caused by allergy) and asthma.

Physical Appearance

Hay fever sufferers often have a characteristic appearance. A horizontal crease across the lower portion of the nose is called the "allergic crease," caused by the "allergic salute," a constant pushing up on the tip of the nose by the palm of the hand prompted by the discomfort of nasal stuffiness.

Dark circles under the eyes are referred to as "allergic shiners." These are probably caused by blockage of blood flow to the tiny veins in the area because of swelling. Blood trapped in the area under the eyes has a very low oxygen content, resulting in the dark blue-black discoloration. There will often be swelling and puffiness of the eyelids, redness of the eyes, and watery discharge from the eyes and nose. Individuals with persistent nasal obstruction often breathe through their mouth, which causes facial abnormalities, such as long faces, flattened cheekbones, pinched nostrils, and raised upper lips. Orthodontic problems arise more frequently in allergic persons because of narrower retracted jaws, overbites, and high arched palates.

See also ASTHMA; HAY FEVER; POLLINOSIS; POLYP, NASAL; RHINITIS.

allergic salute   See ALLERGIC RHINITIS.

allergic shiner   See ALLERGIC RHINITIS.

allergist (allergist-immunologist)   A physician who diagnoses and treats allergic conditions and related disorders. Asthma, hay fever, eczema, and hives are among the illnesses most frequently treated by allergists. Most allergists complete a two-year fellowship in allergy and immunology following a residency in internal medicine or pediatrics. They are then eligible to become board certified in their specialty by passing a comprehensive examination.

See also IMMUNOLOGIST.

allergist-immunologist See ALLERGIST.

allergoids Allergy extracts modified by treatment with the chemical formalin. This modification results in lower incidence of reactions and shorter courses of immunotherapy (allergy shots). While ragweed allergoid has proven to be excellent, no other allergoids are available in the United States. Because most people need multiple extracts for their treatment, use of the singular allergoid may not be practical.

allergy An overreaction by the immune system to a substance called an allergen that does not cause a similar reaction in nonsensitized persons. An allergen is any protein or proteinlike substance recognized by the body as foreign and capable of provoking an allergic response.

Austrian pediatrician Clemens P. Pirquet (1874–1929) first used the term *allergy,* derived from the Greek *allos* ("altered") and *ergia* ("reactivity"), in 1906. He referred both to immunity, which is beneficial, and to harmful hypersensitivity of the immune system as allergy. Today, allergy refers only to the hypersensitivity or injurious effects of the immune system.

Causes

Most individuals inherit the tendency to be allergic from one or both parents. It is not known why some persons develop allergies and others do not. It is thought by some that exposure to viral infections, smoking, or hormones influence a person's propensity for allergy. It is also unknown why some individuals will get hay fever and others asthma, or both.

Types of Allergy

There are four classifications of allergic or hypersensitivity reactions: type I, immediate or immunoglobulin E (IgE) mediated; type II, in which antibodies are directed against cells; type III, in which toxic effects result from antibody and antigen complexes; and type IV, cell-mediated or delayed reactions.

Pollens, animal proteins (dander, saliva, urine, feathers), house-dust mites, molds, drugs, foods, and venoms from insects or reptiles are examples of allergens that can cause immediate, or type I, reactions. After a first exposure, these apparently harmless allergens stimulate the immune system to form IgE antibodies. IgE antibodies are specific to each allergen and attach to the surface of mast cells in the tissues. Upon re-exposure, the recognized allergen combines with its antibodies, rupturing mast cells and releasing biochemical mediators that cause the symptoms of allergy. The most severe form of type I allergic reaction is anaphylaxis.

Prevalence

The most common allergies include allergic rhinitis (hay fever), asthma, eczema, and urticaria (hives). The National Institute of Allergy and Infectious Diseases estimates that 35 million Americans have allergies and about 10 million have asthma. Approximately 80 to 90 percent of adult allergies are caused by inhaled allergens from animals, pollens, molds, or house dust. Foods are responsible for about 20 percent of children's allergies but much less so in adults. A small percentage of allergies is caused by contactants or insect stings.

Treatment

Three main phases of treatment are avoidance of allergen exposure, use of medication, and immunotherapy (or allergy shots). Avoidance of allergy triggers is the management of choice, but it may be difficult or even impossible to achieve. Drugs offer excellent relief from symptoms of allergies and asthma with minimal side effects. Antihistamines, adrenergic agonists or decongestants, beta-agonists and xanthine bronchodilators (theophylline), cromolyn and corticosteroids (derivatives of cortisone) are available in inhaled, oral, and injectable dosage forms. These drugs are among the most widely prescribed of all medicines. Immunotherapy, successfully used to treat allergic rhinitis (hay fever) for many years, is now also recognized as effective treatment for allergic asthmatic patients.

Alternative treatments include homeopathy (natrium muriaticum, or other preparation); kinesiology (balancing, stress reduction counseling, bowel cleansing, etc.); aromatherapy (Roman chamomile, helichrysum, melissa, etc.); hypnotherapy (hypno-healing, neurolinguistic programming, etc.); naturopathy (dietetic management and fasting, applied nutrition, etc.); color therapy (use of blues, greens, and oranges); autogenic training (rebalancing body systems); acupuncture; Ayurvedic medicine (panchakarma and a specialized diet); Chinese and Western herbalism, and auricular therapy (to relieve hay fever symptoms).

See also ALLERGEN; ALLERGY SHOTS; ANAPHYLAXIS; IMMUNOGLOBULINE; MAST CELLS.

Allergy and Asthma Network/Mothers of Asthmatics, Inc. A nationwide, community-based, nonprofit health organization dedicated to eliminating morbidity and mortality due to asthma and allergies through education, advocacy, community outreach, and research. The AAN-MA offers membership, publications (*Allergy & Asthma Health* is the organization's quarterly magazine; *The MA Report* is an eight-page newsletter), news and information, job and volunteer opportunities, marketplace, physician roll-call, outreach programs, and other allergy and asthma-related activities. The AAN-MA may be contacted at:

Allergy and Asthma Network/Mothers of
   Asthmatics, Inc.
2751 Prosperity Avenue
Suite 150
Fairfax, Virginia 22031
(800) 878-4403 or (703) 641-9595
(703) 573-7794 (Fax)
http://www.aanma.org.

allergy shots Allergy immunization or vaccination. According to a July 29, 1999, report by the American College of Allergy, Asthma and Immunology (ACAAI), allergies affect about 38 percent of all Americans, nearly twice as many as allergy experts had believed, and millions of them suffer unnecessarily or rely on medications they don't want to take because they are not aware of other effective treatment options, including allergy shots.

A representative sample of 1,004 adults was surveyed by the ACAAI about their experiences with allergies. According to ACAAI literature, "Thirty-eight percent reported having allergies, while 56 percent said they live in a household in which at least one member, including themselves, has allergies. The number of people affected surprised even allergy experts who thought the incidence of allergies was closer to 20 percent of the population. 'This new data shows us that allergies are almost twice as common as we thought,' said Ira Finegold, M.D., past-president of the ACAAI. 'What's of even greater concern is that the majority of people with allergies don't know about treatment that can bring them relief. A lot of them are either suffering from the symptoms or from medication side-effects.'

"Almost two-thirds of respondents who said they have allergies have never tried or considered allergy shots. . . . Allergy shots are a well-established treatment that naturally desensitizes the immune system. Small amounts of purified extracts of the substance causing allergic reactions are periodically injected and gradually increased until immunity is attained. They are effective against allergic diseases including allergic rhinitis (hay fever), insect sting allergy, and asthma.

"The treatment has a long track record of effectiveness and safety, with the incidence of adverse reactions less than 2/10 of 1 percent. It can be given to children as young as 4 and is safe for pregnant women as long as treatment was begun before pregnancy. Though not well known, allergy shots are viewed positively by those who are familiar with them, especially by those who have had the treatment, according to the survey. The survey also found that 54 percent of respondents would be willing to try allergy shots if the treatment would free them from medication.

"The ACAAI commissioned the national survey as part of a public education campaign to increase understanding of allergy immunization and encourage people who may be helped by this therapy to consider it. The randomized telephone survey was conducted by Opinion Research Corporation (ORC) . . . 502 men and 502 women— 18 years of age and older living in private households in the continental United States. The survey results are projectable to the U.S. population and have a margin of error of plus or minus 2 percent to 4 percent. . . . The only negative perception of allergy shots by a substantial number surveyed was related to cost. More than half answered 'yes' when asked if they thought allergy shots are expensive.

"The perception seems to be that vaccination is a great treatment for allergies but is not affordable," Dr. Finegold said. "In fact, allergy shots often are covered by health plans and the treatment can eliminate the need to buy medications. Overall, it's often less expensive and more effective than relying on medications every day and trying to isolate the allergy-sufferer from the environment. In many cases, the shots eventually can be discontinued, along with allergy medications, and the immunity maintained."

The ACAAI has also created a new consumer education quiz available on its web-site that tests individual knowledge of allergy and treatments, and provides detailed answers. The ACAAI's free brochure, *You Can Have A Life Without Allergies,* is available by calling (800) 842-7777. The brochure explains how allergy shots work and fit into the general management of allergy and asthma.

See also IMMUNOTHERAPY.

altitude sickness   Symptoms including headache, euphoria, shortness of breath, malaise, decreased ability to concentrate, lack of judgment, lightheadedness, and fainting that develop when an individual is in an environment of decreased oxygen, such as high on a mountain. Altitude sickness may cause death in some cases. When lack of adequate oxygen causes euphoria, an individual may be unaware of a potentially dangerous problem. Adaptation to high altitudes is possible over a period of time, perhaps months, depending upon the individual.

Altounyan, Roger E. C.   An Armenian-English physician (1922–87), born in Aleppo, Syria. Altounyan developed disodium cromoglycate, or cromolyn, an anti-inflammatory allergy medication. He first experimented with khella, a substance from the dried fruit of an herb, *Ammi visnaga,* indigenous to Egypt and North Africa, because khella had already been widely used for treating spasms of the intestines, bronchial tubes, uterus,

and arterial smooth muscle of the heart. In addition, Altounyan suffered from atopic dermatitis as a child and later from severe asthma. Using himself as the experimental subject, he investigated 670 synthetic compounds, and in 1967 he recognized the effectiveness of cromolyn.

aluminosis   A chronic inflammation of the lungs as a result of inhaled alum particles. A strong astringent, alum is a double sulfate of aluminum and potassium and aluminum and ammonia. Aluminosis is seen mostly in alum workers.

aluminum chloride   An astringent and antiseptic solution used as an antiperspirant. Aluminum chloride can be irritating and a cause of skin allergy. It also can be toxic if ingested.

Alupent   See METAPROTERENOL.

alveobronchiolitis   Inflammation of the bronchioles and pulmonary alveoli, also known as bronchopneumonia.

See also BRONCHOPNEUMONIA.

alveolitis   An inflammation of the air cells, or alveoli, of the lungs. Allergic alveolitis is a lung disease caused by hypersensitivity to organic dusts that are inhaled, especially by individuals whose occupation involves exposure to various dusts or pollutants.

See also BAGASSOSIS; FARMER'S LUNG; PNEUMONITIS.

alveolus   The air cell, one of many sacs or small hollows at the end of an alveolar duct in the lungs, where gases are exchanged in respiration.

amantadine (Symmetrel)   An antiviral drug that is also used in the treatment of Parkinson's disease. During "flu" epidemics, amantadine may lessen the severity of, shorten the course of, or prevent type A influenza, but it has no effect on influenza B or other viruses. Individuals at risk for severe complications of influenza, including some asthmatics, may benefit from immunization with influenza vaccine and daily doses of amantadine for several weeks until the vaccine becomes effective.

Ambu bag   The trade name for a bag used to help direct air into the lungs by artificial ventilation. The bag is a reservoir for oxygen attached to a one-way flow valve and a face mask that is placed over the mouth and nose of a patient who is not breathing. This resuscitator, also known as a bag-valve-mask resuscitator, is operated manually. A manikin used in teaching cardiopulmonary resuscitation is called an Ambu simulator.

American Academy of Allergy, Asthma and Immunology (AAAAI)   A professional organization of allergists and immunologists that promotes the advancement of scientific study of allergy and immunology both academically and in the practice of medicine. It was established in 1943 with the merger of the American Association for the Study of Allergy and the Association for the Study of Asthma and Allied Conditions.

The AAAAI publishes the *Journal of Allergy and Clinical Immunology.* From time to time the academy issues position statements to clarify confusing issues in the fields of allergy or immunology. An emphasis is placed on aiding the public in seeking competent medical care and avoiding unproven or dangerous techniques for the diagnosis or treatment of these disorders. The majority of fellows and members of the AAAAI are board certified in their specialty. Contact telephone number is (800) 822-ASMA.

American Board of Allergy and Immunology (ABAI)   A conjoint board of the American Board of Internal Medicine and the American Board of Pediatrics, established in 1971 as a nonprofit organization. It is sponsored jointly by the American Board of Internal Medicine (ABIM), the American Board of Pediatrics (ABP), the American Academy of Allergy, Asthma and Immunology (AAAAI), the American College of Allergy, Asthma and Immunology (ACAAI), the American Academy of Pediatrics–Section on Allergy, and the American Medical Association–Section on Allergy. The board consists of an even number of directors. The direc-

tors are nominated by the Sections on Allergy of the American Academy of Pediatrics and the American Medical Association, the AAAAI, ACAAI, and the ABAI itself. The nominees are appointed by the ABIM and the ABP. Each board director is appointed for six years.

Purposes of the ABAI

The major purposes of this organization are (1) to establish qualifications and examine physician candidates for certification as specialists in allergy and immunology, (2) to serve the public, physicians, hospitals, and medical schools by providing the names of physicians certified as allergists and immunologists, (3) to improve the quality of care in allergy and immunology to the public and increase the availability of specialists to deliver such care, (4) to establish and improve standards for the teaching and practice of allergy and immunology, (5) to establish standards for training programs in allergy and immunology, and (6) to provide increased opportunities for physicians wishing to specialize in allergy and immunology.

Certification

The ABAI is interested in candidates who have embarked voluntarily on a graduate program of study with the express purpose of excelling in the practice of the specialty of allergy and immunology. In outlining its requirements, the ABAI hopes to help the candidates select superior educational programs that will develop their competency in allergy and immunology. The ABAI believes that all allergists and immunologists should have a fundamental knowledge of the biological science basic to this discipline. Such knowledge is essential to the continued professional progress of any qualified allergist and immunologist. The ABAI anticipates that adequate knowledge in basic science, as applied to this discipline, will be acquired by the candidates during a post–medical school training program. The ABAI wishes to emphasize that time and training are but a means to the end of acquiring a broad knowledge of allergy and immunology.

The candidate must demonstrate competency to the ABAI in order to justify certification in this discipline. The responsibility of acquiring the knowledge rests with the candidate. The ABAI is responsible for the establishment and maintenance of the standards of knowledge required for certification. Each candidate for certification must satisfy the general and professional qualifications listed below. The candidate must qualify for examination by having passed the certification examination of the ABIM or the ABP. Certification requires three years of postgraduate general training in programs accredited by the Accreditation Council for Graduate Medical Education (ACGME), by presentation of evidence acceptable to the board of directors of at least two years of full-time residency/fellowship or other acceptable training in allergy and immunology programs accredited by the ACGME upon the recommendation of the Residency Review Committee for Allergy and Immunology. These programs are listed in the *Directory of Graduate Medical Education Programs*, published by the American Medical Association, a copy of which may be found in most medical school libraries.

Executive Office

American Board of Allergy and Immunology, A Conjoint Board of the American Board of Internal Medicine and the American Board of Pediatrics

Chairman: Lawrence B. Schwartz, M.D., Ph.D.

Co-chair: M. Louise Markert, M.D., Ph.D.

Executive Secretary: John W. Yunginger, M.D.

Administrative Director: Lynn Des Prez

510 Walnut Street, Suite 1701

Philadelphia, PA 19106-3699

(215) 592-9466

American College of Allergy, Asthma and Immunology (ACAAI)   Formerly the American College of Allergy and Immunology (ACAI), a professional medical organization comprised of 4,000 qualified allergists-immunologists and related health care professionals, founded by physicians and scientists to promote and advance the knowledge of allergy and to assure a high quality of care for patients with allergic disorders. Based in Arlington Heights, Illinois, the college is dedicated to the clinical practice of allergy, asthma, and immunology through education and research.

The ACAAI publishes the monthly scientific journal *Annals of Allergy, Asthma and Immunology*, which is available on-line through December 2000 and thereafter by subscription. *Annals* on-line contains full-text articles, including figures and tables, and text is searchable by keyword, with hyperlinks to MEDLINE. Archives are being built to include full-text articles of back issues since January 1997. Abstracts will be available from earlier publications.

Patient education "Advice From Your Allergist" articles are archived on-line on the following topics: rhinitis, insect sting allergies, urticaria, pregnancy with asthma and allergies, osteoporosis, long-acting bronchodilators, latex hypersensitivity, food allergies, headaches, house-dust allergies, and pet allergies. The website www.annallergy.org provides information about the journal, including instructions to authors, the Editorial Board, and subscription information. The journal received a top rating in a recent readership survey reported by Lippincott Williams & Wilkins and Dataview Research, Inc., scoring its usefulness and comparing it to other medical journals. Additional information on the diagnosis and treatment of asthma and allergic disease is available on the ACAAI public website (http://allergy.mcg.edu).

American Dietetic Association   An organization based in Chicago, Illinois, from which nutritional and dietary information important to individuals with allergies or asthma can be obtained. A list of commonly allergenic foods, including cow's milk, eggs, and wheat, is available. The association may be contacted at:

American Dietetic Association

216 West Jackson Boulevard

Chicago, IL 60606-6995

(312) 899-0040

aminophenols   Chemical derivatives of phenol used in orange, red, and medium-brown hair dyes. Adverse reactions range from mild contact rashes to convulsions from severe absorption or asthma from inhalation.

aminophylline   A bronchodilating drug made up of two components, theophylline and ethylenediamine. Available in both tablet and intravenous forms, aminophylline has been a standard treatment for acute asthma attacks for many years. However, recently, its use has been related to a backup role with the increased use of the beta-agonist bronchodilators. The action of aminophylline is based on the theophylline portion, which is a methylxanthine derivative and has many adverse effects and drug interactions.

See also THEOPHYLLINE.

ammonium carbonate A neutralizing alkaline chemical used as an expectorant in cough syrups, in permanent wave solutions, and in fire extinguishers. It can cause contact rashes.

ammonium iodide A chemical used as an expectorant in cough syrups. It is also used as a preservative and antiseptic by the cosmetic industry.

analgesia (respiratory implications) Drug therapy used to relieve pain. In the case of respiratory disorders, the use of narcotic painkillers such as codeine, morphine, oxycodone, hydromorphone, nalbuphine, pentazocine, and others is contraindicated in the event of acute bronchial asthma and upper airway obstruction. Side effects that may be caused by these drugs are respiratory depression and respiratory arrest, among other conditions.

anaphylactic shock See ANAPHYLAXIS.

anaphylactoid reaction A severe and potentially life-threatening, allergy-like reaction characterized by swelling and constriction of airways caused by the direct release of potent biochemical mediators from cells in the body tissues. As opposed to anaphylaxis, anaphylactoid reaction does not involve immunoglobulin E (IgE) antibodies. Since symptoms of anaphylactoid and true allergic, anaphylactic reactions are indistinguishable, the terms are used synonymously.

Immediate anaphylactoid reactions can result from poisoning after eating fish containing large amounts of histamine. Tuna, mackerel, and mahi mahi are the most common sources. Fish inadequately refrigerated or contaminated by *Proteus morganii* or *Klebsiella pneumoniae* bacteria may also contain dangerously high histamine levels. Allergy-like symptoms—flushing, erythema, itchy eyes, nausea, diarrhea, and headache—may last up to 24 hours and are self-limiting (they eventually disappear on their own). Swiss cheese may cause a similar reaction. Tuberculosis patients taking the drug isoniazid (INH) are highly susceptible to these food reactions.

See also ANAPHYLAXIS.

anaphylaxis (anaphylactic shock) The most severe or extreme type of allergic reaction, which may be life-threatening, characterized by any or a combination of the following symptoms: itching of the throat or skin, hives, dizziness, tightness and swelling in the throat, difficulty breathing, weakness, sudden drop in blood pressure, or unconsciousness. Anaphylaxis ranges from mild itching to collapse and death and, therefore, constitutes a medical emergency. True anaphylaxis occurs after exposure to an allergen to which a person has been previously sensitized.

Prevalence

An estimated four deaths per 10 million people from anaphylaxis occur each year. There are insufficient data to determine increased risk for anaphylaxis, such as age, sex, or ethnic criteria. There does not appear to be a predilection to penicillin or insect-sting anaphylaxis in persons known to have other allergies. However, some studies suggest that allergic individuals do have a higher incidence of anaphylaxis.

In the early 20th century, before the availability of antibiotics, horse-serum antitoxin was used to treat the often fatal diseases such as diphtheria, scarlet fever, tetanus, and tuberculosis. Prior to the penicillin era, horse serum was the most common cause of anaphylaxis.

Penicillin may account for 75 percent of all fatal allergic reactions: an estimated 500 deaths annually in the United States. One fatality occurs for every 7.5 million injections of penicillin; death may also result from oral, inhaled, or topical contact with the drug.

Hieroglyphics depict death from an insect sting 4,000 years ago. In 2640 B.C., the Egyptian pharaoh Menes reportedly died suddenly after being stung by a wasp. Up to 4 percent of the population suffers systemic reactions to stings of bees, wasps, hornets, yellow jackets, and fire ants.

Aspirin and the frequently used arthritis drugs called nonsteroidal anti-inflammatory drugs (NSAIDS), such as ibuprofen, may cause anaphylaxis in as many as 1 percent of individuals. Up to 10 percent of persons with asthma may exhibit anaphylaxis.

Cause

Despite recognition of fatal allergic reactions dating from biblical times, it was not until 1902 that French professors of medicine Charles Richet (1850–1935) and Paul Portier (1866–1962) linked a case of fatal anaphylaxis to a foreign protein injection that had been previously tolerated by a patient. Anaphylaxis occurs when potent biochemicals such as histamine (also called mediators) are released from mast and other special cells in the body tissues and act in a sequence of events affecting various organs. It is now known that there is more than one mechanism for this reaction.

Type I allergy, also called hypersensitivity or IgE-antibody–mediated allergic reaction, is the most common and best understood cause of anaphylaxis. Following initial exposure of a foreign protein or hapten, antibodies develop during a latent period. Anaphylaxis occurs upon re-exposure of this same foreign substance. A hapten, of which penicillin is an example, is a low-molecular-weight and nonallergenic substance until it combines with a larger "carrier" molecule to become allergenic. Hundreds of allergens in drugs (especially antibiotics), foods (the most frequent offenders include eggs, cow's milk, peanuts, fish and shellfish, and tree nuts), food preservatives (especially sulfites), and foreign proteins (including seminal fluid, insulin, and insect and snake venoms) are capable of inducing anaphylaxis in susceptible individuals.

However, other reactions that do not involve antigen-antibody production but stimulate the release of chemical mediators, including histamine, can cause the same symptoms as anaphylaxis. For many years this was referred to as anaphylactoid (anaphylactic-like) reactions. Most allergists feel the term is outdated and refer to all similar reactions as anaphylaxis. Substances capable of inducing these reactions include whole blood, radiocontrast (X ray) media, aspirin, food dyes, and drugs. Trauma, burns, or infections can also induce anaphylactoid reactions.

Signs and Symptoms

An initial sensation of warmth, itching, or tingling begins in the axilla or groin and gradually spreads throughout the body. Sneezing, intense itching, and constriction in the throat may progress to generalized hives and angioedema, or swelling of the face and tongue. Wheezing, shortness of breath, abdominal pain, nausea, vomiting, and diarrhea may follow. A drop in blood pressure, described by some as a feeling of "impending doom," may signal collapse (or shock) and death. Any of these signs and symptoms can occur individually or concurrently. The longer the time interval (or latent period) between the initial exposure to an allergen and the onset of symptoms, the less likely it is that death will occur.

Treatment

Treatment must be initiated at the first signs or symptoms of impending anaphylaxis, since there is no way of anticipating how severe a reaction may become. Epinephrine (adrenaline) given subcutaneously (under the skin) is the drug of choice; if it is given immediately, it may be lifesaving. Antihistamines, bronchodilators, corticosteroids, and oxygen are also administered as needed, but they take much longer to become effective and may not be lifesaving.

Arrange transportation of the patient to the nearest emergency room or other medical facility. A delay of even a few minutes can be fatal. A person may experience a recurrence of anaphylaxis as long as 24 hours after the initial reaction and should be monitored for at least 24 hours.

Prevention

Individuals known to be at risk through a history of a prior severe allergic reaction should carry an adrenaline kit at all times. Identify and avoid a food (rarely more than one) that is thought to be a cause of allergic reaction. Avoidance of a food because another family member has had a serious reaction to it is not necessary. Skin testing for foods can be hazardous and should be avoided if anaphylaxis has occurred; radioallergosorbent test (RAST) blood food testing is safer but often misleading because of false-positive or -negative results.

Specific preventive measures should be taken by persons with cold-induced urticaria (hives), exercise-induced anaphylaxis, and allergy to seminal fluid, venomous insects, drugs, and radiocontrast (X ray) dyes.

See also ADVERSE DRUG REACTIONS.

anapnea   Breathing or regaining the breath.

anergy   The inability of certain individuals to react to a test for hypersensitivity to antigens. Normal individuals almost invariably have positive skin tests to mumps, *Candida* (a common yeast), and tetanus antigens because antibodies to these conditions are present in their blood. However, some skin tests prove negative despite the presence of the antibodies. Several factors influence the possibility of anergy, including the number and type of antigens (bacterial, fungal, or viral) used in the skin test, the characteristics of a positive reaction, and the presence of a mild upper respiratory infection.

Anergy was first noticed when patients with measles lost the ability to react to skin-testing for tuberculosis for a short period of time. Anergy also pertains to one whose skin temporarily does not show a reaction to a tuberculin (e.g., Mantoux) test after receiving a live-attenuated measles, mumps, and rubella (MMR) vaccine. If a tuberculin test is required, it should be administered either before or simultaneously with the MMR vaccine or after three months from the date of the vaccination.

anesthesia for the allergic and asthmatic patient
Alternatives to general anesthesia should be considered for all surgical candidates with allergies or asthma, because any hypersensitivity may be exacerbated by anesthesia drugs with potentially severe results. (The risk of adverse effects of anesthesia, although small, exists even for nonallergic or nonasthmatic normal individuals.) Spinal, epidural, or local anesthesias are excellent choices for many surgical procedures.

Anesthetics, Local
Lotions, creams, ointments, and sprays applied topically in the treatment of local injuries, burns, and insect bites. Other local anesthetics, drugs designed to eliminate sensation only in certain areas of the body, may be injected before minor surgery or repair of skin lacerations, or to numb dental tissues before dental surgery.

Snow may have been the first anesthetic agent used and was recognized for its numbing ability by Hippocrates. Cocaine was isolated in 1860 by Niemann from the *Erythroxylon coca* bush. However, the modern era of a local anesthesia was not entered until 1884, when Sigmund Freud and Karl Koller reported the cocaine's ability to numb the eye for surgical procedures.

Although these agents rarely cause true allergic reactions, they often cause vasovagal syncope (fainting spell brought on by a sudden drop in blood pressure), hyperventilation, palpitations, or anxiety reactions. These are non-immune (nonallergic) adverse reactions resulting from excessive doses or other pharmacologic drug reactions easily confused with allergy.

Patients suspected of having a true type I (immediate) allergic reaction to one of these drugs can be tested by injecting them with minute doses, gradually increasing the dose according to standardized protocol. Drugs may cross-react if they belong to the para-aminobenzoic esters group, such as procaine (Novocain) and tetracaine (Pontocaine). Lidocaine (Xylocaine), bupivacaine, and others do not cross-react and can usually be substituted for the drug suspected of a reaction without the need for the tedious process of testing and desensitization.

Parabens and other preservatives may be responsible for some adverse reactions rather than the anesthetic drug. Local anesthetics are available in individual, preservative-free dose ampules. Benzocaine, although commonly used topically for temporary relief of the conditions listed above, may cause a sensitivity reaction of its own and worsen rather than improve the condition for which it is employed. Many allergists and dermatologists warn against their use on the skin; however, drugs like lidocaine offer temporary relief for ulcers of the mouth, rectal lesions, including hemorrhoids, and painful mucous membranes.

Benzocaine, cyclaine, and tetracaine are used to inhibit the cough reflex before invasive diagnostic tests such as bronchoscopy. Another local anesthetic, benzonatate (Tessalon), is available as a prescription cough suppressant.

High-pressure dental equipment can cause air infiltration into local oral tissues, resulting in swelling and wheezing that may be confused with an allergic reaction.

Local Anesthetic Drugs

Ester Type (contain para-aminobenzoic esters and may cross-react):
benoxinate (Dorsacaine)
benzocaine[1]
butacaine (Butyn)
butethamine (Monocaine)
butylaminobenzoate (Butesin)
chloroprocaine (Nesacaine)[2]
cocaine
cyclomethycaine (Surfacaine)
hexylcaine (Cyclaine)[3]
procaine (Novocain)[4]
proparacaine (Ophthaine)
tetracaine (Pontocaine)[3]

Amide Type (do not contain para-aminobenzoic esters and do not cross-react):
amethocaine[1]
amydricaine (Alypin)
bupivacaine (Marcaine)
dibucaine (Nupercaine)[4]
dimethisoquin (Quotane)
diperodon (Diothene)
dyclonine (Dyclone)
etidocaine (Duranest)
lidocaine (Xylocaine)[5]
mepivacaine (Carbocaine)
oxethazaine (Oxaine)
phenacaine (Holocaine)
piperocaine (Metycaine)
pramoxine (Tronothane)
prilocaine (Citanest)
pyrrocaine (Endocaine)

[1] More likely to cause contact dermatitis.
[2] May be safest because of its short duration of action.
[3] More likely to cause true anaphylaxis.
[4] More likely to cause anaphylaxis or contact dermatitis.
[5] Most widely used and often combined with epinephrine, which may be the cause of adverse effects.

See also SURGERY, RELATED TO ALLERGIC AND ASTHMATIC PERSONS.

aneurysm From the Greek word *aneurysma,* meaning a widening, a dilation occurring due to a weakness in the wall of a blood vessel. In the case of an aortic aneurysm, dyspnea, cough, sputum production, congestion, and other symptoms may appear, and there may be pressure on the trachea, esophagus, veins, or nerves. Aneurysms are often the result of trauma or bacterial and mycotic infection.

angioedema, hereditary A rare inherited disorder (genetically known as autosomal dominant) due to the deficiency or malfunction of a substance called C1-esterase inhibitor usually manifesting in late adolescence or early adulthood. Infected persons have less than 15 percent normal-functioning C1 inhibitor (an inhibitor is a chemical that stops enzyme activity), and family history is positive for this disorder in 85 to 90 percent of patients. Lack of C1 inhibitor results in an activation of the complement system (consisting of components related to how antibodies work in the blood) and the release of chemical mediators that produce the symptoms of angioedema.

The condition is characterized by recurrent episodes of painful swelling of the skin and mucosa of the upper respiratory and gastrointestinal tracts, and the extremities. Hereditary angioedema can be triggered by minor trauma, sudden changes in temperature, infections, and emotional upset. An estimated 25 percent of untreated individuals die of laryngeal edema after dental or throat surgery. Other symptoms include abdominal pain from swelling of intra-abdominal organs, vomiting, diarrhea, and a drop in blood pressure. Unlike idiopathic, or nonhereditary, angioedema, urticaria (hives) and itching do not occur. Diagnosis is made by measuring C1 inhibitor levels, assays that assess functional abnormalities in the presence of normal or near-normal levels of the enzyme, and other complement levels. This life-threatening disease can be treated with synthetic anabolic steroids such as danocrine (Danazol). However, the drug cannot be used in children or adolescents until they have achieved their full growth. Short-term therapy in anticipation of dental or throat surgery includes fresh-frozen plasma given one day prior to surgery. Epsilon-aminocaproic acid and tranexamic acid are drugs sometimes used prior to surgery. Emergency intubation or tracheostomy may be required.

anoxia Lack of oxygen, such as in high altitude anoxia. Anoxic anoxia is caused by a disorder in the lungs' ability to fill with oxygen, which in turn may be caused by decreased oxygen supply, a respiratory obstruction, decreased pulmonary function, or insufficient respiratory movements.

antasthmatic A substance or agent that prevents or relieves the symptoms of asthma.

anthracosilicosis A type of pneumoconiosis characterized by an accumulation of silica and carbon deposits in the lungs as a result of inhaling coal dust.
See also COAL WORKER'S PNEUMOCONIOSIS.

anthracosis Carbon deposits in the lungs from inhaling smoke or coal dust.
See also BLACK LUNG.

anthrax An infectious disease caused by *Bacillus anthracis* that usually attacks cattle, sheep, horses, and goats, but may also be transmitted to humans through contact with animal hair, hides, or waste materials. The disease may target the lungs or loose connective tissue, which may cause malignant edema, necrosis of mediastinal lymph nodes, and pleural effusion. Shock, coma, and respiratory arrest may also occur. Penicillin, tetracyclines, and erythromycin are among the drugs of choice for the treatment of anthrax.

In the fall of 2001 on the heels of the terrorist attacks on the World Trade Center in New York City, anthrax-tainted mail became a major concern for postal workers and the general population. Considered an act of chemical terrorism (also called bioterrorism) committed by yet unknown perpetrators, anthrax spores in a powdered form were found in envelopes and packages. When inhaled by the recipient, there was a possibility of contracting the disease. The first of several victims of inhalation anthrax was American Media photo editor Bob Stevens, of Florida, who died in September 2001. An initial difficulty in diagnosing the disease involved medical professionals who had rarely, if ever, treated cases of anthrax. Now the Centers for Disease Control and Prevention (CDC) in Atlanta, Georgia, releases updated knowledge on the diagnosis and treatment of anthrax.

Believed to have a survival rate ranging from 1 to 15 percent before the terrorism occurred, inhalation anthrax now presents itself with a 60 percent survival rate. Of the 10 individuals who were reported to have contracted the disease, six survived, most likely due to early recognition of symptoms and prompt antimicrobial administration. Some victims of anthrax, aged 43 to 73, complained of various flu-like symptoms, while others experienced non–flu-like drenching night sweats, nausea and vomiting, abdominal pain, and pleural effusion. Of the three types of anthrax—inhalation, cutaneous, and gastrointestinal—inhalation is the most dangerous and life-threatening, particularly because the symptoms, including fever, malaise, nonproductive cough, chest or abdominal pain, nausea, vomiting, and headache, may suddenly subside (called "the anthrax honeymoon"), and treatment may be delayed. However, untreated symptoms of anthrax may lead to acute dyspnea, a widening of the mediastinum (seen in chest X ray/radiograph), diaphoresis, cyanosis, stridor, shock, and death in up to three days. Some victims of anthrax may also develop meningitis. According to reports, all 10 victims showed abnormal chest X rays with pleural effusion, mediastinal widening, or infiltrates.

The incubation period of anthrax may be as brief as two days after contamination to two months. The dearth of information on the incubation period, symptoms, cross-contamination, and methods of infection has prompted the CDC to recommend the use of ciprofloxacin (Cipro) or doxycy-cline for initial intravenous therapy plus other antimicrobial drugs until antimicrobial results are specified. Other antibiotics that may be used include ampicillin, chloramphenicol, clarithromy-cin, clindamycin, imipenem, penicillin, rifampin, and vancomycin, or combinations of various drugs. The use of cephalosporins and trimethoprim-sul-famethoxazole, and the use of penicillin G, ampi-cillin, or amoxicillin alone, are not recommended by the CDC. For those anthrax sufferers who are allergic or cannot take ciprofloxacin or doxycycline for some other reason, high-dose penicillin, such as amoxicillin or penicillin VK may be substituted, and steroids may be necessary if the patient is experiencing respiratory distress or has meningitis. Treatment for children with anthrax may be even more difficult to diagnose, and the CDC urges pedi-atric practitioners to be aware of symptoms that may warrant immediate treatment.

Prophylactic antibiotics have been recom-mended for individuals who may have been ex-posed to aerosolized anthrax spores or to air space shared by a victim of inhalation anthrax. More information is available on the CDC website, www.cdc.gov/ncidod/EID/vol7no6/pdf/jernigan.pdf.

See also ANTIBIOTIC; PLEURA; WOOLSORTER'S DISEASE.

antibiotic   A natural or synthetic substance or agent that inhibits the growth of or destroys microorganisms. In 1939, the first antibiotic—meaning against life—was gramicidin, used by René Dubos to treat infected cattle. Penicillin's clin-ical use came later. A bacteriocidal or bactericidal antibiotic agent kills microorganisms; a bacteriosta-tic antibiotic inhibits their growth. A broad-spectrum antibiotic inhibits or kills a number of microorganisms. Some strains of bacteria were either never affected by antibiotics or have evolved to become resistant to them. This has become a recent problem most likely because the use of antibiotics became so commonplace as to be over-prescribed, and because individuals stopped taking the medication sooner than prescribed (therapy usually spans seven to 10 days) when symptoms subsided or disappeared. Completion of antibiotic

therapy is of utmost importance, even after an ill-ness or infection seems to have gone away.

Also, many patients demand antibiotics for res-piratory or other infections that may in actuality be caused by a virus, not a bacterium, in which case the antibiotic is ineffective and the body develops a tolerance for it that may thwart the effectiveness of an antibiotic prescribed for a future infection. Antibiotics that target certain viruses have been developed.

See also PENICILLIN.

antibody   A substance produced by B cells (lym-phocytes derived from bone marrow) and designed to attack a specific foreign invader called an anti-gen. For example, a cold virus stimulates a B cell to produce an antibody against that specific virus. The immune process involving antibodies is referred to as humoral immunity.

When a B cell encounters its triggering antigen, T cells and other accessory cells collaborate with it to cause the production of large plasma cells. Each plasma cell becomes a factory for producing anti-bodies. Antibodies are Y-shaped protein molecules known as immunoglobulins. Transported through the circulation to the site of inflammation or infec-tion, antibodies neutralize or combine with and identify antigens for attack by other cells or chem-ical mediators.

antibody deficiency disorder   Acquired or con-genital inability to produce all or selective classes of immunoglobulins. Individuals with this disorder have frequent infections or difficulty overcoming them. Examples are X-linked or Bruton's agamma-globulinemia (lack of gamma globulin antibodies in the blood) and common variable or acquired hypogammaglobulinemia (abnormally low level of gamma globulin in the blood).

See also ACQUIRED IMMUNODEFICIENCY SYNDROME; IMMUNOGLOBULIN A; IMMUNOGLOBULIN D; IMMUNO-GLOBULIN G; IMMUNOGLOBULIN M.

anticholinergics   Bronchodilating drugs that block the action of nerve reflexes that constrict muscles of the bronchial tubes in the lungs. Anti-cholinergics take 15 to 20 minutes to become effective, as opposed to faster-acting beta-agonists. Atropine and ipratropium (Atrovent) are examples; only Atrovent is available as a metered-dose inhaler. Adverse effects of anticholinergics, dry mouth and cough, are rarely encountered with ipratropium.

antigen (immunogen) Any substance that, when introduced into the body, is recognized by the immune system and is capable of triggering an immune response. The term *immune* is derived from the Latin *immunis* (free from taxes or free from burden). An antigen can be a bacterium, fungus, parasite, virus, or a part or substance produced by these organisms. Tissues or cells from another individual, except an identical twin, are recognized by the immune system as foreign and, therefore, antigenic.

See also ALLERGEN; IMMUNE SYSTEM.

antigens, cross-reaction among plant families Allergic reactions that occur from exposure to allergens common to more than one plant family. For example, ragweed, a member of the Ambrosiaceae family, has antigens that cross-react with members of the family Compositae. This cross-reaction explains why ragweed-sensitive persons may react when drinking chamomile tea, because chamomile is derived from Compositae. Ragweed-sensitive persons also may react to pyrethrum, an insecticide made from chrysanthemums, another member of the Compositae.

Although hay fever sufferers sometimes experience itching and swelling of the palate after eating melons and bananas during the ragweed season, there is no cross-reactivity between ragweed antigen and the botanical families of melon and banana.

antihistamine Any drug that blocks the effects of histamine, a potent chemical substance produced in the body, and is responsible for the body's allergic responses. For nearly 50 years, antihistamines have been used to prevent or relieve the symptoms of immediate, type I hypersensitivity, or anaphylactic allergic reactions. Characteristic symptoms include sneezing, rhinorrhea (watery nasal discharge), congestion, itching, wheezing, and swelling of tissues. During an allergic reaction, allergens bind to histamine type 1 receptors on the surface of mast cells and basophils, and cause the cells to rupture and release stored histamine and other substances called chemical mediators.

Antihistamines bind to these receptors to prevent allergens from binding, which in turn prevents cell rupture and release of the mediators. Histamine blockade of receptors is competitive, and an inadequate dose or a lapse in timing of a dose of antihistamine may result in poor therapeutic response. Histamine may also be released by other mechanisms during exposure to certain drugs, chemicals, dyes, foods, toxins, alkaloids, venoms, or physical stimuli. Certain foods also contain histamine. Histamine and other released chemical mediators are responsible for the symptoms that occur during anaphylaxis, which may be life-threatening, and antihistamines alone may be inadequate in this situation. The beneficial effects of antihistamines, as well as any adverse ones, are related to their basic chemical structures.

There are five classes of type 1 antihistamines. Some antihistamines such as azatadine have a dual action and also prevent the release of the chemical reactors, thus blocking to varying degrees the cascade of events of allergic reaction. Drugs available in the United States, such as azelastine (Astelin Nasal Spray) and ketotifen (Zaditor Ophthalmic Solution) have traditional receptor blocking abilities, but their greatest antiallergic benefits combat inflammatory late-phase reactions. Since their primary function is against late-phase reaction, azelastine and ketotifen are not really antihistamines by definition. Antihistamines are most effective in seasonal allergic rhinitis or hay fever, slightly less effective for perennial or chronic allergic rhinitis, and least likely to improve symptoms of the nonallergic vasomotor and infectious types of rhinitis. Antihistamines are frequently prescribed with nasal decongestants either separately or combined in one tablet, capsule, or liquid preparation.

There is no evidence that antihistamines are of any benefit for the treatment of colds, despite their inclusion in many over-the-counter and prescription cold remedies. But an indirect benefit may be attributed to the sedative side effect of most antihistamines, especially when the inducement of drowsiness or sleep is desired. The intense pruritus (itching) that accompanies urticaria (hives) and the allergic skin conditions, eczema and contact dermatitis, are relieved to varying degrees by antihistamines. At night, the added benefit of sedation from the first-generation agents such as hydroxyzine (Atarax) may make them more effective. The nonsedating astemizole (Hismanal) is effective for suppressing hives and can be given in a single-daily dose for convenience. H_1 and H_2 antihistamines are sometimes combined in resistant cases of hives. Minor allergic reactions to insect stings, drugs, foods, and allergy immunotherapy (allergy shots) often respond to antihistamines.

When anaphylaxis is impending or has occurred, epinephrine (Adrenalin Chloride) should be administered promptly. Diphenhydramine (Benadryl) or other antihistamines are useful only as a secondary treatment. Prescription and over-the-counter antihistaminic eyedrops relieve itching associated with seasonal allergic conjunctivitis. Antihistamines are sometimes given prophylactically before a blood transfusion in persons with a history of prior transfusion reaction. While antihistamine may reduce the itching and flushing that can occur during a transfusion, it does not prevent the serious reactions possible from receiving blood from an incompatible donor. Many persons experience adverse reactions to radiocontrast (X-ray dye). Such reactions are complex, and there is a higher incidence in allergic individuals. Antihistamines and corticosteroids should be given to anyone who has had a previous reaction.

Sedating properties of antihistamines make them useful as relatively safe, nonprescription hypnotics. One must be warned, however, that overdoses of these drugs may be fatal. Also, tolerance develops quickly, limiting their usefulness for chronic insomnia. Hydroxyzine (Vistaril) and promethazine (Phenergan) are antihistamines often mixed with narcotics such as meperidine (Demerol) to potentiate their effectiveness and also to prevent nausea. Cyclizine (Marezine), meclizine (Antivert, Bonine), and dimenhydrinate (Dramamine) prevent motion sickness and counteract the disabling vertigo of Ménière's syndrome. Side effects vary by incidence. Intensity corresponds to

the class to which a particular antihistamine belongs. The traditional antihistamines cause drowsiness in many individuals because the drug diffuses into the central nervous system from the general circulating blood. Drowsiness varies greatly among individuals, often improving after several days. Great care must be taken when driving or operating dangerous machinery because of impairment of reflexes. Drowsiness intensifies if other sedative drugs or alcohol are used concurrently.

Antihistamines may also disturb coordination and cause dizziness, a feeling of lassitude, fatigue, tinnitus (ringing in the ears), diplopia (double vision), and the inability to concentrate. Instead of sedation from antihistamines, a few individuals, especially infants or toddlers, experience an unexpected excitatory or stimulant effect, at times to the point of insomnia. Seizures, or convulsions, are a potentially serious adverse effect of antihistamines in some individuals predisposed to them, most often children. Sedation is the most frequent side effect of first-generation antihistamines, also referred to as "classic" or traditional antihistamines, such as chlorpheniramine (Chlor-Trimeton) and diphenhydramine (Benadryl). Newer antihistamines such as terfenadine (Seldane), astemizole (Hismanal), and the drugs loratadine (Claritin) and cetirizine are generally nonsedating in most patients.

For many years antihistamines were thought to be contraindicated or harmful to patients with asthma. In fact, most over-the-counter and prescription antihistamines come with a warning against their use by these patients. It was thought that their drying effects would aggravate asthma. Not only has this been disproved, but some antihistamines have mild bronchodilating effects and may actually be beneficial to some asthmatics. Rarely will an antihistamine worsen asthma. The topical use of antihistamines available as over-the-counter remedies for the relief of itching from prison ivy, insect stings, and sunburn should be avoided. These products are skin sensitizers in many persons and frequently cause an allergic contact dermatitis worse than the original condition for which they are recommended.

Anticholinergic, or atropine-like, side effects range from minor dryness of the mucous membranes of the nose, mouth, and throat to constipa-tion, tachycardia (palpitations), excitability, rest-lessness, nervousness, insomnia, irritability, and tremors. Blurred vision could be a potentially seri-ous problem in a person with untreated or inade-quately controlled glaucoma. It is not uncommon for a middle-aged or elderly male to develop a sud-den inability to pass urine (acute urinary retention) after taking an antihistamine. Infrequent gastroin-testinal disturbances include anorexia (loss of appetite), nausea, vomiting, abdominal pain, con-stipation, or diarrhea. The most important advance since the availability of these important drugs in the 1940s has been the development of the "sec-ond-generation" H_1-receptor antihistamines. These newer agents, including terfenadine and astemi-zole, are nonsedating in up to 99 percent of patients because they do not cross the blood-brain barrier in significant amounts. Some rare side effects of nonsedating antihistamines include increased appetite and weight gain in patients taking astemizole and hair loss in a few patients taking terfenadine. A more serious, but fortunately an extremely rare, problem with both astemizole and terfenadine has been the onset of cardiac arrhythmias (irregularities), including ventricular tachycardia and fibrillation, which can be life-threatening. Arrythmias follow doses two or three times the recommended dose. Patients at increased risk have been those also taking the drugs keto-conazole (Nizoral), troleandomycin (TAO), or ery-thromycin, or those with liver diseases such as hepatitis or alcoholic cirrhosis and hypokalemia (a state of low potassium in the blood).

Rare cases of blood disorders, such as agranulo-cytosis (a severe depression of the bone marrow's production of granulocytic white blood cells), leukopenia (low leukocytic white blood cell count), thrombocytopenia (destruction or decreased pro-duction of platelets), and hemolytic anemia (destruction of the red blood cells), are usually reversible when the offending drug is discontinued. Considering the millions of doses of these drugs taken every day, the chances of suffering a serious side effect are slim.

Despite antihistamines' long record of safety, their easy availability makes them popular for sui-cide attempts. The margin of safety for antihista-mines is considerably less for children. The first signs of overdose usually occur within two hours of ingestion: drowsiness, dizziness, unsteady gait, flushing, dilated pupils, and fever; however, chil-dren will often paradoxically appear hyperactive, with hallucinations, toxic psychosis (bizarre behav-ior), and tremors. In adults, seizures, respiratory failure, cardiac arrest, and death may result. There is no perfect antidote for antihistamine overdose. Efforts may include eliminating the drug by induced vomiting in a conscious patient or by pumping the stomach in a lethargic or comatose one. Activated charcoal and strong laxatives called cathartics are also given. The drug physostigmine is sometimes used, but not without risk. It should probably be used only in situations when high tem-perature or delirium does not respond to cooling by hypothermia blankets, fluids, and cold bathing.

Antihistamines may mask the early signs of ana-phylaxis and should not be used to prevent this reaction when administering immunotherapy (allergy shots). Although the use of drugs during pregnancy, especially during the period of organ development in the first trimester, should be lim-ited, the use of an antihistamine may be unavoid-able. Treatment should be based on the same principles for using any drug during pregnancy. Not only must the drug be necessary, but it also should have a long record of use during pregnancy without reported adverse outcomes to the preg-nancy and its use must be monitored by a physi-cian experienced in its use during pregnancy. Chlorpheniramine (Chlor-Trimeton) and tripelen-namine (Pyribenzamine) are the preferred antihis-tamines in pregnancy.

Antihistamines: Chemical Classification and Generic and Trade Names

Amino alkyl ethers (Ethanolamines): clemastine fumarate (Tavist); diphenhydramine hydrochloride (Benadryl)

Ethylenediamines: pyrilamine maleate (generic); tripelennamine citrate or hydrochloride (PBZ)

Alkylamines (Propylamines): brompheniramine maleate (Dimetane); chlorpheniramine maleate (Chlor-Trimeton, Teldrin); dexchlorpheni-ramine maleate (Polaramine); tripolidine hydrochloride (Actidil) [Other antihistamines of this class not generally used for allergic conditions are not listed.]

Phenothiazines: methdilazine (Tacaryl); promethazine hydrochloride (Phenergan); trimeprazine tartrate (Temaril)

Piperidines: azatadine maleate (Optamine); cyproheptadine hydrochloride (Periactin)

Piperazines: hydroxyzine hydrochloride (Atarax, Vistaril); phenindamine tartrate (Nolahist)

Nonsedating: acrivastine (Semprex); astemizole (Hismanal); azelastine (Astelin); cetirizine hydrochloride (Zyrtec); loratadine (Claritin); terfenadine (Seldane).

See also DECONGESTANT; HISTAMINE H$_2$, RECEPTOR AGONIST.

anti-inflammatory An agent or substance that prevents or reduces inflammation, the body's nonspecific immune response to an area that is injured or traumatized. Anti-inflammatory drugs may also relieve pain. Ibuprofen is a popular example of a nonsteroidal anti-inflammatory (trade names include Motrin, Advil, Nuprin, and Rufen). Aspirin (acetylsalicylic acid) is also a nonsteroidal anti-inflammatory (also known as NSAIDs) with painkilling and fever-reducing properties. Some NSAIDs have been known to produce asthma in certain individuals, which contraindicates their use. Bronchospasm, nasal polyps, rhinitis, and hypersensitivity to the particular drug are also contraindications.

antimicrobial An agent or substance that destroys or inhibits the development of microorganisms.

antiseptic An agent or substance that prevents or inhibits the growth of disease-causing microorganisms.

antituberculotic Thwarting or stopping tuberculosis in the body. In the treatment of pulmonary tuberculosis, antituberculars are drugs that inhibit RNA or DNA fats and protein synthesis, which reduces the ability of the tubercle bacillus to replicate.

antitussive An agent or substance that reduces, relieves, or prevents coughing. A centrally acting antitussive acts on the medullary centers of the brain to suppress the cough reflex.

antiviral An agent or substance that inhibits or destroys viruses.

anxiety Feelings including fear and panic or nervousness that may lead to physiological symptoms or discomfort. Breathing difficulties and disorders may cause anxiety in some individuals. Because anxiety is a response to stress or conflict, a person with a respiratory disorder such as asthma or chronic obstructive pulmonary disease may experience symptoms of anxiety during an exacerbation of the disease or after the discontinuation of a medication. Many individuals, with or without respiratory disease, may experience anxiety as shortness of breath or a feeling of being asphyxiated, faintness, heart palpitations, trembling or shivering, increased sweating, a sensation of choking, fear of losing control or dying, chills, numbness, nausea, diarrhea, pains in the chest, and other manifestations.

Very often the family of a person with a respiratory disorder such as asthma may suffer severe anxiety when the person experiences an asthma attack or any situation that causes difficulty breathing. Education, precautions, and strategies prepared ahead of time may decrease the fears of the caregivers.

Those with anxiety disorders not usually induced by a medical problem, such as social phobia, obsessive-compulsive disorder, agoraphobia, posttraumatic stress disorder, panic attacks, or panic disorder, should seek treatment if they develop a respiratory or other medical problem, or if they have an anxiety disorder in addition to a respiratory problem. It is also recommended that physicians check for possible adverse effects of a medication if a patient exhibits symptoms of severe anxiety.

Psychiatric patients with severe respiratory disorders should be monitored carefully so that they can receive the proper medication and comply with proper medical treatment.

apicolysis   A collapse of the apex of the lung induced by surgically creating an opening in the anterior chest wall. This procedure may be performed for a number of reasons based on a physician's assessment of a patient's condition. Symptoms of anxiety may require attention and emotional support. Both during and after the procedure, caregivers must monitor the patient carefully for signs of dyspnea, cyanosis, increased pulse and respiratory rate (which may indicate tension pneumothorax), and signs of mediastinal shift, including severe dyspnea, cyanosis, increased pulse and respirations, distended veins in the neck, and severe, uncontrollable cough.

apnea   A temporary cessation of breathing, which may be caused by failure of the respiratory center of the brain to discharge breathing impulses. Apnea is a symptom of conditions including arteriosclerosis, meningitis, cardiac and renal diseases, or following trauma to the brain. Apneic oxygenation refers to providing oxygen to the upper airway of patients who are not breathing. Apnea monitoring is recommended especially for infants to prevent sudden infant death syndrome. Infants may be placed on an apnea alarm mattress designed to sound an alarm if the infant stops breathing. Sleep apnea, or a cessation of breathing occurring during sleep, may last approximately 10 seconds and recur 30 or more times in a seven-hour period of sleep. This disorder may be caused by an upper airway obstruction, respiratory muscle activity dysfunction, or a combination of factors. Treatment may include surgical correction of an obstruction, the correction of an underlying disease, weight loss, and the prescription of certain drugs.

apneumatosis   Congenital atelectasis.
See also ATELECTASIS.

apneumia   A birth defect in which the lungs are absent. Birth defects may result from chromosomal or genetic abnormalities of one or both parents, and genetic testing may be recommended for those who wish to conceive but may have a family history of genetic problems. Physicians or genetic counselors usually prefer to know the history of at least three generations in a particular family, i.e., causes of death of all parents, siblings, children, aunts, uncles, and grandparents, history of distant relatives if pertinent (such as if they had a genetic disorder), ethnic and racial background, possible intermarriages of relatives, and exposure to drugs that have been known to cause fetal distress or defects. Various testing is also helpful in detecting hereditary disorders. Carrier screening for diseases caused by recessive genes and prenatal diagnosis are among the available methods. Infants born with a physical abnormality such as the absence of lungs are most likely victims of a chromosomal defect or defects in several genes (polygenic). Amniocentesis, ultrasound scanning, and various blood, placental, and fluid tests aid the physician in prenatal diagnosis. Some genetic disorders that are detectable before birth include cystic fibrosis, congenital adrenal hyperplasia, Duchenne's muscular dystrophy, hemophilia A, alpha- and beta-thalassemia, Huntington's disease, polycystic kidney disease, sickle cell anemia, and Tay-Sachs disease.

apneusis   A respiratory abnormality marked by the difficult and prolonged effort to inhale. The condition is the result of surgical removal of the upper portion of the pons in the brain. This procedure may be treatment for a disorder of certain cranial nerves. The pons is fairly centralized in the brain, just above the medulla and in front of the cerebellum. The pons, which works with the medulla to control breathing, connects the spinal cord with the brain and connects other parts of the brain to each other. Located in some of the pons fibers are nuclei for the trigeminal nerves, which govern impulses for chewing and for sensations of the head and face; the abducens nerves, which regulate some movement of the eyeballs; facial nerves, which carry impulses for the production of saliva, the sense of taste, and facial expressions; and part of the vestibulocochlear nerves that are involved with the sense of balance.

apneustic center   The area of the brain stem that regulates respiration.

apple-packer's epistaxis   Nosebleed caused by contact with dyes used in apple-packing trays.
See also EPISTAXIS.

apple-picker's disease   Bronchitis caused by a fungicide used on apples. Bronchitis is an inflammation of the bronchial tubes that causes congestion, pain, and other respiratory symptoms.
See also BRONCHITIS.

apulmonism   A birth defect in which there is an absence of all or portions of a lung.
See also APNEUMIA.

arch, pulmonary   An extension of the fifth aortic arch on the left side of the body into the pulmonary artery.

Aretaeus the Cappadocian   (ca. A.D. 120–180) A Greek physician who wrote treatises on causes, symptoms, and treatments of acute and chronic diseases and is credited with the first valid description of asthma, Aretaeus noted in his writings that exercise or other physical work may induce difficulty breathing and that a "sense of suffocation" may occur when a patient reclines. (Aretaeus also refers to orthopnea, which in modern medicine means respiratory discomfort that can be relieved when an individual either stands or sits erect, with the help of props such as pillows. A person may experience relief, for example, by what is called "two-pillow orthopnea.") Also in the writings of Aretaeus are descriptions of heaviness in the chest, occupational hazards, thickened mucus, coughing and hoarseness, a desire for cold air, expectoration of foamy sputum, and other manifestations of asthma.

Aristocort   See AZMACORT; TRIAMCINOLONE.

Arnold's nerve   The auricular branch of the vagus nerve, which, when stimulated, causes coughing. Originating in the medulla oblongata of the brain,

the vagus is the 10th cranial (head) nerve, which has the widest distribution in the body of any of the other cranial nerves.

arrest, respiratory   The cessation of normal breathing that results in a dangerously low level of oxygen in the blood or a severe increased level of carbon dioxide in the blood. This condition may stem from a number of conditions: chronic bronchitis; emphysema; bronchiectasis; cystic fibrosis; asthma; bronchiolitis; an airway obstruction, or an inhaled or aspirated foreign body, particle, or object; a chest wound; kyphoscoliosis; a drug reaction; acute respiratory distress syndrome; pulmonary fibrosis; fibrosing alveolitis; tumors; sarcoidosis; radiation; burns; myasthenia gravis; muscular dystrophy; polio; Guillain-Barré syndrome; polymyositis; cerebrovascular accident (stroke); amyotrophic lateral sclerosis (Lou Gehrig's disease); an injury to the spinal cord; poor breathing ability due to obesity, sleep apnea, or drug intoxication. In the case of respiratory failure or arrest, oxygen administration and alleviating the cause or causes are the treatments of choice.

arrhinia   A birth defect in which there is the lack of a nose.
See also APNEUMIA.

arterial blood gases (ABGs)   A blood test that determines the body's acid-base balance and the concentrations of the gases oxygen, carbon dioxide, and bicarbonate in the blood. Blood samples are taken from an artery. An ABG test aids in monitoring respiratory failure, because the heart and lungs work to distribute oxygen from inhalation throughout the body via the bloodstream and expel carbon dioxide by exhalation. The normal acid-base balance, also referred to as the pH, or acidity-alkalinity, is 7.39 to 7.41. Asthma, chronic bronchitis, emphysema, diabetes (specifically diabetic ketoacidosis), aspirin poisoning, chronic obstructive lung disease, and symptoms including repeated vomiting may throw ABGs out of the normal range.
See also ASTHMA AND PREGNANCY.

artificial pneumothorax The introduction of air into the pleural cavity by means of the administration of oxygen, nitrogen, or filtered atmospheric air.

artificial respiration See CARDIOPULMONARY RESUSCITATION.

asbestosis A lung disease, a variant of pneumoconiosis, resulting from protracted inhalation of asbestos particles (fibrous particles of magnesium and calcium silicate). Asbestosis occurs among workers who mine, mill, or manufacture the substance and construction workers who are exposed to it through building or demolition. Scarring of the lung tissue caused by inhaling asbestos dust may be severely aggravated by smoking, chronic bronchitis, or other pre-existing respiratory disorders. Inhaled asbestos fibers cause fluid to accumulate in the pleural space (between the two layers of the pleura), or, in some cases, cause cancerous, incurable tumors in the pleura, called mesotheliomas. Only workers trained in the proper techniques for the removal of asbestos should attempt such a task. The incidence of asbestosis has decreased significantly from that of four or five decades ago because of new industrial precautions and preventive measures, but people who were exposed back then to any of the four types of asbestos fibers may begin to exhibit respiratory distress (especially those who smoke) or mesothelioma decades later.

Treatment for asbestosis inhalation includes removing the victim from the contaminated environment, oxygen therapy, the draining of excess fluid from around the lungs, cessation of smoking, and, in some cases, lung transplantation.

See also MESOTHELIOMA.

ascorbic acid A naturally occurring nutrient, also called vitamin C, in citrus fruits and fresh vegetables. It can be synthesized as well, and is important in the maintenance of the body's collagen, bone tissue, and dentin production. Vitamin C, an essential vitamin, prevents scurvy (a nutritional deficiency that results in hemorrhaging of gums and mucous membranes and painful indurations of the muscles), and is considered a natural antibiotic that, when taken prophylactically, boosts the immune system and fights infection.

aspergillosis, allergic bronchopulmonary (ABPA) A pneumonia-like disease caused by an allergic reaction to the mold *Aspergillus fumigatus*. It usually occurs in adult asthmatics.

Signs and Symptoms

This disorder usually involves episodes of fever, shortness of breath, wheezing, and coughing up copious quantities of dark brown, and at times blood-streaked, sputum.

Diagnosis

Because the fungus is ubiquitous (found in healthy persons in small quantities that are harmless), the presence of positive sputum cultures is not sufficient to diagnose this disease. The diagnosis is made in persons meeting the following criteria: (1) episodes of asthma; (2) elevated eosinophils (a type of white blood cell) and total immunoglobulin E (IgE) antibodies in the blood; these values are slightly elevated in most allergic individuals but extremely elevated in persons with this disease; (3) pneumonia-like X-ray findings, which may be temporary; (4) bronchiectasis (destruction of the muscles in the bronchial walls with chronic cough and large amounts of sputum); (5) positive skin tests to the *Aspergillus* fungus; and (6) positive blood tests for antibodies against the *Aspergillus* allergen.

Treatment

Prednisone, a corticosteroid drug, is the treatment of choice. It is used daily, most often for several months, and improvement is usually seen within days. In some cases, recurrences require long-term prednisone use.

Prognosis

If untreated, aspergillosis will damage lung tissues and can be fatal.

See also CORTICOSTEROIDS; PREDNISONE.

asphyxia A life-threatening inability to obtain oxygen, such as in choking, trauma, electric shock, drowning, chest compression, lack of oxygen in the environment, hemorrhage, pharyngeal and retropharyngeal abscesses, paralysis of respiratory muscles, collapsed lung, child abuse, anesthesia, injury of respiratory nerves or centers, and other conditions. Artificial respiration (cardiopulmonary resuscitation) or other treatments may be indicated. Symptoms include difficulty breathing, cyanosis, rapid pulse, sensual and mental impairment, convulsions, and unconsciousness.

aspiration   The act of drawing air or other substance in or out, such as in suction. When an excess of fluid or air, or a foreign body is aspirated into the nose, throat, or lungs upon breathing in, it may be suctioned, or aspirated, out to relieve the undesirable condition. An aspirator is a device designed to evacuate the affected area.

aspirator   See ASPIRATION.

aspirin triad   A condition consisting of asthma complicated by nasal polyps and aspirin sensitivity. However, there are many people with asthma and nasal polyps who can tolerate aspirin, and others with asthma and aspirin sensitivity who do not have nasal polyps. As a rule, it is usually advisable for any person with asthma to use aspirin and related drugs with caution.

Astelin Nasal Spray   Brand name for azelastine, the only antihistamine approved for topical use in the United States.
    See also ANTIHISTAMINE.

astemizole (Hismanal)   A nonsedating (second-generation) antihistamine, prescribed for allergic rhinitis and hives, that may take several days to become effective. Astemizole remains in the body for a prolonged period and may suppress hypersensitivity skin-test results for as long as four weeks. It may not be used simultaneously with the antibiotic erythromycin or in persons with severe liver disease because of the possibility of episodes of cardiac arrhythmias.
    See also ANTIHISTAMINE.

asthma   A chronic lung disease characterized by recurrent attacks of breathlessness, airways (bronchial tubes) that become hyperactive and constrict when exposed to a variety of stimuli or "triggers," obstruction of the bronchioles that is reversible (but not completely in some patients) either spontaneously or with treatment, and inflammation of the airways. *Asthma* derives from the Greek word for "panting." According to the American Lung Association, more than $3.2 billion are spent annually for in-patient hospital services and a total of $11.3 billion per year: $7.5 billion in direct costs and $3.8 billion in indirect costs.

The basic cause of asthma is not yet known. The airways of the asthmatic are hyperactive (twitchy) and overly responsive to environmental changes or stimuli called triggers. Triggers result in wheezing and coughing that some researchers think may be set off by an abnormal reaction to sensory nerves in the lungs. As the attack progresses, chemical mediators are released from cells lining the bronchioles, causing inflammation that leads to contraction of airway muscle, production of mucus, and swelling in the airways.

Asthma can be classified as either extrinsic (triggered by outside influences such as allergy) or intrinsic (from within). Each asthmatic reacts to a different set of triggers. Identification of a person's personal triggers is a major step toward learning to control asthma attacks. Although episodes can sometimes be triggered by strong emotions, asthma is not caused by emotional factors, such as a troubled parent-child relationship. However, researchers at the Children's National Medical Center in Washington and the National Jewish Center for Immunology and Respiratory Medicine in Denver have found a relationship between family stress and the onset of asthma by age three in genetically predisposed children. Three factors—marital discord, prolonged maternal depression, and parental problems in day-to-day care of the child—significantly increased asthma predisposition in genetically at-risk children from 17 percent (if one or none of these stress factors was present) to 42 percent (if at least two of the risk factors were present). Asthma is a disease, not a psychogenic illness or a sign of emotional instability.

There are great variations in asthma severity from person to person and in the individual asthmatic from time to time. Symptoms range from mild to severe and can become life-threatening. The frequency of episodes ranges from one occurrence in a lifetime to daily attacks. The individual attack may be short-lived, lasting from a few minutes to a few hours, or continuous, with daily symptoms for days or weeks. A severe, constant state of asthma is referred to as "status asthmaticus." The symptoms of asthma are a major cause of sleep disturbances and time lost from school and work. Although asthma cannot be cured, the symptoms can almost always be controlled with proper treatment.

In one study of more than 300 asthma patients, researchers found that only 54 percent accurately estimated the severity of their asthma and 27 percent overestimated the severity. The 20 percent who underestimated the severity of their asthma were considered to be at a greater risk for suffering a life-threatening attack. Experts selected to serve on the National Asthma Education Program have developed guidelines for the treatment of asthma. The four basic steps are:

1. Education of the patient and family
2. Control of the environment
3. A comprehensive drug regimen that may include immunotherapy (allergy shots)
4. Objectively monitoring progress.

The goals of therapy are to maintain normal or near-normal activity levels including exercise; maintain normal or near-normal lung function test results; prevent coughing, shortness of breath, waking up at night, and loss of time at school or work; prevent the need for emergency room visits or hospitalizations; and avoid medication side effects.

The National Asthma Education Program emphasizes an understanding of asthma by each patient and family members. An educated patient is better able to anticipate and, thus, avoid situations that might trigger or worsen asthma.

Other guidelines include identification of triggers at home, school, or work; development of effective and simple drug regimens for the patient to follow; close monitoring of medication dosage adjustments; monitoring effectiveness of advised environmental control measures; monitoring symptoms objectively with doctor's office spirometry and home peak flow meters, devices that accurately measure breathing status; identifying high-risk individuals and providing psychological support utilizing mental health and social services personnel; preparation, frequent review, and revision as necessary of a crisis management plan for the patient and his or her family; aggressive, prompt treatment of acute episodes; and primary care coordinated with a specialist in asthma.

Recognizing Asthma

Asthma may resemble, and can be confused with or might coexist with, other respiratory problems such as emphysema, bronchitis, and lower respiratory tract infection. At times, the only symptom of asthma is a persistent cough, usually at night. In some individuals, coughing and wheezing may occur only with exercise.

In infants and children, symptoms suggestive of asthma must be differentiated from many other conditions that cause wheezing. The sudden onset of unremitting wheezing in an infant or small child may point to an obstruction of the large airways by a foreign body lodged in the trachea, bronchus, or esophagus until proven otherwise. Laryngo-tracheobronchomalacia is a congenital disorder involving the softening of cartilage that may be associated with asthma and increased incidence of respiratory infections during a child's first two years.

Croup, caused by a respiratory virus, or acute epiglottitis, a serious bacterial infection that can threaten life, can be confused with asthma because inspiratory wheezing is common to both. Cystic fibrosis (CF) may coexist with asthma and should be suspected in any infant with failure to thrive (poor growth) and recurrent respiratory infections. In older children and adolescents, CF should be suspected in asthmatic patients who have had recurrent pneumonia.

Mitral valve prolapse, which occurs commonly in slender adolescents (females more than males) and causes chest pain during strenuous exercise, may be confused with exercise-induced asthma. It is characterized by a systolic click heard in the mitral area with a stethoscope; diagnosis is confirmed by an echocardiogram. Hyperventilation syndrome may be misdiagnosed or coexist with asthma, especially in adolescents. The patient typically appears anxious and breathless but without wheezing. A complaint of tingling of the fingers and toes is common. Treatment consists of reassurance and having the patient rebreathe into a paper bag to elevate carbon dioxide levels. Recurrences may require psychological counseling and, possibly, antianxiety drugs.

In adults, asthma is often confused with the other common lung diseases, emphysema and chronic bronchitis, which to some degree act like asthma. The hallmark of the three lung diseases is airway obstruction. The principal difference in the conditions is the degree of reversibility of the airway obstruction. A patient with asthma should have normal airflow between attacks. Chronic bronchitis is characterized by obstruction to varying degrees but usually is not completely reversible with treatment. The obstruction found in patients with emphysema is irreversible by definition. However, most patients fall between these strict limits.

Asthma may be hard to diagnose and is greatly underdiagnosed. To distinguish asthma from other lung diseases, doctors rely on a combination of the patient's medical history (the patient's recount of his or her symptoms and past disorders), a thorough physical examination, and certain tests: measurement of airflow into and out of the lungs, chest X rays, blood tests, and skin tests. Sometimes, challenges with methacholine (a drug that constricts the bronchi in persons with asthma) are indicated.

Asthma Screening

The American College of Allergies, Asthma and Immunology's (ACAAI's) Nationwide Asthma Screening Program is an assessment tool used to identify individuals who may be at risk for asthma and its complications. Now in its fourth year, the program has screened more than 20,000 people and referred more than half of them to professionals for diagnosis. The screenings are conducted by allergists, physicians who are asthma specialists, free of charge at shopping malls, civic centers, health fairs, and other accessible locations throughout the country. During a screening, adults who are experiencing breathing problems complete a 20-question Life Quality Test developed by the ACAAI. A special test is available for the parents of children up to age eight, called the Kids' Asthma Check. In addition, participants in the screenings take a special lung function test that involves blowing into a tube and meet with a physician to determine if they should seek a thorough examination and diagnosis. People who already know they have asthma may also speak with a specialist at the screenings.

The following Kids' Asthma Check questions for children ages one through eight require a yes or no answer:

Symptoms and Signs of an Asthma Attack

It is unusual to have a sudden life-threatening attack of asthma without warning signs. Usually the signs of an impending asthma attack manifest hours or even days before a full-blown attack develops.

Every asthma patient should have an emergency strategy preplanned with his or her physician. The

QUESTIONNAIRE FOR ASTHMA IN CHILDREN	YES	NO
1. When walking or playing hard with friends, my child has trouble breathing or coughs.		
2. When walking up hills or stairs, my child has trouble breathing or coughs.		
3. When running or playing sports, my child has trouble breathing or coughs.		
4. Sometimes my child wakes up at night with coughing or trouble breathing.		
5. Sometimes my child has trouble taking a deep breath.		
6. Sometimes my child makes wheezing sounds.		
7. Sometimes my child complains of pain or tightness in the chest.		
8. Sometimes my child coughs a lot.		
9. Being outdoors or around dust or pets makes my child's breathing worse.		
10. It's hard for my child to breathe in cold weather.		
11. It's hard for my child to breathe when people smoke or there are strong odors.		
12. Colds make my child cough or wheeze.		

National Asthma Education Program recommends the use of peak flow meters to follow the progress of an asthma attack. There are inexpensive portable devices to measure the peak flow (airflow in the bronchial tubes). Use of a peak flow meter can be a valuable guide with which to follow a person's progress. Worsening of asthma can usually be detected in time to take corrective measures.

Because individuals vary, *patients should know their own signs of an impending attack.* The initial sign may be itching of the face or throat, a feeling of tightness in the chest, and mild wheezing. This is the time to act to prevent progressive or sudden worsening of the attack. *Early intervention is the key to preventing the need for emergency treatment and asthma fatalities.*

Extrinsic asthma is a form of asthma caused by allergens found in the environment, such as seasonal or perennial allergens such as house-dust mites, but can be triggered by a perennial allergen. A greater percentage of children (up to 85 percent) than adults (about 50 percent) suffer from extrinsic asthma. Extrinsic asthmatics usually have positive skin or radioallergosorbent tests (RAST), but not every asthma patient suffers from allergies.

Foods may be blamed as a cause of asthma. Foods were cited for allergic reactions by patients almost four times as often as allergic rhinitis. However, most experts feel the true incidence of food-induced asthma is much less frequent. In double-blind food challenges (tests in which a suspected allergenic food or placebo is given to a patient and monitored for reaction), symptoms of asthma could be confirmed only in 25 to 33 percent of the children.

Most cases of food hypersensitivity stem from milk allergy in early infancy. Many adverse food reactions are probably caused by food additives or preservatives such as sulfites, bisulfites, and metabisulfites.

Intrinsic asthma may be caused by factors other than allergy. Intrinsic asthma occurs in less than 50 percent of adults and in about 15 percent of children with asthma. Some children from infancy experience wheezing triggered only by viral respiratory infections. Other children and adults suffer asthma triggered by irritants, emotional factors, and other nonallergenic stimuli. Many of those with intrinsic asthma have nasal polyps and sensitivity to aspirin. Skin tests for allergy are usually negative in these persons, but it is possible to have both intrinsic and extrinsic asthma.

Nocturnal Asthma

Nocturnal asthma refers to the occurrence of symptoms of asthma during the night. Nearly 40 percent of asthmatics experience nightly symptoms; approximately 64 percent have episodes three nights a week, and about 75 percent at least one night per week. Asthma attacks seem to occur most often between 10 P.M. and 7 A.M., peaking at about 4 A.M. When several things simultaneously trigger asthma, results can be severe. The most devastating asthma attacks that lead to respiratory arrest and possibly death most often occur between midnight and 6 A.M.

During sleep, mucus secretions accumulate in the bronchial tubes, and the backup, or reflux, of stomach acid may spill over into the lungs, causing irritation and inflammation of lung tissue. The circadian fall in the body's production of cortisone and adrenaline and the rise of other chemicals, such as histamine, further worsen the situation during the night. In addition, the cell counts of neutrophils and eosinophils (cells that release mediators of inflammation) are higher in patients with nocturnal symptoms. Timing medications to coincide with peak effectiveness and times of greatest need can greatly reduce symptoms and allow patients to sleep through the night.

Medications for Asthma

Medications are prescribed when the symptoms of asthma cannot be prevented by controlling the environment or other triggers such as a viral respiratory infection. The medicines used depend on the frequency and severity of symptoms and may be therapeutic or preventive, or both.

Bronchodilators are chosen for their ability to prevent or reverse airway obstruction. They include beta-adrenergic agonists such as albuterol, metaproterenol, and pirbuterol; methylxanthines such as theophylline; and the anticholinergics atropine and ipratropium.

Anti-inflammatory agents interrupt the development of bronchial inflammation and also act to prevent asthma attacks. These drugs include corti-costeroids (cortisone-like drugs), cromolyn, and others that are still investigational.

Beta-agonists alone may be all the therapy necessary for mild, episodic asthma. Metered-dose inhalers (MDIs) on an as-needed, or "PRN," basis are the first line of therapy. These drugs are also taken before exercise or sports to prevent symptoms. Their prolonged use at regular four- to six-hour intervals has been associated with some diminished occurrences of asthma, and the recommended three to four doses a day should rarely be exceeded. Overuse of beta-agonists has been associated with increased risk of death from asthma.

Oral dosage forms of beta-agonists are also available as short-acting (six to eight hours duration of action) or sustained-release (lasting up to 12 hours) tablets. When both dosage forms of beta-agonists are taken simultaneously, the MDI is reserved for acute episodes or prior to exercise.

Theophylline is the most widely used methylxanthine. It is available in tablet, capsule, and liquid forms, which are short- or long-acting, and for many years was the prime drug for the treatment of asthma. A related drug, aminophylline, is available for intravenous use but is rarely used orally. Theophylline and aminophylline have come under scrutiny because of the frequency of adverse effects, especially in infants.

The 1991 asthma expert panel report from the National Institutes of Health (see the 1997 report below) relegates the methylxanthine drugs to a secondary or tertiary role behind beta-agonists and the anti-inflammatory medications. The methylxanthines are thought to inhibit phosphodiesterases, enzymes implicated as a cause of asthma. These drugs dilate constricted bronchioles. Long-acting forms are most useful in preventing nighttime awakening from asthma. In addition, they reduce respiratory muscle fatigue and have a mild degree of anti-inflammatory activity. Close monitoring of blood levels can usually avoid the most serious complications of these drugs.

The inhaled anticholinergic ipratropium, an atropine-like drug, is a weak bronchodilator that also blocks reflex bronchoconstriction by inhaled irritants. Although it is less effective than other bronchodilators, ipratropium lacks side effects and is useful in the few individuals who cannot tolerate other drugs.

Corticosteroids are the most effective anti-inflammatory drugs for the treatment of asthma. They can be given orally as tablets or liquids, by injection, or topically as aerosol MDIs. Despite the fear of adverse effects, systemic corticosteroids, when used appropriately early in an asthma attack, prevent progression and lessen the need for emergency room visits and hospitalizations, and they may be lifesaving. In severe asthmatics, they may be required daily or on alternate days.

Inhaled corticosteroids are safe and effective as preventive therapy and are first-line therapy for anyone with frequent symptoms of asthma. In recommended doses, side effects are usually limited to local irritation of the pharynx, though this can be prevented by rinsing the mouth after each use or by using a spacer device. Spacers allow active medication to be inhaled, while irritating larger particles settle in the chamber of the spacer. In addition to reducing adverse effects, they allow poorly coordinated persons, often including young children, to use MDIs effectively.

Cromolyn sodium is a preventive, anti-inflammatory drug causing no serious side effects, administered by MDI or nebulizer. It is most effective in children.

Prevalence

According to a March 1999 report by the U.S. Centers for Disease Control and Prevention, asthma now affects more than 14 million Americans, approximately double the rate of 20 years ago. The asthma rate for children age four and younger has increased 160 percent between 1980 and 1994. The incidence of asthma seems to be equally distributed among males and females, but blacks have a 4.4 percent rate of asthma, while whites have a 4.0 percent rate. Increases have been reported in all ages, races, and in both sexes. Individuals with asthma require more than 100 million days of restricted activity per year. African Americans are three times as likely to die from asthma as are whites of all ages; however, this incidence increases five times in individuals ages 15 to 44. The asthma death rate doubled for children ages five to 14.

According to the American Academy of Allergy, Asthma and Immunology, nearly one in 10 American children have asthma, and the reason for that is still unknown. One theory for the increase is the result of spending more time indoors where we are exposed to more potent allergens. Studies are now being conducted to better understand the inflammatory response to allergens and the fundamental regulators of the entire process. The studies are focused on identifying the basic abnormality that causes asthma and the genes that direct the allergic process, developing more advanced patient-education, medicine, and treatments, including asthma self-management techniques, and refining emergency measures for asthma attacks.

In the December 1999 issue of the *Annals of Allergy, Asthma and Immunology,* asthma "far exceeds other causes of occupational pulmonary disease, with an estimated 5 percent of all adult asthma cases workplace-related, and some 250 causative agents implicated."

The American Lung Association says the rate of asthma in the United States will likely double by the year 2020. The association supports the findings and recommendations of the report released by the Pew Environmental Health Commission at the Johns Hopkins School of Public Health entitled "Attack Asthma: Why America Needs a Public Health Defense System to Battle Environmental Threats." The report calls for the creation of a national asthma tracking system within five years, development of an action plan to coordinate the efforts of federal agencies responsible for responding to the nation's asthma problem, expanded investment in asthma prevention research, and implementation of a comprehensive public education campaign for the public and health care providers.

John M. Corruthers, Jr., president of the American Lung Association, said the association "will continue to work with the 17 million Americans who have asthma and establish a foundation for significantly reducing the number of people who develop asthma in the future."

Asthma-Related Death

In the United States, minorities from inner-city neighborhoods have a much higher proportion of deaths as a result of asthma than do urban whites. In Chicago in a five-year period, 90 percent of all asthma deaths were persons in minority groups, although minorities accounted for only 40 percent of the total population.

In the past decade, the greatest increase in deaths occurred in those older than 65 years of age. Nonwhites are almost three times as likely to die from asthma as whites. However, despite recently increased asthma deaths, the number of such deaths in the United States—approximately 14 people per day (more than 5,000 per year), according to the *Statistical Abstracts of the United States*—is one of the lowest numbers of asthma deaths in the world. Factors that increase risk for a fatal attack of asthma include age over 65, ethnicity (nonwhite race), previous life-threatening asthma attack(s), hospital admission for asthma within the last year, psychological and psychosocial problems, lack of access to medical care, and abuse of asthma drugs.

In the past decade (1990–2000), the greatest increase in asthma deaths is seen in older age groups. There has also been a significant trend in deaths among those from five to 34 years of age during the same period.

African Americans have almost three times the rate of asthma deaths as Caucasians for all ages. However, in age group 15 to 44, the rate increases to five times the rate for Caucasians.

Persons who have required intubation and a respirator for respiratory failure, or who have suffered respiratory acidosis in the past, are at increased risk to die from a similar episode. Persons hospitalized within the previous year for asthma were more likely to die from asthma, as well as those with more than two hospitalizations for severe asthma and patients on oral corticosteroid therapy.

There is an association between children dying suddenly from asthma and prior expressions of hopelessness, despair, and a wish to die. Unemployment, alcohol abuse, recent family loss, recognizable depression, and schizophrenia increase the risk of sudden and unexpected death from asthma for adults.

Many poor families in urban neighborhoods lack a regular family doctor or asthma specialist. Treatment is often delayed until the patient's diagnosis is status asthmaticus (severe unrelenting asthma). Patients usually seek emergency room medical care only during a crisis. In rural areas, a similar situation can arise because of the great distance to a medical facility or lack of a specialist. Lack of prevention and knowledge of asthma may prevail in any environment.

A Canadian study, based on health insurance records of 12,300 asthma patients between 1978 and 1987, demonstrated twice the risk of a fatal or near-fatal asthma attack in patients overusing certain medications. The use of twice the maximum recommended dose of a beta₂-agonist MDI was considered the causative factor in this increased risk.

Risk Factors for Asthma-Related Death

- Past history of sudden severe exacerbations.
- Prior intubation for asthma.
- Prior admission for asthma to an intensive care unit.
- Two or more hospitalizations for asthma in the past year.
- Three or more emergency care visits for asthma in the past year.
- Hospitalization or an emergency care visit for asthma within the past month.
- Use of more than 2 canisters per month of inhaled short-acting beta₂-agonist.
- Current use of systemic corticosteroids or recent withdrawal from systemic corticosteroids.
- Difficulty perceiving airflow obstruction or its severity.
- Comorbidity, as from cardiovascular diseases or chronic obstructive pulmonary disease.
- Serious psychiatric disease or psychological problems.
- Low socioeconomic status and urban residence.
- Illicit drug use.
- Sensitivity to *Alternaria.*

Special Considerations for Infants

- Assessment depends on physical examination rather than objective measurements. Use of

accessory muscles, paradoxical breathing, cyanosis, and a respiratory rate of greater than 60 are key signs of serious distress.

- Objective measurements such as oxygen saturation of higher than 91 percent also indicate serious distress.
- Response to beta₂-agonist therapy can be variable and may not be a reliable predictor of satisfactory outcome. However, because infants are at greater risk for respiratory failure, a lack of response noted by either physical examination or objective measurements should be an indication for hospitalization.
- Use of oral corticosteroids early in the episode is essential but should not substitute for careful assessment by a physician.
- Most acute wheezing episodes result from viral infections and may be accompanied by fever. Antibiotics are generally not required.

Sources: Kallebnach et al., 1993; Rodrigo and Rodrigo, 1993; Suissa et al. 1994; Greenberger et al., 1993; O'Hollaren et al., 1991.

See also ACIDOSIS, RESPIRATORY; APPENDIX I; ARTERIAL BLOOD GASES; ASTHMA AND PREGNANCY; ASTHMA CAMPS; BETA-ADRENERGIC AGONISTS; BRONCHITIS, CHRONIC; CORTICOSTEROIDS; CROMOLYN SODIUM; CROUP; CYSTIC FIBROSIS; EMPHYSEMA; EPIGLOTTITIS; EXERCISE-INDUCED ASTHMA; IMMUNOTHERAPY; IPRATROPIUM; OCCUPATIONAL ASTHMA; PEAK FLOW METER; SPIROMETER; TRIGGER, ASTHMA; THEOPHYLLINE.

Asthma and Allergy Poster Child From 1983 to 1993, the Asthma and Allergy Foundation of America (AAFA) sponsored a national, annual contest in which a child with a documented history of asthma and allergies, as well as other certain qualities, was selected to represent all children who wish to overcome their illness. Poster children were judged to be outgoing and articulate, and would participate in AAFA-sponsored events. Past national poster children are: Lanny Bert Powell (Greenville, S.C.), 1983; Reggie Smith (Baltimore, Md.), 1984; Ann Cordrey (Cincinnati, Ohio), 1985; Jamie Noland (Ft. Collins, Colo.), 1986; Scott Halverson (Omaha, Nebr.), 1987–88; Chele Williams (Newport News, Va.), 1989; Jennifer Carol Price (Midland, Tex.),

1990; Chris Dulman (Michigan), 1991–92; and Amanda Johnston (Portland, Oreg.), 1993.

The AAFA may be contacted at:

Asthma and Allergy Foundation of America
1125 15th Street NW, Suite 502
Washington, DC 20005
(800) 7-ASTHMA

asthma and pregnancy   Asthma is present in at least 4 percent of all pregnancies and may occur in as many as 10 percent. Asthma may occur for the first time during pregnancy. Preexisting asthma may worsen or improve during pregnancy. About one-third of pregnant women with asthma worsen during pregnancy, one-third continue unchanged, and one-third improve.

General Treatment Principles of Asthma During Pregnancy

- Asthma is a chronic condition with acute exacerbation or attacks; close monitoring by both patient and doctor is necessary to detect subtle changes throughout pregnancy.

- Prevention of attacks is of utmost importance. Identify and avoid triggers, and optimize measures to reduce the presence of indoor allergens, such as furry pets, dust mites, and molds. *Especially avoid tobacco smoke.* Use air-conditioning during pollen seasons to reduce exposure. Use preventive drugs daily exactly as prescribed.

- Anticipate or intervene early during an attack. Use a peak flow meter to detect subtle changes in breathing and have a plan to act before attacks become severe or catastrophic.

- Although using as few medications as possible is generally desirable during pregnancy, normal breathing and oxygen levels must be maintained in the mother to assure normal oxygen supply to the fetus. Inhaled drugs are preferred, but if they are not totally effective, systemic drugs should be used to achieve normal lung function.

- Disorders that aggravate asthma, such as sinus infections, nasal allergies, and heartburn, should be treated promptly so they will not trigger asthma.

Adverse Effects

Whether a pregnant woman's asthma worsens, remains the same, or improves, uncontrolled asthma can produce serious complications for mother and fetus. Maternal complications from asthma include preeclampsia (a toxemia of pregnancy), gestational hypertension, hyperemesis gravidarum (severe nausea and vomiting during pregnancy), vaginal hemorrhage, toxemia, and induced and complicated labor. Fetal complications include increased risk of fetal death, diminished growth, prematurity, low birth weight, and neonatal hypoxia. The more severe the asthma, the greater the risk, but even mildly uncontrolled asthma is a risk. When asthma is well controlled, even if medications are required, the outcome of pregnancy should be the same as those experienced by a nonasthmatic mother.

PREFERRED DRUGS FOR THE TREATMENT OF ASTHMA DURING PREGNANCY

Drug Type	Specific Drug
anti-inflammatory	beclomethasone (Beclovent, Vanceril) cromolyn sodium (Intal) prednisone
bronchodilator	inhaled beta$_2$-agonist: albuterol (Proventil, Ventolin), metaproterenol (Alupent), pirbuterol (Maxair), terbutaline (Brethaire) theophylline (Constant-T, Quibron, SloBid, Slo-Phyllin, Theo-Dur, Theo-24, Theolair, Theovent, Uniphyl; serum levels must be monitored to avoid toxicity)

Effect on Fetal Oxygen Supply

During pregnancy, changes occur in the mother's body, unrelated to asthma, that cause a mild sensation of shortness of breath in many normal women. However, these "normal" changes affect neither the supply of oxygen to the fetus nor the results of breathing tests that are used to measure the severity of asthma in the mother.

During an asthma attack, the mother's body utilizes available oxygen, reducing the amount supplied through the placenta to the fetus. A small fall in oxygen concentration that would result in only minimal to moderate distress to the mother can be catastrophic to the baby.

Goals of Therapy and Treatment

Traditionally, asthma was viewed as an intermittent acute illness. Symptoms were due to constriction of the bronchioles, and the goal of drugs was to reverse this spasm. Since scientists have determined the importance of lung inflammation in asthma, the goal of treatment is not only to improve symptoms during an attack but also to prevent symptoms from recurring. Treatment of asthma during pregnancy follows the same principles as for the nonpregnant individual. Avoidance of asthma triggers may reduce the need for drugs. When drugs are needed, the preventive anti-inflammatory cromolyn and corticosteroid inhalers are especially useful, safe, and effective.

Monitoring Mother's Breathing Status

For pregnant patients with asthma, objective measurement of lung function is essential. This can be done in the doctor's office with spirometry or a peak flow meter. Inexpensive hand-held peak flow monitors can be used at home or in the workplace to detect changes that may indicate the onset of an asthma attack. The peak flow meter may detect changes before symptoms are apparent.

Fetal Monitoring

For pregnant women with asthma, fetal evaluation is based on objective measurements such as sonography (ultrasound), electronic fetal heart rate monitoring, and by subjective means, such as the mother's assessment of fetal kicks ("kick count"). Sonography from 12 to 20 weeks provides a guide to fetal growth and should be followed frequently in cases where asthma is moderate or severe to detect growth retardation.

Effects of Asthma Drugs

In considering the possible effects of drugs and disease on pregnancy, it is important to keep in mind the incidence of adverse pregnancy outcomes in the general population. Congenital anomalies (birth defects) occur in 3–8 percent of all newborns, and of these only 1 percent or fewer are attributable to drug exposures.

Both animal and human data are studied to evaluate the safety of drugs. If studies in animals, where huge doses are used during testing, are reassuring, the potential for effects in humans is low. However, animal data do not always give complete information. It may not be possible to know whether the effects of a drug on the newborn were caused by the use of excessive doses by the mother, the disease process itself, or other multiple factors. Human studies rarely include large numbers of patients exposed to a particular drug. Therefore, drugs that have been used for many years without a significant number of reported adverse effects are considered most reliable.

Immunotherapy

Immunotherapy (allergy shots) may prevent asthma symptoms triggered by allergies, therefore reducing the need for drugs. Desensitization by injecting minute amounts of allergy extracts for cat dander, dust mites, molds, and pollens is generally safe and effective. The principal concern for giving immunotherapy during pregnancy is the same as in nonpregnant individuals, to avoid anaphylaxis (the most severe form of allergic reactions). Because a severe reaction may threaten the lives of both mother and fetus, injections of allergy extracts must be given cautiously and doses are usually not increased or sometimes slightly decreased during pregnancy. It is generally recommended that allergy immunotherapy not be initiated during pregnancy, because it takes several months for any benefit to be evident and doses must be given in increasing amounts during the early stages of treatment.

Influenza ("Flu") Vaccine

Annual flu vaccine is recommended for all patients with moderate or severe asthma. Influenza vaccine is based on a killed virus, and there is no evidence of risk to mother or fetus.

Physical Activity

Physical activity should be encouraged and no different from that of a nonasthmatic pregnant woman. If necessary, pretreatment with a beta-agonist metered-dose inhaler such as albuterol or cromolyn five to 60 minutes before exercise should be used.

PREFERRED DRUGS FOR THE TREATMENT OF ALLERGY OR RESPIRATORY INFECTIONS COMPLICATING ASTHMA DURING PREGNANCY

Drug Type	Specific Drug
antibiotics	amoxicillin
antihistamine	chlorpheniramine (Chlor-Trimeton) tripelennamine (Pyribenzamine)
anti-inflammatory	cromolyn sodium (Nasalcrom nasal spray) beclomethasone (Beconase, Vanceril)
cough	dextromethorphan, guaifenesin (Robitussin)
decongestant	oxymetazoline (Afrin) nasal
spray or drops	pseudoephedrine (Sudafed) (must be used sparingly to avoid rebound worsening of nasal congestion)

Summary

Pregnant women with asthma need specific treatment. Nondrug measures are preferred such as improving the environment to avoid known trigger-allergens or irritants such as tobacco smoke. Drugs with many years of safe use are the best choice. A panel of experts from the National Institutes of Health strongly recommends that asthma be as aggressively treated in pregnant women as in nonpregnant women.

See also EXERCISE-INDUCED ASTHMA; PEAK FLOW; PEAK FLOW METER; RHINITIS MEDICAMENTOSA; SPIROMETER.

[Adapted from the National Asthma Education Program's report Management of Asthma During Pregnancy (NIH Publication No. 93-3279A, October 1992).]

asthma camps   These recreational facilities provide a safe, medically supervised, and enjoyable experience for children with asthma who would otherwise be unable to attend camps. According to the American Lung Association, there are currently more than 130 children's asthma camps in the nation and the number is growing. The Consortium on Children's Asthma Camps (CCAC) has established parameters for the operation of asthma camps. The Consortium was established in 1988 to coordinate camp activities of national organizations involved in the care of children with asthma. According to CCAC,

the purpose of the Consortium is to promote the quality of medical care delivered at existing asthma camps; to provide parameters for educational goals; to promote the development of new asthma camps, and to develop initiatives to target high-risk children and give them the opportunity to attend asthma camp. The Consortium is composed of representatives from the American Academy of Allergy, Asthma and Immunology, the American Lung Association, the American Thoracic Society, the American Academy of Pediatrics, and the Asthma and Allergy Foundation of America. The current chairman is Sherwin Gillman, a practicing allergist in Orange County, California.

The key objectives of asthma camps include:

1. improving a child's ability to self-manage asthma through a creative yet systematic approach to asthma education;
2. introducing children with asthma to a full camp/outdoors experience;
3. gathering valuable information on the effectiveness of various means of asthma education;
4. teaching asthma management in a fun and engaging way, leading to improved patient compliance;
5. providing health care volunteers with an opportunity to utilize and hone their professional skills in a fun, unusual environment;
6. providing a forum for all relevant audiences for teaching and learning optimum asthma management practices.

The Inner City Asthma Camp Initiative

In 1993, the national Consortium on Children's Asthma Camps launched Phase I of the Inner City Asthma Camp Initiative:

to meet the growing needs of inner-city children with asthma. The goals of this phase of the initiative were to develop and implement educational programs to take place both before and after asthma camp, and to involve not only camp attendees but their families as well; to identify and recruit for these programs disadvantaged children, ages 9–12, who have asthma and live in urban areas, and to increase knowledge of, change attitudes about, and gain more control over asthma among inner-city children who have the disease and their parents, guardians, or adult caregivers.

Five asthma camps participated independently in Phase I, which included a study to evaluate the effectiveness of asthma camps in teaching inner-city children and their families about the disease and how to manage it better.

Results of the study determined that, after participating in camp and pre- and post-camp activities, children reported fewer symptoms of asthma, and their ability to manage asthma increased. They also indicated that the camp experience expanded their knowledge of asthma and improved family communication. Most of the children in the study said they enjoyed the camp experience and found it helpful. (A complete copy of the study *Effectiveness of Asthma Camps for Inner City Families* by Stephen C. Weisberg, M.D., David H. Olson, Ph.D., and Richard J. Sveum, M.D., is available from the Consortium.)

Asthma Roadways, Phase II, of the initiative (July 1995–November 1999) elected the following goals: to reduce asthma-related hospitalizations; to reduce asthma-related emergency room visits; to decrease symptom days, and to improve the quality of life, related to asthma, in the target population. Asthma Roadways was designed to encourage children with asthma and their families to interact effectively, which, it is hoped, will help them gain control over asthma by setting individual and family goals; learn more about asthma and environmental controls; reduce family stress related to asthma; improve family communication about asthma and increase overall satisfaction of individuals within families.

In 1999, the Consortium sought to create comprehensive and consistent national guidelines and standards for the set-up, operation, and evaluation of resident and day asthma camps. In March 1999 a website was launched with links to all sponsors. In addition to a database of all asthma camps in the country, the *Parameters for Medical Policies and Procedures for Children with Asthma* was published in 1996, and the book for children *I'm Going to Asthma Camp* was published in 1997. For more informa-

tion, visit http://www.lungusa.org/asthmacamps/about.htm.

Camp Broncho Junction

Camp Broncho Junction, formerly in Red House, West Virginia, was a pioneering, 16-year effort. The founders, the late Dr. Merle S. Scherr and his late wife, Lois, conducted psychological evaluations of the campers in the areas of behavioral and sociopsychological adjustment and provided a sharp profile not only of the individual patients but also of the group as a whole. Clinical psychologists and psychiatrists, testing with the California Test of Personality, and counselors' ratings implemented psychological evaluation through personal interviews. The results point toward a more realistic and positive integration of the children's physical problems into their total lifestyle. When the children were separated into two groups, those with severe asthma and those with the least severe asthma, improvement was especially striking in the most severe group. Group therapy sessions with children and families and weekend therapy sessions also contributed to patient improvement.

asthma-friendly schools The National Heart, Lung, and Blood Institute, the National Asthma Education and Prevention Program, and the School Asthma Education Subcommittee developed the following questions to determine what constitutes asthma-friendly schools.

Children with asthma need proper support at school to keep their asthma under control and be fully active. Use the questions below to find out how well your school assists children with asthma:

1. Is your school free of tobacco smoke all of the time, including during school-sponsored events?
2. Does the school maintain good indoor air quality? Does it reduce or eliminate allergens and irritants that can make asthma worse? Allergens and irritants include pets with fur or feathers, mold, dust mites (for example, in carpets and upholstery), cockroaches, and strong odors or fumes from such products as pesticides, paint, perfumes, and cleaning chemicals.

3. Is there a school nurse in your school all day, every day? If not, is a nurse regularly available to the school to help write plans and give guidance for students with asthma about medicines, physical education, and field trips?
4. Can children take medicines at school as recommended by their doctor and parents? May children carry their own asthma medicines?
5. Does your school have an emergency plan for taking care of a child with a severe asthma episode (attack)? Is it made clear what to do? Who to call? When to call?
6. Does someone teach school staff about asthma, asthma management plans, and asthma medicines? Does someone teach all students about asthma and how to help a classmate who has it?
7. Do students have good options for fully and safely participating in physical education class and recess? (For example, do students have access to their medicine before exercise? Can they choose modified or alternative activities when medically necessary?)

If the answer to any question is no, students may be facing obstacles to asthma control. Asthma that is out of control can hinder a student's attendance, participation, and progress in school. School staff, health care professionals, and parents can work together to remove obstacles and to promote students' health and education.

Contact asthma organizations for information about asthma and helpful ideas for making school policies and practices more asthma-friendly. Federal and state laws are there to help children with asthma. Asthma can be controlled; expect nothing less.

asthmatic bronchitis   See ASTHMA.

Atarax   The trade name for the antihistamine hydroxyzine hydrochloride, also known as Vistaril Parenteral.
See also ANTIHISTAMINE.

atelectasis   A partial or total collapse of the lung that may be caused by mucous plugs, excessive secretions, foreign-body obstruction, or compression of the bronchus by enlarged lymph nodes, tumors, or aneurysms. Atelectasis in varying degrees is present during asthma attacks, particularly in children. Symptoms range from none to breathlessness. The X-ray appearance of atelectasis may be confused with the markings, or infiltrates, in the lungs associated with pneumonia.
See also PNEUMOTHORAX.

atmiatrics (atmotherapy)   Therapeutic treatment with medicated vapors.

atmotherapy   See ATMIATRICS.

atomizer   See NEBULIZER.

atresia, pulmonary   A congenital condition in which the pulmonary valve between the pulmonary artery and the right ventricle of the heart is closed.

Aufrecht's sign   Named for the German physician, Emanuel Aufrecht (1844–1933), who first defined it, a diminished breathing sound heard through a stethoscope that indicates stenosis (constriction) of the trachea or windpipe.

auscultation   The act of listening to bodily sounds, usually through a stethoscope in order to determine any abnormalities. Chest sounds are heard both anteriorly and posteriorly, and patients are typically requested to take deep breaths in and out, and cough.

autoimmune disease   See ACQUIRED IMMUNE DEFICIENCY SYNDROME.

autotuberculin   Tuberculin, or the soluble cell substance prepared from the tubercle bacillus that causes tuberculosis, made by taking cultures of an individual's own sputum.

Ayerza's syndrome   Named for the Brazilian physician, Abel Ayerza (1861–1918), a condition of pulmonary insufficiency marked by difficulty breathing, chronic cyanosis (blue coloration of skin and mucous membranes), erythrocytosis, spleen and liver enlargement, and bone marrow hyperplasia.

Ayurvedic medicine The ancient Hindu medical system, named from the Sanskrit words *ayu* (lifespan) and *veda* (knowledge). Through yoga, herbal remedies, massage therapy, pulse diagnosis, and other factors, Ayurveda medicine seeks to integrate mind and body for optimal wellness.

Azmacort Metered-dose asthma inhaler containing the cortisone-like anti-inflammatory drug triamcinolone. This unique inhaler comes with a white barrel-shaped device called a spacer. Spacers assure that even individuals with less than perfect coordination receive an adequate dose of the drug.

See also CORTICOSTEROIDS; INHALED MEDICATIONS; INHALER; SPINHALER.

Bacillus anthracis   See ANTHRAX.

bacteria   Living microscopic organisms composed of a single cell and lacking chlorophyll. Structurally, a bacterium bears some resemblance to the human cell. Parts of one bacterium include the nuclear region (or chromosomes), or "central intelligence" in which DNA dictates the characteristics of the cell; ribosomes, which carry RNA and units of protein in the cell's cytoplasm; and the cell membrane and the cell wall, which carry proteins, fats, and sugars. Bacterial infections, especially those affecting the respiratory and integumentary systems, may trigger or intensify conditions of allergy and asthma, or be mistaken for them.

The three major categories of bacteria are spherical or ovoid, such as micrococci, diplococci, staphylococci, streptococci, and sarcinae; rod shaped, or bacilli, such as coccobacilli and streptobacilli; and spiral, or spirilla, such as spirochetes and vibrios.

Because bacteria have no chlorophyll and do not photosynthesize the way plants do, they derive their nutrients from organic material, parasites, soil, or nonliving organic matter. Bacteria are considered pathogenic if they are capable of causing disease in their host, but many bacteria are nonpathogenic and perform beneficial functions in the human body and the environment, especially in the nitrogen cycle of the soil. Aerobes are bacteria that thrive on atmospheric oxygen; anaerobes can live without oxygen. Most bacteria reproduce asexually by binary fission, or splitting into two parts.

Certain species of rod-shaped bacteria form spores, which are encapsulated bacterium cells in a resting or dormant stage. While in this stage, spores resist heat, cold, dehydration, disinfectants, and other attempts to destroy them.

Bacteria generally have flagella, or whiplike tails, for motility, and most form colonies that can flourish in soil, water, organic matter, humans, animals, and plants. In humans, undesirable bacteria usually succumb to antibiotic treatment.

See also ANTIBIOTIC.

bagassosis   A form of hypersensitivity pneumonitis. This allergic pneumonia-like disease is caused by the inhalation of bagasse dust, the dusty fibrous waste of sugarcane after the sugar-containing sap has been removed.

See also HYPERSENSITIVITY PNEUMONITIS.

bag-valve-mask resuscitator   See ARTIFICIAL RESPIRATION.

baker's asthma   An occupational lung disease caused by repeated exposure to flour, especially wheat, an airborne allergen. There is usually no related allergy to ingested bakery products. In one study, 10 percent of exposed bakers selected randomly developed asthma. The bakers were exposed an average of 17.4 years before symptoms developed.

Immunotherapy (allergy shots) may be effective treatment for the inhaled food allergen causing baker's asthma. This type of therapy is not recommended when the food allergen exposure is from oral ingestion.

Baker's rhinitis is an allergic condition of the upper respiratory tract caused by repeated exposure to flour, usually airborne wheat allergen.

bambuterol   A beta-agonist (bronchodilating) drug chemically related to terbutaline. Bambuterol has a direct action in lung tissue; little of the active

41

drug is absorbed into the bloodstream, therefore minimizing the possibility of side effects. It also has the advantage of requiring only one daily dose.

See also BETA-ADRENERGIC AGONISTS.

barosinusitis A condition characterized by pain and inflammation in one or more of the nasal sinuses when they have ascended or descended in response to a change in environment, such as being in an airplane when a sinus outlet is blocked.

barrel chest Enlarged chest diameter attributable to conditions including chronic obstructive pulmonary disease (COPD), chronic bronchitis, and emphysema.

basic life support Part of cardiopulmonary resuscitation (CPR) and emergency cardiac care that attempts to prevent respiratory or circulatory arrest and provides means for external support of those functions.

See also CARDIOPULMONARY RESUSCITATION; BAG-MASK-VALVE RESUSCITATOR.

beclomethasone (Beconase, Beconase AQ, Vancenase, Vancenase AQ, Beclovent, Vanceril) A corticosteroid drug used as a nasal spray for the prevention of allergic rhinitis and as a metered-dose inhaler for the prevention of asthma. Beclomethasone's anti-inflammatory action, considered safe for use during pregnancy, is also prescribed for the treatment of nonallergic nasal polyps and rhinitis medicamentosus. However, the drug is typically more effective for allergic rather than nonallergic disorders. Some authorities recommend cautious use in persons with active tuberculosis, bacterial, systemic fungal, or viral infections, recent nasal injury or surgery, nasal infection, or ocular herpes simplex. For hay fever, beclomethasone may take a week or more before reaching full effectiveness; in nonallergic conditions, it may take three weeks to prove either effective or noneffective.

Severe asthma should be stabilized by using oral corticosteroids before a beclomethasone inhalant can elicit preventive, anti-inflammatory benefits. Most asthma authorities now advocate the use of this and other anti-inflammatory metered-dose inhalers as first-line maintenance therapy in persons with mild to moderate asthma.

See also AEROSOL; CORTICOSTEROIDS; CORTICOSTEROID NASAL SPRAYS.

Beclovent See BECLOMETHASONE.

bends Bubbles of nitrogen that get into the blood and tissues in the event of a rapid decrease in air pressure. The condition (common among deep-sea divers) causes pain in the limbs and abdomen. It occurs also when a person ascends too fast after a period of exposure to increased air pressure while under water. The treatment is to restore normal air pressure via a hyperbaric chamber so the patient may slowly regain normal pressure.

See also CAISSON DISEASE; DECOMPRESSION ILLNESS.

benign pneumoconiosis Conditions such as siderosis (from the inhalation of iron oxide), baritosis (inhalation of barium), and stannosis (inhalation of tin particles) that show up in a chest X ray but actually do not cause symptoms or dysfunction of the lungs.

berylliosis Poisoning typically affecting the lungs, caused by beryllium particles (beryllium is a metallic element) that may be inhaled or contracted under the skin. The particles result in fibrosis and granulomata.

Beryllium is used today mainly in the aerospace industry, but it used to be mined for use in the electronics and chemical industries, particularly in the manufacture of fluorescent light bulbs.

The lung inflammation from beryllium fumes or dust is different from other occupational lung diseases because it seems to affect only those with a hypersensitivity to beryllium, although symptoms may not appear for one or two decades after even a brief exposure to the substance. It has been reported, too, that people living near beryllium refineries have also developed berylliosis. Potentially fatal, acute berylliosis may manifest suddenly with coughing, dyspnea, weight loss, and eye and skin irritation. Chronic berylliosis is characterized by abnormal tissue forming in the lungs and enlarged lymph nodes, and involves the individual's history of exposure to beryllium and subsequent events in his or her medical history, such as changes in the chest X ray. The disease may be mistaken for other lung diseases, such as sarcoidosis, and may require other diagnostic testing.

Treatment consists of corticosteroid medications and ventilator support, and proper and prompt treatment may lead to recovery in a week to 10 days. If lungs have been severely damaged over a long period of time or over the course of many flareups of the chronic form of the disease, there may be concurrent cardiac problems, including heart failure.

beta-adrenergic agonists Drugs, also known as beta-agonists, that act as bronchodilators to relieve spasms of the bronchi during an asthma attack. These potent drugs act by stimulating the $beta_2$-receptors on smooth muscle in the bronchial tree.

Alpha-adrenergic receptor stimulation causes a constriction of blood vessels and may raise blood pressure and heart rate. Beta-adrenergic stimulation primarily affects the airways or air passages. There are two types of receptors, $beta_1$ and $beta_2$. Drugs that act only on $beta_2$-receptors have fewer side effects and are the most frequently used in treating patients with asthma.

More than 5,000 years ago, the ancient Chinese treated asthma with *ma huang*, an herbal remedy that contains the beta-agonist ephedrine. Epinephrine (adrenaline) is a hormone that affects both alpha and beta receptors, and because of its rapid onset of action, it is a useful emergency drug. Within minutes after being injected into the subcutaneous tissues, it induces relief of severe bronchoconstriction and can usually prevent or reverse anaphylaxis if given promptly. Thus, epinephrine can be a truly lifesaving drug. Because of its alpha-adrenergic properties, however, it tends to cause a jittery feeling and heart palpitations in many individuals.

Albuterol, an example of a selective $beta_2$ drug, with sufficiently rapid onset of action for all but the most extreme situations, has relatively few adverse stimulatory effects and is available in a wide variety of dosage forms.

A Canadian study of more than 12,000 patients over a 1-year period through 1977 raised some questions about the safety of beta-agonists. The Canadian data suggest that merely taking twice the usual dose of $beta_2$ from an inhaler more than doubles the risk of death from an asthma attack.

The drug fenoterol (Berotec) is twice as potent as any $beta_2$ drug available in the United States.

Asthma Medication Safe When Taken as Directed (Palatine, Illinois, Aug. 9, 1991)

Drugs known as $beta_2$-agonists are safe and effective for the treatment of asthma, and patients taking the medication should continue despite recent reports of potentially fatal side effects associated with overuse of the drugs, according to a national professional organization of physicians specializing in the treatment of asthma.

The American College of Allergy, Asthma and Immunology said $beta_2$-agonists are the drugs of choice for the treatment of acute, intermittent, and exercise-induced asthma and are safe if taken as prescribed. $Beta_2$-agonists belong to a class of drugs called bronchodilators and are often administered through an inhaler.

"We have been successfully and safely using $beta_2$-agonists to treat asthma for more than 10 years," said Dr. Edward O'Connell, president of the college. "As with any drug, there can be side effects if the patient exceeds the prescribed dosage, and we caution patients not to do this."

O'Connell also cautioned against discontinuing medication and said patients should discuss concerns about recent reports with their physicians. About 10 million Americans suffer from asthma, a disease that causes wheezing, coughing, and difficulty in breathing, and claims about 4,600 lives each year. $Beta_2$-agonists relieve the symptoms of asthma attacks by relaxing and expanding the lung airways.

The FDA is considering a review of $beta_2$-agonists because of reports that taking twice the prescribed dose might be fatal. "The danger for asthmatics is that if the prescribed dose of $beta_2$-agonists does not bring relief, the patient may try taking more of the drug," O'Connell said.

"Patients who are not getting relief from the prescribed dose of medication should never increase the dosage on their own," O'Connell said. "They should talk with their doctors about supplementing with other drugs or switching to a different treatment plan. The essential thing is to develop a treatment plan only under the direction of the doctor."

The 3,600-member American College of Allergy, Asthma and Immunology is a national organization of physicians who specialize in the treatment of asthma and other allergic diseases. Board-certified allergists complete a three-year residency in either pediatrics or internal medicine and a two-year fellowship study in allergy and immunology.

—Press release from the American College of Allergy, Asthma and Immunology issued in August 1991.

BETA-AGONISTS AVAILABLE IN THE UNITED STATES

	Dosage Forms Available
albuterol (Proventil, Ventolin)	1, 3, 4
bitolterol (Tornalate)	3
epinephrine (Adrenalin, Primatene)	2, 3, 4
isoetharine (Bronkometer Bronkosol)	3, 4
isoproterenol (Isuprel)[1]	1, 2, 3, 4
metaproterenol (Alupent, Metaprel)	1, 3, 4
pirbuterol (Maxair)	3
terbutaline[2] (Brethaire, Brethine, Bricanyl)	1, 2, 3

orally=1; injectable=2; metered-dose inhaler (MDI)=3; nebulizer solution=4 (Not all brands are available in all dosage forms.)
[1] Rarely used for the treatment of asthma because of adverse effects.
[2] Terbutaline ampules for injection may be used as a nebulizer solution.

beta-adrenergic receptors See BETA-ADRENERGIC AGONISTS.

beta-blocking agents Drugs used to treat heart problems, high blood pressure, migraine headaches, and glaucoma. The most serious side effect of beta-blockers is constriction of the bronchial tubes, which can cause or worsen an asthma attack in an allergic or asthmatic person. Epinephrine (adrenalin chloride), the drug of choice for the treatment of severe allergic reactions or anaphylaxis, may be ineffective in persons taking beta-blocking drugs. Beta-blockers should be avoided by those with asthma or severe allergies.

WARNING: BETA-BLOCKING AGENTS MUST NEVER BE USED IN ANY PATIENT RECEIVING ALLERGY IMMUNOTHERAPY OR ALLERGY SHOTS and must be used very cautiously, if at all, in any allergic or asthmatic patient. Examples of beta-blocker medications (capsules, tablets, or eye-drops) are (brand names in parentheses):

acebutolol (Sectral)
atenolol (Tenormin)
atenolol + chlorthalidone (Tenoretic)
betaxolol hydrochloride (Betoptic) eyedrops
carteolol (Cartrol)
labetalol (Normodyne or Trandate)
labetalol + hydrochlorothiazide (Nonnozide or Trandate HCT)
levobunolol (Betagan) eyedrops
metoprolol (Lopressor)
metoprolol + hydrochlorothiazide (Lopressor HCT)
nadolol (Corgard)
nadolol + bendroflumethiazide (Corzide)
penbutolol (Levatol)
pindolol (Visken)
propranolol (Inderal)
propranolol + hydrochlorothiazide (Inderide)
timolol (Blocadren)
timolol (Timoptic) eyedrops
timolol + hydrochlorothiazide (Timolide)

beta-receptors See BETA-ADRENERGIC AGONISTS.

biopsy The removal of a tiny portion of live tissue for medical analysis leading to a diagnosis. Tissue may be obtained by aspiration through a needle or other methods.

bioterrorism The use of toxic substances, particularly biological agents classified by the Centers for Disease Control and Prevention (CDC) that may be deliberately aerosolized and inhaled, constituting an act of war. Among the highest risks to national security according to transmissibility and threat to life are smallpox, anthrax, *Yersinia pestis* (which causes bubonic, septicemic, and pneumonic plague), botulism, tularemia, and viral hemorrhagic fevers. Other somewhat lower risks include Q fever, brucellosis, glanders *(Burkholderia mallei),* castor bean toxin (ricin toxin), *Staphylococcus* enterotoxin B, Nipah virus, and hantaviruses.

Bioterrorism, with "weapons" including bacteria, viruses, and poisons, has an extensive history that dates back to the 12th century. According to a *Nursing Spectrum* article (December 17, 2001, Vol. 13, No. 25 NY/NJ) on biological weapons by Richard Stilp, R.N., M.A., C.H.S.P., corporate director of safety for Orlando Regional Healthcare, "In 1346, the Tatar army hurled the corpses of those soldiers who died of the plague over the Kaffa City walls, infecting residents who were defending the city. Some of those who left Kaffa may have started the Black Death pandemic that spread throughout Europe. Russian troops used this same tactic against Sweden in 1710. Biological warfare also occurred during the French and Indian War (1754–63) when an Englishman, Sir Jeffrey Amherst, gave smallpox-laden blankets to Native Americans who were loyal to the French. The Native Americans sustained epidemic casualties as a result."

The most recent instances of bioterrorism occurred concurrently with the terrorist attacks on the United States on September 11, 2001, with the destruction of the World Trade Center in New York City and damage to the Pentagon in Washington, D.C. As the news media reported the details of these events, letters containing powdery anthrax spores were sent through the mail to media and political offices. Stilp wrote that at least 17 countries have developed an anthrax weapon program in the knowledge that the spores can sustain their viability for more than 40 years. "In 1970, the World Health Organization (WHO) concluded that the release of 50 kilograms of aerosolized anthrax upwind of a population of 5 million could lead to an estimated 250,000 casualties and 100,000 deaths," he explained.

Preventive measures include the prophylactic administration of appropriate antibiotics if infection is suspected, the development of immunizations, and education of health care professionals as well as the lay public on the prevention, detection, and treatment of diseases transmitted through terrorism.

See also ANTHRAX; BOTULISM; TULAREMIA.

bird breeder's lung   An adverse reaction in certain individuals caused by contact with birds, particularly their excrement, including pigeons and parakeets. Symptoms—chills, fever, shortness of breath, and coughing—may be acute or delayed and subside when contact is no longer occurring.

black death   See BUBONIC PLAGUE.

black lung   See COAL WORKER'S PNEUMOCONIOSIS.

blast injury   An injury attributable to a sudden, severe change in air pressure.
See also ALTITUDE SICKNESS.

block, air   Air that leaks from one of the passageways of the respiratory system and collects in connective lung tissue. This causes an obstruction of the normal air flow.

blowing exercise   Blowing into a tube attached to a bottle of water, which is attached to another bottle so the air pressure from one projects the water into the other. This exercise is designed to increase intrabronchial pressure and help expand the lung.

blue baby   A newborn whose blood is not properly oxygenated, thus causing cyanosis, or bluish coloration of the skin and mucous membranes. In some cases, this condition may be a congenital anomaly in which the blood travels directly from the right to the left side of the heart without reaching the lungs.

Bostock, John   British physician (1773–1846) credited with coining the term *hay fever,* which he believed was "produced by the effluvium from new hay." In his writings "Case of a Periodical Affection of the Eyes and Chest" and "Of the Catarrhus Aestivus, or Summer Catarrh," Bostock described in accurate detail common symptoms of hay fever as heat, fullness, redness, and itching in the eyes, sneezing with the discharge of mucus, difficulty in breathing, a quickened pulse, restlessness, perspiration, and loss of appetite.

botulism   A life-threatening condition caused by a neurotoxin called botulinum, caused by the spore-forming bacillus *Clostridium botulinum,* that is usually associated with ingestion of improperly canned and, thus, contaminated food. However, botulinum may be intentionally aerosolized, which would pose a serious threat to the public. Symptoms include paralysis of respiratory muscles and upper and lower extremities, diplopia, dysphonia, dysphagia, and dysarthria. The Centers for Disease Control and Prevention (CDC) maintains a supply of an antitoxin to fight cases of botulism, and if detected early, most individuals afflicted with the toxin recover.

See also BIOTERRORISM.

Bouchut's respiration   Exhalation longer than inhalation in children with asthma or bronchopneumonia, named for French physician Jean A. E. Bouchut (1818–91).

Bovet, Daniele   Swiss-born Italian scientist (1907–92), who discovered antibacterial sulfanomides and, with Ernest Fourneau in 1933, succeeded in synthesizing the first series of antihistamines. Bovet won the Nobel Prize in physiology or medicine in 1957.

bradykinin   A potent chemical mediator whose vasodilating action plays a role in asthma, pulmonary edema, and anaphylaxis. This slow-moving kinin, a term for a group of polypeptides, influences contraction of smooth muscle, promotes hypotension, increases blood flow in small blood capillaries, and sparks the pain reflex.

bradypnea   Excessively slow respirations.

brass founder's ague   Tremors resulting from the inhalation of toxic fumes or from zinc or brass poisoning.

See also BRASS POISONING.

brass poisoning   The adverse effect of inhaling the fumes of zinc and zinc oxide. Although rarely fatal, brass poisoning damages tissue in the respiratory system and may result in dryness and burning in the respiratory tract, cough, headache, and chills. Inhaling humidified air often relieves the symptoms.

breath, bad   Malodorous air expelled from the mouth. Also called halitosis, bad breath is usually caused by the ingestion of foods containing potent oils, such as onions and garlic, strong-smelling beverages, and other liquid substances, or the fermentation of food particles lodged between teeth. Proper toothbrushing, flossing, and regular dental hygiene prevent bad breath in most cases. Deodorant mouthwashes, gargles, sprays, mints, lozenges, and gum are available. Although not the cause of intestinal disorders, halitosis may indicate a systemic disease. For example, renal failure causes the breath to take on the characteristic smell of urine. An abscess on the lung creates bad breath. Liver disease may cause the breath to smell mousy. Severe diabetes may cause an acetone (nail polish remover) breath odor.

People who think their breath smells bad when it does not may be suffering from psychogenic halitosis. Schizophrenics or people with paranoid or obsessive feelings of being dirty or smelly or the sense of "rotting inside" may believe they have offensive breath.

Breath Enhancer   A device to facilitate the use of aerosol metered-dose inhalers for poorly coordinated persons with asthma.

breath-holding attacks   Arrested breathing, cyanosis (turning blue), rigidity and extension of the arms and legs, and possible loss of consciousness that starts with a child's crying and, subsequently, the child's body goes limp, he or she resumes breathing and becomes alert. Breath-holding attacks cease of their own accord before the child reaches school age. Voluntary or involuntary breath-holding on the part of a child may be part of a tantrum or tactic used to get parents' attention and an attempt to manipulate their behavior and responses. Psychological counseling may be recommended for both the child and parents.

breathing The process of respiration, that is, the taking in (inhaling) of oxygen into the lungs and the expelling (exhaling) of carbon dioxide. The normal exchange of these gases is essential to life. Certain breathing patterns characterize a variety of conditions, including *asthmatic breathing,* or prolonged wheezing heard throughout the chest cavity; *bronchial breathing,* or harsh breathing sounds accompanied by a high-pitched expiration; *Cheyne-Stokes breathing,* or periods of apnea followed by increased depth and frequency of respirations; *cogwheel breathing,* or a respiratory murmur often associated with bronchitis and incipient tuberculosis; *continuous positive-pressure breathing,* or a method of artificially assisting respiration; *intermittent positive-pressure breathing,* or a mechanism that administers air or oxygen for assisting respiration; *Kussmaul breathing,* or very deep, gasping seen in cases of severe diabetic acidosis and coma; and *shallow breathing,* which occurs in cases of acute lung disease when chest walls are thickened, when ribs are fractured thus inhibiting deep breathing, in pleurisy, emphysema, and other respiratory disorders.

See also RESPIRATORY SYSTEM.

breathing exercises A series of deep breathing techniques to build up lung capacity and to help an individual with respiratory disorders to relax and breathe as normally as possible. The Eastern practice of yoga includes breath control and rhythmic, deep breathing, which are geared to overall physical and mental improvement.

Asthmatic children often respond to relaxation breathing techniques when they feel an asthma attack coming on, and in some cases, the full-blown attack can be avoided. Essentially, one is advised to inhale through the nose, filling the belly and then the chest with air, and to exhale through the mouth and contract the muscles in the abdomen. Breathing exercises may also be done with a spirometer, a plastic tube containing plastic balls. As one blows air into the mouthpiece of the tube, the balls rise. This encourages deep breathing, which helps clear the lungs and oxygenate the entire body. Physicians prescribe spirometry for patients with bronchitis, pneumonia, and other, especially chronic, lung diseases.

Brethaire See TERBUTALINE SULFATE.

Brethine See TERBUTALINE SULFATE.

Bricanyl See TERBUTALINE SULFATE.

Bromfed See BROMPHENIRAMINE.

brompheniramine (Bromfed, Dimetane, Dimetapp) A mildly sedating, commonly used antihistamine of the alkylamine class. Brompheniramine is available alone or in combination with a decongestant in prescription and over-the-counter allergy preparations.

See also ANTIHISTAMINE.

bronchadenitis Inflammation of bronchial glands.

bronchi The two large branches extending from the trachea, or windpipe, into the lungs, forming what is commonly known as the "bronchial tree." Because each bronchus is an airway, a buildup of mucus, an infection, physical and chemical irritants, swelling of the bronchial mucosal lining, excess calculi, or a foreign body or obstruction can cause choking, bronchitis, bronchoedema, lung abscess, and pneumonia. A bronchoscope is an instrument through which the bronchi can be examined. Bronchopulmonary disorders are those that involve both bronchi and lungs, such as bronchial pneumonia.

See also BRONCHIOLES; RALE.

bronchial asthma A common term for asthma.
See also ASTHMA.

bronchial breathing Harsh breathing associated with high-pitched expiration (tubular breathing).

bronchial challenge A diagnostic breathing test.
See also SPIROMETER.

bronchial crises Paroxysms of coughing in locomotor ataxia.

bronchial glands   Mucous or mixed glands in the bronchi or bronchioles.

bronchial tree   See BRONCHI.

bronchial washing   Cleansing of one or both bronchi, or the process of irrigating the bronchi for the collection of cells for diagnostic testing.

bronchiarctia   A narrowing or constriction of a bronchial tube.

bronchiectasis   Dilation or irreversible widening of a bronchus or bronchi, usually chronic and involving a secondary infection, such as bronchopneumonia, chronic bronchitis, tuberculosis, and whooping cough or other damage to the bronchial wall. The bronchial wall has several varying layers corresponding to each segment of airway and is lined by an inner mucosa and submucosa that serve to protect airways from harmful particles and substances. Structural layers provide elastic, cartilage, and muscle fiber, while blood vessels and lymphoid tissue nourish and maintain the bronchial wall. When parts of the wall are inflamed or destroyed in bronchiectasis, mucus production increases and promotes bacterial growth, and the general protective structure breaks down. The damage may extend to the alveoli of the lungs and result in bronchopneumonia, scarring, and dysfunctional lung tissue. Inflammation and an increase in blood vessels in the bronchial wall may also result in coughing up blood and airway blockage that inhibits oxygen distribution.

Bronchiectasis may be acquired or congenital, and on one or both sides of the chest. An underlying disease, such as allergic bronchopulmonary aspergillosis, may also be the cause. Frequent occurrences of pneumonia may be a sign of bronchiectasis. The most common cause is chronic or recurring infection; other conditions, including abnormal immune response, birth defects of the airways, and a predisposing factor such as bronchial obstruction, may lead to bronchiectasis as well. Symptoms include coughing, difficulty breathing, the production of foul secretion and sputum that

separates into three layers, the bottom layer containing pus cells, a greenish middle layer, and a layer of froth on top. Treatment includes antibiotics, postural drainage, and bronchodilating aerosols.

Saccular bronchiectasis refers to dilated bronchi that are irregularly shaped or shaped somewhat like a sac. Varicose bronchiectasis refers to dilated bronchi that look like varicose, or herniated, veins, and an irregular dilation also found in cystic fibrosis.

Preventive measures reduce the incidence of bronchiectasis: immunizations against measles and whooping cough; influenza and pneumococcal vaccines; early use of antibiotics in the case of pneumonia or tuberculosis; appropriate use of corticosteroid and other anti-inflammatory drugs if allergic bronchopulmonary aspergillosis and other disorders are present; avoidance of noxious fume, gas, dusts, and smoke; avoidance (in infants and children) of aspiration of foreign objects; avoidance of oversedation that leads to respiratory depression; prompt medical attention to neurological symptoms, including coughing or vomiting after eating, difficulty swallowing, and impaired consciousness; avoidance of using mouth or nose drops such as mineral oil at bedtime, and diagnosis by bronchoscopy and treatment of any obstruction in the bronchus before an extreme condition arises.

bronchiloquy   Strange vocal sounds as a result of a bronchus covered with consolidated lung tissue.

bronchiocele   A dilatation, swelling, or tumor located in a bronchus, one of the two large branches of the trachea or windpipe. This may indicate a number of bronchial disorders, including chronic bronchiectasis.
See also BRONCHIECTASIS.

bronchiolectasis   Dilation of the bronchioles.
See also BRONCHIECTASIS.

bronchioles   The smaller subdivisions of the bronchial tree in the thorax, so named because the bronchi and bronchioles resemble a tree trunk and its roots. The bronchioles bring air from the trachea, the upper part of the windpipe, to the lungs and participate in the exchange of gases (oxygen and carbon dioxide) in the breathing process. Bronchial glands are mucus-producing organs in the bronchi and bronchioles. (The Greek word for windpipe is *bronchus*.) Among disorders of the bronchioles are bronchitis, bronchiolitis, and bronchopneumonia.

See also BRONCHIOLITIS; BRONCHITIS.

bronchiolitis   An acute inflammatory disease of the bronchioles, or small airways, in infants in which excessive mucus production results in airway obstruction. This obstruction leads to tachypnea (rapid shallow breathing), with a respiratory rate of 50 to as high as 80 breaths per minute, hypoxemia (reduced oxygen content of the blood), and hyperinflation (overinflated lungs).

Bronchiolitis occurs more often in winter and spring months, usually during the first six months of life. It predominantly affects males and may occur in epidemics. During outbreaks, respiratory syncytial virus and parainfluenza are most often the cause, but the bacterium *Mycobacterium pneumoniae* can cause bronchiolitis in older children and bronchioles may be contused with asthma. X rays, blood gas studies, and physical examination findings are virtually identical. Both illnesses are often caused by viral respiratory infections in infants, although allergy testing in the older child may help to confirm the diagnosis. Congestive heart failure can also be mistaken for both bronchiolitis and asthma in the infant.

Treatment of acute bronchiolitis is based on improving hypoxemia, preventing dehydration, and administering bronchodilating drugs and corticosteroids. Antibiotics are probably of no value unless there is suspicion of a secondary bacterial infection. Recovery usually occurs within two weeks, but bronchiolitis can be fatal. Some believe that infants with bronchiolitis have a greater chance of developing asthma later on in life. However, it may be difficult to determine if the original diagnosis of bronchiolitis was correct or if the infant was actually having an initial attack of asthma.

See also RESPIRATORY SYNCYTIAL VIRUS.

bronchiospasm   See BRONCHOSPASM.

bronchiostenosis   Constriction or narrowing of a bronchial tube.

bronchitis   An infection or inflammatory disease in the bronchi and bronchioles caused by viral or bacterial germs, allergy, or irritating dust and fumes. It may be an acute infection or a chronic process. Typical symptoms may include coughing, wheezing, shortness of breath, chills, fever, fatigue, and excessive sputum. Infectious bronchitis, which occurs most often in winter months, may be caused by microorganisms such as *Mycoplasma pneumoniae* and *Chlamydia*, and recurring infections stemming from chronic sinusitis, bronchiectasis, allergies, and in children, enlarged tonsils and adenoids. Irritative bronchitis involves inhalation or exposure to various chemical dusts and fumes such as ammonia and strong organic solvents, air pollution such as ozone and nitrogen dioxide, or cigarette and other smoke.

Treatment includes drinking adequate fluids, taking aspirin or acetaminophen to reduce fever, and, in certain cases in which a bacterial infection is evident, antibiotics, including tetracycline, ampicillin, trimethoprim-sulfamethoxazole, erythromycin (when *Mycoplasma pneumoniae* is suspected), and amoxicillin (for children). Sputum tests provide the information for proper diagnosis in the event of severe bronchitis. Chest X ray may be necessary to rule out the development from bronchitis to pneumonia. In mild cases, patients recover fully, although bronchitis may be life-threatening to the elderly and individuals with chronic heart or lung disease.

See also BRONCHITIS, CHRONIC.

bronchitis, chronic   A disorder characterized by excessive mucus production in the bronchial tree with a persistent productive cough. By definition it lasts at least three months of the year for at least two consecutive years.

Chronic bronchitis may or may not be related to asthma. Persons with chronic asthmatic bronchitis have a long history of cough and mucus production and develop wheezing as the disease progresses.

Chronic asthma with obstruction is characterized by a prolonged course of wheezing and late onset of a chronic productive cough.

Chronic bronchitis is often confused with emphysema, an expansion of the air spaces in the lungs resulting in destruction of the alveoli, or air sacs. In chronic obstructive lung, or pulmonary, disease (COLD, COPD), the flow of air in and out of the lungs is blocked as a result of chronic bronchitis or emphysema, or both. In asthma without chronic obstruction, the blockage is present only during an attack. However, in chronic obstructive lung disease, some obstruction exists at all times.

Approximately 20 percent of adult males have chronic bronchitis, although only a small number become disabled because of it. Chronic bronchitis is less common in females. Individuals who smoke, have allergies, or are frequently exposed to irritants or pollution in the environment may also suffer the disease.

See also BRONCHITIS; EMPHYSEMA.

bronchoalveolar lavage   The use of sterile saline solution to "wash" the lungs of secretions, cells, and protein from the lower respiratory tract. A fiberoptic bronchoscope introduces the fluid into the lung, and this treatment may be for diagnostic purposes or to treat patients with cystic fibrosis, pulmonary alveolar proteinosis, and severe asthma with bronchial obstruction due to a mucus plug.

bronchoblennorrhea   Chronic bronchitis characterized by large amounts of thin sputum.

bronchocele   A dilation or swelling of a part of a bronchus.

bronchoconstriction   See BRONCHOSPASM.

bronchodilating drugs   Also known as bronchodilators, first-line medications that block the constriction of bronchial tubes during an asthma attack. Bronchodilators include beta-agonists, such as albuterol, and xanthine derivatives, such as theophylline. The exact mechanism by which these drugs exert their beneficial effects is unknown. These drugs are available as metered-dose inhalers, solutions for injection or inhalation, or as oral tablets, capsules, and syrups.

See also BETA-ADRENERGIC AGONISTS; THEOPHYLLINE.

bronchodilator   See BRONCHODILATING DRUGS.

bronchoedema   Swelling of the mucosa of the bronchial tubes that constricts the airways and makes breathing difficult.

bronchofiberscope   An instrument also known as a fiberoptic endoscope used to examine the bronchi.

bronchography   The introduction of a radiopaque substance into the trachea or bronchial tree for the diagnostic purposes of x-raying the lung or a portion of the lung. A bronchogram, or X ray of the lung, may be obtained during a bronchography.

broncholithiasis   Calculi (stones) developed in the bronchi causing an obstruction or inflammation.

bronchomycosis   An infection in the bronchi or bronchial tubes caused by a fungus, typically of the genus *Candida*.

bronchopathy   Any disease involving the bronchi or bronchioles.

bronchoplegia   Muscle paralysis of the walls of the bronchial tubes.

bronchopneumonia   Lung inflammation (pneumonia) complicated by the concurrent inflammation of the terminal bronchioles and alveoli. Caused by various pneumococci, Group A hemolytic streptococci, varieties of staphylococci, *Klebsiella pneumoniae*, *Francisella tularensis*, and various forms of other bacteria, viruses, rickettsiae, and fungi, bronchopneumonia is characterized by productive coughing (i.e., cough with expectoration of sputum), short and shallow respirations (50 to 75 breaths per minute), and sometimes cyanosis (blue coloration of the mucous membranes due to lack of oxygen). In children, the temperature may reach to 105 degrees Fahrenheit, and the fever may last two to three weeks. In the elderly, the fever (if any) may be 100 to 101 degrees Fahrenheit with only a slight cough and a small amount of sputum, but weakness, chest pain, chills, and sore throat may be evident.

The treatment of choice includes antibiotic therapy, bed rest, increased fluids, a soft diet, painkilling medication, oxygen (for cyanosis), and treatment of shock symptoms if they present. Complications of bronchopneumonia include lung abscess, empyema, pericarditis, paralytic ileus, and atelectasis.

See also PNEUMONIA.

bronchopulmonary aspergillosis, allergic (ABPA)
Pneumonia-like disease caused by an allergic reaction to the mold *Aspergillus fumigatus*. It usually occurs in adult asthmatics.

Signs and Symptoms
This disorder usually involves episodes of fever, shortness of breath and wheezing, and coughing up copious quantities of dark brown, and at times blood-streaked, sputum.

Diagnosis
Because the fungus is ubiquitous (found in healthy persons in small quantities that are harmless), the presence of positive sputum cultures is not sufficient to diagnose this disease. The diagnosis is made in persons meeting the following criteria: (1) episodes of asthma; (2) elevated eosinophils (a type of white blood cell) and total immunoglobulin E (IgE) antibodies in the blood; these values are slightly elevated in most allergic individuals but extremely elevated in persons with this disease; (3) pneumonia-like X-ray findings, which may be temporary; (4) bronchiectasis (destruction of the muscles in the bronchial walls with chronic cough and large amounts of sputum); (5) positive skin tests to the *Aspergillus* fungus; and

(6) positive blood tests for antibodies against the *Aspergillus* allergen.

Treatment
Prednisone, a corticosteroid drug, is the treatment of choice. It is used daily, most often for several months, and improvement is usually seen within days. In some cases, recurrences require long-term prednisone use.

Prognosis
If untreated, aspergillosis will damage lung tissues and can be fatal.

bronchopulmonary dysplasia A chronic lung disease of premature infants that develops after a period of intensive respiratory therapy. Dysplasia refers to abnormal formation of tissue.

bronchopulmonary lavage Irrigation of the bronchi and bronchioles to remove abnormal or excessive secretions.

bronchorrhagia Hemorrhage (profuse bleeding) in the bronchial tube.

bronchorrhea An abnormal secretion, which may be offensive to others, from the mucous membrane in the bronchi.

bronchorrhoncus From the Greek word *rhonchos,* meaning "snore," a rale heard in the bronchial passageway.

bronchoscopy An examination of the bronchi through a device called a bronchoscope. The instrument is inserted into the trachea and down to the bronchi so the physician can diagnose a bronchial abnormality.

bronchosinusitis The simultaneous inflammation and infection of the bronchi and sinuses.

bronchospasm Also called bronchiospasm, sudden narrowing or constriction of the bronchial tubes during an asthma attack or in persons with bronchitis. Bronchospasm is also referred to as bronchoconstriction.

See also ASTHMA; BRONCHITIS.

bronchospirochetosis A type of bronchitis caused by spirochetes, or microorganism of the order Spirochaetales. Bronchopulmonary spirochetosis is also known as hemorrhagic bronchitis.

bronchostaxis Profuse bleeding, or hemorrhage, from a bronchial wall.

bronchostomy From the Greek word *stoma*, or mouth, the surgical creation of an opening into a bronchus.

bronchotomy A surgical incision made into a bronchus, the larynx, or trachea, usually in order to open an airway.

Bronkaid Mist The trade name for epinephrine, USP.

Bronkephrine The trade name for ethylnorepinephrine hydrochloride, USP.

Bronkodyl See THEOPHYLLINE.

Bronkometer See ISOETHARINE.

Bronkosol See ISOETHARINE.

bubonic plague (black death) Named from the Greek word for gland, *bubo*, and the Latin *plaga*, meaning stroke or wound, bubonic plague is most famous for its epidemic proportions in Europe during the Middle Ages, hence the term "black death." Plague is an acute, extremely contagious disease caused by *Yersinia pestis*, a microorganism found in infected rats, mice, squirrels, and prairie dogs. It is mainly transmitted to humans by way of a rat flea bite, and results in enlarged lymphatic glands, adenitis or pneumonia, and symptoms of severe poisoning. Symptoms include high fever, a staggering gait, restlessness, delirium or confusion, shock,

and coma. Even though it may be fatal, a mild form of plague is known as ambulatory; pneumonic plague refers to extensive lung involvement. In hemorrhagic plague, one of the severe forms of the disease, there is bleeding into the skin. Bubonic is the most common form of plague characterized by the formation of buboes, or swollen lymph nodes. Untreated bubonic plague causes death between the third and fifth day from the onset of symptoms in 60 percent of its victims. (Tuberculosis, caused by a *Mycobacterium*, is sometimes called "white plague.")

Plague infections occur most frequently in the United States in the Southwest, including Arizona, California, Colorado, and New Mexico. Recent outbreaks have been limited to an individual case or small clusters of people. In addition to infected flea bites, plague may be transmitted by the droplets of an infected person's cough or sneeze.

Pneumonic plague occurs when the lungs are infected by the plague bacteria.

Symptoms

High fever, chills, rapid heartbeat are signs of the plague, and in most cases, a severe headache, with a cough developing within a day or so from the time of exposure to the bacteria. The sputum becomes bloody and eventually turns uniformly foamy, resembling raspberry syrup. If untreated, a victim may die within two days of the onset of symptoms.

Prevention

Rodent control and use of insect repellent are key, especially to travelers to areas in which there are reported incidences of plague infection. Prompt treatment, i.e., within 24 hours, is also important when plague infection is suspected. Treatment includes streptomycin, tetracyclines, and chloramphenicol, and individuals with pneumonic plague must be isolated to prevent spreading the disease. A plague vaccine is available and is made by adding the preservative chemical formaldehyde to kill specific plague bacilli.

budesonide (Rhinocort, Pulmocort) Corticosteroid available in the United States as a nasal spray for allergic rhinitis and in other countries as a metered-dose inhaler for asthma. Budesonide has a greater potency than many similar drugs.

See also CORTICOSTEROID METERED-DOSE INHALERS; CORTICOSTEROID NASAL SPRAYS.

butane   See INHALANT ABUSE.

byssinosis   An allergic lung disease caused by occupational exposure to an unknown allergen in the dust from the processing of cotton, flax, hemp, or sisal. Symptoms of shortness of breath and wheezing gradually intensify upon increased exposure and may lead to respiratory failure. Smoking increases the risk of permanent lung damage. Byssinosis is largely preventable by wearing a face mask and treating raw textiles before manufacturing. Because these measures are ignored in developing countries, the incidence of this disease is greater there than in the United States. Government compensation is available in the United States for those afflicted with byssinosis.

Bronchodilating drugs, either aerosol inhalers or tablets, and removal of exposure to the harmful dusts are the treatment of choice.

See also OCCUPATIONAL ASTHMA.

cachexia The condition of being in bad health, malnourished and wasting that may occur in the course of chronic catastrophic disease, including advanced pulmonary tuberculosis. In addition to prescribed medical therapy, treatment consists of rest, good hygiene and nutrition, prevention of skin breakdown, pain, and fractures, maintenance of elimination, and emotional support.

caisson disease Pain in the joints, skin irritation, a burning sensation in the lungs, coughing, and various neurological disturbances caused by a sudden or rapid reduction in environmental air pressure. Caisson disease—named from the French word *caisse*, meaning "box"—is frequently seen in aviators and deep-sea divers. Also known as the bends or decompression illness, caisson disease is characterized by nitrogen bubbles forming in the tissue space and small blood vessels when a diver comes to the surface of the water after being 30 or more feet below in an environment of compressed air, or a pilot ascends rapidly from sea level to an elevation of 18,000 feet or higher. Treatment includes use of a hyperbaric chamber for recompression and then a gradual decompression.

See also BENDS.

canal, pharyngeal The tubular opening from the sphenoid bone to the palatine bone that contains the sphenopalatine vessels.

canal of Lambert The connecting points between bronchioles and alveoli in the lungs, which may help prevent collapse of the lung.

See also ATELECTASIS.

cancer, lung A form of disease characterized by the uncontrolled growth of cells (derived from normal cells) and subsequent malignancy that is capable of killing the host by spreading from the original site to other parts of the body. Cancer is named from the Greek word *karkinos,* meaning crab. It is estimated that 200 different types of cancers exist, most of which, like the crab's slow movement, have an insidious onset.

See also LUNG CANCER.

candidiasis An infection by the yeastlike fungus of the species *Candida albicans* affecting various parts of the skin or mucous membranes, including the bronchi and lungs. Oral nystatin, ketoconazole, or clotrimazole may be prescribed for localized infections, and systemic infections may be treated with amphotericin B and other medications.

cannabis The hemp plant, *Cannabis sativa,* from which the dried flowering tops are processed into a preparation that, when inhaled or ingested, may cause euphoria and, according to some reports, pain relief, antiemesis (particularly the important constituent called delta-9-tetrahydrocannabinol, or THC, in the treatment of cancer), and alleviation of the symptoms of glaucoma. Cannabis is also known as marijuana, which can be smoked. In addition to possibly exacerbating psychoses, such as schizophrenia, marijuana is a "gateway" drug known to cause psychological dependence, and the inducement of toxic delirium, among other ill effects. Cannabis that is smoked may lead to respiratory disorders. Although it has not been proven that heavy and chronic marijuana use causes lung cancer and other serious pulmonary impairments, marijuana contains some of the same harmful components as tobacco smoke. Smoking marijuana is often concurrent with cigarette smoking, which increases the risk of respiratory disease.

See also HASHISH; TOBACCO.

cannula, nasal Flexible tubing inserted into the nostrils that provides oxygen at 1 to 6 liters per minute. The tubes that go approximately 1 centimeter into each nostril are connected to a common tube and an oxygen source.

capacity, vital The volume of air that can be forcibly exhaled from the lungs after a full inhalation.

Caplan's syndrome Named for British physician Anthony Caplan (1907–76), a type of rheumatoid arthritis with severe fibrosis of the lung, found in coal miners and others with forms of pneumoconiosis. The syndrome is a rare disorder in which scar nodules develop in the coal miner's lung as well as in the lungs of people who have been exposed to coal dust even if they do not suffer from black lung.

See also COAL WORKER'S PNEUMOCONIOSIS.

capnography The record made of the level of carbon dioxide in the exhaled air of patients connected to a ventilating device.

capreomycin sulfate A tuberculostatic drug (Capastat).

See also TUBERCULOSIS.

carbinoxamine An antihistaminic drug, commonly combined with a decongestant, used to treat allergic rhinitis (hay fever) conditions. It is available in oral formulations as Rondec (Abbott) or as a generic brand. Carbinoxamine may cause drowsiness.

See also ANTIHISTAMINE.

carbon dioxide [CO_2] A colorless, odorless gas exhaled during respiration that is the result of carbon oxidation that takes place in the tissues. Blood levels of CO_2 increase during hyperventilation, characterized by shortness of breath, tingling of extremities, and, at times, vomiting, elevated blood pressure, and disorientation.

See also ARTERIAL BLOOD GASES; CARBON DIOXIDE INHALATION; CARBON DIOXIDE POISONING; HYPERVENTILATION.

carbon dioxide inhalation A 5 to 7.5 percent level of carbon dioxide and oxygen used for patients to inhale as a way to stimulate respiration (particularly in individuals with pulmonary disease) and as part of or sequel to the administration of artificial respiration.

See also CARBON DIOXIDE.

carbon dioxide poisoning The intake of excessively high levels of carbon dioxide, characterized by extremely deep breathing, a feeling of pressure in the head, acid taste in the mouth, ringing in the ears, a slight burning sensation in the nose, and possibly near respiratory arrest and unconsciousness. The treatment is administration of oxygen.

See also CARBON DIOXIDE.

carbon monoxide Known as CO, a colorless, tasteless, odorless, and insidiously poisonous gas produced as a result of imperfect combustion and oxidation. Engine exhaust gas is a common source of CO, and it is also found in coal mines (from the incomplete combustion of coal), sewers, cellars, and gasoline motors. Smoking tobacco, which impedes the level of oxygen in the bloodstream, increases the blood's level of CO. In turn, night vision may be affected.

Carbon monoxide detectors, similar to smoke detectors, have been developed for household use to prevent poisoning.

See also CARBON MONOXIDE POISONING.

carbon monoxide poisoning The intake of excessively high levels of carbon monoxide in a brief period of time or the effect of inhaling small amounts over an extended period of time may cause poisoning. Inhaling fumes while in a closed car with the motor running, or using a gasoline motor in an enclosed area may cause the CO to combine with the hemoglobin and thereby cut off the body's oxygen supply.

Poisoning symptoms vary and may include a "cherry red" skin color, weakness of muscles, pounding heart, headache and throbbing in the temples, nausea, dilated pupils, ringing in the ears, and rapid pulse. Treatment of choice is the administration of 100 percent oxygen. Complications that may arise include cerebral edema, muscular spasms, blindness, paralysis, and other neurological disturbances.

See also CARBON MONOXIDE.

carbon tetrachloride poisoning   The result of inhaling excessive levels of carbon tetrachloride (CCl$_4$), a clear liquid with an odor similar to that of ether. Inhaling even a small quantity may cause death by damaging the liver and kidneys. Symptoms include eye, nose, and throat irritation, headache, nausea, visual disturbance, confusion, ventricular fibrillation, and depression of the central nervous system. Treatment includes the administration of oxygen, lavage with saline solution, and the removal of clothing contaminated with the chemical.

carcinogen   Any chemical or substance that induces the risk of developing cancer in animals or humans. Carcinogenesis refers to the origin of cancer.

carcinoma, alveolar cell   A malignant tumor that develops in the lung. A carcinoma specifically occurs in epithelial tissue and they frequently metastasize through the bloodstream or the lymph system.

See also CANCER, LUNG.

carcinoma, bronchogenic   A bronchogenic carcinoma is malignant and develops in the bronchi.

See also CANCER, LUNG.

carcinoma, oat cell   A tumor that develops in the bronchus and contains tiny cells shaped like oats.

See also CANCER, LUNG.

Cardarelli's sign   Named for Italian physician Antonio Cardarelli (1831–1926), a throbbing movement of the trachea, or windpipe, to one side, which may accompany an aortic aneurysm.

cardiac asthma   Severe shortness of breath caused by fluid in the lungs that produces bronchospasm and wheezing. This condition results from an inability of the left chambers of the heart to pump adequately, that is, congestive heart failure. Cardiac asthma is accompanied by hyperventilation, a state of rapid breathing, and the person appears to be having an asthma attack. Primary treatment involves heart drugs such as diuretics, digitalis, and ACE inhibitors. Bronchodilators are sometimes helpful.

cardiopneumograph   A device that records the motions of the heart and lungs for diagnostic purposes.

cardiopulmonary arrest   The sudden cessation of breathing and blood circulation, indicating the need for cardiopulmonary resuscitation and/or other methods that may revive the victim.

See also CARDIOPULMONARY RESUSCITATION.

cardiopulmonary resuscitation   Commonly referred to as CPR, a method to try to restore breathing and heart function, i.e., to provide oxygen as quickly as possible to all the vital organs of a breathless victim. A CPR assessment is the first step to determine the victim's state of consciousness; in three to five seconds, a caregiver must lift the jaw and remove any liquid or solid material in the mouth to make sure the airway is open. It is also best to remove the victim's dentures at this time. (If the victim has sustained trauma of the head and neck, care must be taken not to move the victim unless it is absolutely necessary.) Next, the caregiver should observe the chest for breathing movements and listen for breaths. If there is no rise and fall of the chest or evidence of breathing, CPR may be started.

To begin CPR, the caregiver kneels over the victim at the shoulder, tilts back the head and lifts the chin (unless spinal injury is suspected, in which case, one simply brings the jaw forward). Once the airway is open, the caregiver gently pinches the victim's nostrils closed, takes a deep breath and places the lips to form a seal over the victim's mouth. (If the victim is an infant, the caregiver creates a seal over the nose and mouth.) The caregiver then gives two full breaths lasting one to one-and-a-half seconds, watching carefully that the victim's chest rises with each ventilation. A bag-valve-mask or other device may also be used to prevent the spread of disease between caregiver and recipient of CPR. The caregiver must also assess the victim's circulation by taking the carotid-artery pulse (between the groove of the trachea and the strap muscles in the neck). If there is a pulse but no sign of breathing, continue mouth-to-mouth resuscitation by administering one breath every five seconds, or 12 breaths per minute. If there is still no pulse, the victim is suffering cardiac arrest and chest compressions over the lower part of the sternum (breastbone) should be started.

With fingers either interlocked or extended and using the heel of the hands placed over the notch where the ribs meet the sternum in the middle of the chest, the caregiver should compress straight down on the sternum approximately an inch-and-a-half to two inches on an adult victim, an inch to an inch-and-a-half on a child, and half an inch to an inch on an infant. After each rhythmic compression, the chest should return to its natural position. Eighty to 100 compressions per minute (at least 100 per minute for an infant) should be applied. CPR should not be interrupted for more than seven seconds. IT IS IMPORTANT FOR SOMEONE TO CALL 911 OR A LOCAL EMERGENCY NUMBER WHILE CPR IS BEING GIVEN SO EMERGENCY MEDICAL PERSONNEL CAN REACH THE VICTIM AND TAKE HIM OR HER TO THE HOSPITAL.

When the victim begins to breathe on his own, stop chest compressions. Check with community health facilities and organizations for complete CPR instructions and emergency measures. Everyone capable of learning CPR should be certified.

carrier   A person, animal, insect, substance, or other agent capable of spreading a disease organism without showing signs of having the disease itself.

See also INFECTION CARRIERS.

case-control study   A method of examining disease and disease processes by way of two groups, one of those who have a disease—referred to as cases—and one of those who do not—referred to as controls. Information is obtained from each group and analyzed. The method is useful in epidemiology. The first case-control study involved English chimney sweeps who developed cancer of the scrotum. Researchers hypothesized that the nature of their work had something to do with the incidence of scrotal cancer among their group as opposed to the rate of scrotal cancer in the general public. Epidemiologists also use the case-control study to determine other characteristics of disease processes, such as frequency of occurrence, risk factors, circumstances of exposure, and the differences between the cases and the controls.

cast, bronchial   Hardened segments of bronchial secretions that accumulate and take on the shape of the bronchial tubes. Bronchial casts may be seen in the sputum of asthma or bronchitis patients. Cast material consists of substances thrown off during the course of pathological conditions (the products of effusion). The substances may also mold themselves to nasal, tracheal, esophageal, renal, urethral, intestinal, and vaginal passages.

catarrh   Inflammation of mucous membranes characterized by a dry cough and severe coughing spells with little or no expectoration, especially in the aged with emphysema or asthma.

catheter, pulmonary artery   A tube that is passed into the pulmonary artery for the purpose of measuring pressures in the artery, wedge pressure in the pulmonary capillaries, and heart function.

cavernous rale   Hollow spaces in the respiratory tract that produce a bubbling sound. Cavernous respiration refers to a hollow sound heard when there is a lung cavity.

See also RALE.

cavity, pleural   The space between the parietal pleura, serous membranes that extend from the roots of the lungs and cover the pericardium to the chest wall and backward to the spinal cord, and the visceral pleura, which invests the lungs and enters the interlobar fissures. The pleura pulmonalis refers to the membranes investing the lungs and fissures between the lobes. Pleurae secrete a lubricating substance that decreases friction between the structures of the lungs during respiratory movements.

Pleural effusion refers to fluid escaping into the chest cavity between the visceral and the parietal pleura and may be seen in a chest X ray if the fluid measures more than 300 milliliters. Pleural fibrosis, which occurs with pulmonary tuberculosis, means the pleura thickens and obliterates the pleural cavity, making respiratory movements difficult. Pleuralgia is the medical term for pain occurring in the pleura or in the side.

See also PLEURISY.

cell-mediated immunity Immune protection provided by the direct action of immune cells such as macrophages. This differs from humoral (bodily fluids) immunity, which chiefly involves B cells and antibodies. The macrophage ingests the antigen, digests it, and then displays antigenic fragments on its own surface. The macrophage then binds to a group of genes called a major histocompatibility complex (MHC). This combined structure attracts a T cell's attention. A T cell whose receptor fits this antigen-MHC complex binds to it and stimulates the macrophage to secrete interleukin-1. Interleukin-1 in turn activates other T cells and starts a series of biochemical processes that may result in certain subsets of T cells becoming cytotoxic, or killer, cells. The T killer cells track down viral-infected body cells. When the infection has been eradicated, suppressor T cells shut down the immune response.

cephalosporin A group of antibiotics called cephalosporin C, derived from the fungus *Cephalosporium,* which are used to treat a wide range of infections that may be resistant to the penicillins. Cephalosporins kill bacteria by interfering with the development of the bacterial cell wall and production of proteins by the organism. Older, or first-

generation, cephalosporins are sometimes ineffective against some bacteria that produce a defensive enzyme, beta-lactamase, which inactivates the antibiotic before it can kill the bacteria. The newer second- and third-generation drugs in this group are more effective against these infections, including sinusitis and bronchitis. Trade names include Keflex, Duricef, Velosef, Ceclor, Ceftin, and Suprax. Many other cephalosporins are available in injectable forms for serious infections.

cerebral anoxia A condition in which there is a severe lack of oxygen supply to the brain usually caused by cardiopulmonary arrest. Irreversible brain damage may result within a few minutes if the anoxia remains untreated.

See also CARDIOPULMONARY RESUSCITATION.

chalcosis Poisoning caused by copper deposits in the lungs and tissues.

chalicosis A form of pneumoconiosis, or silicosis, a respiratory tract disorder associated with the inhalation of dust from stonecutting.

See also PNEUMOCONIOSIS.

Charcot-Leyden crystals Six-sided, double-pointed crystals (solid formations made by salts, water, and other substances of the body) found on microscopic examination of sputum from asthma and bronchitis patients. The crystals are also found in the feces of patients with certain inflammatory conditions of the bowels, including ambiasis. Named for French neurologist Jean M. Charcot (1825–93) and German physician Ernst V. von Leyden (1832–1910), these colorless and sometimes needlelike protein crystals are produced by eosinophil cells.

chemical warfare Another term for biological warfare referring to the tactics of combatants that include the release of toxic chemicals. The substances—gases, defoliants, herbicides, etc.—are capable of producing lung, nerve, skin, and eye irritation, blindness, paralysis, hallucinations, and deafness.

See also BIOTERRORISM.

chest (thorax) The area between the frontal base of the neck and the diaphragm, named from the Greek word *thorax,* which means chest. The anterior surface of the chest is located above and over the clavicles, or collarbones, over and above the sternum, or breastbone, over the breast, or mammary, area, between the third and sixth ribs on either side, and the area above the lower border of the 12th rib on either side. The posterior (rear) surface includes the entire area of the scapulae, or shoulder blades, and the side regions include above the sixth rib and under the arms.

In patients with advanced pulmonary emphysema, the chest becomes rounded out like a barrel and is called a barrel-shaped thorax. The bony thorax refers to the skeletal structure including the thoracic vertebrae, 12 pairs of ribs and the breastbone. In individuals with large pleural effusions, the chest becomes an obliquely oval shape and is known as Peyrot's thorax. The long, flat chest of patients with constitutional visceroptosis (a dropped or downward displacement of one of the organs enveloped in a body cavity such as the thorax) is known as thorax paralyticus. The chest houses the lungs, heart, pleural cavity, pulmonary artery and veins, the thoracic aorta, vena cava, thymus gland, lymph nodes, trachea, bronchi, mediastinum, thoracic duct, and esophagus.

chest expansion, normal The upward movement of the chest as air is taken into the lungs.

Cheyne-Stokes respiration See BREATHING.

chill Shivers, coldness, pallor, body tremors, and chattering of teeth associated with infections or diseases, including pneumococcal pneumonia and malaria. Chills may be caused by a disturbance in the temperature-regulating center of the hypothalamus, the part of the brain that controls certain metabolic activities, such as water balance, sugar and fat metabolism, and inhibiting and releasing hormones.

chin-lift airway technique See CARDIOPULMONARY RESUSCITATION.

chiropractic A widely acclaimed discipline eschewing drugs and surgery and favoring hands-on manipulations, referred to as adjustments, of the spinal cord. Modern chiropractic follows tenets expressed in 1895 by Daniel David Palmer, of Iowa, based on the teachings of Hippocrates, who believed all illnesses had their sources in the spine. According to chiropractic, when vertebrae are subluxated, or dislocated or misaligned, the person experiences any number of ailments, including allergy, headaches, and back pain. Although there is a great deal of anecdotal testimony to their effectiveness, chiropractic techniques and theories have not been scientifically proven. Since symptoms of allergy and asthma often wax and wane, improvement following spinal manipulation may be falsely attributed to chiropractic. Because emotional stress triggers asthma (although it is not its cause), a placebo effect may result from chiropractic treatments. However, chiropractic as a system of health care thrives on the premise that the relationship between the spinal column and the nervous system is significant, and that normal transmission and expression of nerve energy are key elements in the healing and maintenance of the body. The main approach is that vertebral subluxation causes stress, which when removed will lead to the body's capacity of setting intrinsic healing mechanisms in motion. The American Chiropractic Association is the major organization for chiropractic physicians.

Chlamydia psittaci A microorganism that causes a disease in birds and lower mammals that may be transmissible to humans. In an accidental human host, the illness takes on an influenza-like form or may be a severe type of pneumonia.

See also PSITTACOSIS.

chloral hydrate poisoning An adverse effect of excessive amounts of chloral hydrate, a sedative and hypnotic drug, that causes respiratory depression that may require assisted respiration.

chloroformism The potentially lethal inhalation of chloroform, an antiseptic and local anesthetic, as recreational drug abuse. A clear liquid with an etherlike odor, chloroform was used in the early days of medicine as anesthesia by having the patient inhale it, usually by placing a piece of cloth or gauze soaked in the chemical over the person's nose and mouth, a practice that is now obsolete. Developed in 1838, chloroform was chemically referred to as $CHCl_3$ and was also used as a solvent and a veterinary antiseptic. Chloroform as a singular substance is not readily available today. Other substances, including nail polish remover, rubber cement, nitrite room deodorizers, gasoline, and paint thinner, are among the numerous abused inhalants in popular use today, particularly by teenagers.

See also HUFFING; INHALANT ABUSE.

choana   From the Greek word meaning funnel, a funnel-shaped opening at the back of the nostrils (posterior nares) leading to the pharynx.

choke, choking   The condition of impaired breathing and circulation of air to the brain attributable to a compression or obstruction in the trachea or larynx. A spasm in the larynx as a result of inhaling an irritating gas or anything that constricts the neck may also cause interference in the airway. If a person is choking on food or an object, the Heimlich maneuver may relieve complete airway obstruction. Signs of true choking include panic, inability to speak or make noise, cyanosis, and fainting. If the forced air pressure of the Heimlich maneuver does not work, a surgical intervention may be necessary to restore breathing.

See also HEIMLICH MANEUVER.

cholesterohydrothorax   A pleural effusion in which the fluid contains cholesterol.

See also CAVITY, PLEURAL.

cholohemothorax   Abnormal presence of bile and blood in the thoracic cavity.

chorditis   Inflammation of the vocal cord (also called the spermatic cord). Chorditis nordosa refers to tiny white nodules that form on one or both vocal cords and accompanying hoarseness. Usually this is a condition in singers or others who overuse

their voice. Resting the voice is the treatment of choice, but surgery to remove the nodules may be necessary in severe cases.

chronic obstructive pulmonary disease   Known commonly by its acronym COPD, or COLD (chronic obstructive lung disease), a condition in which there is persistent blockage of airflow into or out of the lungs because of chronic bronchitis or emphysema or both, or chronic asthma or chronic bronchiolitis. In all forms of COPD, air gets trapped in the lungs, which then leads to a decrease in the number of capillaries in alveoli walls and the impairment of the exchange of oxygen and carbon dioxide between the alveoli and the bloodstream. Eventually carbon dioxide becomes elevated, and the oxygen level is dramatically reduced. A history of persistent dyspnea (difficulty breathing) on exertion, with or without a chronic cough, and less than one-half the normal breathing capacity are the main diagnostic criteria for COPD.

In the United States, approximately 14 million people suffer from COPD, according to the *Merck Manual of Medical Information, September 2000,* and it is "secondary only to heart disease as a cause of disability that makes people stop working, and the fourth most common cause of death. More than 95 percent of all deaths from chronic obstructive pulmonary disease occur in people over age 55. It affects men more frequently than women and is more often fatal in men. It's also fatal more often in whites than in nonwhites and in blue-collar workers than in white-collar workers." Merck also says COPD may be an inherited tendency, and that smoking or working in an environment where there are chemical fumes or nonhazardous dust may increase the risk of COPD. Also, approximately 10 to 15 percent of smokers develop COPD. As they age, their lung function decreases more rapidly than that of nonsmokers.

Symptoms of COPD include a "smoker's cough," bringing up mucus, common colds that frequently become chest colds (during which sputum may turn yellow or green because of pus), wheezing, and, as the disease progresses, shortness of breath when carrying out normal activities of daily living, possible severe weight loss, and swelling of the legs.

In mild asthma, inflammation that thickens the bronchial walls, constriction of the muscles in the bronchial tubes, or obstruction by excessive mucus is present only during an attack. However, in the case of severe asthma, there is usually a degree of chronic obstruction that is reversible to varying degrees with treatment.

Chronic bronchitis is often confused with emphysema, an expansion of the air spaces resulting in destruction of the alveoli, or air sacs in the lungs. Approximately 20 percent of adult males have chronic bronchitis, although only a small number are disabled because of it. It is less common in females and most common in smokers, but allergies and other irritants, pollution from the environment, and occupational exposure can be causes. Pure emphysema is rare and is not reversible with treatment. The degree of obstruction found in chronic bronchitis is often greater than that found in most asthmatics but less than that in emphysemics.

In rare cases, a deficiency of the protein alpha$_1$-antitrypsin, produced naturally by the body and which prevents neutrophil elastase (an enzyme) from injuring the lung's air sacs, or alveoli, may also be the cause of emphysema. Individuals who inherit the deficiency develop emphysema by early middle age, particularly in smokers. Young people who develop emphysema are tested for the deficiency by way of a blood test.

The main treatment is cessation of smoking, use of bronchodilating drugs, avoiding exposure to airborne irritants, and avoiding dehydration. Antibiotics may be used in the presence of bacterial infection, and oxygen therapy and exercise programs may improve the quality of life for COPD patients. For those with the alpha$_1$-antitrypsin deficiency, intravenous infusions of the protein may be required. Lung transplantation may also be an option in certain patients. People with COPD have an increased risk of developing lung cancer.

See also BRONCHITIS; BRONCHODILATORS; CANCER, LUNG; EMPHYSEMA.

Churg-Strauss syndrome (allergic angiitis and granulomatosis)

A combination of symptoms first reported in 1951 in association with a cluster of 13 cases of severe asthma. Patients have fever, extremely elevated eosinophil counts in their blood, and vasculitis. In addition, they generally have a long history of allergies, usually allergic rhinitis (hay fever) that progresses to asthma. A vasculitis, an inflammatory condition of blood vessels, evolves that may affect almost any organ but most often targets the heart, lungs, skin, central nervous system, muscles and bones, kidneys, or gastrointestinal tract. The person may develop nasal polyps, which cause obstruction of the nasal passages and sinusitis. The most serious complications result from vasculitis.

About one-third of patients have abnormal chest X rays that resemble those seen in cases of pneumonia. If the skin is involved, rashes, hives, bumplike lesions called nodules, or large areas of bruising may occur. Abdominal obstructions and perforations cause pain and diarrhea. Myocardial infarctions (heart attacks) or inflammation of the heart muscle can result in heart failure. Brain and nerve involvement often leads to strokes and is a major cause of serious disability or death. Kidney impairment leads to hypertension (high blood pressure). Symptoms of arthritis and muscle cramping may be present. Churg-Strauss syndrome may begin with a feeling of malaise but may progress quickly with severe weight loss.

The American College of Rheumatology lists six criteria for diagnosing this condition:

(1) asthma; (2) eosinophil count increasing to 10% of white blood cells; (3) a mononeuropathy or polyneuropathy (singular or multiple degeneration of nerves resulting in weakness); (4) pneumonialike fluid accumulation seen in chest X rays; (5) abnormality of the sinuses; and (6) characteristic blood vessel biopsy. The presence of four or more of these criteria highly suggests Churg-Strauss.

Cortisone is the treatment of choice, but other immunosuppressive drugs are sometimes used. Five-year survival was greater than 60 percent in 1977, the last year data are available.

chylopneumothorax The condition of chyle and air in the pleural space. Chyle is a milky alkaline fluid, found in the intestine, consisting of absorbed fats and the products of the digestive process. Chylothorax refers to chyle present in the pleural cavities.

chylothorax   See CHYLOPNEUMOTHORAX.

cigarette smoke   Fumes from a burning cigarette, which are not in themselves allergenic, although tobacco smoke is an irritant to persons with asthma and nasal or eye allergy. In the past some practitioners have skin-tested and given immunotherapy (allergy shots) to patients believed to be allergic to tobacco smoke, but there is no scientific rationale for this treatment.

See also LUNG CANCER; PASSIVE SMOKING; TOBACCO.

circulation, pulmonary   Blood from the veins entering the right atrium of the heart that then passes through the tricuspid valve and into the heart's right ventricle to the pulmonary artery. Each of the artery's two branches then goes into a lung and its capillaries, where, by way of hemoglobin in the red corpuscles, the venous blood takes up oxygen from inspired air. The red arterial blood then goes back to the heart through the four pulmonary veins, two from each lung going into the heart's left atrium. When the blood enters the atrium, it is fully oxygenated.

Citelli's syndrome   Named for Salvatore Citelli, an Italian laryngologist (1875–1947), a condition characterized by insomnia or drowsiness seen accompanying infected adenoids or sphenoid sinusitis in children.

clapping   Also called cupping or tapping, percussion of the chest using a cupped hand as a method of loosening secretions in patients with respiratory disorders such as tuberculosis involving excessive mucus and congestion.

Clara cells   Named for Max Clara, the Austrian anatomist born in 1899 who identified them, the cells in the epithelium of the bronchioles that provide secretions for the respiratory tract.

clean room   A room or environment in which the air—its temperature, pressure, humidity, and purity—is controlled. A filter may be used to remove 99.97 percent of all particles 0.3 microns (1 micron = 1/25,000 inch) and larger. Clean rooms are used in research and for individuals suffering from severe allergy or chronic infection due to immune system deficiency.

cleft palate   A congenital anomaly in which there is a fissure, or elongated opening, in the roof of the mouth (palate) that creates a passageway between the mouth and the internal portions of the nose.

clubbing   Enlargement of the tips of the fingers or toes and loss of the normal angle at the nail bed, frequently caused by lung or other diseases or a hereditary factor.

coal worker's pneumoconiosis   Commonly known as black lung, a lung disease caused by the inhalation and accumulation of coal dust in the lungs. After the coal dust collects around the bronchioles, it spreads to other parts of the lung and eventually causes spots that may be detected on a chest X ray. A more serious form of the disease may occur in 1 to 2 percent of individuals who have simple black lung. Even long after exposure to coal dust has ended, lung tissue and blood vessels may suffer the effects of progressive massive fibrosis, or severe scarring. The scars measure at least a half-inch in diameter, and the fibrosis then causes coughing and debilitating shortness of breath, especially in coal miners who have been exposed to coal dust for more than 10 years.

There is no cure for black lung, but drugs that help keep airways patent and free of secretions may be of help. Prevention is the key: adequate suppression of coal dust at the worksite; chest X ray every four to five years; transfer of workers at risk for progressive massive fibrosis to an area where coal dust levels are minimal; cessation of cigarette smoking; and avoidance of toxic exposure to industrial pollutants.

cocaine hydrochloride poisoning, acute The toxic effect of applying or inhaling cocaine hydrochloride, a topical anesthetic derived from the shrub *Erythroxylon coca* of Bolivia and Peru. Street names for the drug include crack, snow, gold dust, toot, coke, and lady. Symptoms after an initial stimulating effect are irregular respirations, tachycardia, hallucinations, vomiting, muscle spasms, chills or fever, restlessness, incoherence, dilation of pupils, seizures, coma, and death from respiratory arrest. Treatment includes intravenous diazepam (Valium), an emetic (or gastric lavage if the drug was ingested), succinylcholine chloride if convulsions interfere with breathing, oxygen, and artificial respiration. If a victim survives for three hours after the onset of symptoms, he or she is likely to recover.

coccidioidomycosis Also known as granuloma, valley fever, desert rheumatism, and coccidioidal, a disease affecting the respiratory organs in its acute (primary) form, caused by the fungus *Coccidioides immitis*. The progressive form of the disease may involve any part of the body and is considered grave and often fatal. The primary type does not require treatment. For patients with pulmonary disease, ketoconazole may be prescribed to inhibit the infection and suppress symptoms. However, amphotericin B is the only drug that is effective against the progressive form.
See also GRANULOMATOSIS, WEGENER'S.

codeine poisoning An overdose of codeine, an alkaloid obtained from opium, that causes serious and potentially fatal depression of respiration and heart rate.

cogwheel respiration See BREATHING.

coin test A diagnostic test for pneumothorax, or collapsed lung. A coin is placed on the chest over a suspected area of the lung and struck by another coin. If a metallic ringing sound is heard, a cavity containing air is underneath. Physicians now order X rays to confirm the diagnosis.

COLD The acronym for chronic obstructive lung disease.

See also CHRONIC OBSTRUCTIVE PULMONARY DISEASE.

cold, common A respiratory infection caused by a virus including sneezing, nasal discharge and congestion, sore throat, and coughing, all of which are often confused with or coexist with allergy symptoms. Viral colds can also trigger asthma; shortness of breath and wheezing may persist for a prolonged period following resolution of the viral infection. Some patients have asthma symptoms only when they "catch" a cold.

cold-induced rhinorrhea A runny nose that occurs upon exposure to cold air. It is not an allergy and does not respond to antihistamines, but it may be prevented by using a mixture of atropine sulfate and saline solution as a nasal spray.

columna nasi Another term for the nasal septum.
See also NOSE.

coma From the Greek *koma*, meaning deep sleep, an abnormal stupor from which the victim cannot be aroused. Occurring as a result of illness, acute infection or bacterial intoxication, inhalation of gases or fumes, or injury, coma may require basic life support as treatment. A patient's airway must be kept patent, and all vital signs and bodily functions must be monitored. Adequate ventilation and oxygenation are also among the top priorities for a patient in a coma. There are several types of coma, including diabetic, hepatic, uremic, vigil, apoplectic, alcoholic, hypoglycemic, Kussmaul's, and irreversible (brain death).

communicable disease Any infection or malady that is transmissible from one body to another.

concha, nasal Part of the anatomical structure of the nose, one of three bones shaped like scrolls, hence the name from the Greek word meaning shell, that project from the lateral wall of the nasal cavity. The superior, middle, and inferior conchae all protrude over an opening, or meatus.

congestion, pulmonary   An abnormal amount of blood in the pulmonary vascular bed, usually associated with heart failure.

coniofibrosis   Pneumoconiosis caused by the inhalation of asbestos, silica, or other dust, which produces fibrosis in the lung.

coniosis   Any illness, ailment, or anomaly caused by the inhalation of dust.

coniosporosis   Asthma and pneumonitis caused by inhaling the spores of the fungus *Cryptostroma corticale* or *Coniosporium corticale*. Essentially a hypersensitivity reaction, coniosporosis occurs in workers who strip the bark of trees under which the fungi grow.

cor pulmonale   A dysfunction of the heart's right ventricle caused by lung disease or disorders of the pulmonary vessels or chest wall. Long periods of time spent at high altitudes may also result in cor pulmonale.

corticosteroid metered-dose inhalers   Various asthma inhalers containing cortisone derivatives possessing anti-inflammatory properties useful in the prevention of asthma symptoms.

See also CORTICOSTEROIDS.

corticosteroid nasal sprays (beclomethasone, budesonide, dexamethasone, flunisolide, fluticasone, mometasone furoate, triamcinolone)   Derivatives of the hormone cortisone that relieve symptoms of nasal congestion and excessive discharge from allergic rhinitis (hay fever). They may also give relief for vasomotor rhinitis (nonallergic nasal congestion) and may have a beneficial effect on small nasal polyps.

Also called "steroid" nasal sprays, these medications may take one to two weeks to become effective and may be prematurely discarded by uninformed patients as ineffective. These are considered maintenance medications, and since their effectiveness does not accumulate, they must be used continuously. Because only a minimal quantity of the active drug is absorbed from the nasal passages into the bloodstream, there is little chance for side effects. Use in children, however, must be closely monitored.

See also CORTICOSTEROIDS.

corticosteroids   Naturally occurring (or synthetically manufactured) hormones produced by the adrenal glands, located next to the kidneys. Although corticosteroids do not initiate cellular or enzymatic activity, they are essential for many functions necessary for life, including the regulation of carbohydrate, protein, and fat metabolism, and salt and water balance.

Natural and synthetic corticosteroids play a vital role in fighting allergic and inflammatory reactions. Although these drugs can be lifesaving, they also may produce very deleterious effects with large doses or prolonged therapy. Corticosteroids differ from dangerous anabolic steroids, which are often used illegally by athletes to enhance bodybuilding.

Antiallergy Effects

The cortisone-like drugs have the ability to interfere with allergic antigen-antibody reactions. This most likely occurs by blocking the inflammatory tissue injury that results from the release of chemical mediators from mast and basophilic cells. Prostaglandin production is also suppressed by these drugs. In addition, these drugs suppress all types of delayed hypersensitivity or cell-mediated immune reactions. This is especially useful for preventing tissue transplant rejections from occurring.

Metabolic Effects

Hydrocortisone removes glycogen stores in the liver and raises blood sugar levels. In corticosteroid-treated patients, diabetes mellitus usually develops only in those with a latent diabetic tendency and rarely raises glucose to dangerous levels in normal patients.

Hydrocortisone in physiologic or normal quantities is essential for normal muscle contraction. However, large doses or prolonged therapy causes a negative nitrogen balance by increasing amino acid production from protein, with depletion of body protein. This in turn causes severe muscle wasting, or atrophy, and weakness. A similar effect on bone results in osteoporosis with decreased bone matrix and removal of bone calcium. This process also interferes with normal growth in children. Aseptic necrosis is another serious adverse effect of high-dose corticosteroid therapy. Hydrocortisone in high doses also causes a redistribution of the body's fat stores with thinning of the extremities and increased disposition in the face and trunk. Thinning of subcutaneous tissue may occur

Estimated Comparative Daily Dosages for Inhaled Corticosteroids

ADULTS

Drug	Low Dose	Medium Dose	High Dose
Beclomethasone dipropionate 42 mcg/puff 84 mcg/puff	168-504 mcg (4-12 puffs – 42 mcg) (2-6 puffs – 84 mcg)	504-840 mcg (12-20 puffs – 42 mcg) (6-10 puffs – 84 mcg)	>840 mcg (>20 puffs – 42 mcg) (>10 puffs – 84 mcg)
Budesonide Turbuhaler 200 mcg/dose	200-400 mcg (1-2 inhalations)	400-600 mcg (2-3 inhalations)	>600 mcg (>3 inhalations)
Flunisolide 250 mcg/puff	500-1,000 mcg (2-4 puffs)	1,000-2,000 mcg (4-8 puffs)	>2,000 mcg (>8 puffs)
Fluticasone MDI: 44, 110, 220 mcg/puff	88-264 mcg (2-6 puffs – 44 mcg) OR (2 puffs – 110 mcg)	264-660 mcg (2-6 puffs – 110 mcg)	>660 mcg (>6 puffs – 110 mcg) OR (>3 puffs – 220 mcg)
DPI: 50, 100, 250 mcg/dose	(2-6 inhalations – 50 mcg)	(3-6 inhalations – 100 mcg)	(>6 inhalations – 100 mcg) OR (>2 inhalations – 250 mcg)
Triamcinolone acetonide 100 mcg/puff	400-1,000 mcg (4-10 puffs)	1,000-2,000 mcg (10-20 puffs)	>2,000 mcg (>20 puffs)

CHILDREN

Drug	Low Dose	Medium Dose	High Dose
Beclomethasone dipropionate 42 mcg/puff 84mcg/puff	84-336 mcg (2-8 puffs – 42 mcg) (1-4 puffs – 84 mcg)	336-672 mcg (8-16 puffs – 42 mcg) (4-8 puffs – 84 mcg)	>672 mcg (>16 puffs – 42 mcg) (>8 puffs – 84 mcg)
Budesonide Turbuhaler 200 mcg/dose	100-200 mcg	200-400 mcg (1-2 inhalations – 200 mcg)	>400 mcg (>2 inhalations – 200 mcg)
Flunisolide 250 mcg/puff	500-750 mcg (2-3 puffs)	1,000-1,250 mcg (4-5 puffs)	>1,250 mcg (>5 puffs)
Fluticasone MDI: 44, 110, 220 mcg/puff	88-176 mcg (2-4 puffs – 44 mcg)	176-440 mcg (4-10 puffs – 44 mcg) OR (2-4 puffs – 110 mcg)	>440 mcg (>4 puffs – 110 mcg) OR (>2 puffs – 220 mcg)
DPI: 50, 100, 250 mcg/dose	(2-4 inhalations – 50 mcg)	(2-4 inhalations – 100 mcg)	(>4 inhalations – 100 mcg) OR (>2 inhalations – 250 mcg)
Triamcinolone acetonide 100 mcg/puff	400-800 mcg (4-8 puffs)	800-1,200 mcg (8-12 puffs)	>1,200 mcg (>12 puffs)

NOTES:

■ **The most important determinant of appropriate dosing is the clinician's judgment of the patient's response to therapy.** The clinician must monitor the patient's response on several clinical parameters and adjust the dose accordingly. The stepwise approach to therapy emphasizes that once control of asthma is achieved, the dose of medication should be carefully titrated to the minimum dose required to maintain control, thus reducing the potential for adverse effect.

■ See figure 3-5c for an explanation of the rationale used for the comparative dosages. The reference point for the range in the dosages for children is data on the safety of inhaled corticosteroids in children, which, in general, suggest that the dose ranges are equivalent to beclomethasone dipropionate 200-400 mcg/day (low dose), 400-800 mcg/day (medium dose), and >800 mcg/day (high dose).

■ Some dosages may be outside package labeling.

■ Metered-dose inhaler (MDI) dosages are expressed as the actuator dose (the amount of drug leaving the actuater and delivered to the patient), which is the labeling required in the United States. This is different from the dosage expressed as the valve dose (the amount of drug leaving the valve, all of which is not available to the patient), which is used in many European countries and in some of the scientific literature. Dry powder inhaler (DPI) doses (e.g., Turbuhaler) are expressed as the amount of drug in the inhaler following activation.

Estimated Clinical Comparability of Doses for Inhaled Corticosteroids

Data from in vitro and clinical trials suggest that the different inhaled corticosteroid preparations are not equivalent on a per puff or microgram basis. However, it is not entirely clear what implications these differences have for dosing recommendations in clinical practice because there are few data directly comparing the preparations. Relative dosing for clinical comparability is affected by differences in topical potency, clinical effects at different doses, delivery device, and bioavailability. *The Expert Panel developed recommended dose ranges (see figure 3-5b) for different preparations based on available data and the following assumptions and cautions about estimating relative doses needed to achieve comparable clinical effect.*

■ **Relative topical potency using human skin blanching**
The standard test for determining relative topical anti-inflammatory potency is the topical vasoconstriction (MacKenzie skin blanching) test.
The MacKenzie topical skin blanching test correlates with binding affinities and binding half-lives for human lung corticosteroid receptors (see table below) (Dahlberg et al. 1984; Högger and Rohdewald 1994).
The relationship between relative topical anti-inflammatory effect and clinical comparability in asthma management is not certain. However, recent clinical trials suggest that different in vitro measures of anti-inflammatory effect correlate with clinical efficacy (Barnes and Pedersen 1993; Johnson 1996; Kamada et al. 1996; Ebden et al. 1986; Leblanc et al. 1994; Gustafsson et al. 1993; Lundback et al. 1993; Barnes et al. 1993; Fabbri et al. 1993; Langdon and Capsey 1994; Ayres et al. 1995; Rafferty et al. 1985; Bjorkander et al. 1982; Stiksa et al. 1982; Willey et al. 1982).

Medication	Topical Potency (Skin Blanching)*	Corticosteroid Receptor Binding Half-Life	Receptor Binding Affinity
Beclomethasone dipropionate (BDP)	600	7.5 hours	13.5
Budesonide (BUD)	980	5.1 hours	9.4
Flunisolide (FLU)	330	3.5 hours	1.8
Fluticasone propionate (FP)	1,200	10.5 hours	18.0
Triamcinolone acetonide (TAA)	330	3.9 hours	3.6

* Numbers are assigned in reference to dexamethasone, which has a value of "1" in the MacKenzie test.

■ **Relative doses to achieve similar clinical effects**
Clinical effects are evaluated by a number of outcome parameters (e.g., changes in spirometry, peak flow rates, symptom scores, quick-relief beta$_2$-agonist use, frequency of exacerbations, airway responsiveness).
The daily dose and duration of treatment may affect these outcome parameters differently (e.g., symptoms and peak flow may improve at lower doses and over a shorter treatment time than bronchial reactivity) (van Essen-Zandvliet et al. 1992; Haahtela et al. 1991)
Delivery systems influence comparability. For example, the delivery device for budesonide (Turbuhaler) delivers approximately twice the amount of drug to the airway as the MDI, thus enhancing the clinical effect (Thorsson et al. 1994; Agertoft and Pedersen 1993).
Individual patients may respond differently to different preparations, as noted by clinical experience.

Clinical trials comparing effects in reducing symptoms and improving peak expiratory flow demonstrate:
BDP and BUD achieved comparable effects at similar microgram doses by MDI (Bjorkander et al. 1982; Ebden et al. 1986; Rafferty et al. 1985).
BDP achieved effects similar to twice the dose of TAA on a microgram basis.
FP achieved effects similar to twice the dose of BDP and BUD via an MDI on a microgram basis (Gustaffson et al. 1993; Fabbri et al. 1993; Barnes et al. 1993; Dahl et al. 1993; Ayres et al. 1995).
BUD by Turbuhaler achieved effects similar to twice the dose delivered by MDI, thus implying greater bronchial delivery by the delivery device (Thorsson et al. 1994; Agertoft and Pedersen 1993).

■ **Bioavailability**
Both the relative potency and the relative bioavailability (systemic availability) determine the potential for systemic activity of an inhaled corticosteroid preparation. As illustrated here, the bioavailability of an inhaled corticosteroid is dependent on the absorption of the dose delivered to the lungs and the oral bioavailability of the swallowed portion of the dose received. As illustrated here, the bioavailability of an inhaled corticosteroid is dependent on absorption of the dose to the lungs and the oral bioavailability of the swallowed portion of the dose received.

Absorption of the dose delivered to the lungs:
Approximately 10 to 30 percent of the dose from the MDI is delivered to the lungs. This amount varies among preparations and delivery devices.
Nearly all of the amount delivered to the lungs is bioavailable.
Oral bioavailability of the swallowed portion of the dose received:
Approximately 80 percent of the dose from the MDI without a spacer/holding chamber is swallowed.
The oral bioavailability of this amount varies:
Either a high first-pass liver metabolism or the use of a spacer/holding chamber with an MDI can decrease oral bioavailability, thus enhancing safety (Lipworth 1995).
The approximate oral bioavailability of inhaled corticosteroids has been reported as: BDP 20%; FLU 21%; TAA 10.6%; BUD 11%; FP 1% (Chaplin et al. 1980; Check and Kaliner 1990; Clissold and Heel 1984; Davies 1993; Harding 1990; Heald et al. 1995; Martin et al. 1974; Mollman et al. 1985; Szefler 1991; Wurthwein and Rohdewald 1990).

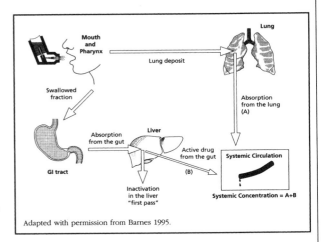

Adapted with permission from Barnes 1995.

Although few clinical trials are available that compare systemic activity among preparations (Kamada et al. 1996), studies have found:
As suggested by one cross-over comparison study, BDP, FLU, and TAA appear to have equivalent dose-dependent systemic activity, as measured by 24-hour urinary free cortisol excretion (McCubbin et al. 1995).
Inconsistent results comparing BDP and BUD. Some show equivalent systemic activity (Kamada et al. 1996; Prahl 1991; Prahl et al. 1987); others show BUD having slightly less systemic activity than BDP (Barnes and Pedersen 1993; Pedersen and Fuglsang 1988; Bisgaard et al. 1988).
FP had greater adrenal suppression at doses of 400 to 2,000 micrograms than BUD in equivalent microgram doses delivered by MDI and accompanied by mouth washing to prevent oral bioavailability (Clark et al. 1996). This confirms that there are differences in microgram potencies among preparations and that absorption through the lung can result in systemic activity.

with resulting red or purple striae and ecchymosis, or bruises. Sodium and water retention also occurs, but potassium is lost. Blood pressure elevation may occur with high-dose therapy.

Hormonal Changes

When used for a prolonged time, corticosteroids may suppress the production of the pituitary hormone corticotropin (ACTH). ACTH secretion stimulates the adrenal glands for the natural production of cortisone. If the adrenal glands atrophy, they may fail to respond adequately to a crisis such as an acute illness, like an asthma attack or the stress of surgery, and if an extra dose of the drug is not administered, the patient may die. Some women develop hirsutism (excessive hair production), and acne is more common as a result of breakdown products of androgens, or male hormones, from prolonged use of corticosteroids, but rarely do these drugs affect menstrual function.

Anti-inflammatory Effects

One of the beneficial roles of anti-inflammatory drugs is to assuage reactions in asthma and arthritis; this same ability to suppress inflammation may have a deleterious effect on wounds by interfering with the healing process. The ability to suppress inflammation may be so great that the warning signs and symptoms of a major complication may be missed until there are serious consequences, such as a bleeding peptic ulcer or a severe infection. There may be an increased incidence of gastric or duodenal ulcers in corticosteroid-treated patients.

Central Nervous System and Behavioral Changes

Hydrocortisone stimulates the central nervous system and may cause seizures, especially in children with a seizure disorder. High-dose therapy may induce psychotic behavior, including hallucinations and delusions. Depression or alternately euphoria, insomnia, and agitation may result. Effects cannot be predicted by prior personality qualities.

Rarely, increased intracranial pressure develops, resulting in a condition called "pseudotumor cerebri."

Effects on the Eyes

Topical corticosteroid eyedrops are frequently prescribed to treat allergic eye conditions, but they can cause a dangerous increase in intraocular pressure and other serious adverse effects that may lead to blindness. They should be prescribed only after evaluation by a physician well trained in their use.

Uses

Corticosteroids are mainstays for allergy and asthma treatment and are often lifesaving. In addition, they are effective therapy for arthritis, eye diseases, skin diseases, and many other diseases. Corticosteroids are available by injection, orally, and topically as creams, gels, ointments, lotions, solutions, aerosolized metered-dose inhalers, skin sprays, and nasal sprays.

The potential for adverse effects is great with prolonged systematic use. Use of alternate-day dosing can greatly lessen this potential, but not completely. When allergy patients have been stabilized, they are usually candidates for aerosol corticosteroid therapy to prevent attacks by keeping inflammation under control. Corticosteroid nasal sprays play a similar preventive role for nasal allergies.

Contraindications to the Use of Corticosteroids

In early 1992, the Food and Drug Administration (FDA) warned about the use of corticosteroids in patients not immune to chicken pox (varicella) or other reduced-immunity illnesses. Several deaths have occurred in otherwise normal, asthmatic children who contracted chicken pox while being treated with corticosteroids. These drugs should be used only if no alternative exists.

Corticosteroids absolutely must be avoided in the presence of herpes simplex infection of the eyes. They must be used cautiously in patients with coexisting diseases, including diabetes mellitus, hypertension, peptic ulcer disease, osteoporosis, diverticulitis, psychotic conditions, renal insufficiency, and congestive heart failure (except in certain inflammatory conditions such as rheumatic heart disease), and following some recent surgical intestinal procedures. Some references recommend against the use of corticosteroids during pregnancy; however, the use of prednisone should not be withheld in patients with asthma and other serious diseases.

Use of these drugs in patients with tuberculosis was once considered an absolute contraindication. However, in life-threatening situations they can be used in combination with antituberculosis drugs.

WARNING: The risk of using corticosteroids must always be weighed against the risk of not using them.

coryza spasmodica See HAY FEVER.

CO$_2$ therapy See CARBON DIOXIDE INHALATION.

cough A reaction, or reflex, of the upper respiratory tract to correct an irritation or blockage of the airways. Dust or other particles, fumes, smoke, gases, and viral and bacterial infections cause the sudden, expulsive rumble characterizing a cough. Some coughs, such as whooping cough, create high-pitched sounds, whereas the inflammation of the upper respiratory tract, especially when children have croup, creates a narrowing of the airways and a barking cough.

When an object becomes lodged in the larynx, or voice box, the cough mechanism is triggered to help expel the object and stop a person from choking. Coughing is also the body's way of expelling mucus, phlegm, or other irritant, in which case it is called a productive cough. A dry, or unproductive, cough, which does not result in expulsion of a substance, may be caused by bronchospasm (a sudden narrowing of the bronchi), featured in asthma, allergic reactions, or infection.

Causes of chronic coughing include smoking and/or lung disease, a foreign object trapped in a bronchus, and anxiety or nervousness. Other causes of cough include upper airway obstruction or irritation; infections; irritation or structural abnormalities; or other disorders of the epiglottis and larynx such as vocal cord paralysis, polyp, or tumor; tracheomalacia; external compression by lymph nodes, tumor, or vascular ring; intraluminal obstruction by foreign body, mucus plugs, inflammation or tumor; bronchospasm of asthma, chronic bronchitis, or emphysema; cysts; congenital malfor-

mation; inflammation from allergic diseases such as hypersensitivity pneumonitis; interstitial lung diseases; congenital heart disease; congestive heart failure; gastroesophageal reflux; hiatus hernia; edema; hysteria; paralysis; adverse effects of drugs such as the ACE inhibitor antihypertensives (benazepril, captopril, enalapril, fosinopril, lisinopril, quinapril, and ramipril) or drug toxicity; smoke from tobacco or fires; noxious fumes or gases; organic dusts containing allergens such as dust mites, animal allergens, industrial allergens, scents in perfumes and household or commercial cleaning agents; aerosol products; cold; humidity; and dryness.

Types of coughs include 1) aneurysmal, described as brassy and clanging, as in individuals with an aneurysm; 2) asthmatic, i.e., more closely resembling difficulty breathing; 3) brassy, such as the cough in individuals who have pressure on the left recurrent laryngeal nerve; 4) bronchial, such as that which occurs in individuals with bronchiectasis or bronchitis and is accompanied by the production of sputum; 5) diphtherial, i.e., a brassy cough and labored breathing as a result of laryngeal diphtheria; 6) dry, in which there is no accompanying moisture; 7) effective or productive, which refers to the expectoration of exudates; 8) hacking, such as repeated coughing associated with pulmonary tuberculosis; 9) harsh, referring to the metallic-sounding cough heard in patients with laryngitis; 10) moist, or a loose cough that produces mucus or exudates; 11) paroxysmal, i.e., in whooping cough and bronchiectasis patients; 12) pulmonary, i.e., hard, painful coughing such as patients with pneumonia experience; 13) reflex, which refers to a cough that is a result of irritation of Arnold's nerve, the middle ear, pharynx, stomach, or intestine; 14) uterine, i.e., a reflex cough caused by an irritation of the uterus or other female organ; and 15) whooping, also known as pertussis, described as a paroxysmal cough with a whooping sound made upon inspiration.

An antitussive refers to a drug that inhibits or suppresses a cough.

See also COUGH, EAR; WHOOPING COUGH.

cough, ear A reflex cough resulting from an ear infection, irritation, or foreign body lodged against the tympanic membrane (eardrum).

cracked pot sound The sound, similar to that of striking a cracked pot, during percussion to diagnose a pulmonary cavity.

crackles Rales or abnormal lung sounds including coarse crackles, which are longer, louder, and low-pitched, and fine crackles, which are soft, short, and high-pitched.
 See also RALE.

crepitation A crackling sound, such as a rale heard in pneumonia patients, or the grating sound caused when the ends of broken bones rub against another bone or surface.
 See also RALE.

crepitus redux A rale or any abnormal sound heard through a stethoscope placed on the chest, that signals the recovery stage in pneumonia patients.
 See also RALE.

cromolyn sodium (disodium cromoglycate, Intal, Nasalcrom, Opticrom) A drug that prevents the release of histamine and other chemical substances from mast cells in the eye, nose, and lungs, therefore preventing allergy symptoms and asthma. This drug is often discarded by patients who underestimate its benefit because it is very slow-acting and requires up to two months to exert its full effectiveness. However, cromolyn is a first-line treatment for respiratory allergies and asthma. It also has almost no side effects and is safe to use during pregnancy.

crossed finger airway technique A technique for removing debris or foreign material from the mouth of a person about to receive cardiopulmonary resuscitation.
 See also CARDIOPULMONARY RESUSCITATION.

croup A disease characterized by a metallic cough, often described as a "seal-like" bark, with hoarseness that occurs when breathing in. It is accompanied by thick mucus in the nose and throat, dyspnea, laryngeal spasm, and, at times, by the formation of a membrane. Catarrhal croup refers to acute catarrhal laryngitis.
 Croup is most commonly caused by a viral infection during infancy or early childhood, and is generally a benign condition. However, when accompanied by high fever, it may be caused by a dangerous bacteria, *Haemophilus influenzae*. Unless antibiotics are started early, the bacterial form of croup may lead to the life-threatening complication known as acute epiglottis. The less severe forms of croup can be treated by breathing warm, humid air in a steamed-up shower or small bathroom.

crowing A harsh, crow-like sound produced when air is taken into the lungs.

Curschmann's spirals Named for German physician Heinrich Curschmann (1846–1910), coiled spirals of mucus seen frequently in the sputum of asthma patients.

cyanosis Blue coloration of the mucous membranes caused by lack of oxygen supply.
 See also BLUE BABY.

cyclic adenosine 3′, 5′-monophosphate (camp, cyclic AMP) A substance whose presence is essential for stabilization of mast cells in body tissues, which along with basophils are responsible for the symptoms of allergy. It is also deficient in asthmatics. Drugs such as epinephrine and theophylline increase camp-inhibiting mast cell degranulation and are useful for the treatment of asthma.

cyclosporin An immunosuppressant drug used to prevent or suppress organ transplant rejection. Researchers at the National Heart and Lung Institute in the United States and the Royal Brompton Hospital in London are investigating cyclosporin as an alternative to dangerously high levels of corticosteroids required by the most severe asthma patients. Although some individuals in one study group had a significant improvement in lung function and less frequent acute episodes of asthma, cyclosporin can cause serious kidney problems and is still considered experimental therapy.

cyst, alveolar   An air cyst or sac, formed when alveoli (air sacs) in the lungs dilate and rupture.

cystic fibrosis (CF)   Among the most common fatal inherited diseases, an autosomal recessive genetic disorder. CF affects the exocrine secretory glands of the respiratory and digestive systems.

Often called "sixty-five roses" by children afflicted with the disease, CF's excessive production of thick, sticky mucus causes a chronic cough, wheezing, and plugging of the bronchial tubes. Trapped bacteria cause recurrent respiratory infections. Mucus also blocks the pancreatic secretion of digestive enzymes, causing malabsorption of nutrients and foul bulky stools, with failure to gain weight and thrive, a common finding in young children.

This disorder is often confused with asthma, pneumonia, or other respiratory diseases when symptoms first appear, usually in infancy. Mild cases may escape recognition until adulthood. Gastrointestinal symptoms may be confused with celiac disease or other disorders. Diagnosis is confirmed by a positive sweat chloride test.

Since CF was first recognized as a disease in 1938, it has been estimated to occur in one in 2,000 to one in 1,600 live white births in the United States, but only one in 17,000 blacks. About one in every 20 persons carries the CF recessive gene. Genetic counseling is advisable when a previous pregnancy resulted in CF. Prenatal diagnosis and carrier state of parents can be established by DNA genetic markers.

Until recently the prognosis for CF patients was poor, with very few patients surviving childhood. However, newer antibiotics and aggressive physical therapy to help drain the mucus from the airways by a technique called postural drainage, and the use of pancreatic enzymes and nutritional supplements, can greatly improve the outlook. Males generally outlive female patients, with half of patients living past age 21. Respiratory failure is the leading cause of death. The discovery of the CF gene on the long arm of chromosome 7 gives hope for the possibility of a cure for this disease utilizing gene therapy within a few years.

death rattle   A rattling sound, or rale, produced in the throats of patients who are dying. The sound is caused by excess mucus and the absence of the cough reflex.

decompression illness   See BENDS.

decongestant   A class of drug or other agent that acts against nasal or bronchial congestion. Also known as alpha-adrenergic agonists, decongestants may be used topically as nasal spray or drops, and orally in capsules, tablets, or syrups.

decortication, pulmonary   The surgical removal of a segment of surface lung tissue or a pleura. Decortication is used as a treatment, though rarely, for severe pleural effusion when there is difficulty accomplishing the drainage of pus from the area.

degree of asthma severity   The ranges or the levels of asthma from asymptomatic to fatal, with the majority of cases described as mild to moderate.

Chronic Mild Asthma

Persons with chronic mild asthma have no abnormalities in baseline pulmonary lung tests, or spirometry, between asthma attacks. During attacks, airflow rates fall 20 percent below their predicted normal values. Asthma symptoms are usually triggered by exercise; exposure to irritants or allergens such as pollens, animals, or house-dust mites; or respiratory infections. Treatment prior to exposure is usually effective in preventing symptoms. Inhaled beta$_2$-agonists are usually the only therapy necessary to control attacks, and they are used on an as-needed (PRN) basis only.

Chronic Moderate Asthma

In this category, asthma symptoms are not controlled by the occasional use of a beta$_2$-agonist. There may also be a frequent need for beta$_2$-agonists, possibly more than twice a week. Symptoms in this group may be most apparent at night or, as in mild asthma, may be triggered by the environment or exercise. The lungs function at 60 to 80 percent of the predicted range for a person's age, sex, and height, indicating a compromise in airway flow.

The National Asthma Education Program's *Guidelines for the Diagnosis and Management of Asthma* recommends the use of an anti-inflammatory agent in any person with moderate or severe asthma. Anti-inflammatory drugs include inhaled cromolyn sodium or inhaled corticosteroids. These safe and effective medications reduce the frequency and severity of asthma attacks and the need for oral corticosteroids.

Nighttime awakening may necessitate the addition of long-acting bronchodilating drugs such as theophylline or albuterol. Occasional short bursts of oral corticosteroids are needed, but not on a daily or frequent basis. Individuals rarely require urgent emergency room visits.

Chronic Severe Asthma

Individuals whose asthma is not controlled by maximal drug doses and who may be at risk for life-threatening asthma attacks show a pulmonary function less than 60 percent of baseline. Airflow varies widely during attacks. These persons may require long-term use of daily or every-other-day oral corticosteroids.

See also ASTHMA; CORTICOSTEROIDS.

demand valve manually cycled resuscitator   A type of resuscitator (trade names include Robershaw valve and Elder valve) that uses high-low oxygen that is cycled by pushing a button and watching the chest of the patient rise.

depressant, respiratory   A drug that lessens the frequency and depth of breathing.

depression   A neurotic or psychotic disorder characterized by lethargy, loss of interest in socializing, sex, work and other activities of daily living, weeping and/or pervasive sadness, insomnia, inability to concentrate, and other symptoms. When asthma and depression occur simultaneously, both conditions can intensify, according to Nancy J. Rubin, Psy.D., of the University of Alabama School of Medicine in Tuscaloosa. Rubin reported in the American Medical Association's *Archives of Family Medicine* that people with depressive disorders or symptoms tend to have physical, social, and role-functioning difficulties comparable to the difficulties of those who suffer from one or more of the eight major chronic illnesses, including lung disease. One association involves the effect of depression on the respiratory system. A depressed person enters a psychological state of nonaction, associated with decreased energy expenditure, decreased ventilation, low oxygen consumption, and skeletal relaxation. These conditions further complicate asthma, a disorder already characterized by compromised ventilation and borderline blood gas values.

Another theory involves dysfunctional brain mechanisms associated with depression. One group of researchers speculates that neurotransmitter imbalances found in asthma and depression may combine to worsen both conditions. However, the correlation of brain dysfunctions and asthma is not fully understood.

Formal assessment by a mental health professional of the patient with severe asthma is recommended as part of the standard medical assessment.

dexamethasone (Decadron)   An anti-inflammatory derivative of cortisone.

See also CORTICOSTEROIDS.

dexchlorpheniramine (Polaramine)   An antihistaminic drug used in the treatment of allergic disorders. This drug is moderately sedating and has few side effects.

dextromethorphan   Non-narcotic synthetic derivative of levorphanol similar in structure and effectiveness to codeine as a cough suppressant. Dextromethorphan is found combined with antihistamines, decongestants, and expectorants in many prescription and over-the-counter allergy and cold remedies, including Benylin DM, Delsym, Mediquell, Pertussin, and Robitussin DM.

This antitussive (cough-suppressing) drug is the safest available. It rarely causes minor adverse effects, such as mild nausea or dizziness, and is the cough suppressant of choice during pregnancy.

diaphragm   From the Greek word *diaphragma,* or partition, the musculomembranous structure that separates the abdomen from the thoracic cavity. When a breath is taken in, the diaphragm contracts and moves downward to make room for the lungs to expand. Upon exhalation, it rises to its normal inverted-basin shape. Originating at the sixth ribs (anterior intercostals) and the 11th and 12th ribs posteriorly, the diaphragm is the major inspiratory muscle that helps draw air into the lungs, aids in defecation and childbirth by its capacity to increase intra-abdominal pressure during exhalation with the glottis closed, and its spasmodic activity during hiccoughs or sneezing.

diffusion   The action of gaseous, liquid, or solid molecules of a substance to travel from an area of high concentration to an area of lower concentration.

Dilor   See DYPHILLINE.

Dimetane   See BROMPHENIRAMINE.

Dimetapp   See BROMPHENIRAMINE.

diphenhydramine (Benadryl)   An antihistaminic drug used to treat the symptoms of allergic rhinitis (hay fever) and urticaria (hives), including sneezing, runny rose, nasal congestion, itchy eyes and pruritus (itching). It is given by injection as a secondary treatment for severe allergic anaphylactic reactions (epinephrine, or adrenaline, must be used as the primary drug in this severe, shock-like, life-threatening condition), which may occur in persons allergic to bee stings or certain foods.

Diphenhydramine is also useful as a cough suppressant, for the prevention and treatment of motion sickness, and for parkinsonism. It is widely available topically in creams or lotions for the relief of itching. However, many allergists and dermatologists advise against this use because of frequent adverse effects. The principal side effect is sedation, and it is often prescribed as a nonhabituating hypnotic in the treatment of insomnia.

diphtheria A contagious and sometimes life-threatening infection by the bacterium *Corynebacterium diptheriae* spread by moist droplets coughed into the air by an infected person. The microorganism multiplies and causes inflammation in the mucous membranes of the mouth and throat, and certain types of the bacterium produce a toxin that may damage the heart and brain. Because of the effectiveness of the diphtheria-tetanus-pertussis (DTP) vaccine, diphtheria is rare in the United States and other developed countries, with fewer than five cases since 1980. Current instances of the disease have been reported in countries of the former Soviet Union, including Russia. Although anyone may be affected, the disease is mostly seen in children younger than 10.

The Schick test, developed by the Hungarian-born pediatrician Bela Schick (1877–1967), determines the degree of an individual's immunity to diphtheria. The test involves an intradermal injection of 0.1 milliliters of dilute diphtheria toxin, which is one-fiftieth of the minimum lethal dose (MLD) that would kill a small guinea pig within four days. A red, inflamed spot at the site of injection appearing after three or four days indicates a positive test. Little or no reaction to the injection constitutes a negative result and therefore an immunity.

Symptoms include a mild sore throat and pain with swallowing, nausea, vomiting, chills, head-ache, low-grade fever, swollen lymph nodes in the neck, runny nose, laryngitis, difficulty breathing, rapid heart rate, and prostration. In nasal diphtheria, a higher fever is usually present. Also, there may be inflamed adenoids, a blood-tinged discharge from the nose, and bad breath. Named from the Greek *diphthera*, or membrane, the disease is characterized by the false membrane on a mucous surface and at times affecting the skin. The pseudomembrane appears yellowish-white or gray and adheres to the tonsils or pharyngeal walls. If a child develops mild diphtheria, a pseudomembrane may never appear. Also, diphtheria carriers are able to spread the disease but manifest no symptoms themselves.

Treatment involves hospitalization, usually in the intensive care unit (ICU) in order to monitor breathing and heart function, and the intravenous administration of the diphtheria antitoxin, which is made from horse serum. A patient may be allergic to the antitoxin, in which case he or she must be desensitized before receiving the drug. Penicillin, ampicillin, and erythromycin are also used to fight the bacterium. Three consecutive negative cultures after the completion of antibiotic therapy indicate that the bacterium has been eliminated.

When the larynx is severely affected and an airway becomes obstructed, intubation or surgery (tracheotomy) may be necessary. Nerve damage may result if the condition is not treated promptly.

Diphtheria victims may also develop skin lesions, especially where crowded conditions and poor hygiene prevail, myocarditis (inflammation of the heart muscle) and rarely, disturbances of the eye. Recovery from diphtheria may take many weeks.

diphtheria-pertussis-tetanus toxoid vaccine See DIPHTHERIA.

disinfectant Any chemical that kills bacteria, especially vegetative microorganisms. Examples are chlorine, fluorine, iodine, silver nitrate, sulfurous acids, alkalies, formaldehyde, 70 percent alcohol, salts of heavy metals, cresols, phenol (carbolic acid), benzoic and salicylic acids and their sodium salts, thymol, potassium permanganate, boric acid, chloride of lime, and iodoform.

disodium cromoglycate   See CROMOLYN SODIUM.

Dittrich's plugs   Small particles, named for German pathologist Franz Dittrich (1815–59), made of pus, detritus, bacteria, and fat globules in fetid sputum.

diver's paralysis   See BENDS.

doxapram hydrochloride (Dopram)   A drug that stimulates respiration.

drainage, negative pressure   In the treatment of pneumothorax (collapsed lung), the use of a tube promoting negative air pressure (suction) so that excessive or abnormal fluids, blood, pus, or secretions may be drained. A drainage tube is a device that allows those substances to flow out of a wound or abscess.

drainage, postural   The use of gravity to help remove secretions from the nose, bronchi, sinuses, and lungs by placing the patient in a position in which his head is lower than his feet. Tapping or cupping on the patient's back may also aid in the procedure.

drainage tube   A hollow cylindrical device that may be inserted into the body in order to draw pus, blood, serum, or other fluid out of an area of a wound or infection in which fluid has accumulated. When drainage is required in the chest cavity, the tube is attached to a suctioning device. Typically, chest drainage may also involve the suctioning of air from the pleural space while preventing air from being sucked back in. Chest tubes are inserted into the pleural space for this procedure.

Drinker respirator   The apparatus, commonly known as the "iron lung," that presses upon a patient's thoracic area in order to produce alternating positive and negative air, as in the normal breathing process. The device was invented by Philip Drinker, born in 1894, an American engineer in industrial hygiene. The iron lung became widely used for the treatment of poliomyelitis, to which some individuals are predisposed through adverse reaction to routine immunizations and the removal of tonsils, and other nose and throat operations. Bronchopneumonia has been known to develop in rare cases of severe poliomyelitis.

drip, postnasal   A discharge flowing from the postnasal region (behind the nose) to the throat, caused by allergic or vasomotor (nonallergic) rhinitis or chronic sinusitis.

droplet infection   The result of inhaling infected microorganisms, usually spread by an infected person's cough or sneeze into the air. The common cold is typically transmitted by droplets.

drops, nose   Any medication or solution sprayed or dropped into the nostrils and nasal cavity.

drowning   The cessation of breathing and heart function as a result of immersion in water or a spasm in the glottis that stops air or water from getting into the lungs (dry drowning). Near-drowning refers to recovery from severe oxygen deprivation and subsequent lung damage after being underwater for a long time.

An individual who is submerged in cold water may survive because of the "diving reflex" such as that discovered in seagoing mammals. Very cold water slows the heart rate and redirects the blood from the extremities and intestines back to the heart and brain. It also cools the body tissues, which then do not require as much oxygen as warm ones do. Victims of near-drowning may, however, experience impaired breathing and abnormal volume and content of the bloodstream well after the actual crisis. Also, submersion in and inhalation of fresh water may have a damaging effect on the lungs, and salt water draws fluid from the bloodstream into the lungs.

Treatment includes resuscitation techniques if the victim is not breathing and hospitalization to ensure the reoxygenation of the blood and maintenance of vital signs. Antispasmodic medication may be necessary to keep airways patent. Corticosteroids may be given to reduce lung inflammation, and antibiotics may be necessary in the case of infection. Hyperbaric chamber therapy may be required. Even with modalities to prevent brain damage, some victims of near-drowning sustain permanent neurological impairment.

See also CARDIOPULMONARY RESUSCITATION.

duct, thoracic Another term for the left lymphatic duct, or channel, that drains the left side of the body above the diaphragm and the entire body below the diaphragm.

dyphylline (Dilor, Lufyllin) A bronchodilator drug derived from xanthine and related to theophylline, used for the treatment of asthma.

dyspnea Difficulty breathing, also called air hunger, which may be painful and caused by a respiratory disorder or extremely strenuous exercise. Cyanosis, or blue coloration, indicates lack of sufficient oxygen in the blood in individuals experiencing dyspnea. Inspiratory dyspnea refers to difficulty breathing because of some blockage or interference with the individual's ability to take in air. Expiratory dyspnea is usually seen in asthma and bronchitis patients, with wheezing and pain upon exhaling air. A shortness-of-breath attack that occurs at night and awakens an individual is known as paroxysmal nocturnal dyspnea and may be caused by heart failure and pulmonary pressure. In the past, this type of dyspnea was called cardiac asthma, which is erroneous.

Eaton-Lambert syndrome   Named for American physician Lee McKendree Eaton (1905–58) and American physiologist Edward Howard Lambert (b. 1915), a myasthenia syndrome characterized by muscle weakness, hyporeflexia, and autonomic dysfunction, frequently associated with oat cell carcinoma of the lung.
   See also CANCER, LUNG.

ECHO virus   A virus of the group of approximately 30 viruses whose acronym stands for Enteric Cytopathogenic Human Orphan, associated with acute respiratory infection, myocarditis, enteritis, pleurodynia, and nonbacterial viral meningitis.

edema, pulmonary   From the Greek *oidema*, or swelling, an accumulation of fluid in the lungs as a result of heart failure, in which more blood enters the pulmonary circulation than is released. In general, edema refers to any excessive amount of fluid in body tissues. Laryngeal edema typically occurs along with an anaphylactic allergic reaction that requires prompt treatment before it causes airway obstruction. Edema of the glottis refers to the cough, loss of voice, and feeling of suffocation when the submucosa of the larynx becomes infiltrated with excessive fluid.

electrophrenic respiration   A type of artificial breathing technique in which electrodes providing intermittent electrical stimuli are applied over the phrenic nerves in the neck. This is used for patients with respiratory center injury.

ELISA (enzyme-linked immunoabsorbent assay)
A method for detecting antigens, antibodies, and hormones through immunological and enzymatic activity.

Elixophyllin   A trade name for theophylline.
   See also THEOPHYLLINE.

embolism, pulmonary   A blood clot or obstruction of a blood vessel in the pulmonary artery or a branch of the artery, usually as a result of thrombosis, or blood clot, in a vein in the leg or pelvis. An embolus may also be an air bubble or consist of fat, amniotic fluid, bone marrow, or a tumor fragment. Anticoagulants such as heparin are used as prophylaxis before and after surgery and as treatment for thrombus formation. Acute dyspnea, chest pain, coughing, anxiety, and rapid breathing are often associated with pulmonary embolism. In addition to dextran (a plasma volume expander) and graduated compression elastic stockings, supplemental oxygen and mechanical ventilation may be required.
   An embolus may be diagnosed through chest X ray, electrocardiogram, a lung perfusion scan, lung ventilation scan, and pulmonary arteriography.
   Approximately 10 percent of patients with pulmonary embolism sustain a certain amount of lung-tissue death (also called pulmonary infarction), and large clots may cause sudden death. Treatment of a pulmonary embolism involves oxygen therapy and, if necessary, pain-killing medication, in addition to anticoagulants, thrombolytics (drugs such as streptokinase and urokinase that break up the clot), and surgery (pulmonary embolectomy).

emphysema   A chronic lung disease named from the Greek word *emphysan*, meaning "to inflate," and characterized by difficulty in breathing, especially shortness of breath due to enlarged and damaged air sacs (alveoli) found at the ends of thin-walled air passages called bronchioles. Almost always, emphysema is caused by cigarette smoking; smoke as well as other pollutants stimulate the release of alveolar chemicals, which impede the oxygen and carbon dioxide exchange necessary for normal maintenance of the body's metabolism. The lungs become progressively inefficient, which may result in pulmonary hypertension (increased blood pressure in the pulmonary artery), cor pulmonale (enlargement and/or failure of the heart's right ventricle), edema (swelling due to excess fluid in the tissues), and chronic bronchitis (inflammation of the bronchial tubes). In mild cases this disorder may be confused with asthma.

Symptoms of emphysema may not emerge until the disease is well under way. Initial signs include shortness of breath on exertion, such as climbing stairs, which gradually worsens until a person is short of breath even at rest. The chest may become barrel-shaped because air becomes trapped outside the lungs and pushes out the thorax. Coughing and wheezing may be present, too. When cor pulmonale develops, oxygen deficiencies cause edema of the legs, and a person looks blue or purplish. These persons are called "blue bloaters." Individuals who breathe rapidly but retain normal coloring are referred to as "pink puffers." In advanced emphysema, breathing becomes increasingly difficult. Chest X rays and pulmonary function tests determine the extent of the lung damage and breathing capacity.

Emphysema is one of the causes of chronic obstructive pulmonary disease (COPD), which affects approximately 14 million people in the United States, second only to heart disease that results in disability.

Treatment includes bronchodilating, diuretic, and corticosteroid drugs, nebulizers, and oxygen administration. In addition, patients are advised to avoid air pollutants, stop smoking, prevent respiratory infections with good pulmonary hygiene, lose weight if obese, improve nutritional status, and increase oral fluid intake. Smaller meals help reduce pressure on the diaphragm, which makes it easier to breathe. Breathing exercises also may help to increase breathing efficiency and expiratory functional capacity, keep small airways patent, and educate the patient on the dangers of increased oxygen intake and other proper procedures in relation to ventilation therapy for hypoxic drive.

See also CHRONIC OBSTRUCTIVE PULMONARY DISEASE.

employment opportunities for individuals with allergies and asthma   Occupations or professions in which persons afflicted with allergic disorders or asthma can function in an environment free from occupational allergens or pollutants. An example of an inappropriate choice for an asthmatic person might be a zookeeper, pet shop employee, veterinarian, or farmer.

See also OCCUPATIONAL ASTHMA.

empyema   A type of pleural effusion, the presence of pus in the pleural space that occurs when pneumonia or a lung abscess spreads into the space. Other causes of empyema are an infection from a chest wound or surgery, esophageal rupture, or an abdominal abscess. Thoracic empyema, i.e., caused by the pus-forming pneumococci, may require surgical drainage. Pus in the pleural cavity, also called pyothorax, stems from a primary infection and may involve chills, fever, gray, sweaty skin, poor appetite, chest pain, cough, emaciation, and dyspnea. Treatment of the primary infection is key. Interlobular empyema refers to pus occurring between the lobes of the lung.

E-Mycin   See ERYTHROMYCIN.

encephalitis   An inflammation of the brain that may be a result of influenza or other diseases, including rabies, measles, smallpox, and viral infections. Treatment consists of therapy for the primary cause and physical and emotional support of the patient, such as monitoring vital signs, hydration, motor function, sleep patterns, and behavior.

endobronchitis   Inflammation of the smaller bronchi.

See also BRONCHITIS.

endotracheal tube　A tube with an inflated cuff surrounding it placed in the trachea, or windpipe, to prevent aspiration of a foreign substance or object into the bronchus and to keep the airway patent.

endotracheitis　An inflammation of the mucosa of the trachea.

ephedrine (Ephedrine, Ephedrine Sulfate, Neo-respin)　A sympathomimetic drug, similar to adrenaline but less powerful, that dilates bronchial muscles, contracts nasal mucosae, and elevates blood pressure. In the past, ephedrine was important in the treatment of asthma. An alkaloid originally derived from a species of *Ephedra*, a genus of shrubs, it was used in ancient Chinese medicine as an antipyretic (fever reducer) and diaphoretic (perspiration or sweat inducer). Later, its actions were rediscovered, and it was produced synthetically for oral or parenteral administration. Side effects may include tremors, anxiety, insomnia, headache, dizziness, confusion, hallucinations, convulsions, central nervous system depression, palpitations, dyspnea, nausea and vomiting, urinary retention, and chest pain.

epidemic　A massive outbreak of an infectious disease in a particular geographical area.

epiglottitis　An inflammation of the epiglottis, a slender, leaf-shaped, cartilaginous structure with an outer mucous membrane at the opening of the larynx, or voice box. When a person swallows, the epiglottis covers the larynx to prevent food or liquid from entering the airway. The inflammation, commonly experienced as a sore throat, fever, and a barking cough, may lead to cyanosis (blue coloration of skin), drooling, and coma, and may be fatal. In extreme cases, a tracheostomy may be necessary to reopen the airway. Treatment includes antibiotic therapy.

epinephrine (Adrenalin Chloride, Asthma Haler, Asthma Nefrin, Bronitin Mist, Bronkaid Mist, Epinal, Epinephrine HCl, Epinephrine Pediatric, Epipen Jr., Epitrate, Eppy/N, Glaucon, Medihaler-Epi, Micro-Nefrin, Nephron Inhalant, Primatene Mist, S-2 Inhalant, Sus-Phrine, Vaponefrin)　Also called adrenaline, one of the two active hormones, along with norepinephrine, produced by the adrenal glands, which sit on top of the kidneys (hence the combination of the Greek words *epi*, meaning upon, and *nephros*, or kidney). Epinephrine has long been used as a vasoconstrictor, especially to prolong the action of local anesthesia, a cardiac stimulant, a topical application for the eye, a bronchiolar relaxant, and as a treatment for asthma attack.

epipharynx　The portion of the pharynx, or throat, that connects with the nose. Another term for epipharynx is rhinopharynx.

episodic asthma　Symptoms of asthma occurring only sporadically, such as during an acute upper respiratory infection, or cold, or upon exposure to a specific trigger. In the interim, there is no shortness of breath or wheezing, and lung function studies are normal.

epistaxis　A nosebleed, or hemorrhage from the nose, caused by trauman to membranes or structure of the nose or by skull fracture, various diseases, and high altitudes. It may also occur after surgery. Allergy and asthma patients may suffer nosebleeds as a result of violent, repeated sneezing, picking or blowing the nose, or dryness of the mucous membranes. Rhinitis and sinusitis may also cause epistaxis. To treat a nosebleed, have the patient sit upright and help him or her lean forward to spit out blood in order to prevent nausea and vomiting swallowed blood and to prevent aspiration of fluid into the trachea. Pinch the nostrils against the nasal septum for five to 10 minutes while the patient breathes through the mouth. Cold compresses applied over the nose and at the nape of the neck and applying pressure across or under the upper lip may be helpful. Other treatment includes local epinephrine use; if required, balloon tamponade, posterior packing of the nasal cavity, and cauterization of the bleeding vessel are also treatments. Increased humidity may help if dryness caused the nosebleed.

Epstein-Barr virus Named for English pathologists M. A. Epstein (b. 1921), and Y. M. Barr (b. 1932), a type of herpesvirus thought to be the cause of infectious mononucleosis. Discovered in 1964, the virus is also associated with Burkitt's lymphoma in South African children and nasopharyngeal carcinoma in Asian populations. The Epstein-Barr virus first affects cells in the nasal lining and spreads to the white blood cells called B lymphocytes that produce antibodies. Infectious mononucleosis has been known to be common among teenagers and young adults, who come in contact with the virus by kissing or intimate relations with an Epstein-Barr–infected individual, hence the term "the kissing disease." Approximately 50 percent of all children in the United States have had an Epstein-Barr virus infection before the age of five, and the virus affects people of all ages.

Symptoms of infectious mononucleosis include fever, sore throat, and enlarged lymph nodes. Also associated with the disease is a pronounced fatigue, which may last for weeks or months. The spleen and liver may become enlarged, a skin rash may develop, and serious complications such as encephalitis, seizures, meningitis, nerve and behavioral abnormalities may require further treatment. Sometimes an enlarged lymph node may press on the airway; lung congestion may also develop but may not cause symptoms.

The Epstein-Barr virus has been suspected of causing chronic fatigue syndrome, a debilitating disorder that affects adults between 20 and 40 years of age, but it has not been proven. Treatment frequently includes antibiotic therapy and rest. In the case of a severe swelling of the airway, a corticosteroid may be prescribed.

esophageal obturator airway A tube that is inserted into the esophagus to block vomitus and keep the airway patent for optimal lung ventilation.

ethmoiditis An acute or chronic inflammation of ethmoid cells (the air cells or space in the ethmoid bone, which open into the nasal cavity) accompanied by headache, pain between the eyes, and a nasal discharge.

eupnea Normal breathing.

exercise-induced asthma The onset of coughing, wheezing, shortness of breath, and a feeling of tightness or pains in the chest following exercise. Exercise endurance is limited and should be anticipated in all asthma or respiratory disorder patients. Symptoms usually begin after three to five minutes of strenuous exercise. They may be minimal, occurring only with extremes of effort, or severe enough to require emergency treatment. The presence of cold weather, air pollution, hay fever-causing pollens, or a coexisting cold or sinus infection may lessen the degree of exercise needed to cause symptoms. Although the exact cause of exercise-induced asthma is unknown, it is thought by experts to be related to water loss from the bronchial tubes and increased concentration of the remaining fluid in the lining of the bronchi, provoking smooth muscles in the airways to constrict. Well-conditioned athletes may experience symptoms only at the extremes of their abilities; however, even Olympic medal-winning athletes often require asthma drugs to restore their breathing to normal. Diagnosis is suggested by a history of the symptoms. Exercise-induced asthma is confirmed by a decrease of at least 15 percent in lung function after an exercise challenge. Lung function can be documented by using either an inexpensive peak flow meter or a more sophisticated computerized spirometer. Swimming, downhill skiing, gymnastics, and karate are sports less likely to trigger asthma, but some well-known professional football and basketball players have asthma.

The use of two or three puffs of a beta-agonist bronchodilator metered-dose inhaler (MDI), such as albuterol, pirbuterol, terbutaline, and metaproterenol, or two to four puffs of the anti-inflammatory drug cromolyn sodium 10 to 15 minutes before the start of exercise will prevent exercise-induced asthma in the majority of patients. Alternative drugs include the MDI ipratropium, an anticholinergic (two to three puffs 20 to 30 minutes before exercise), or albuterol; metaproterenol syrup, astemizole, or terfenadine one hour before exercise may be effective. Albuterol and cromolyn are often combined for resistant individuals.

Allergy and lung specialists urge the participation of all students and adults in exercise programs. Students should be excused from gym classes only if they are having symptoms on the day of activity and should not be given blanket excuses.

See also ASTHMA.

expectorant   A substance or agent that stimulates the ability to remove bronchopulmonary mucus from the lungs, bronchial tubes, and throat. Expectorants may be sedative or stimulating. Ammonium carbonate and ammonium chloride are rarely used today, but they were frequently found in cough medicines. Guaifenesin (Robitussin), iodinated glycerol (Organidin), and ipecac may be used alone or in combination with cough suppressants. Proof of their effectiveness has been questioned by some experts.

expectoration   The act of ridding the mouth of saliva or the throat of sputum, mucus, or exudates from the bronchi or lungs by spitting.

expiration   Breathing out, or expelling air from the lungs. A duration of expiration, or exhalation, longer than inspiration may indicate emphysema, asthma, or other respiratory pathology. In active expiration, one uses muscles including those of the abdominal wall. Passive expiration occurs without muscular effort, but rather with the elasticity of lung and chest tissues and the weight of the chest wall.

expiratory center   Part of the medulla's respiratory center in the brain that controls expiratory movements.

exsufflation   The expulsion of air from the lungs that is accomplished by natural force or mechanical exsufflator.

extracorporeal membrane oxygenator   Known as an ECMO, a device outside the body that oxygenates blood and returns it to the body, particularly in patients suffering acute respiratory failure.

face (cyanotic; flushing)　The visage of a person suffering from respiratory or other disorders, either cyanotic (blue) or flushing (pink or red). Cyanosis indicates deficient oxygenation of the blood, such as in the case of asthma, whooping cough, pulmonary tuberculosis, croup, tracheal obstruction, asphyxia, drug poisoning, emphysema, or cardiac maladies. Flushing, or hyperemia, is often attributable to pulmonary tuberculosis, alcoholism, febrile, and other diseases. A swelling of the face from edema is seen in cases of pneumothorax, mediastinal tumors, and aneurysm.

See also EDEMA, PULMONARY.

failure, respiratory　The inability of the lungs to function because of a disease of the lung tissue, or weakness or paralysis of the muscles of the respiratory system.

falling drop　A clinking sound heard during auscultation with a stethoscope over large cavities in which there is air or fluid, such as in hydropneumothorax.

farmer's lung　A pneumonia-like allergic lung disease from exposure to bacteria-like microorganisms called actinomycetes. These organisms thrive in silos when the water content of the hay exceeds 28 percent. Emptying a silo often causes an attack.

See also PNEUMONITIS.

fascia, endothoracic　The fibrous membrane separating the pleura of the lung from the diaphragm and the inside of the chest, or thoracic, cavity.

faucitis　Inflammation of the fauces, or the constricted opening that leads from the mouth to the throat.

fexofenadine (Allegra)　Metabolite, or derivative, of the popular nonsedating antihistamine Seldane. Unlike Seldane, fexofenadine bypasses the liver and avoids the drug interactions that can cause potentially life-threatening heart irregularities. Allegra is effective for the treatment of sneezing, runny noise, itching, and other allergy symptoms.

fibrosis, pulmonary　Abnormal scar tissue that forms in the connective tissue of the lungs as a result of an inflammation, pneumonia, or pulmonary tuberculosis. The most common causes include the inhalation of dusts, such as silica, carbon, metal, asbestos, molds, and bird droppings; immune system disorders such as rheumatoid arthritis, scleroderma, systemic lupus erythematosus, and polymyositis; inhalation of gases, fumes, and vapors, especially chlorine and sulfur dioxide; therapeutic or industrial radiation, and drugs and poisons, including gold, methotrexate, sulfonamides, penicillamine, cyclophosphamide, busulfan, nitrofurantion, amiodarone, and paraquat.

Idiopathic pulmonary fibrosis refers to an unknown cause of scarring in the lung, but symptoms and diagnosis may be determined by the extent of the lung damage, the disease process, and the manifestation of complications such as infection or heart failure. Coughing, loss of stamina, shortness of breath, weight loss, loss of appetite, fatigue, chest pain, cyanosis, and finger clubbing may develop. Chest X ray, arterial blood gas tests, and pulmonary function tests may confirm the condition of fibrosis. If the scarring is not too extensive, a corticosteroid such as prednisone may be prescribed, along with oxygen therapy, medication to treat infection if necessary, and drugs for heart failure. In severe cases of fibrosis, lung transplantation may be an option.

Variants of idiopathic pulmonary fibrosis include desquamative interstitial pneumonia and lymphoid interstitial pneumonia (which involves the lower lobes of the lung and may be secondary to HIV infection in children and adults). Both variants have been known to respond to corticosteroid therapy.

fibrothorax The development of scar tissue that causes the two pleural surfaces of the lung to stick to each other.

fistula, pulmonary arteriovenous The congenital condition in which a fistula, or abnormal channel between an artery and a vein, forms in a pulmonary artery in the lung and then communicates with a pulmonary vein. The connection of the two vessels causes blood to bypass the oxygenation process. An arteriovenous fistula may also be acquired after birth, or as a result of an injury to an artery and vein in close proximity to one another. It may also be subsequent to kidney dialysis or other medical treatment in which a vein is pierced repeatedly and clotting and scar tissue develop. Small congenital fistulas can be excised surgically or destroyed by laser coagulation therapy; large acquired fistulas, which can cause heart failure if untreated, must be surgically corrected.

flames, inhalation of Severe irritation of the nose, throat, windpipe, and lungs as a result of exposure to flames or smoke. Coughing, choking, difficulty breathing, facial and nasal burns, elevated carboxyhemoglobin, and shock are among the initial symptoms that may lead to adult respiratory distress syndrome (ARDS), pulmonary complications, upper airway obstruction, and carbon monoxide poisoning.

flatness Heard on auscultation with a stethoscope, the sound produced by the presence of fluid in the thoracic cavity.

flint disease Also known as chalicosis, a type of pneumoconiosis resulting from the inhalation of dust from stone cutting.

See also CHALICOSIS; PNEUMOCONIOSIS.

Flonase Brand of fluticasone, a corticosteroid for topical use as a nasal spray for the prevention of nasal allergy symptoms.

Flovent Brand of fluticasone, a corticosteroid for topical use as a metered-dose inhaler for the prevention of asthma symptoms. It is available in three strengths.

flow meter A device that measures the flow of a liquid or gas, including the respiratory gases oxygen and carbon dioxide.

Floyer, Sir John British physician (1649–1734) who designed a 60-second pulse watch that made it possible to study the pulse and respiratory rates as they are affected by sex, age, emotional state, temperature, climate, diet, drugs, and disease. Floyer also estimated blood volume according to an individual's body weight. An asthmatic, Floyer wrote of his increased difficulty in breathing in the presence of tobacco smoke, dust, and other changes in the air as a sequel to ingesting certain foods, performing exercise, and experiencing emotional changes. Floyer is credited as the first to observe that asthma and predisposition to asthma are hereditary. In addition, he dissected a "broken-winded mare," and his findings provided the first description of a lung physically deteriorated by emphysema.

flunisolide (Aerobid, Nasalide) A corticosteroid for topical use as a nasal spray and metered-dose inhaler for prevention of nasal allergy symptoms and asthma.

fluticasone (Flonase, Flovent) Corticosteroid for topical use as a nasal spray and metered-dose inhaler for the prevention of nasal allergy and asthma symptoms.

flu vaccine See INFLUENZA.

forced expiratory time (FET) The amount of time one needs to strongly exhale a certain volume of air, called the forced expiratory volume (FEV). Spirometers are the devices that measure lung volumes and flow rates during forced breathing tests for the diagnosis of laryngeal or tracheal blockage, and other abnormalities.

formaldehyde A poisonous, foul-smelling, colorless gas that when dissolved in water is used as a preservative for animal tissues. Formaldehyde is found in abundance in our environment. Also a by-product of the combustion of gasoline and diesel, and from cigarette smoke, gas, wood stoves, and kerosene heaters in the home or workplace, this gas is an irritant to the respiratory system. Formaldehyde is also widely used in building materials, especially in mobile homes. Urea formaldehyde foam insulation was injected into the walls of homes until 1977, when it was replaced by safer materials. Plywood, molded plastics, and carpeting are additional sources of formaldehyde. It has been blamed as a cause of the strange symptoms referred to as "mobile home syndrome." Although there is no evidence that formaldehyde causes allergy, it is a frequent cause of contact dermatitis.

4-Way Nasal Spray A topical, vasoconstricting drug generically known as naphazoline hydrochloride. Other trade names are Privine HCL, Albalon Liquifilm, and Vasocon.

fraction of inspired oxygen Abbreviated as FiO_2, the percentage of oxygen in the air taken into the lungs. More than 50 percent oxygen indicates toxicity in air provided to patients through ventilation devices for extended periods of time.

Freeman, John British physician (1877–1962) who investigated tests for immunity and contributed to the development of therapeutic immunization. He served as director of the clinic for allergic disorders and bacteriological services at St. Mary's Hospital in London for many years. Freeman also published *Hay Fever, a Key to the Allergic Disorders,* which he dedicated to his colleague Leonard Noon, who died from tuberculosis.

fremitus Tremors or vibrations in the chest that can be felt by placing a hand on the chest. Tactile and vocal fremitus refers to vibrations felt through the chest wall of a person who is speaking, and tussive fremitus may be felt when a person coughs. This type of auscultation may help determine the symptoms of pleural effusions, emphysema, abnormal growths on the lung, and obstruction in a bronchus that may lead to collapse of the lung.

friction rub, pleural The sound produced during respiration by inflamed pleural surfaces, frequently heard on auscultation of patients who have a newly developed pleurisy.

Friedländer's bacillus Named for German physician Carl F. Friedländer (1847–87), the *Klebsiella pneumoniae,* a species of bacteria that causes pneumonia and is also known as a secondary invader in conditions including bronchitis and sinusitis.

fumes Irritating vapors, such as smoke fumes and ammonia gas, that may cause sneezing, coughing, choking, tightness in the chest, and shortness of breath or trigger an attack in an asthmatic person.

ganglia, thoracic   The eleven or twelve sympathetic nervous tissue masses located in the thorax or chest.

gas, lung irritant   Chlorine, phosgene, and other gases that cause burning sensations in the eyes, nose, and throat and may trigger asthma or cause bronchitis and pneumonia.

gas, suffocating   Phosgene or diphosgene, or any gasses made with chlorine that cause severe irritation of the bronchi and lungs. Inhalation of these so-called war gases may result in pulmonary edema and other respiratory disorders.

gas exchange, impaired   See ARTERIAL BLOOD GASES.

gasoline poisoning   The toxic result of inhaling gasoline, a distillation of petroleum that may contain poisonous additives such as tetraethyl lead or tricresol phosphate. Some people are poisoned by gasoline during an attempt to siphon the substance from a gas tank by suctioning it through a tube. Putting the suctioning end of the tube in one's mouth may lead to inhalation or swallowing the gas. Symptoms include headache, nervousness, dyspnea, cyanosis, pulmonary hemorrhage, and other disturbances. Treatment involves getting the victim into fresh air, administering oxygen and carbon dioxide, or cardiopulmonary resuscitation if necessary, removal of gasoline-soaked clothing, and cleaning of gas-contaminated skin. Every precaution should be taken to keep the victim away from sparks, open flames, or potential explosive substance or circumstance.

gastrointestinal reflux and asthma   A flow of acidic gastric juices from the stomach into the esophagus (also called heartburn or reflux esophagitis) because the muscle at the junction of the esophagus and stomach does not function well enough to keep the stomach contents from backing up into the esophagus or the throat. The juices may also flow into bronchial tubes and cause asthma symptoms or aggravate preexisting asthma. One of the adverse effects of theophylline, an effective, widely used drug for the treatment of asthma, is reflux esophagitis. Drugs used to treat reflux esophagitis include Tagamet and Zantac. However, Tagamet may increase blood levels of theophylline and therefore should be avoided in patients for whom theophylline products are prescribed.

gastropulmonary   A term used to denote any condition or concern involving both the stomach and the lungs.

gating, respiratory   A radiological procedure that attempts to reduce image discrepancies that may be caused by involuntary movement, such as during a certain stage of the respiratory process. Respiratory gating refers specifically to images collected repeatedly during a patient's respiration cycle.

general adaptation syndrome (G.A.S. syndrome) The body's overall response to stress as described by Austrian-Canadian endocrinologist Hans Selye (1907–82). Selye noted that the response consists of three stages, the alarm reaction (also known as "fight or flight"); the resistance or adaptive stage; and the exhaustion stage. A consequence of the exhaustion stage may be the body's inability to fight disease, and certain types of asthma may manifest.

See also ASTHMA.

glands, bronchial   Mixed glands, i.e., glands that produce both a clear, watery (serous) secretion and a viscous (mucous) secretion, located in the submucosa (connective tissue) of the bronchi and bronchial tubes.

glossitis   From the Greek *glossa,* meaning tongue, an inflammation of the tongue causing symptoms that may include tenderness, pain, localized ulcers, swelling, burning, dark and furry patches, intensified sensitivity to certain foods, elevated temperature, edema, thickened saliva, and malaise. In the case of acute glossitis, edema in the tongue may lead to asphyxia, for which a tracheostomy may be necessary to create an airway. Glossitis is frequently treated with antiseptic mouthwashes, anesthetic oral solution, bland or liquid diet, and, if necessary, surgery.

glossopharyngeal breathing   Taught to patients with inspiratory muscle weakness, a breathing technique in which one takes "gulps" of air and closes his or her mouth in order for the gulped air to reach the lungs. This technique increases the patient's air intake.

glucocorticoids, inhaled   Named from the Greek *gleukos,* or sweet, and *cortex,* or shape, a class of adrenal cortical hormones that combat stress and promote protein and carbohydrate metabolism.

glue sniffing   The act of deliberately inhaling the fumes of glue or solvent chemicals such as benzene, toluene, and xylene for the effect of an altered state of consciousness. The practice can be fatal.

See also INHALANT ABUSE.

Goodpasture's syndrome   Named for American pathologist Ernest William Goodpasture (1886–1960), a rare, often fatal disease—also known as progressive glomerulonephritis, hemoptysis, and hemosiderosis—characterized by bleeding into the lungs and eventually failure of the kidneys and respiratory system. The cause of Goodpasture's syndrome, which typically affects young men, is unknown, but it has been established that in individuals with the syndrome, certain antibodies appearing in the filtering apparatus of the kidneys and of the lungs' alveoli and capillaries are responsible for causing the deleterious inflammation and malfunction of those organs. Considered an allergic disorder, Goodpasture's syndrome causes the presence of protein and blood in the urine, abnormal areas in both lungs, a specific pattern of antibodies in kidney tissue, anemia attributable to the rapid loss of blood, shortness of breath, and coughing up blood. Treatment includes high intravenous doses of corticosteroids and cyclophosphamide, removal, cleaning (of undesirable antibodies), and return of blood to the circulation, supplemental oxygen, blood transfusions, renal dialysis, and possibly kidney transplant. Early treatment is essential to prevent permanent damage to the kidneys and lungs.

goundou   An African word referring to the enlargement of nasal bones as a result of yaws or syphilis infection. Other colloquial descriptions of the condition include "big nose" or "dog nose."

grain allergies   Symptoms of allergy caused by allergens found in flour, often leading to occupational asthma in up to 10 percent of bakers or those exposed to flour on a regular basis.

See also OCCUPATIONAL ASTHMA.

Grancher's disease   Named for French physician Jacques J. Grancher (1843–1907), a disease known also as splenopneumonia. Splenization refers to any change in tissue, such as lung tissue, that creates a resemblance to tissue of the spleen. Grancher's sign, heard on auscultation of the lungs, is the high-pitched murmur that occurs when a patient with Grancher's disease exhales.

See also PNEUMONIA.

granulomatosis, Wegener's   Named for F. Wegener, a German pathologist of the 20th century, a rare and potentially fatal disease that involves inflammation of blood vessel walls of the sinuses, nasal passages, lungs and airways, kidneys, and skin. In some cases, only respiratory system structures are affected. The inflammation may be so severe that lung tissue is at risk of being destroyed. The vasculitis (swelling and inflammation of the vessel walls) is accompanied by granulomatous lesions throughout the respiratory tract and by glomerulonephritis, a kidney disorder. Granulomas are grain-like tumors that factor into the disease, affecting the skin and the other organs.

Possibly attributable to allergic reactions but generally of unknown cause, Wegener's syndrome may or may not be evidenced by symptoms including fever, fatigue, weight loss, shortness of breath, chest pain, coughing, purulent rhinitis, sinusitis, polyarthalgia, nasal septum ulcerations, and signs of renal dysfunction. After early diagnosis by chest X ray showing areas of the lung that appear to be cancerous, the syndrome is treatable with cyclophosphamide (an immunosuppressive drug) and corticosteroids, or, if there are intolerable side effects from the cyclophosphamide, with azathioprine. Untreated or not treated promptly, the disease may cause death within a year of detection.

grass pollen allergy Hay fever symptoms related to the seasonal exposure of more than 4,500 plant species of the family Gramineae in North America and approximately 9,000 grass species worldwide. Grasses cover roughly 20 percent of the world's surface. These monocotyledonous, herblike, mostly anemophilous (having windborne pollen) plants reach their peak of pollination in temperate climates of North America from mid-May to mid-July. In tropical and subtropical regions, however, pollens may be present throughout the year. The grass flowers are open for only a few hours a day during the pollinating season. The pollen grains are viable for less than one day. A majority of hay fever sufferers experience symptoms when there is a concentration of pollen grains approaching 50 per cubic meter. The weather is largely responsible for pollen counts, with rain washing the air clean and higher winds blowing the pollens away.

See also HAY FEVER.

green tobacco sickness A nonallergenic, toxic disorder occurring in tobacco harvesters from absorption of dissolved nicotine from wet tobacco exposure.

See also TABACOSIS.

grindelia An American flowering, resinous herb known as gum weed whose dried leaves and stumps are used in making a remedy for bronchitis as well as a topical preparation for poison ivy rash.

grinders' disease See SILICOSIS.

grippe See INFLUENZA.

growing out of allergies and asthma Disappearance of childhood allergic symptoms and asthma upon reaching puberty. Generally the more severe the symptoms in childhood, the more likely the continuance during adolescence and adulthood. Usually the tendency for hyperreactivity of the airways remains for a lifetime, although often there are no symptoms. The tiny bronchioles of infancy widen profoundly with age, and therefore a greater triggering stimulus is required to cause wheezing or shortness of breath.

British studies have established that most asthma begins during childhood. As many as 11 percent of all children experience asthma symptoms at least once. Eighty-five percent, or the vast majority, have mild asthma, and 50 percent stop wheezing once they achieve adulthood and almost all have milder attacks. Children, whose asthma develops after the age of six months and who do not have allergies, have the best chance to outgrow their asthma tendency by adulthood.

guaifenesin (Robitussin) An expectorant drug used singly to loosen thick mucus or to help expel mucus and in conjunction with cough suppressants.

Guillain-Barré syndrome Named for French neurologists Georges Guillain (1876–1961) and J. A. Barré (1880–1967), a type of polyneuritis allegedly caused by an autoimmune attack of the nerves' myelin sheath. Severe weakness occurs in the muscles that support the respiratory system, and a respirator or tracheostomy may be necessary to sustain the life of the patient. The prognosis is good provided there is prompt and appropriate treatment, which includes corticosteroids, immunosuppressive drugs, physical therapy, plasma-pheresis, infusion of autoimmune globulin, and other measures.

gustatory rhinitis The nasal congestion and inflamed mucous membranes that follow smelling or tasting a substance to which an individual may or may not be allergic.

Habitrol   See NICOTINE PATCHES.

hacking cough   A dry and recurrent cough.
See also COUGH.

Haemophilus influenzae   See INFLUENZA.

Haemophilus **influenza type b infections**   See
INFLUENZA.

halitosis   See BREATH, BAD.

Hamman-Rich syndrome   Named for American
pathologists Louis Hamman (1877–1946) and
Arnold Rich (1893–1968), another term for idiopathic pulmonary fibrosis.
See also FIBROSIS, PULMONARY.

Hamman's disease   Named for American pathologist Louis Hamman (1877–1946), another term
for spontaneous mediastinal emphysema.
See also EMPHYSEMA.

Harrison's groove   Named for British physician
Edwin Harrison (1779–1847), a groove or
depressed area of the lower chest caused by the
pulling of the diaphragm, usually seen in infants
afflicted with an airway obstruction or rickets.

hashish   The Arabic word for the extract of the
female hemp plant, *Cannabis sativa,* to be smoked or
chewed for its mind-altering effect. The gummy,
concentrated resin extract is made from the plant's
flowers, stalks, and leaves. Also called "hash" and
"charas," the substance is often used to make marijuana cigarettes (joints). Despite its reputation for
inducing euphoria and intensified perception, frequent smoking of marijuana can cause bronchitis,
lung cancer, and any disorder caused by using cigarettes made from tobacco. Although marijuana
has not been conclusively proven to be physically
addictive, it may cause psychological dependence
and lead the user toward addiction to other illegal
drugs.
See also CANNABIS; TOBACCO.

hay fever   A common name for allergic rhinitis or
nasal allergy, also known as coryza spasmodica.
The term originated in England when symptoms
were observed as they occurred simultaneously
with the harvesting of hay. However, exposure to
hay does not usually produce the characteristic
sneezing, runny and stuffy nose, or itchy, watery
eyes, and does not cause fever. Seasonal hay fever
occurs in the spring and fall with exposure to pollinating trees, grasses, and weeds in susceptible
persons. Perennial hay fever affects some allergic
individuals and occurs year-round from exposure
to animal danders, house-dust mites, and molds.

An estimated 22 million Americans suffer from
seasonal allergies and spend approximately $225
million for 8.4 million doctor visits and testing,
$300 million on prescription drugs, and $2 billion
on over-the-counter medications. These individuals suffer six million days of bed rest, 28 million
days of restricted activity, 3.5 million days out of
work, and 2 million lost school days.

A Type I hypersensitivity reaction also known as
pollinosis and vasomotor rhinitis, this disease of the
nasal mucosa and upper airways may also be
caused by airborne fungus spores. Coughing and
asthmatic symptoms may occur. In addition to

treatment by antihistamine or corticosteroid medication in the form of nasal sprays, nose drops, pills, or liquid, the patient may benefit from air-filtration systems, air masks, nasal filters, removal of the irritating allergen, and, if required, hypersensitivity testing and desensitization.

See also BOSTOCK, JOHN.

headache, histamine   Headache that appears to be a direct result of histamine given by injection or ingested through certain wines containing histamine.

See also HISTAMINE.

heartburn   A burning pain typically arising between the esophagus and stomach and possibly radiating through the chest, neck, and throat often as the result of gastroesophageal reflux disease (GERD). Nearly one-third of the American population suffers from GERD, the backward flow of the stomach's contents into the esophagus. The lower esophageal sphincter valve, the muscle at the base of the esophagus and stomach that is supposed to block food from getting back into the esophagus, may be weak in individuals with GERD, though anyone may experience occasional heartburn. Also, GERD patients may be breathing in gastric fluids that irritate the lungs, and in addition to heartburn, they may have asthma. Heartburn, indigestion, and regurgitation may trigger asthma.

Heartburn is usually treated with antacids and lifestyle modifications, but there is a surgical option for those with severe heartburn called Nissen fundoplication, in which the upper portion of the stomach is wrapped around the esophagus to create a new sphincter valve and thus reduce reflux.

heart-lung machine   Also known as a heart-lung bypass, a device designed to support the functions of both the heart and lungs when an individual's body is unable to pump and deoxygenate blood in the normal exchange of blood gasses (oxygen and carbon dioxide).

Heimlich maneuver   Named for American physician H. J. Heimlich, born in 1920, a lifesaving technique for expelling a foreign object from a person's throat or windpipe. The three basic steps of the maneuver are: 1) standing behind the victim and putting your arms around his waist; 2) making a fist with one hand and putting it between the victim's navel and rib cage while the other hand supports the intended thrust of the fist, and 3) pressing with the fist with a quick and forceful upward thrust, to create a burst of air pressure that will send the blockage out the victim's mouth. This technique should be used only if a person is choking. The name "Heimlich sign" has been given to the natural instinct of a choking victim to grasp his throat with the thumb and index finger. In the event that the victim is alone, he may thrust the midsection of his body (between navel and rib cage) against a counter top, chair, table, or other strong, stable object to simulate the thrust a rescuer would provide. Most adults can effectively use the back of a chair to press against for self-administration of the Heimlich. The maneuver may also be performed if the victim is lying on his back. Instructions for the Heimlich maneuver are usually posted in restaurants and other public places and are available through most local first-aid squads.

Heiner's syndrome   A chronic lung disease, characterized by cold-like symptoms, caused by allergy to cow's milk. Hypoventilation, that is, the reduction of the rate and depth of breathing, may occur in conjunction with other respiratory disorders, such as chronic obstructive lung disease, and with various obstructions in the respiratory tract. Less severe blockage may occur as an allergic reaction to cow's milk. The condition usually improves with the elimination of cow's milk protein from the diet.

See also HYPOVENTILATION SYNDROME.

helium   A low-density gas often mixed with air or oxygen for the treatment of respiratory disorders including air pressure-related problems such as caisson disease. Helium and air administered to individuals subjected to high atmospheric pressure helps reduce the time they need to adjust to varying air pressure.

See also BENDS.

hemithorax   A term referring to half of the chest.

hemlock poisoning Intoxication caused by the ingestion of the oil extracted from the unripe fruit of the hemlock, a species of evergreen plant, *Conium maculatum.* If respiratory failure occurs, the patient must be treated with artificial respiration and oxygen therapy.

hemopleura The presence of blood in the pleural space.

See also HEMOTHORAX.

hemopneumothorax The presence of blood and air in the pleural cavity.

hemoptysis From the Greek words *haima,* or blood, and *ptyein,* meaning to spit, the expectoration of blood from the mouth, larynx, trachea, bronchi, or lungs through a coughing attack. The sputum becomes salty-tasting, red, and frothy. Hemoptysis may be the result of hemorrhage, respiratory disease, or a lung infection caused by the parasitic fluke *Paragonimus westermani.* Treatment includes the application of ice packs over the chest, bedrest, sedatives, and other medication and procedures, depending upon diagnosis.

hemorrhage, lung The bright red, frothy blood coughed up as a result of a lung disease or other respiratory disorder.

hemothorax The presence of blood in the pleural cavity caused by ruptured blood vessels as a result of pneumonia, pulmonary tuberculosis, traumatic injury, or malignancy.

hepatopulmonary The term used in reference to both the liver and the lungs.

Hering-Breuer reflex Named for German physiologist Heinrich Ewald Hering (1866–1948) and Austrian physician Josef Breuer (1842–1925), the reflex inhibition of breathing in as a result of pressoreceptor-nerve stimulation when the lungs are inflated.

hernia, diaphragmatic The protrusion or "dropping" of part of the diaphragm into the stomach through the esophageal hiatus. The hernia may be congenital, esophageal, or acquired (traumatic), the latter possibly caused by debilitating illness, weakness, tumors, physical exertion, or strenuous, chronic coughing. Hernia may also be characterized by an organ or part of an organ projecting into the diaphragm. Treatment may include surgery.

See also HERNIA, PHRENIC.

hernia, phrenic The rupture or abnormal protrusion of an organ through the diaphragm into a pleural cavity.

heroin toxicity Poisoning from heroin, a morphine-derived narcotic drug, in which there is pulmonary edema and a decrease in respiration that may require artificial resuscitation and oxygen therapy. Treatment also may include the administration of a drug that stimulates the respiratory system, such as doxapram hydrochloride. Heroin toxicity is life-threatening.

hiccough, hiccup A short cough or sound on inspiration caused by the sudden closure of the glottis after a spasm that lowers the diaphragm. Also known as singultus, hiccups may be the result of indigestion, respiratory irritation, growths within the pleural cavity, hysteria, cerebral lesions, or alcoholism. Prolonged hiccups often require treatment, including inhaling carbon dioxide (breathing into a paper bag), antiemetic drugs, nasopharyngeal stimulation with a rubber tube, or placing some granulated sugar in the hypopharynx. In severe cases, the phrenic nerve may need to be anesthetized.

hilitis Inflammation occurring at the root of the lungs at the fourth and fifth dorsal vertebrae level.

Hippocrates Greek physician who lived ca. 460–375 B.C., considered by many "the father of modern medicine." Among his major tenets are that physicians should observe all, evaluate honestly, assist nature, work for the good of the patient, treat the whole person and not simply the illness, and, above all, do no harm. Modern chiropractic also employs Hippocrates' idea that all illness stems from anomalies of the spine. In Hippocrates' writings, he described, for example, the symptoms of pulmonary edema: "Water accumulates; patient has fever and cough; the respiration is fast; the feet become edematous; the nails appear curved and the patient suffers as if he had pus inside, only less severe and more protracted. One can recognize that it is not pus but water. . . . If you put your ear against the chest you can hear it seethe inside like sour wine."

Hippocrates also wrote that some foods known to be safe and healthful for most people caused illness in some, possibly, he speculated, because of a "poison" in the food, such as cheese, to which some people were particularly sensitive.

hippus, respiratory The condition characterized by the pupils of the eye dilating during inspiration and contracting during expiration.

Hismanal See ASTEMIZOLE.

histaminase An enzyme found throughout the body that counteracts histamine.
See also HISTAMINE.

histamine A natural substance liberally distributed throughout the body (especially in the skin, heart, lungs, gastrointestinal mucosa, the brain, and other organs) and a major substance released by mast cells of the tissues to initiate an allergic reaction. Inflammation, excess acid production in the stomach, constriction of the bronchi in the lungs, red flushing of the skin (as occurs with a burn), red rashes, decrease in blood pressure, and headache are among the symptoms characteristic of histamine release. Antihistamines are substances that counteract histamine.
See also ANTIHISTAMINE.

histamine H_1, receptor antagonist An alternate term for antihistamine.

histamine H_2, receptor antagonist A drug that blocks the effects of the chemical histamine by competing for receptor sites on the surface of cells in the stomach, thus preventing the secretion of gastric acid in the treatment of peptic ulcers. H_2-blocking drugs available in the United States include cimetidine (Tagamet), ranitidine (Zantac), nizatidine (Axid), and famotidine (Pepcid). Traditional antihistaminic drugs, called H_1-receptor antagonists, differ from H_2 agents by blocking the allergic symptoms caused by histamine primarily in the respiratory system and skin. H_1 and H_2 antihistamines are sometimes combined for the treatment of hives.

H_2-antagonist drugs rarely have adverse effects; however, cimetidine causes a rise in theophylline levels and should be used with caution in asthmatic patients taking both drugs. The other drugs in this class are probably free of this problem.
See also ANTIHISTAMINE.

histamine headache See HEADACHE, HISTAMINE.

histoplasmosis A fungal respiratory infection characterized by acute shortness of breath, coughing, fever, pains in the joints, potential adrenal gland failure, and other symptoms if the disease goes untreated or becomes chronic. Infection may be caused in susceptible or immunocompromised individuals who inhale the spores of the fungus *Histoplasma capsulatum,* found in soil (especially when contaminated by fecal material of birds or bats) in the southern and central United States, regions of South America, Africa, and Asia. In severe cases ulcers may appear in the gastrointestinal tract, and the spleen and liver may become enlarged. Other aspects of the disease may include weight loss, leukopenia, anemia, and adrenal necrosis. Histoplasmosis may be fatal. Treatment with antifungal medications is usually effective. Histoplasmosis is not an allergic disorder, but it may easily be mistaken for symptoms of allergy or asthma.

hoarseness A raspy or rough-sounding voice caused by an inflammation of the throat and vocal cords. Among the causes are allergy to certain foods, chemical irritants, tobacco, and alcohol. Persistent hoarseness may be a sign of benign or malignant polyps in the throat.

holistic medicine   A recognized discipline of Western medicine that incorporates some theories of Eastern medicine and the recognition of the patient as both a physiological and psychological being. Holistic practitioners believe that psychological factors affect well-being and disease processes. They employ various techniques, including relaxation, guided imagery and visualization, and hypnosis, along with conventional methods of treatment appropriate to the ailment, and they advocate the patient's participation in his or her own healing.

See also HIPPOCRATES.

homeopathy   An alternative treatment system based on the theory that "like cures like," that is, if a substance causes a symptom, it can conversely cure it when taken in a highly diluted form or in minute quantity. Remedies are made from plant, animal, and mineral sources and are available at health food stores and pharmacies. Homeopathy relates to desensitization techniques to treat allergic patients. Depending upon the patient's complaints, homeopathic remedies are reported to have had positive effects against allergies, sore throats, arthritis, indigestion, colds and flu, chronic pain, and infections.

home remedies   Actions that individuals can take on their own to help combat allergies, asthma, and other ailments and augment treatments prescribed by the physician. According to some experts, one can seal bedding in plastic liners to keep mattresses free of dust and dust mites, get rid of carpeting, use fungicides in damp areas of the house, avoid fireplace fires, install air-conditioning, maintain a sensible diet and avoid foods that may be allergenic, and other such measures. Other home remedies involve herbalism, a practice that relies on the use of various herbs as combatants of disease. For example, a syrup made with rhubarb, water, and sugar and then diluted with four inches of water to one inch of syrup is said to have a soothing effect

when taken by individuals with emphysema. Home remedies do not substitute for professional care.

hormone   A natural substance produced in an organ or gland that, when conveyed by the bloodstream, stimulates either increased or decreased functioning in various parts of the body. Among the most commonly known hormones are thyroid hormone, parathormone, cortisone, estrogen, testosterone, progesterone, human growth hormone, insulin and glucagons, adrenocortical hormone, ACTH (adrenocorticotropic hormone), and gastric hormone. Cortisone-like synthetic hormones, known as corticosteroids, are often used in the treatment of asthma because they act against inflammation.

See also CORTICOSTEROIDS.

house-dust mites   Microscopic members of the class Arachnida, subclass Acari. Species known to be important as allergens are *Dermatophagoides pteronyssinus* (skin-eating, feather-loving), *D. farinae, D. microceras, Euroglyphus maynei,* and *Blomia tropicalis.*

Many asthma experts consider dust mites to be the single most important allergen associated with asthma. Two principal groups of allergens of considerable importance are digestive enzymes, one group of them found in high concentrations in the fecal pellets, and a second group found in both fecal pellets and mite bodies.

Two micrograms of *Der p* I (mite allergen) per gram of dust is considered a risk factor for sensitization and the development of asthma in susceptible individuals. A concentration of 10 micrograms of allergen per gram of dust is a risk factor for triggering acute asthma in these persons.

Prevalence

House-dust mite exposure is especially great in the Gulf Coast region and Pacific Northwest of the United States, the United Kingdom, northern Europe, Australia, New Zealand, Brazil, and Japan. Dust mites require high humidity, moderate temperatures, and a food source that includes human skin scales.

In the United Kingdom, an estimated 80 percent of asthmatic children are sensitive to house-dust mites. When placed in a dust-mite-low environment, such as a hospital ward or a high-elevation, mountainous region, sensitive individuals invariably improve. Unfortunately, it takes several months for the condition to improve; as soon as allergic individuals were placed in their former environment, the asthma returned.

Dust Mite Control

Removal of the dust mite from the environment by either killing them with acaricides, benzyl benzoate or tannic acid, or changing environment is an effective measure.

The relative humidity in bedrooms should be kept below 60 percent. Uncarpeted floors are best, but treatment of carpets with acaricides is recommended. Vacuum cleaners with double bags may be beneficial, but most vacuuming increases airborne levels of mites. HEPA filters on vacuum cleaners are of little or no value. Covering mattresses, box springs, and pillows, and hot washing of bedding can reduce mite allergen levels significantly.

Dust mites were discovered in 1964. House-dust mites are microscopic (approximately one-third of a millimeter in length), sightless, eight-legged arthropods that are natural inhabitants of our indoor environment. These mites are not an indicator of uncleanliness and do not transmit human diseases. However, they are a major cause of asthma, allergic rhinitis (hay fever), and atopic dermatitis (eczema).

The most important house-dust mite allergens result from proteins in the mite's digestive tract excreted in the fecal waste rather than the mite itself. The tiny fecal particles break down to an extremely fine powder that sticks to surrounding absorbent materials. The allergen-containing powder becomes airborne when carpets are walked on, upholstery is disturbed by sitting or rising, shaking out blankets and quilts, or airing out rooms.

The growth and reproduction of house-dust mites are dependent on a food supply, relative humidity, and temperature. They feed on human and animal dander (flakes, scales, or dandruff) and other materials such as fiber and feathers. The average human sheds up to 1.5 grams of skin particles per day. The mites thrive at temperatures between 68 degrees and 84 degrees Fahrenheit and a relative humidity of 65 to 80 percent.

Distribution

Moist areas such as the South, the Gulf Coast region, and the Pacific Northwest present excellent breeding grounds for these microscopic organisms. House-dust mites mature and breed from May to October and may be responsible for triggering as many as 44 percent of acute asthma attacks in these areas. Since the dust mites do not thrive where relative humidity is above 90 percent or below 33 percent, they are rarely found in dry climates over 3,600 feet above sea level.

There are 47 recognized species in 17 genera of the family Pyroglyphidae. Species common in temperate and tropical regions are *Dermatophagoides, Euroglyphus, Hirstia, Malayoglyphus, Pyroglyphus,* and *Sturnophagoides. Dermatophagoides* or *Euroglyphus* species can be found in most homes in North America, Western Europe, Japan, New Zealand, and Australia.

House-Dust Mite Control

The highest number of dust mites are found in bedding, upholstered furniture, and carpeting. They also inhabit pillows, quilts, children's stuffed animals, and areas where pets sleep. They are rarely found in hospitals.

It has been established that a level of 100 dust mites per gram of dust is a risk factor for sensitization and the development of asthma in susceptible persons. A level of 500 mites per gram of dust is considered a major risk factor for the development of acute asthma in a sensitized individual.

Bedrooms are usually the chief target of avoidance measures for dust mites because of the allergic individual's continuous exposure. Asthma has been demonstrated to improve in mite-free environments. The following measures have been found to reduce dust mite exposure by tenfold or more: (1) covering mattresses and other bedding with encasings designed to prevent dust mites from penetrating them; (2) hot washing of all bedding at least every 10 days; (3) removal of carpets and upholstered furniture; (4) reduction of humidity, and (5) use of acaricides. Other measures include replacing cloth curtains with blinds, vacuuming and dusting with a moist cloth every week, organizing and rotating clothes in your closet and dresser by season, and storing out-of-season clothes in plastic tubs, according to Gerald Vanderpool, M.D., past president of the American Association of Certified Allergists. More information on allergen barrier encasings is available at www.allergydirect.com or by calling (877) 283-2323.

Test kits are available to measure the quantity of dust mites in a particular room. After treatment to reduce the mite population, tests can be repeated to determine the success or failure of the measures taken.

Immunotherapy

When avoidance measures are unsuccessful or impossible to achieve, standardized allergen extracts for *Dermatophagoides* subspecies *farinae* and *pteronyssinus* are available in the United States for immunotherapy.

Huang-ti Legendary ruler of China in the 25th century B.C., according to Chinese historians, known as the "Yellow Emperor" because he reigned under the influence of the earth, whose elemental color was believed to be yellow. Huang-ti (Huangdi) is considered the author of the oldest recorded canon of internal medicine called the *Nei ching su wen*. In this work, Huang-ti conducts a discussion between himself and his physician-minister Ch'i Po on the physical and mental aspects of health and disease. The *Nei ching* is valued today by many for its observations on "noisy breathing," serving as the original description of asthma.

huffing Slang term used by youths to describe the inhalation of airplane glue, aerosol gas, solvents, gasoline fumes, and other noxious substances in order to achieve euphoria, or a "high." Because the exact contents of these substances may be unknown by the user, they have the potential of causing a life-threatening allergic reaction or of masking symptoms of asthma. If inhalant abuse is suspected, a hotline has been established to help: (800) 788-2800.

See also INHALANT ABUSE.

humidifiers Devices that increase the humidity in a building or room by blowing moisture into the air, including ultrasonics, cool-mist impeller types, evaporative units, and steam vaporizers. Humidifiers may be part of a centralized or portable heating/air-conditioning unit. These units have the potential to cause harm because they may promote the growth of molds and distribute them as an aerosol into the local environment. Even if the units are kept mold free, increasing the relative humidity of a room may stimulate growth of molds and dust mites. Steam vaporizers are considered by some experts to have the lowest potential of contamination of the humidifying units in light of the fact that the steam kills many offending microorganisms. (However, the danger of burns exists if this type of unit is knocked over or the steam comes into direct contact with skin.)

The Environmental Protection Agency discovered that ultrasonic units, which claim to kill microorganisms by ultra-high-frequency sound waves, can nonetheless send out particles of dead bacteria and molds into the room air. Evaporative units on central heating systems, some with tanks in which water stays warm, have also been criticized as potential breeding harbors for bacteria.

Commercial units may be sources of microorganisms, such as actinomycetes and fungi, that may cause the allergic lung disease hypersensitivity pneumonitis. Severe sinusitis has also been linked to contaminated humidifiers. One report describes "humidifier fever," a syndrome characterized by flu-like symptoms including fever, chills, cough, headache, and malaise. It was first recognized when large numbers of office and factory employees became ill and the origin of their illness was central humidifying systems contaminated by microorganisms. After the systems were cleaned, affected individuals recovered. According to research scientists at the University of Michigan, all humidifiers are contaminated, leading to warnings of possible health hazards issued by the federal Consumer Products Safety Commission. Some research indicates that humidifying dry air is of little or no health benefit because oral and nasal passages are designed to stay moist under all environmental conditions.

humidity The amount of moisture, or water vapor, in the air, ranging from 100 percent humidity (air completely saturated with moisture) to small percentages. An extremely humid atmosphere may seem oppressive to some individuals; those with allergies or asthma may experience discomfort in cold, dry air, often an asthma trigger. In addition, dust mites and molds thrive in humidity greater than 60 percent. The ideal humidity for persons with allergies is 25 to 40 percent; higher relative humidity may be irritating to the respiratory system. Humidification of the air from swimming pool water is excellent for moisturizing bronchial tubes, and the slow, deep breathing during swimming can be beneficial to asthmatics.

hunger, air Shortness of breath, breathlessness, dyspnea.
See also BREATHING; DYSPNEA.

hydroconion An atomizer that produces a fine spray.
See also AEROSOL.

hydrogen A highly flammable, colorless, odorless, tasteless gas that occurs in water (hydrogen oxide, or H_2O) and in nearly all organic compounds. Hydrogen is also present in all acids and as a component of all carbohydrates, proteins, and fats. The most abundant element in the universe, it occurs in a quantity of only 0.00005 percent of Earth's atmosphere.

hydropneumatosis Liquid and gasses found in body tissues that cause edema (swelling) and emphysema.
See also EMPHYSEMA.

hydropneumothorax A collapse of a lung or lungs in which gas and fluids have accumulated in the space surrounding the lungs (pleural cavity).
See also PNEUMOTHORAX.

hydrorrhea Excessive watery discharge from the nose, eyes, or other body parts. This symptom may be suggestive of allergic rhinitis (hay fever).
See also RHINORRHEA.

hydrothorax An accumulation of fluid in the pleural cavity that is non-inflammatory. Patients with hydrothorax may exhibit symptoms including dyspnea, lack of vesicular breath sounds, and flatness over the buildup of fluid.

hyperbaric oxygen therapy A treatment using a hyperbaric chamber of oxygen to combat various problems such as bends (caisson disease), carbon monoxide poisoning, smoke inhalation, and acute ischemia of tissues. Hyperbarism involves exposure to greater than atmospheric pressure, often the case of deep-sea divers and miners. Hyperbaric oxygen is oxygen that is one-and-a-half to three times absolute atmospheric pressure. The chamber itself is large enough to accommodate a patient and a team of medical professionals, and its pressure may be increased if more oxygen is necessary to treat the specific needs of the patient.
See also BENDS.

hyperinflation An excess amount of air in the lungs.

hyperpnea Rapid breathing or increased respiratory rate, such as that after exercise, or deeper than normal breathing during normal activity. Hyperpnea may be experienced at high altitudes or as a result of pain, drug reaction, hysteria, fever, heart disease, or respiratory disorder.

hypersensitivity pneumonitis (HSP) Also known as extrinsic allergic alveolitis, an allergic lung disease caused by repeated exposure to organic dusts or other offending agents. In an acute case, flu-like symptoms may include cough, shortness of breath, fever, chills, sweating, headaches or generalized pains, malaise, and nausea with onset from two to nine hours after exposure. Symptoms peak between six and 24 hours and last from several hours to several days.

A subacute form that may gradually worsen over a period of days to several weeks may be much more severe, with shortness of breath progressing to the point of cyanosis and requiring hospitalization.

CAUSES OF HYPERSENSITIVITY PNEUMONITIS

Disorder	Source
Aspergillosis	*Aspergillus* spores
Bagassosis	Moldy sugarcane
Bible printer's lung	Moldy typesetting water
Bird breeder's lung	Avian droppings or serum
Budgerigar fancier's lung	Parakeets
Chicken handler's lung	Chickens
Pigeon breeder's lung	Pigeons
Turkey handler's lung	Turkeys
Cephalosporium hypersensitivity	Contaminated sewage
Cheese washer's lung	Cheese mold
Coffee worker's lung	Coffee dust
Corn farmer's lung	Corn dust
Detergent lung	Detergents (*Bacillus subtilis* enzyme)
Drug-induced	Amiodarone, gold, procarbazine
Duck fever	Duck feathers and proteins
Epoxy resin lung	Heated epoxy resin
Familial hypersensitivity pneumonitis	Contaminated wood dust in walls
Farmer's lung	Moldy hay or grain
Furrier's lung	Hair dust
Humidifier air-conditioner lung	Thermophilic actinomycetes, amoebae
Laboratory technician's lung	Rat urinary proteins
Malt worker's lung	Moldy malt, malt dust
Maple bark stripper's lung	Moldy maple bark
Miller's lung	Grain contaminated by wheat weevils
Mummy handler's lung	Cloth wrappings of mummies
Mushroom worker's lung	Mushroom compost
Paint refinisher's disease	Automobile spray painting (diisocyanates)
Paper mill worker's lung	Moldy wood pulp
Paprika slicer's lung	Moldy paprika
Pituitary snuff syndrome (snuff taker's lung)	Bovine and porcine proteins
Plastic worker's lung	Plastics, varnish (diisocyanates)
Rat lung	Rat urinary proteins
Sauna taker's disease	*Pullularia* in sauna water
Sequoiosis	Moldy wood from maple logs, moldy redwood dust
Smallpox handler's lung	Smallpox scabs
Streptomyces hypersensitivity pneumonia	Contaminated fertilizer
Suberosis	Moldy cork dust
Summer type	House dust contaminated with *Trichosporon cutaneum*
Tea grower's lung	Tea plants
Thatched roof disease	Dried grasses and leaves
Wheat weevil's disease	Infested wheat flour
Wood joiner's lung	Sawdust
Wood pulp worker's lung	Moldy logs
Wood trimmer's disease	Moldy wood trimmings

The chronic form has an even more gradual onset with increasing cough, shortness of breath, fatigue, and weight loss over several months.

Diagnosis is based on a history of exposure to a recognized allergen and confirmed by positive skin tests, finding antibodies in the blood to that allergen, and biopsy. Chest X-ray findings range from normal to severely abnormal.

The diagnosis may be confused with immune deficiency diseases, pulmonary mycotoxicosis (atypical farmer's lung), toxic organic dust syndrome (grain fever), idiopathic interstitial fibrosis (cryptogenic fibrosing alveolitis), cystic fibrosis, silofiller's lung, psittacosis, eosinophilic pneumonias, allergic bronchopulmonary aspergillosis, collagen vascular diseases, granuloma-vasculitis syndromes, or sarcoidosis.

hyperventilation Rapid breathing resulting in diminished carbon dioxide levels in the bloodstream. Tingling or numbness in the extremities, muscle spasms, and a feeling of anxiety may simulate, or in some cases trigger, an asthma attack.

hypnosis Techniques including guided deep relaxation, trance or altered state of awareness, suggestions, ideas, and imagery performed by a hypnotherapist, psychologist, psychiatrist, or various certified health professionals with patients suffering from asthma, allergies, respiratory disorders, and other health-related ailments. According to Susan Bendersky Sacks, R.N., M.S.N., C.S., in an article in *Nursing Spectrum,* March 19, 2001, "Research studies have shown that hypnosis can significantly improve pulmonary function tests, increase compliance, decrease hospital admissions and medication requirements, and in some cases, result in discontinued medication altogether. Proposed explanations include: Hypnosis decreases bronchospasm and airway resistance by influencing cerebral metabolism and the vagal and sympathetic pathways; hypnosis decreases bronchoconstriction by activating the release of neurotransmitters that stabilize IgE-mediated mast cells; hypnosis creates the perception of reduced airway resistance; hypnosis reduces anxiety and increases coping and compliance with conventional treatment." In addition to reporting that hypnosis as a technique is controversial, Sacks emphasizes that "hypnotic trance is attained solely by the control of the patient, while the hypnotherapist functions as a consultant, facilitator, and guide. . . . Myths and misconceptions about hypnosis are prevalent and often deter interested patients from seeking treatment. Patients commonly fear being controlled and manipulated into revealing secrets and engaging in embarrassing behaviors. . . . The truth is that patients can never be coerced into displaying unwanted or unnatural behaviors or disclosing personal information. During hypnosis, the patient is aware of everything that is said and is able to guard private issues." More information is available at copeconsultants@hotmail.com or from the American Society of Clinical Hypnosis at www.asch.net.

hypocapnia Abnormally low level of carbon dioxide in the blood.

hypoepinephria A decrease in epinephrine secretion in the body.

hypostatic pneumonia Pneumonia occurring in a patient, usually elderly or severely debilitated, who does not move enough to ward off alveolar fluid congestion, poor aeration or collapse of the lungs, and capillary pooling. The congestion creates an opportunity for infection to set in. Preventive measures should be taken for immobile patients.

hypoventilation syndrome Abnormally diminished respiration with reduced depth of inspiration and rate. It is characterized by cyanosis (skin or nail beds that appear blue), clubbing of the fingers, decreased oxygen content with a subsequent increase in red blood cells and blood hemoglobin (in the body's attempt to improve the oxygen supply to the tissues), and an increase in carbon dioxide (level builds up because of the inability to exhale adequately).

Hypoventilation occurs with the severe chronic obstructive lung diseases such as chronic bronchitis and emphysema, and from massive body obesity (also called pickwickian syndrome). Severe obstruction of the upper respiratory tract, which may occur in cases of extremely enlarged tonsils or adenoids, may result in diminished breathing during sleep; it usually improves with adenoidectomy. Less severe blockage may occur in cow's milk allergy (also called Heiner's syndrome), and this usually improves with elimination of cow's milk protein from the diet.

See also CHRONIC OBSTRUCTIVE PULMONARY DISEASE; HEINER'S SYNDROME.

hypoxemia Lack of sufficient oxygen in the blood.

hypoxia Lack of sufficient oxygen circulating to body tissues.

hysteria A state of severe anxiety that can involve emotional and physical symptoms, uncontrollable laughter, crying, or fear reactions. Individuals who experience severe shortness of breath may become so stressed as to be hysterical. The term, derived from the Greek word *hystera*, or womb, was once applied to a woman's disorder; contemporary terms for such anxiety include conversion, dissociative, or somatization disorders, and psychoneurosis.

idiopathic pulmonary fibrosis A lung disease secondary to interstitial pneumonitis or fibrosis characterized by dyspnea, weakness and fatigue, anoxia, rapid respirations, progressing to cyanosis, clubbed fingers, and heart failure. Corticosteroids, cyclophosphamide, other antibiotics, and oxygen therapy are among the treatments of this disease, which is usually fatal four to five years after its onset.

See also HAMMAN-RICH SYNDROME.

idiosyncrasy An individual's unexpected abnormal response to a food, drug, or other usually non-allergenic substance.

ID tags See MEDICAL ALERT BRACELETS AND NECKLACES.

IgE-mediated reactions An alternate term for immediate allergic reactions.

See also HYPERSENSITIVITY; IMMUNOGLOBULIN E.

illuminating gas A combination of combustible gases such as hydrogen and carbon monoxide, which can be poisonous. Resuscitation may be necessary as treatment.

Ilosone See ERYTHROMYCIN.

imagery A technique using mental pictures, sounds, odors, tastes, feelings, and other sensory experiences in order to understand and resolve psychological and physical problems. Imagery is also employed as a relaxation technique.

immediate hypersensitivity An alternate term for immediate allergic reactions.

See also HYPERSENSITIVITY.

immune complex A cluster of interlocking antigens and antibodies found in the bloodstream and usually cleared away by cells known as phagocytes, which "consume" and destroy other cells recognized as invaders. When this process fails, immune complexes may be deposited in, injure, and cause inflammation in tissues, such as kidney, lung, skin, joints, and walls of blood vessels. Diseases in which these complexes are involved include those in the category of type III hypersensitivity (antigen-antibody complement reactions): drug-induced systemic lupus erythematosus, serum sickness, nephritis, and bacterial endocarditis.

immune complex assay Methods of detection of circulating clusters of antigens and antibodies, or immune complexes, that are used to measure disease activity in patients with vasculitis, systemic lupus erythematosus, some malignancies, and other diseases. Immune complex assay is of doubtful importance in allergy diagnosis.

See also IMMUNE COMPLEX DISORDERS.

immune complex disorders A group of diseases associated with failure of the complement system and other components of the immune system. Immune complexes are aggregations or clusters of interlocking antigens and antibodies. Usually, these complexes are removed from the circulation by large phagocytic cells (macrophages) in the spleen and Kupffer cells in the liver. Research suggests that deficiencies of certain components of the complement system or complement receptors disrupt this process, allowing circulating immune complexes to accumulate inappropriately in certain organs such as the kidneys, lungs, skin, joints, or blood vessels and interfering with their function. An example is systemic lupus erythematosus ("lupus"). In this autoimmune disease, a continuous supply of autoantibodies overloads the immune system's ability to remove the immune complexes. Immune complexes also play an important destructive role in many other diseases, including infections such as viral hepatitis, malaria, and allergic lung disorders such as farmer's lung.

immune system A complex network of specialized cells and organs that protect the body against attacks by foreign invaders such as infections. When the immune system is intact, it fights off pathogenic, or disease-causing, bacteria, viruses, fungi, and parasites. When it is weakened or fails, the results can range from a minor allergy such as hay fever to the usually fatal acquired immunodeficiency syndrome, or AIDS.

The immune system protects by barring the entry of, or destroying, dangerous foreign organisms while fostering peaceful coexistence of protective or beneficial organisms. The immune response requires a complex but cooperative interplay between the various cells of the system, including effector lymphocytes (killer T cells, antibody-producing B cells, mast cells), regulating lymphocytes (T-helper and T-suppressor cells), and phagocytes. Many other factors, some not yet understood by scientists, are involved in the control of and response to immune stimuli. The immune system is further influenced by genes that determine the body's ability to respond to an antigen. Mutation, congenital or acquired, of certain genes may impair our response not only to allergens and infectious microorganisms but to cancerous cells as well.

Tissues and Organs of the Immune System

Immune system components are scattered throughout the body. Bone marrow, thymus, spleen, tonsils, adenoids, lymph nodes, the appendix, and Peyer's patches in the small intestine are known as lymphoid organs, named for their ability to produce, develop, or control white blood cells, or lymphocytes.

There are two major types of lymphocyte: B cells and T cells. Bone marrow is soft tissue in the hollow shafts of long bones. The marrow produces all blood cells, including mature B cells. T cells migrate to the thymus, a gland located behind the breastbone, where they multiply and mature. In a process called "T-cell education," these cells become immunocompetent—that is, they develop the ability to evoke an immune response and learn to distinguish self from nonself cells. B and T cells circulate throughout the blood vessels and lymphatics, a network similar to blood vessels.

Clusters of lymph nodes, located in the neck, armpits, abdomen, and groin, contain collections of B and T lymphocytes and other cells capable of engaging antigens and causing an immune response.

The spleen is a scavenger of the immune system. An encapsulated, highly vascular, fist-sized organ in the left upper portion of the abdomen, the spleen contains two distinct regions of tissues, the red and white pulp. Red pulp disposes of worn-out blood cells. Red pulp also contains immune cells called macrophages, which trap and destroy microorganisms in blood passing through the spleen during the circulatory process. White pulp contains lymphoid tissue similar to that of the lymph nodes and is similarly subdivided into compartments specializing in different types of immune cells. Patients with a nonfunctioning spleen or who have had the spleen surgically removed are highly susceptible to infections. The tonsils and adenoids in the respiratory tract and the appendix and Peyer's patches in the digestive tract are nonencapsulated clusters of lymphoid tissue in the body's main ports of entry—the mouth, nose, and anus.

Lymph is a clear fluid that travels through the lymphatic vessels, bathing the body tissues. Lymph, along with lymphocytes, macrophages, other cells, and foreign antigens, drains out of tissues and seeps across the thin walls of lymphatic vessels to be transported to lymph nodes, where antigens can be filtered out and attacked by immune cells. Other lymphocytes enter and exit the nodes from the bloodstream. Tiny lymphatics feed into larger and larger channels, like small creeks joining larger streams and rivers. At the base of the neck, large lymphatic vessels merge into the thoracic duct, where its contents are emptied into the bloodstream to begin the cycle again.

Self and Nonself

The ability of the immune system to distinguish between self and nonself is vital to its function. All body cells have distinctive molecules that allow them to be recognized as "self." When the immune system malfunctions, it may attack its own body. This occurs in diseases such as rheumatoid arthritis and systemic lupus erythematosus, which are referred to as autoimmune disorders.

Antigens, Allergens, or Immunogens

Any substance capable of triggering an immune response is called an antigen, allergen, or immunogen. An antigen can be a bacterium, fungus, parasite, virus, or a part of a substance produced by those organisms. However, not all antigens are capable of causing an antibody response, and some may provoke a cellular, or delayed hypersensitivity, response or even tolerance. Tissues or cells from another individual, except an identical twin, are also antigenic, that is, recognized as foreign.

The structure of antigenic molecules varies from proteins, polysaccharides, lipids, or nucleic acids. The molecular weight of antigens ranges from less than a thousand to several million daltons (a unit of mass = approximately 1.65×10^{-24}) but must reach a threshold size in order to stimulate an immune response. Although the exact size required for allergenicity is unknown, the larger the size of a molecule, the better the chance that it will invoke a reaction. From the human organism to the smallest and simplest microbes, all cells have structures called epitopes on their surfaces that are characteristic and unique to that cell. Epitopes enable the immune system to recognize foreign cells and are the smallest antigenic structure capable of recognition by an antibody. Most cells carry different kinds of epitopes, which may number up to several hundred, on their surface. However, these epitopes differ in their immune-stimulating capabilities.

Haptens are molecules too small to elicit an immune response in themselves. However, when haptens are coupled to a carrier immunogenic mol-

ecule, usually a protein or synthetic polypeptide, they can cause a very strong allergic response. Penicillin is one of many drugs that are haptens that bind with serum protein. This complex molecule then stimulates an allergic reaction to the penicillin or other drug. Other examples are the allergic responses to plant substances or metals that cause rashes upon contact with skin. The sensitizing allergens in poison ivy, oak, and sumac are haptens that combine with proteins in the skin. Upon subsequent exposure to these substances, antibodies in the skin react, causing the often debilitating contact dermatitis. Antigens such as pollen grains or cat dander are categorized as allergens because of their ability to provoke an allergic response in susceptible individuals. The first time an allergic individual is exposed to an allergen, the immune system responds by making a corresponding antibody. The antibody molecules are called immunoglobulin E (IgE). IgE molecules attach to the surfaces of mast cells in tissues or basophils in the circulatory system.

Multiple factors determine the potential for an immune response. Among these are foreignness and chemical structure of the antigen. The genetic disposition of the exposed individual and the method of exposure—by injection, orally, skin or mucous membrane contact, or inhalation—affect the strength of immune response.

Cells of the Immune System

The immune system maintains a huge array of cells, some always present and others manufactured upon demand. Some cell types control general body defenses, while others target specific, highly selective targets. A competent immune system relies on the interactions of many of these cells by direct contact or by the release of chemical messengers by some.

When mast cells or basophils with IgE antibodies on their surface encounter specific allergens, they release biochemical substances called mediators. Mediators include histamine, heparin, prostaglandins, and leukotrienes. These chemicals cause allergic symptoms—wheezing, sneezing, runny nose, watery eyes, and itching. The most serious response of the immune system is anaphylaxis, characterized by edema or swelling of body tissues and a sudden, dangerous decrease in blood pressure that can be life-threatening.

Antibodies

Immunoglobulins, commonly called antibodies, are protein molecules produced and secreted by B cells (lymphocytes manufactured in the bone marrow) designed to attack a specific foreign invader called an antigen. The resulting antibody is capable of binding, or attaching, to that specific antigen. For example, a cold virus stimulates a B cell to produce an antibody against that specific virus. When a B cell encounters its triggering antigen, T cells and other accessory cells collaborate with it to cause the production of large plasma cells. Each plasma cell becomes a factory for producing antibodies. Transported through the circulation to the site of inflammation or infection, antibodies neutralize or combine with and identify antigens for attack by other cells or chemical mediators.

All antibodies have a common Y-shaped molecular structure consisting of two light (L) and two heavy (H) polypeptide chains bound together by two disulfide linkages or bridges. The resulting light and heavy chain section is called the fragment antigen binding, or Fab. A third portion of the immunoglobulin, Fc fragment, does not combine with antigen. The Fc portion of the antibody binds to cells, fixes complement, and allows for placental transfer. The five classes of immunoglobulins (Ig) identified in humans are IgA, IgM, IgD, IgE, and IgG. These immunoglobulins are distinguished by the structure of heavy chains called, respectively, τ, α, μ, ζ, and Σ. The two types of light chains are kappa (k) or lambda (L). IgG is the predominant human antibody and along with the other immunoglobulins has special roles in maintaining body defenses.

Genes direct the manufacture of all body protein molecules including antibodies. (Insulin is another example.) Although there is a limited number of genes, the immune system apparently can produce an unlimited number of antibodies. The DNA segment of most genes is fixed; however, antibody genes are constructed from fragments of DNA scattered throughout the genetic material. A B cell sorts through the available material, arranging and rearranging these fragments and piecing them together to form a new gene that with the antibody it encodes is unique. Each B cell proliferates, or clones, identical antibody-producing cells. As the cells continue to multiply, mutants arise that allow for the selection of antibodies that target specific antigens. This process enables antibodies to respond to an enormous range of antigens. T cells, or T lymphocytes, are processed by the thymus gland, act directly by attacking viruses and fungi, and are involved in transplantation rejection reactions. T cells react with specific antigens similar to antibodies. There are three types of T lymphocytes: "killer" T cells, which directly attack antigens; "helper" T cells, which help the killer cells; and "suppressor" T cells, which regulate the killer cells' activity and stop their action when an infection has been controlled.

Phagocytic white blood cells destroy invading foreign microbes by directly engulfing them. Most phagocytes are macrophages, large mononucleated cells derived from monocytes, which are produced and mature in the bone marrow. After a few days, they leave the general circulation and enter various tissues. Other phagocytic cells include Langerhans cells of the skin, dendritic cells, keratinocytes, and brain astrocytes. These cells affect chemotaxis (cell movement) by engulfing foreign antigens, ridding the body of dead tissues and cells. In the process of phagocytosis, these cells process the antigen and present an immunologically active antigen to the T lymphocytes. The macrophages are not antigen-specific like lymphocytes. Microphages consume bacteria.

Complement is a complex series of blood proteins whose action "complements" the action of antibodies. The complement system comprises about 25 proteins that coat bacteria or immune complexes. This coating facilitates their ingestion and destruction by phagocytes. Complement also destroys bacteria by puncturing their cell membranes.

When the complement system is activated by either the "classic" or an "alternative pathway" (also called the "proteolytic" or "properdin" pathway), an inflammatory response occurs. Immune complexes, consisting of IgG or IgM classes of immunoglobulin antibodies combined with antigen, activate a pathway targeting an invading substance. During this process, the enzyme C1 esterase sets off a cascading-type reaction against the invader. The "proteolytic" alternative, or "properdin" pathway, can be activated without the presence of antibodies.

The complement system not only aids in the body's defense against infection but also helps protect against immune-complex diseases. However, if there is a deficiency of certain components of the system or cell receptors are deficient, the complement can actually induce immune-complex disorders such as serum lupus erythematosus. Serum complement levels are often measured to help diagnose hereditary angioedema, bacterial endocarditis, acute glomerulonephritis, serum sickness, systemic lupus erythematosus, and other autoimmune diseases.

A deficiency in any component of the immune system may result in an immune deficiency disorder. In some cases there are no clinical manifestations, but in others recurrent, minor, or life-threatening infections may occur.

See also IMMUNOGLOBULIN A; IMMUNOGLOBULIN D; IMMUNOGLOBULIN E; IMMUNOGLOBULIN G; IMMUNOGLOBULIN M.

immunity   The quality of being protected from, or resistant to, infection, disease, and any "invasion" imposed on the body. Being immune involves the ability of the immune system—consisting of white blood cells manufactured by the bone marrow, thymus, lymph, and other structures—to prevent or fight an infectious disease. Natural resistance or immunity refers to the human body's rejection of certain cells, such as those causing Texas cattle fever, which cannot live in human tissues. Immunity is described in various ways: natural, passive, humoral, and cell-mediated (cellular).

See also ACTIVE IMMUNITY; IMMUNITY, PASSIVE.

immunity, passive   The protection from disease afforded by way of antibodies received by an infant from its mother through the placenta or breast milk, or antibodies conveyed by injecting immune serum globulin (gamma globulin) from an individual known to be immune to a certain disease into a susceptible individual. Passive immunity is short-lived, but immediate protection against an infection.

Serum from immune individuals or animals is pooled to achieve a highly concentrated suspension of antibodies against a specific infection such as hepatitis or tetanus. Immediate tetanus protection can be administered to a non-immunized person by injecting human tetanus immunoglobulin. Horse-derived equine tetanus antitoxin is rarely used because of the frequent occurrence of severe adverse reactions.

immunodeficiency disease   A defect or insufficiency of one or more components of the immune system resulting in an inability to fight off infections. A variety of immunodeficiency disorders can be inherited, acquired through infection or other illness, or caused by an adverse reaction to certain drugs.

Some children are born with abnormal B-cell components and lack the ability to produce immunoglobulins or antibodies. These defects may be absolute, as in agammaglobulinemias, or partial, as in hypogammaglobulinemias. Injections of immunoglobulins can protect these children against infections. Children who lack T cells as a result of abnormal or missing thymus glands can be treated by thymus transplantation. Rarely, an infant lacks all immune defenses, which is referred to as severe combined immunodeficiency disease (SCID). These are the so-called bubble children who often live for years in germ-free rooms. Bone marrow transplants have cured a few of these children.

Acquired immunodeficiency syndrome, or AIDS, is caused by the human immunodeficiency virus, or HIV. In AIDS, a virus destroys helper T cells, allowing microorganisms that are normally harmless to cause life-threatening infections. These are referred to as "opportunistic infections."

See also ACQUIRED IMMUNODEFICIENCY SYNDROME; IMMUNODEFICIENCY DISEASE, SEVERE COMBINED (SCID).

immunodeficiency disease, severe combined (SCID)   A genetic disorder of the immune system giving rise to what has been called "bubble babies"—children who are afflicted with SCID and require a highly protective environment to avoid contracting potentially fatal infectious diseases. Approximately one-third of SCID victims have shown a deficiency of the enzyme adenosine deaminase, which may be a cause of SCID. Enzyme replacement therapy treatments involve injections of the drug pegademase bovine.

SCID is considered the most severe immunodeficiency disorder; victims lack adequate quantities of B lymphocytes and antibodies, and their T lymphocytes are either deficient or not functioning. SCID that afflicts infants usually begins with pneumonia and thrush (an oral fungal infection), and if untreated, an infant may not live into a second year. Diarrhea and other infections such as pneumocystitis pneumonia may also develop during infancy. Treatment options include antibiotics, immunoglobulin, and bone marrow or umbilical cord blood transplantation.

immunofluorescence, direct   A test to detect antibodies in tissue specimens used to aid in the diagnosis of glomerulonephritis, systemic lupus erythematosus, Goodpasture's syndrome, pemphigoid, pemphigus, and dermatitis herpetiformis, and herpes simplex infections.

immunofluorescence, indirect   A test to measure the presence and quantity of antibodies in body fluids. It is especially useful in detecting autoantibodies in diseases including diabetes mellitus, thyroiditis, myasthenia gravis, chronic active hepatitis, systemic lupus erythematosus, systemic sclerosis, pernicious anemia, pemphigus, and bullous pemphigoid.

immunogen   Any substance capable of triggering an immune response. Immunogens may also be called antigens or allergens. An antigen can be a bacterium, fungus, parasite, virus, or a part of a substance produced by those organisms.

immunoglobulin A (IgA) (secretory antibody)   The primary immunoglobulin in body orifices, or entrances. IgAs are concentrated in body fluids such as the bronchial and intestinal secretions,

especially tears and saliva. IgA recognizes invading microorganisms in the mucous membranes as foreign protein. It combines with these invaders in antigen-antibody reactions to prevent viral and bacterial infections such as brucella, diphtheria, and poliomyelitis. IgA deficiency is the most common primary immunodeficiency, occurring in about one in 400 to 800 individuals, and more frequently in those with allergy. Most persons with low IgA levels produce sufficient IgM antibodies to provide an adequate defense against infections. However, IgA deficiencies are commonly associated with chronic lung infections, autoimmune diseases, especially rheumatoid arthritis and systemic lupus erythematosus, gastrointestinal disorders, hepatitis, and some malignant tumors. There are no known cures, and treatment is directed at the underlying disease or infection. Human immune globulin contains only minimal levels of IgA and is of no value in treating IgA deficiency disorders. In addition, IgA may cause anaphylaxis in persons with this deficiency.

See also IMMUNOGLOBULIN G.

immunoglobulin D (IgD)   A class of antibodies found in very small concentrations in human serum. IgD antibodies, first discovered in the 1960s, are found on the surface of lymphocytes. Although the IgD antibody's exact role has yet to be defined, it seems to play a role as a specific surface receptor in the immune response.

immunoglobulin E (IgE)   Antibodies manufactured by the immune system that play an important role in primary type I hypersensitivity, or immediate allergic, responses. Once called "reaginic antibodies," these antibodies are normally present in very small quantities. Allergic individuals generally have higher total IgE levels in their blood. However, other diseases can also be associated with very high levels of IgE antibodies.

Skin-sensitizing, anaphylactic antibodies are of this type. IgE antibodies' unique biologic properties are based on their ability to bind with special receptors on mast cells and basophils in body tissues. People differ in their ability to develop an IgE response to common allergens in the environment. The tendency to produce IgE antibodies is genetic.

When IgE antibodies specific to a previously sensitized allergen are reexposed to that allergen, cells degranulate and chemical mediators of anaphylaxis and type I reactions are released.

DISORDERS ASSOCIATED WITH ELEVATED SERUM IgE LEVELS

Acral dermatitis
Allergic diseases (severely elevated levels in allergic bronchopulmonary aspergillosis)
Bone marrow transplantation (immediately post-transplantation)
Bullous pemphigoid
Celiac disease (gluten-sensitive enteropathy)
Drug-induced interstitial nephritis
IgE myeloma
Infectious mononucleosis
Job-Buckley syndrome
Kawasaki disease
Laënnec's cirrhosis
Minimal change nephritis
Parasitic infections
Polyarteritis nodosa
Pulmonary hemosiderosis
Selective IgA deficiency
T-cell deficiency (DiGeorge syndrome, Wiskott-Aldrich syndrome, Nezelof syndrome)
Wegener's granulomatosus

Serum levels of IgE antibodies can be measured as "total IgE" or to identify specific allergens. This measurement is performed by a method called radioallergosorbent tests (RAST). Testing for allergen-specific IgE by RAST is useful when skin testing is unreliable because of generalized skin disease or dermatographia, or if the patient is unable to discontinue antihistamines.

immunoglobulin E (IgE) assay (total IgE, PRIST, RIST)   A quantitative test measuring immunoglobulin E antibodies in the blood serum to assess an individual's tendency to have allergies. An elevated level of IgE antibody in blood obtained from the umbilical cord at birth correlates with an increased risk of the development of allergy in later life. Persons with high total IgE levels are usually sensitive to many allergens, but an individual can be sensitive to specific IgE allergens and have a low total IgE level. Furthermore, allergic bronchopulmonary aspergillosis, parasitic infections, and other

rare diseases can cause extreme elevations in total IgE. There may be elevations of circulating IgE antibodies in some persons with food allergies, but the Allergy Council on Scientific Affairs of the American Medical Association considers this test investigational and experimental.

The Paper Radioimmunosorbent Test and Radioimmunosorbent Test (both blood tests) are methods of measuring total IgE. In 1981, the Immunology Unit, a committee of the World Health Organization, recommended against the measurement of total IgE as a screening test for allergy.

RELATIONSHIP OF IgE LEVELS TO DIAGNOSIS OF ALLERGY

Total IgEU/ml	Predictability of Allergic Tendency
>100	Multiple allergens highly likely
25–100	Intermediate
<25	Low probability of allergy

RADIOALLERGOSORBENT LEVELS (TRADITIONAL METHOD)

RAST Class	Level of Antigen-Specific IgE
4	Very high
3	High
2	Moderate
1	Low
1/0	Very low
0	Below detection

immunoglobulin E (IgE) immune complexes   The percentage (up to 50 percent) of immunoglobulin E (IgE) circulating in the bloodstream in immune-complex form. The relevance of these complexes to allergy is unknown.

immunoglobulin G (IgG)   The most common antibody in human serum, found throughout the circulatory system and other body tissues. IgG immunoglobulins enjoy a relatively long half-life (the time required for half the amount of a specific substance to be eliminated or to disintegrate in the body) of 23 days and readily cross the placenta.

Antibodies of this class are involved in the immune system's defense against bacterial, viral, parasitic, and some fungal infections. Receptors for IgG are found on the surface of monocytes, on polymorphonuclear leukocytes, or polys, on reticuloendothelial cells in the spleen and liver, and on some lymphocytes. IgG antibodies also activate complement.

immunoglobulin G (IgG) subclasses   Minor differences in molecular structure among a specific class of antibodies. Two IgA and IgD and four IgG immunoglobulin subclasses have been discovered. The minor variations, however, may result in significant differences in the function of these subclasses. Repeated infections may occur in individuals who have normal levels of total IgG but absent or reduced levels of one or more of the subclasses. Such persons fail to develop antibody responses to naturally occurring infections or to vaccines.

immunoglobulin M (IgM)   The largest antibody molecules of the immune system, found almost exclusively in the circulation. IgM is the major antibody of the early humoral response to foreign invaders, particularly to nonprotein bacterial antigens. Although its large molecular size prohibits transfer through the human placenta, its structure allows for IgM's ability to agglutinate, or clump, particles of bacteria and red blood cells and fix, or attach, to complement.

immunoglobulins   Another term for antibodies.

immunologist   A physician who diagnoses and treats disorders of the immune system, such as acquired immunodeficiency syndrome, or AIDS. Many immunologists are also allergists, but some are nonphysician scientists who do not care for patients. Upon completion of medical school, a two- or three-year residency in pediatrics or internal medicine, and a two-year fellowship in allergy and immunology, these doctors are then eligible for a board-certification examination in their specialty.

immunology   The study of immunity and immune responses, which are the bodily processes whose main function is to maintain a constant internal environment and to protect the body from, and/or help the body fight, the invasion of disease-causing microorganisms. The field of immunology evolved from the ancient Chinese practice of variolation as early as the 11th century, in which intradermal applications of powdered smallpox scabs were used to prevent smallpox.

immunopathology   The study or science of the body's immune reactions to disease-causing, or pathogenic, microorganisms.

immunopolysaccharide   Antigenic substances obtained from the bodies of specific infectious bacteria that have the ability to stimulate the production of antibodies to protect against that particular infection. Immunizations against pneumococcal pneumonia and *Haemophilus influenzae* (cause of meningitis in infants) are examples of polysaccharide vaccines.

immunostimulant   Any foreign agent, including allergens, microbes, or vaccines, that will cause the production of antibodies.

immunosuppressant   Any agent, such as cancer-fighting drugs, that inhibits the immune response.

immunotherapy (allergy shots)   A series of injections of solutions of allergenic extracts administered to a person suffering from allergies. By gradually injecting increasing doses of specific allergens to which that individual has been shown to be sensitive, the individual is expected to develop a tolerance to those allergens and experience few or no symptoms upon environmental exposure.

Mechanism of Action

Researchers believe a positive response to allergy immunotherapy requires an increase in immunoglobulin G (IgG)-blocking antibody, which is capable of blocking allergic reactions mediated by IgE antibodies. Five changes in the immune response have been recognized in persons receiving immunotherapy: (1) a rise in blood levels of

IgG-blocking antibodies; (2) a suppression of the usual seasonal rise in IgE antibodies followed by a slow decline in the level of specific IgE antibodies during continued immunotherapy; (3) an increase in levels blocking IgA and IgG antibodies in body secretions; (4) a diminished ability of basophilic cells to react to allergens; and (5) a tempering of the reactivity of lymphocytic cells in contact with allergens *in vitro* (tests performed in a test tube or an artificial environment). An individual may be sufficiently protected from allergy without demonstrating all five postulates.

Treatment Course

Treatment usually begins once or twice weekly until a maintenance dose is achieved. Therapy is usually continued at monthly intervals for three to five years. In most persons, however, symptoms eventually recur, and treatment is sometimes repeated. Immunotherapy usually requires six to 12 months of regular injections; if there is no beneficial response within two years, it is generally recommended that treatment be discontinued.

Allergens included in immunotherapy are based on skin or blood tests and a detailed medical history of the patient to determine a person's sensitivity to a particular allergen or multiple allergens. Many individuals show positive tests to substances that are not the cause of their allergy symptoms. Allergens not directly responsible for triggering an individual's symptoms should not be included in the solution. Allergy immunotherapy is a consideration when avoidance of offending allergens and medications are ineffective. Immunotherapy has been shown to be effective for allergy symptoms associated with grass, tree, and weed pollens, house-dust mites, cat dander, and certain molds. Stinging insect venom immunotherapy is also highly effective.

House-dust mixture is prepared from dust collected by beating carpets or vacuuming. Responsiveness is related to the presence of cat and dog dander, house-dust mites, cockroaches, and other allergens in the preparation. But variation in potency and effectiveness of batches of extract does not permit standardization, and the availability of house-dust extract may eventually be withdrawn by the Food and Drug Administration.

immunotherapy, oral The administration of an allergen extract liquid by mouth, a method of immunotherapy now being investigated by researchers at the Johns Hopkins Asthma and Allergy Center. Administering an allergen dose 100 times that of a typical injected dose of ragweed antigen to patients resulted in clinically significant improvement of hay fever symptoms, such as sneezing, nasal congestion, and itchy eyes. Side effects have been minimal; a few patients show a mild worsening of symptoms, abdominal cramps, or a tightness in the throat. These adverse effects cleared up with slight reduction in dosage of the allergen.

Oral immunotherapy has been shown to be effective against allergy through the body's increased ability to promote an IgG-blocking antibody response.

immunotransfusion Transfusion of blood from a donor who has antibodies against a specific infection from having been inoculated with bacteria from the recipient patient or from the specific infection, or who has recently recovered from that infection.

infarction, pulmonary Necrosis, or death, of part of a lung because blood supply to the area has halted. Pulmonary embolism is usually the cause of the infarct, and treatment includes oxygen therapy, reduction of pain, and restoring the circulatory system.

infection carriers From the French word *carier,* meaning to bear, an individual who has no symptoms of infection but may be able to transmit it to others. Carriers may be human, animal, or substances, such as blood and bodily fluids. Microorganisms may also be carried by insects or intermediary hosts such as soil and water. Human carriers may asymptomatically harbor parasites or pathogenic microorganisms, a prime example of which is "Typhoid Mary." Mary Mallon was an Irish domestic in the United States during the 1930s. When members of the family for whom she worked contracted typhoid fever, it was discovered that she was the carrier and that her questionable hygiene led to her spreading of the bacterium *Salmonella typhi.* The bacterium lives in the carrier. If a carrier handles food without applying fastidious cleanliness measures, as did Mallon, the bacterium may be transmitted. She spread typhoid fever throughout New York City before she died in 1938.

In addition to asymptomatic contact carriers, there are incubationary carriers, or those who have just become infected by a pathogenic microorganism and have not yet gone through the incubation period, and convalescent carriers, or those who have recovered from the illness but in whose body the disease-causing organism still remains. Proper handwashing, especially before and after using the toilet, is essential in preventing the spread of disease.

A genetic carrier refers to a parent-child transmission of a mutant, disease-causing gene. Prenatal genetic testing is available to determine prospective parents' risks.

One of the most volatile of carriers is an individual with an active infection from which he or she is suffering. Avoiding contact with the individual is the primary means of prevention. In hospital units that specialize in highly infectious diseases, methods for isolation, such as gloves, gowns, masks, and preventive techniques, are employed.

infection, respiratory tract (RTI)   An invasion of the body's respiratory tract or organs by pathogenic, or disease-producing, microbes and the symptoms that occur from the presence of these bacteria, viruses, parasites, or fungi, or from toxins produced by these organisms. An infection may also be present without detectable symptoms.

inflammation   Redness, heat, and pain associated with cellular injury upon the exposure to allergens or pathogens and occurring when white blood cells migrate to a traumatized or hypersensitive area of the body. Inflammation is a major contributing factor to chronic asthma. After each exposure to an allergen or pathogen that results in inflammation in lung tissues, the tissues attempt to repair themselves. This leads to subepithelial fibrosis, thickened noncellular (basement) membranes that may be permanent and occur very early in the course of

asthma. Anti-inflammatory therapy is a mainstay of asthma treatment. Cromolyn sodium (Intal), nedocromil sodium (Tilade), and corticosteroids by metered doses are used to prevent inflammatory changes in the lungs. However, systemic corticosteroids, by injection or orally, are often required in moderate to severe cases. The inflammatory changes that occur with allergic skin disorders such as contact dermatitis result in the itching, burning, and rashes characteristic of these conditions.

influenza   Derived from the Italian word meaning influence, an acute, highly contagious infection of the respiratory tract caused by the influenza virus. Numerous forms of the virus have been identified, such as types A, B, and C, and subtypes, including human, swine, equine, and avian. The virus has a great capacity to vary, which is why epidemics of one form of flu may occur in populations that have already been exposed to a different form.

Nicknamed the "flu," influenza causes sudden fever of 101 to 103 degrees Fahrenheit, chills, headache, muscle pain (particularly in the back), sore throat, sneezing, coughing, lack of appetite, and other symptoms that last usually from two to seven or eight days. Nausea, vomiting, and diarrhea may sometimes accompany the infection, but the term "stomach flu" may actually describe gastrointestinal illnesses caused by other microorganisms.

Most flu sufferers recover completely, but some develop secondary nasal infections of the sinuses, middle ear, and lungs, pneumonia or other complications that may be life-threatening. More than 100,000 hospitalizations and 200,000 deaths throughout the nation occur each year. The most susceptible members of the population are the elderly, individuals with chronic medical problems, and infants, although medical sources also claim that healthy, young adults may be very susceptible. Spread by discharges from the nose and mouth of infected individuals, the influenza virus is the only organism that still causes acute epidemics in America.

In 1918, there was an influenza pandemic—the "Spanish flu"—that caused the greatest flu-related mortality rate. Approximately 500,000 people died in the United States, and 20 million died through-out the world. The flu became so dramatic that a book by Gina Kolata, *Flu: The Story of the Great Influenza Pandemic of 1918 and the Search for the Virus That Caused It,* has been published. In 1957–58, the "Asian flu" caused 70,000 deaths in America. In 1968–69, the "Hong Kong flu" took the lives of 34,000 in America.

Flu-virus A subtypes are identified by two viral proteins: hemagglutinin (H) and neuraminidase (N). Flu A viruses may undergo changes called "antigenic drift." This means a virus mutates and gradually changes, enabling the virus to escape the efforts of a person's immune system and cause a permanent susceptibility to influenza. Another "drift"—known as an antigenic "shift"—is charac-terized by a sudden change in the hemagglutinin and/or the neuraminidase proteins, which pro-duces a new strain of influenza virus. Unlike influenza A viruses, influenza B viruses shift only through the slower process.

According to the *Morbidity and Mortality Weekly Report* of March 23, 2001, printed by the U.S. gov-ernment, influenza activity was summarized from October 1, 2000, to March 10, 2001. "Influenza increased in December and January and peaked at the end of January," the report says. "The most fre-quently isolated viruses were influenza A (H1N1); however, influenza B viruses have been co-circu-lating and appear to be increasing. . . . The World Health Organization (WHO) collaborating labora-tories and National Respiratory and Enteric Virus Surveillance System (NREVSS) laboratories tested 64,840 specimens for influenza, and 8,386 (13 per-cent) were positive. Of these, 4,885 (58 percent) were influenza type A and 3,501 (42 percent) were influenza type B. Of the 4,885 influenza A viruses identified, 1,826 (36 percent) were subtyped: 1,746 (96 percent) were A (H1N1) and 80 (4 percent) were A (H3N2). The percentage of specimens posi-tive for influenza injections, an indicator of influenza activity, peaked at 24 percent during the week ending January 27, 2001. For the week end-ing March 10, 6 percent of tested specimens were positive for influenza."

The report also says the Centers for Disease Con-trol and Prevention (CDC) antigenically character-ized 436 flu viruses since October 1, although state and territorial epidemiologists report that flu activ-ity peaked during the weeks ending February 3 and 10, 2001, when 28 states reported regional or widespread activity. "This peak was lower than those reported during the 1997–98, 1998–99, and 1999–2000 seasons, when 46, 43, and 44 states reported regional or widespread influenza activity, respectively. . . . As reported by the 122 Cities Mor-tality Reporting System, the percentage of total deaths that resulted from P&I (pneumonia and influenza) remained below the epidemic threshold each week since October 1. During the previous three, the percentage of deaths attributed to P&I was above epidemic threshold for 10 consecutive weeks each season." The CDC reports flu data October through May and is available by telephone at (888) 232-3228, the fax information system at (888) 232-3299 (request document number 261100), or on the web at http://www. cdc.gov1/ ncidod/diseases/flu/weekly.htm.

Influenza A (H3N2) viruses predominated throughout the world for the third consecutive sea-son during 1999–2000, according to the American Medical Association, and the influenza vaccine should be effective against the viruses. In addition, the AMA reported that the 2000–01 season was the first for which flu vaccination is recommended for everyone 50 years or older.

Influenza A (H3N2) outbreaks occurred in Tu-nisia, China, Albania, Austria, Belarus, Belgium, Bulgaria, Croatia, Czech Republic, Denmark, Fin-land, France, Germany, Hungary, Iceland, Ireland, Israel, Italy, Latvia, Netherlands, Norway, Poland, Portugal, Romania, Russian Federation, Slovakia, Spain, Sweden, Switzerland, Ukraine, United King-dom, United States, and Canada, with sporadic cases reported in Argentina, Australia, Brazil, Republic of Cyprus, Egypt, Greece, Guam, French Guyana, India, Republic of Syria, Taiwan, Thailand, Turkey, and the Federal Republic of Yugoslavia. Influenza A (H1N1) cases occurred in the Hong Kong SAR of China, Japan, and Spain, with isolates of the same virus sporadically occurring in Ar-gentina, Australia, Belgium, Brazil, Canada, Chile, China, France, Germany, Iceland, Italy, Latvia, Philippines, Portugal, Russian Federation, Saudi Arabia, Singapore, South Africa, Spain, Thailand, United Kingdom, United States, and Vietnam.

Influenza B incidences were low, but some cases were reported in Argentina, Australia, Brazil, Canada, China, Croatia, Czech Republic, Egypt, Finland, France, Germany, Hong Kong SAR of China, Hungary, Iceland, Israel, Italy, Japan, Republic of Korea, Madagascar, Malaysia, New Caledonia, New Zealand, Norway, Philippines, Russian Federation, Singapore, Senegal, South Africa, Spain, Sweden, Syria, Taiwan, Thailand, Tunisia, United Kingdom, United States, Vietnam, and the Federal Republic of Yugoslavia.

Type C infections usually cause a mild respiratory illness or no symptoms, thereby posing no real threat to public health like the A and B viruses.

Many aspects of the influenza viruses remain a mystery for researchers. Treatment is mainly bedrest, forcing fluids, analgesics, antipyretics, and nasal decongestants. Antibiotics are not treatment for flu unless there is another bacterial infection present. Amantadine or rimantadine given early may help prevent or treat influenza A infection.

Vaccination against influenza is available. According to the CDC, flu can be prevented by an annual vaccine and is specifically recommended for people 50 years and older and people of any age who have chronic heart, lung, or kidney disease, people with diabetes or severe forms of anemia, and those who are immunosuppressed. In addition, the vaccine is recommended for nursing home or chronic care facility residents, women who will be more than three months pregnant during the flu season, and children and teenagers who are receiving long-term aspirin therapy and are at risk of developing Reye's syndrome following a bout with influenza. Health caregivers and others in contact with individuals in the high-risk groups should also be vaccinated. Travelers may risk exposure to influenza depending upon the time of year and their destination. Flu occurs year-round in the tropics, April through September in temperate regions of the Southern Hemisphere. In temperate zones of both Northern and Southern Hemispheres, travelers may risk exposure during the summer months. Because flu vaccine may not be available during the summer in North America, individuals wishing to travel should consult with their physicians. Antiviral medications may be advised for prevention or treatment of flu contracted outside the United States.

An article in *Blended Medicine,* published by Rodale in July 2000, reported that a passenger with the flu took a five-hour flight, and three days later 72 percent of the other passengers contracted the disease. Alternative methods of prevention and treatment include (1) consume only liquids for a day or two after the onset of symptoms, because minor dehydration may make the flu worse; (2) Echinacea, an herb reported to boost the immune system; (3) Sambucol, a sweet medicinal syrup made from elderberries reported to reverse symptoms; and (4) see a doctor for prescription amantadine or rimantadine.

Students, particularly those residing in institutional settings such as dormitories, are urged to be vaccinated to reduce the possibility of both suffering and transmitting the disease.

Misconceptions about the flu vaccine include that it is not effective, it will cause the disease it is supposed to prevent, or that severe allergic reactions will occur. However, the only flu vaccine produced and licensed in the United States is made from killed influenza viruses that cannot cause infection. The risk of an allergic reaction or other adverse side effect is extremely small. Soreness at the site of the injection may last a day or two, but it is usually mild and does not impair normal functioning. Children who have never been exposed to flu virus may experience a fever and some achiness after the vaccination; these symptoms may last one or two days. The possibility of developing Guillain-Barré syndrome (GBS), a severe paralytic disease, is also extremely rare and may occur in individuals who are severely allergic to any type of vaccine or to eggs, because the flu viruses used in the vaccine are grown in hens' eggs. Such an allergy should be reported before vaccination. Although an estimated one or two cases of GBS per million persons vaccinated may be related to the flu vaccine, the risk of severe influenza is much greater and can be prevented by the vaccine.

More information on the flu vaccine is available through http://www.cdc.gov/epo/mmwr or http://www.cdc.gov/nip/publications/VIS/default.htm or by calling the toll-free number 888-CDC-FACT (888-232-3228).

inhalant abuse Potentially lethal sniffing, snorting, or otherwise taking in through the nose or mouth the fumes of substances including adhesives (toluene, ethyl acetate, hexane, and trichloroethylene, among others), aerosols (butane, propane, fluorocarbons), solvents and gases (acetone, petroleum distillates, esters, mixed hydrocarbons), cleaning agents (tetrachloroethylene, xylene, chlorohydrocarbons), dessert sprays such as whipped cream (nitrous oxide), and room deodorizers containing alkyl nitrite, butyl nitrite, and isopropyl nitrite. Because they are easily accessible, these substances may be abused by teenagers, though they are less abused by this group than marijuana and alcohol. Products' fumes may be inhaled by spraying the substance into a plastic bag and sniffing it or inhaled directly from the container. Rapid intoxication occurs, and, in some cases, cardiac arrhythmia or severely depressed breathing may cause death even on the first experience, often called "huffing." If one also lights a match while inhaling dangerous fumes, the fumes may ignite and cause a fire that would spread quickly through the nose and mouth and into the lungs, causing life-threatening internal burns. Some noxious sprays create a seal, or a coating on the lungs that prevents oxygen from going into the bloodstream, causing asphyxiation.

Habitual inhalant abuse may also lead to brain, heart, lung, kidney, liver, and bone marrow damage. The inhalation of amyl nitrite, used therapeutically to relieve chest pain in patients with coronary artery disease, should not be used recreationally for the enhancement of sexual pleasure. Inhalation of any nitrite may have extremely dangerous effects on blood pressure and heartbeat. Although the recovery rate from inhalation abuse is among the most dismal of any substance abuse, treatment for inhalation abuse includes medical and psychosocial therapy.

See also HUFFING.

inhalant allergies Symptoms of hay fever and asthma triggered by contact of the respiratory system with allergens, including pollens, house-dust mites, fungi, and animal dander, that have been inhaled through the nose or mouth.

inhalation anthrax See ANTHRAX.

inhalation challenges The administration of a specific substance to determine an individual's reaction to that substance, also known as provocative testing. In conjunctival, nasal, or bronchial challenge, the mucosae of the eyes, nose, or lungs are directly exposed to an allergen to determine that person's sensitivity to a particular allergen. Methacholine is a substance frequently used to determine reactivity of the bronchioles as an aid in the diagnosis of asthma. (Oral challenges confirm or reject the diagnosis of food allergy.)

Direct provocative testing is the most sensitive test for allergy. The principal disadvantage of a challenge is its ability to induce a serious allergic response. Therefore, these tests should be performed only if clearly necessary in a carefully monitored setting. Other disadvantages include difficulty in standardizing test materials and measuring responsiveness quantitatively.

inhalation therapy The act of breathing in medicines dissolved in water vapors or gasses through devices such as nebulizers and aerosolized metered-dose inhalers. Inhalation therapy is a mainstay of treatment for patients with asthma and other lung disorders.

inhaled medications Drugs dissolved in water vapors or gasses and administered by metered-dose inhalers or nebulizers for the treatment of asthma and other lung disorders. Inhaled drugs include albuterol (Proventil, Ventolin), metaproterenol (Alupent), pirbuterol (Maxair), terbutaline (Brethaire), and cromolyn sodium (Intal).

See also AEROSOLS; BETA-ADRENERGIC AGONISTS; INHALATION THERAPY.

inhaler A small device, usually made of plastic, containing medication for the relief of allergy and asthma symptoms and other respiratory problems. Patients should be taught to use the various types of inhalers according to the manufacturer's instructions and the desired dosage of medicine to be inhaled.

See also ASTHMA.

Steps for Using Your Inhaler

Please demonstrate your inhaler technique at every visit.

1. Remove the cap and hold inhaler upright.
2. Shake the inhaler.
3. Tilt your head back slightly and breathe out slowly.
4. Position the inhaler in one of the following ways (A or B is optimal, but C is acceptable for those who have difficulty with A or B. C is required for breath-activated inhalers):

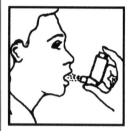 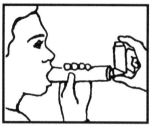 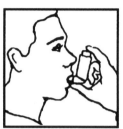 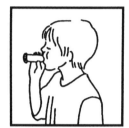

A. Open mouth with inhaler 1 to 2 inches away.

B. Use spacer/holding chamber (that is recommended especially for young children and for people using corticosteroids).

C. In the mouth. Do not use for corticosteroids.

D. NOTE: Inhaled dry powder capsules require a different inhalation technique. To use a dry powder inhaler, it is important to close the mouth tightly around the mouthpiece of the inhaler and to inhale rapidly.

5. Press down on the inhaler to release medication as you start to breathe in slowly.
6. Breathe in slowly (3 to 5 seconds).
7. Hold your breath for 10 seconds to allow the medicine to reach deeply into your lungs.
8. Repeat puff as directed. Waiting 1 minute between puffs may permit second puff to penetrate your lungs better.
9. Spacers/holding chambers are useful for all patients. They are particularly recommended for young children and older adults and for use with inhaled corticosteroids.

Avoid common inhaler mistakes. Follow these inhaler tips:
- Breathe out *before* pressing your inhaler.
- Inhale *slowly.*
- Breathe in through your mouth, not your nose.
- Press down on your inhaler at the *start* of inhalation (or within the first second of inhalation).
- Keep inhaling as you press down on inhaler.
- Press your inhaler only *once* while you are inhaling (one breath for each puff).
- Make sure you breathe in evenly and deeply.

NOTE: Other inhalers are becoming available in addition to those illustrated above. Different types of inhalers may require different techniques.

---

inspiration   Taking in air (inhalation), or breathing in.

See also BREATHING.

inspirator   A respirator or inhaler.

Instep International   A website that promotes the Buteyko asthma relief system, consisting of breathing techniques based on asthma severity and other information. The Australian Buteyko Asthma Trial was founded in 2000 by the Australian Association of Asthma Foundations. You may contact Instep International ACN 008207789; P.O. Box 2094, Townsville, 4810 Australia. Phone: (+61) 747 255 972. Or visit www.nqnet.com

insufficiency, pulmonary valvular   A condition characterized by the failure of the pulmonary valve between the right atrium and right ventricle of the heart to close properly.

insufficiency, respiratory   Dysfunction of the respiratory system, or a condition characterized by inadequate exchange of oxygen and carbon dioxide necessary for optimal functioning of the body.

See also BREATHING.

insufflation   The inspiration of a powder or vapor into the lungs or other body cavity. Examples of insufflation drugs for the treatment of asthma include cromolyn sodium and albuterol powders.

See also INHALATION THERAPY.

intermittent positive pressure breathing apparatus (IPPB) Device that forces air into the lungs during inspiration but allows normal exhalation. This type of breathing assistance, formerly used to treat chronic bronchitis or patients with emphysema, should generally be avoided in these as well as asthmatic patients because lung tissues may be seriously injured by excessive pressure from the device.

interstitial lung disorders (ILD) A roster of approximately 200 diseases characterized as chronic, nonmalignant, noninfectious diseases of the lower respiratory tract. They cause inflammation and disturbances in the walls of the alveoli, which hinders the lungs in transferring oxygen from the alveoli to the pulmonary capillaries and causes difficulty breathing. Some of the causes of ILD include inhaling toxic dusts, fumes, vapors, aerosols, drugs and poisons, and radiation.

See also DYSPNEA.

ipratropium (Atrovent) Atropine-like drug with bronchodilating properties useful for treating bronchospasm in patients with chronic obstructing lung disorders, such as chronic bronchitis, and occasionally asthma. The drug is especially effective in smokers or former smokers. Atrovent is available as both a metered-dose inhaler and solution. The latter is suitable for addition to nebulizers, where it can be combined with albuterol. The drug has virtually no adverse effects. There is also an Atrovent nasal spray effective against the runny noses of common colds and allergies. Combivent is the trade name for a combination of ipratropium and salbutamol.

iron lung An artificial respiration device for patients with paralyzed respiratory muscles.

irrespirable Term used to describe any vapor, gas, or atmospheric condition unfavorable to breathing or incapable of being inhaled.

irritant Any substance or agent that causes inflammation or adverse reaction either topically, such as skin reactions, or systemically, affecting internal body systems. Irritants trigger allergies and asthma even though they may not be considered allergens. Examples are dust, perfumes, insecticides, cleaning chemicals, cold air, paints and varnishes, smoke (especially tobacco smoke) or fumes, pollutants, and ozone.

isoetharine (Bronkometer, Bronkosol) A selective, beta-adrenergic agonist bronchodilating drug used for the treatment of asthma by inhalation.

See also BETA-ADRENERGIC AGONISTS.

isolation Another term for quarantine, or limitation of the activity and social interaction of patients with communicable diseases. Isolation techniques protect health care personnel and patients who are immunosuppressed.

isoniazid (INH) An antibacterial drug, also known as isonicotinic acid hydrazide, used mainly for the treatment of tuberculosis. Trade names include Cotinazin, Dinacrin, and Nydrazid.

isoproterenol A beta-adrenergic agonist bronchodilating drug (trade names include Duo-Medihaler, Isuprel, and Medihaler-Iso) formerly in wide use for the treatment of asthma by inhalation. However, isoproterenol has a greater potential for causing tremors and a feeling of nervousness than newer beta-agonist drugs such as albuterol or pirbuterol.

isthmus, pharyngonasalis The opening between the nasopharynx and the oral pharynx.

Jimson weed Another name for stramonium, an atropine derivative formerly used in the treatment of asthma and the active ingredient in Asthmador Cigarettes.

juxtangina Inflammation of the muscles of the throat or pharynx.

kaolinosis Pneumoconiosis resulting from the inhalation of kaolin particles. Kaolin is a clay powder (hydrated aluminum silicate, also known as China clay) used as an absorbent.

Kartagener's syndrome A congenital disorder (also called immotile colia syndrome) inherited as an autosomal recessive trait that is characterized by a structural abnormality of the cilia, hairlike projections from the surface of epithelial cells that line the respiratory system. Normal cilia propel mucus, dust, and other debris, preventing excessive accumulation in the nasal passages, sinuses, and bronchi. The defective cilia do not move normally or at all, and the thick mucus that builds up obstructs the sinuses, eustachian tubes, and lungs, causing chronic sinusitis and bronchitis. Nasal polyps are also common.

Kartagener's syndrome may also be complicated by incomplete or total situs inversus (reversal of body organs including the heart) and fertility problems in both sexes—especially immotile sperm in males. The syndrome occurs in an estimated one in 50,000 births. Symptoms usually occur within the first year of birth and require frequent antibiotics as well as bronchodilator and decongestant medications.

ketotifen An oral drug with antihistaminic properties used prophylactically to prevent symptoms of asthma. Ketotifen appears to be only mildly effective and may take as long as one to three months to demonstrate an effect. Ketotifen is sedative but otherwise has few adverse side effects.

Klebsiella pneumoniae A cause of pneumonia, bronchitis, sinusitis, and other respiratory infections.
See also PNEUMONIA.

Klebs-Löeffler bacillus Named for T. A. Edwin Klebs (1834–1913) and German bacteriologist Friedrich Löeffler, also Löffler (1852–1915). The diphtheria-causing bacillus is now called *Corynebacterium diphtheriae*.

Koch, Robert German physician (1843–1910) who won the Nobel Prize for his study of anthrax. Educated in Göttingen, he also did basic research that showed the reduced reaction of previously infected animals to being reinfected by the same infectious agent. Koch based his study on the inoculation of guinea pigs with tuberculosis and was startled to find that the reduced reaction also occurred if the original exposure had been to bacilli killed by exposure to extreme temperatures or certain chemicals. His scientific findings are also called Koch's *Grundversuch,* or Koch's phenomenon.

koniosis From the Greek word *konis,* meaning dust, any adverse reaction or disease caused by dust. Koniology is the study of dust and its effects. A koniometer is an instrument to measure the amount of dust in the air.
See also CONIOSIS; PNEUMOCONIOSIS.

Korányi's sign Named for Hungarian physician Friedrich von Korányi (1828–1913), a sign of pleural effusion determined by increased resonance upon percussion of a patient's dorsal spine.
See also PLEURAL EFFUSION.

Kronig's area Named for German physician Georg Kronig (1856–1911), a section over the thoracic cavity (chest) and lungs that resonates.
See also RESONANCE.

Kussmaul's breathing See BREATHING.

L

Laborde's method   Named for French physician Jean B. V. Laborde (1830–1903). Rhythmic traction movements made on a patient's tongue to stimulate the respiratory center when asphyxiation is evident.

Laënnec's pearls   Round, gelatinlike mucous particles or "pearls" found in the sputum of patients with asthma. These particles were first described by Rene T. Laënnec, French physician (1781–1826) and inventor of the stethoscope.

la grippe   A French term for influenza.
     See also INFLUENZA.

laryngeal reflex   A cough that results from irritation of the larynx (voice box) or fauces (the constricted opening from the mouth that includes the oral pharynx, the glossopalatine arch, and the pharyngopalatine arch).

laryngeal vertigo   Dizziness and fainting that occurs during a coughing spell in a patient with chronic bronchitis. Laryngeal vertigo is also known as tussive syncope.

laryngemphraxis   Obstruction of the larynx.

laryngismus   Spasm of the larynx that occurs during a severe allergic reaction.

laryngismus stridulus   Also known as child crowing, a spasm that briefly causes closure of the glottis and is followed by a noisy inspiration.

laryngitis   Inflammation of the larynx, or voice box, the musculocartilaginous upper end of the windpipe (trachea) lined with mucous membrane. Characterized by a sore throat and hoarseness or temporary inability to speak (aphonia), laryngitis may be caused by improper use or overuse of the voice, exposure to wet and cold, extension of a nose or throat infection, or inhalation of irritating vapors or dust. Although the larynx is part of the respiratory system, which is often affected by allergic symptoms, allergies themselves are not generally a cause of laryngitis. Patients with persistent hoarseness should be evaluated for polyps or other disorders of the vocal cords.

laryngoceles   Outpouchings filled with air that form from the larynx's mucous membrane. They can produce a visible, egg-shaped lump in the neck and cause hoarseness and airway obstruction. Musicians who play wind instruments often suffer from laryngoceles, which can also fill with mucuslike fluid and become infected. Surgical removal is the typical treatment.

laryngoplegia   Paralysis of the muscles in the larynx, caused by brain tumors, strokes, nerve damage (stemming from tumors, neurotoxins, injury, or a viral infection) and demyelinating diseases. Symptoms of laryngoplegia include difficulty speaking, swallowing, and breathing, a hoarse, breathy voice, abnormal-sounding or weak voice, and high-pitched sounds on respiration. The usual treatments are surgical repair, removal, or tracheostomy, which creates a permanent or temporary opening in the windpipe. Arytenoidectomy serves to widen the airway between vocal cords.

laryngorhinology   The study of diseases of the larynx and nose.

laryngorrhea   Excessive mucus discharge from the larynx.

laryngospasm   Sudden muscular contractions, or spasms, of the larynx.

laryngotracheobronchitis   Inflammation of the larynx, trachea, and bronchi.

larynx   The vocal cords, or voice box, the part of the respiratory system located at the upper end of the trachea below the root of the tongue. The larynx, a Greek word meaning the "upper part of the windpipe," is made of nine cartilages bound by an elastic membrane and lined with mucous membrane. When moved by muscles and aided by air pressure, the mouth, and the tongue, the larynx produces sounds, including speech.

According to the American Lung Association, the incidence rate for cancer of the larynx has decreased 20 percent between 1973 and 1997, although incidences among white and black women have slightly increased. The 1997 statistics show that in 11.5 per 100,000 black males, the incidence is 88 percent higher than it is in 6.1 per 100,000 white males.

Larynx cancer is one of the most common types of head and neck cancer and is usually associated with abuse of alcohol and cigarettes. One of the symptoms of larynx cancer is hoarseness, especially chronic hoarseness that lasts for more than two weeks, which requires medical attention. Difficulty swallowing, pain, and a lump in the neck may also indicate laryngeal cancer. Treatment is surgery or radiation therapy for early-stage cancer, but advanced cancer may require partial or total removal of the larynx (laryngectomy) and radiation. When the vocal cords are removed, speaking or making sounds must be accomplished through the use of esophageal speech, in which a person is instructed to inhale into the esophagus and produce sound upon exhalation; a tracheoesophageal fistula, a surgically inserted valve between the windpipe and the esophagus that can help produce sound when a person inhales; or an electrolarynx, a device that is held against the neck to help an individual produce sound. All these methods tend to sound artificial.

Other problems associated with the vocal cords are polyps, nodules, contact ulcers, and one- or two-sided paralysis.

See also LARYNGOPLEGIA.

laughing gas   Nitrous oxide gas inhaled for use as a temporary general anesthetic.

See also INHALANT ABUSE.

learning disabilities and theophylline   Behavioral changes and inattentiveness that are attributed to the use of theophylline as treatment of childhood asthma, resulting in poor performance in school.

See also THEOPHYLLINE.

lecithin-sphingomyelin ratio   A method of determining the maturity of the lungs in a fetus, the ratio of lecithin to sphingomyelin in the amniotic fluid. In the process of development, fetal lungs (after the 34th week of gestation) becoming more mature produce more lecithin—a type of fatty substance known as phospholipids, than sphingomyelin—one of the phosphorus-containing sphingolipids found in nervous tissue and blood. If a fetus is delivered before the lungs produce more lecithin than sphingomyelins, there is a high risk of the infant's having hyaline membrane disease.

Leeuwenhoek's disease   Named for Dutch microbiologist Anton van Leeuwenhoek (1632–1723), a disorder known also as respiratory myoclonus, which stems from an abnormality in the respiratory control system in the brain stem. The disorder is characterized by shortness of breath and epigastric pulsations caused by involuntary contractions of the diaphragm and other proximate respiratory muscles. Treatment may include the drug diphenylhydantoin and surgical section of the phrenic nerve, which arises in the cervical plexus, goes into the chest and then to the diaphragm.

See also DIAPHRAGM.

Legionnaire's disease A type of pneumonia caused by the gram-negative bacillus *Legionella pneumophila*, named for a group of people who contracted the disease during a 1976 convention of the American Legion in Philadelphia, Pennsylvania. Also known as legionellosis, the disease may include dry cough, muscle pain, shortness of breath, confusion, headache, fever, fatigue, and sometimes gastrointestinal symptoms such as diarrhea. If untreated, cardiovascular collapse may occur. The bacillus can be inhaled from droplets from air conditioners, humidifiers, water cooling towers, faucets, shower heads, evaporative condensers, whirlpool spas, decorative fountains, ultrasonic mist machines (used to mist produce in supermarkets), and respiratory therapy equipment that is contaminated, but there is no direct contagion between individuals. Treatment of choice consists mainly of the antibiotics azithromycin, fluoroquinolones (trovafloxacin, sparfloxacin, pefloxacin, levofloxacin, ofloxacin, and grepafloxacin), tetracycline, and erythromycin, preferably administered immediately after diagnosis, or rifampin. Patients who are immunocompromised or have had a prolonged illness and respiratory failure caused by pneumonia or nosocomially acquired disease prior to infection with the Legionnaire's bacillus often have an approximately 50 percent higher risk of dying. Recovery rate is slow.

Legionnaire's disease may be indistinguishable from other forms of pneumonia caused by bacteria, and chest radiographs may not be totally reliable in the diagnosis. The presence of *Legionella pneumophila* in sputum, blood, and urine specimens may indicate Legionnaire's disease or Pontiac fever, a self-limited illness that does not include pneumonia. Risk factors that point to a possible diagnosis of Legionnaire's disease are recent travel, recent plumbing repairs in one's home, smoking, diabetes, kidney or liver failure, a systemic malignancy or immunosuppressive disorder, use of corticosteroids, alcohol abuse, and exposure to aerosol-producing devices.

It is estimated that Legionnaire's disease accounts for 1 to 8 percent of all cases of pneumonia and 4 percent of fatal pneumonias contracted by individuals while they are hospitalized. The death rate is about 20 percent.

leishmaniasis An infection caused by a species of *Leishmania*, a genus of parasitic flagellate protozoa named for Sir William B. Leishman, a British medical officer (1865–1926). In the form of American leishmaniasis, the organism mainly affects the nasal cavities, mucocutaneous membranes, and pharynx.

leprosy, tuberculoid A form of a chronic disease caused by the *Mycobacterium leprae*, also known as Hansen's disease, characterized by asymmetrical nerve lesions and skin anesthesia. The infection in this form resembles tuberculosis. Treatment includes dapsone or a combined chemotherapy of dapsone, rifampin, and clofazamine. In severe cases, corticosteroids or thalidomide may be administered. Individuals who have undergone three months of dapsone or clofazamine therapy, and those who have taken rifampin for three days are not considered infectious and isolation is not necessary. As opposed to the obsolete idea that leprosy is incurable, the prognosis is good if the patient receives proper therapy.

leukocyte histamine release assay Another name for basophil degranulation and histamine release.

leukocytes White blood cells produced in bone marrow, lymph nodes, and cells lining capillaries in organs such as the spleen. There are two types of leukocytes: granulocytes, which have granules on their cytoplasm, and agranulocytes, which do not have granules. Granulocytes include juvenile neutrophils, segmented neutrophils, basophils, and eosinophils, and agranulocytes include lymphocytes (produced in lymph nodes) and monocytes, all of which participate in helping the body fight infection and in the inflammatory processes that occur during allergic reactions. Leukocytes of all types circulate throughout the body, especially to troubleshoot in areas where there are injured tissues or infections. The normal adult white blood count is approximately 4,000 to 10,000 leukocytes per cubic millimeter of blood. Leukopenia refers to fewer than 4,000 white blood cells; leukocytosis is indicated by a count greater than 10,000.

A white blood cell differential count, which examines the various types of leukocytes in the circulating blood and other body secretions, helps diagnose many medical disorders, including allergies and infections. For example, bacterial infections usually cause an increased number of total white blood cells, whereas viruses may slightly increase, decrease, or maintain a normal count. Bacterial infections most often result in an increase in polymorphonuclear cells (also called neutrophils, polys, or segs) relative to the increase in total white cells. Viral infections may cause an increase in the number of leukocytes. The presence of more than 5 percent eosinophils in the white blood count frequently suggests an allergic or parasitic disorder.

leukotrienes   Potent biochemicals produced and secreted by various types of immune cells such as macrophages, mast cells, eosinophils, basophils, and monocytes, along with other chemical mediators (natural substances in the body that act like drugs), including histamine. Leukotrienes and other substances including prostaglandins, collectively called eicosanoids, are fatty acids derived during the metabolism of arachidonic acid, an essential component of the cell membrane. Certain leukotrienes may be held partly accountable for effects of asthma such as bronchospasm or constriction, increased airway hyperresponsiveness to triggers, increased microvascular permeability (the ability to pass substances through the walls of tiny blood vessels), and excessive production of mucus. These chemicals may be 100 to 1,000 times more potent and exert a more prolonged effect than histamine in contracting the smooth muscle of airways. The presence of leukotrienes may also be a reason that antihistaminic drugs, which block the action of histamine, do not fully alleviate allergic reactions.

Zafirlukast (Accolate) is the first of a class of drugs effective for the treatment of leukotriene-mediated reactions. Accolate antagonizes or blocks the effects of LTD_4 (a type of leukotriene) and is useful to prevent inflammatory changes that occur in mild to moderate asthma. It is not known if the effects of these agents will be an additive to other inflammatory drugs such as corticosteroids. Accolate is approved for the treatment of mild to moderate asthma. There do not appear to be any serious adverse effects.

Zileutron (Zileutrol) inhibits, or prevents, the action of 5-lipoxygenase, and may have additive effects to inhaled corticosteroids.

Leutrol   See ZILEUTRON.

licorice   A flavoring, demulcent, and mild expectorant derived from the root of the plant *Glycyrrhiza glabra*. Licorice may be included in cough medicines.

ligament, pulmonary   A fold of pleura located from the root of the lung to the base of the medial surface of the lung.

lingulectomy   The surgical removal of the lingula, a tongue-shaped projection from the upper lobe of the left lung.

lobar pneumonia   An inflamed condition in one or more lobes of the lung.
See also PNEUMONIA.

lobes of lungs   Segments, or large divisions, of the lungs consisting of the superior and inferior lobes of the left lung, and the superior, middle, and inferior lobes of the right lung.

lobules of lungs   The smaller parts of the lungs, including the respiratory bronchiole and its branches, known as the alveolar ducts, alveolar sacs, and alveoli.

locations ideal for asthma and allergy patients
Geographic areas considered to provide improved living conditions, depending upon the specific allergens to which an individual is sensitive. Some people feel the need to move from their present homes to avoid allergens indigenous to that area, but climates and geographic characteristics can change in time, causing previously favorable areas

to become havens for new allergens and pollutants. For example, Arizona was once thought to be an ideal climate for asthmatics. However, pollutants (including the introduction of pollinating plants and grasses by the incoming new residents) and environmental changes such as urbanization and irrigation have turned populated areas of this state into high-risk zones. In addition, the stress of moving and new environmental exposures may intensify asthma and allergy symptoms.

loratadine   An antihistamine (trade name Claritin) with a lower potential for sedation than traditional allergy drugs. Introduced in the United States in 1993, loratadine is taken once daily on an empty stomach.

Lucas-Championnière's disease   Pseudomembranous bronchitis (related to croupous bronchitis, inflammation of the bronchi including some of the symptoms of croup: difficulty breathing and spasm of the larynx), named for French surgeon J. M. M. Lucas-Championnière (1843–1913). This condition may be confused with asthma.

See also BRONCHITIS.

lung   The main organs of the respiratory system. The lungs are two spongelike structures located in the chest within the rib cage that provide life-sustaining oxygen to the body. Lungs contain air sacs, called alveoli, that accommodate air taken into and expressed out of the lungs by inhalation and exhalation, respectively, during which oxygen is transmitted to the bloodstream and carbon dioxide is expelled.

In the process of breathing, air from the atmosphere enters the trachea, or windpipe, and passes into the two large bronchi, each branching into a lung on either side, then to the smaller bronchi and bronchioles. The entire structure resembles a tree. The lungs, which move upon inhalation and exhalation, are encased by pleurae, protective membranes that allow each lung to expand and contract. (In the event of pleurisy, these membranes swell and rub against each other, causing pain during respiration.) The right lung is divided into three lobes, or sections, and the left lung is divided into two lobes. In the adult male, the approximate weight of the right lung is 625 grams, and the left lung 570 grams. The lungs contain 300 million alveoli, with a respiratory surface of about 70 square meters.

In the left lung is the cardiac depression, an indentation that accommodates the heart. Pulmonary circulation describes blood traveling from the heart to the lungs and back to the heart. The primary lung function is to bring air in contact with the blood to add oxygen and remove carbon dioxide. Respirations in adults average at 18 per minute, and the total capacity of the lungs ranges from 3.6 to 9.4 liters in adult males and from 2.5 to 6.9 liters in adult females. Nerve supply to the lungs consists of parasympathetic fibers by way of the vagus (cranial) nerve and sympathetic fibers from the anterior and posterior pulmonary plexuses. The main blood vessels are the bronchial and pulmonary arteries and the pulmonary veins.

Diseases of the lung include bronchial asthma, tumors, and anomalies caused by injury to the lungs. Many diagnostic procedures include chest X ray, pulmonary function tests, bronchoscopy, biopsy of lung tissue, blood tests, and sputum analysis.

See also BREATHING.

lung abscess   The formation of pus in the lung that causes high fever, sweats, pallor, loss of appetite, chest pain, dyspnea, coughing, foul-smelling, purulent expectoration, cavernous breathing, and possibly bubbling rales. Lung abscess is usually caused by bacteria from the mouth or throat that is then inhaled into the lungs, especially when an individual's immune system is impaired for some reason, such as unconsciousness attributable to anesthesia, sedation, or substance abuse, or if a person has pneumonia, an infected pulmonary embolus, a blood infection, a lung tumor, or a neurological disorder. With proper treatment, which, depending upon the severity and size of the abscess, may include draining the abscess, respiratory therapy, dietary measures, surgery, and oral or intravenous antibiotic therapy, the prognosis is fair. Lung abscess causes death in approximately 5 percent of the cases, particularly if a patient has lung cancer, an impaired immune system, or other pre-existing serious condition.

See also BREATHING.

lung cancer   Cancer manifesting in the trachea, air sacs, and structures of the lungs of the respiratory system, or originating in lung cells and then metastasizing to other parts of the body, such as the lymphatic system and bloodstream. According to the American Lung Association, lung cancer is the leading cause of death from cancers in the United States, and incidence and mortality have continued to increase since the 1930s. Lung cancer accounts for 28 percent of all deaths from cancer. Approximately 156,900 deaths were estimated for the year 2000. The lung cancer rate in 1997 was 54.4 per 100,000. In 1987, lung cancer surpassed breast cancer as the prime cause of cancer mortality among women, largely attributed to the fact that more women are smoking cigarettes. Incidence is declining in men (80 per 100,000) and rising in women (42 per 100,000).

Cigarette smoking is the most significant cause of lung cancer in America, with an estimated 87 percent of all lung cancer incidences resulting from smoking. According to the Surgeon General's latest report, in 1998 there were 47.2 million smokers in the United States: 24.8 million male, 22.4 million female. For both sexes combined, the percentage of lung cancer deaths attributed to smoking increased between 1990 and 1995. However the National Cancer Institute says men's lung cancer rates have been steadily declining from a high of 87 men per 100,000 in 1984 to 70 men per 100,000 in 1996, while lung cancer deaths among women have increased 600 percent over the past 50 years and now account for a quarter of women's cancer deaths, surpassing both breast and ovarian cancer statistics. According to estimates from National Vital Statistics, 1994, 126,999 people of both sexes and all ages died in 1990, and in 1995 the number grew to 151,075. The National Cancer Institute's calculated lifetime risk of dying from lung cancer includes smokers and nonsmokers. Based on statistics set forth between 1995 and 1997, 7.62 percent of males of all races and 4.77 females of all races risk dying from lung cancer. It is also the most common form of cancer among African-American men and women.

Other causes of lung cancer include occupational hazards, such as exposure to asbestos, radiation, arsenic, chromates, nickel, chloroethyl ethers, radon gas, mustard gas, coke-oven emissions, etc., and pre-existing diseases such as fibrosis, tuberculosis, or cancer that has spread from the skin, kidney, thyroid, stomach, bone, rectum, or other part of the body to the lung.

Many lung cancers begin as small cell (or oat cell) lung cancer (SCLC) and nonsmall cell lung cancer (NSCLC) in the bronchial lining, in the trachea, or in the bronchioles or alveoli. SCLC, making up approximately 20 percent of all lung cancers, is mostly attributable to smoking. The other 80 percent of lung cancers are the nonsmall varieties including squamous cell carcinoma, adenocarcinoma, and large-cell undifferentiated carcinoma. Less common lung cancers include carcinoid tumors, hamartomas, sarcomas, lymphomas, and adenoid cystic carcinomas, which may warrant special treatment regimens.

The diagnosis of lung cancer usually involves chest X rays, CT scans, bronchoscopy, pulmonary function tests, needle biopsy, and sputum analysis after a person complains of symptoms such as chest pain, a persistent cough or hoarseness, blood in the sputum, shortness of breath, and significant weight loss. However, once these symptoms appear, the disease may be well advanced and perhaps beyond a curable stage. Diagnostic tests for early detection of lung cancer, a low-dose helical or spiral CT scan among them, are being developed, along with new combinations of chemotherapy, immunotherapy, and drugs that can stop tumor blood vessels from thriving.

Treatment of lung cancer includes surgery, typically followed up by chemotherapy and radiation depending upon the type of cancer and effectiveness of having removed the diseased portion of tissue. Cancers such as small-cell lung cancer may respond to chemotherapy, but there exists the possibility of drug resistance after repeated treatments. Surgery or radiation may be combined with chemotherapy, and in the event that a cure is not accomplished, symptoms may respond well to palliative therapy. Radiation therapy is significant in treating and often curing early-stage non–small-cell lung cancer. One of the newest treatments still under investigation is dose-intensity chemotherapy, which is used to treat recurring tumors that have become resistant to the drug to which they

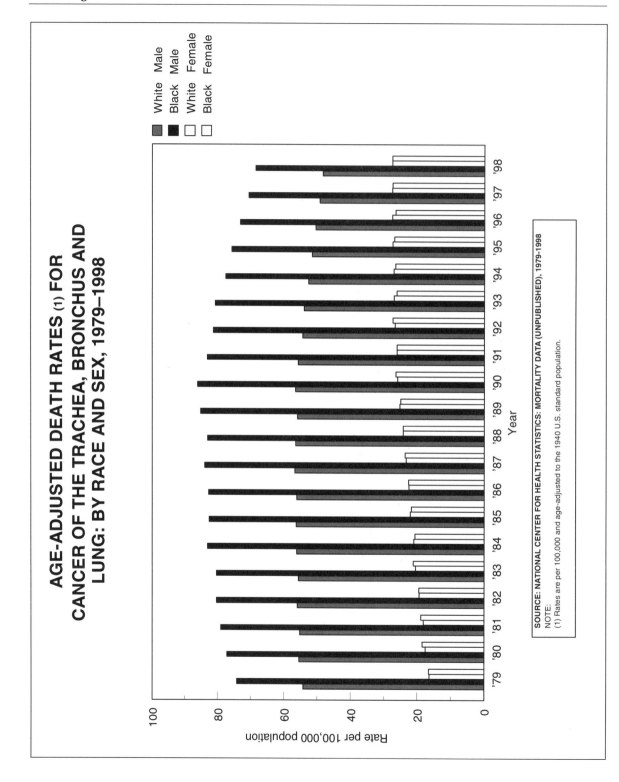

AGE-ADJUSTED DEATH RATES (1) FOR CANCER OF THE TRACHEA, BRONCHUS AND LUNG: BY RACE AND SEX, 1979–1998

White Male
Black Male
White Female
Black Female

Rate per 100,000 population

Year

SOURCE: NATIONAL CENTER FOR HEALTH STATISTICS: MORTALITY DATA (UNPUBLISHED), 1979-1998
NOTE:
(1) Rates are per 100,000 and age-adjusted to the 1940 U.S. standard population.

DEATH RATES FOR MALIGNANT NEOPLASMS OF THE RESPIRATORY SYSTEM (1) BY AGE, 1998

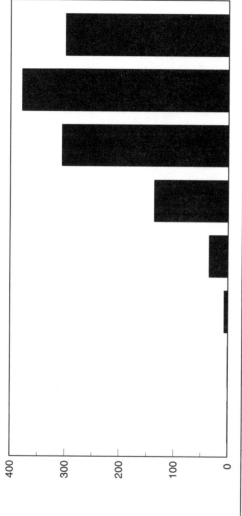

RATE PER 100,000 RESIDENT POPULATION

AGE GROUP	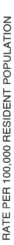 *	15-24	25-34	35-44	45-54	55-64	65-74	75-84	85 and up
RATE		0.0	6.8	8.1	33.3	131.4	296.7	387.7	289.9

SOURCE: NATIONAL CENTER FOR HEALTH STATISTICS: REPORT OF FINAL MORTALITY STATISTICS, 1998
NOTE:
(1) Includes lung, larynx and other respiratory cancers.
*Represents data greater than zero but statistically unreliable

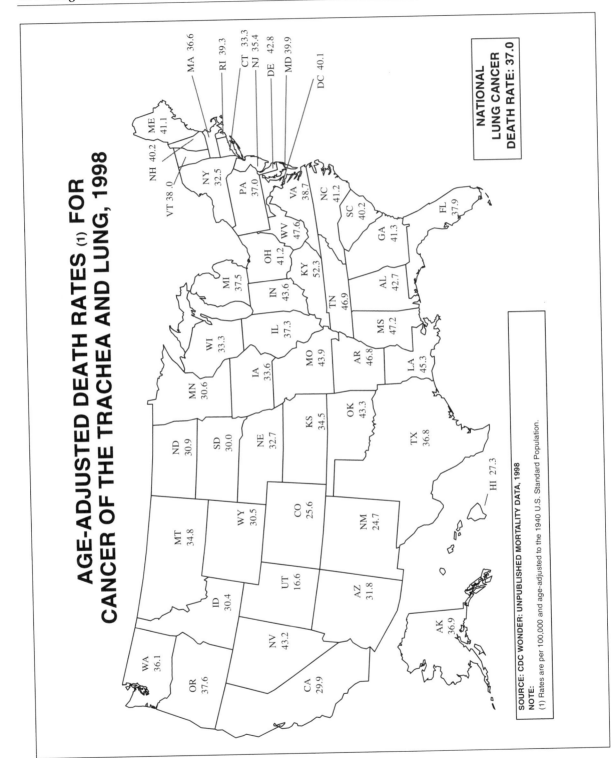

AGE-ADJUSTED DEATH RATES (1) FOR CANCER OF THE TRACHEA AND LUNG, 1998

NATIONAL LUNG CANCER DEATH RATE: 37.0

MA 36.6
RI 39.3
CT 33.3
NJ 35.4
DE 42.8
MD 39.9
DC 40.1

ME 41.1
NH 40.2
VT 38.0
NY 32.5
PA 37.0
VA 38.7
NC 41.2
SC 40.2
GA 41.3
FL 37.9

WV 47.6
OH 41.2
KY 52.3
TN 46.9
AL 42.7

MI 37.5
IN 43.6
IL 37.3
MS 47.2

WI 33.3
IA 33.6
MO 43.9
AR 46.8
LA 45.3

MN 30.6
KS 34.5
OK 43.3
TX 36.8

ND 30.9
SD 30.0
NE 32.7

HI 27.3

MT 34.8
WY 30.5
CO 25.6
NM 24.7

ID 30.4
UT 16.6
AZ 31.8

WA 36.1
OR 37.6
NV 43.2
CA 29.9

AK 36.9

SOURCE: CDC WONDER: UNPUBLISHED MORTALITY DATA, 1998
NOTE:
(1) Rates are per 100,000 and age-adjusted to the 1940 U.S. Standard Population.

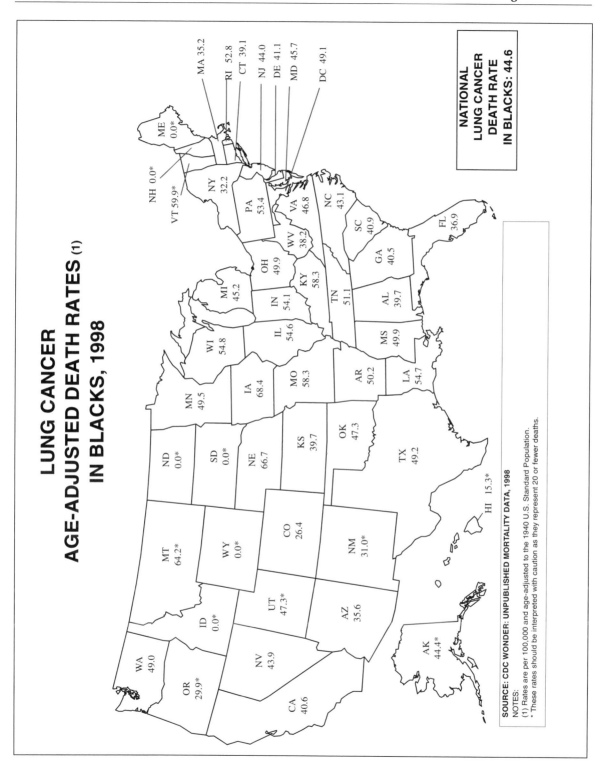

LUNG CANCER
AGE-ADJUSTED DEATH RATES (1)
IN BLACKS, 1998

NATIONAL
LUNG CANCER
DEATH RATE
IN BLACKS: 44.6

ME 0.0*
NH 0.0*
VT 59.9*
MA 35.2
RI 52.8
CT 39.1
NY 32.2
NJ 44.0
DE 41.1
MD 45.7
DC 49.1
PA 53.4
WV 38.2
VA 46.8
NC 43.1
SC 40.9
GA 40.5
FL 36.9
OH 49.9
KY 58.3
TN 51.1
AL 39.7
MI 45.2
IN 54.1
IL 54.6
MS 49.9
WI 54.8
IA 68.4
MO 58.3
AR 50.2
LA 54.7
MN 49.5
NE 66.7
KS 39.7
OK 47.3
TX 49.2
ND 0.0*
SD 0.0*
CO 26.4
NM 31.0*
MT 64.2*
WY 0.0*
ID 0.0*
UT 47.3*
AZ 35.6
NV 43.9
WA 49.0
OR 29.9*
CA 40.6
AK 44.4*
HI 15.3*

SOURCE: CDC WONDER: UNPUBLISHED MORTALITY DATA, 1998
NOTES:
(1) Rates are per 100,000 and age-adjusted to the 1940 U.S. Standard Population.
* These rates should be interpreted with caution as they represent 20 or fewer deaths.

AGE-ADJUSTED LUNG AND BRONCHUS CANCER INCIDENCE RATES BY SEX AND RACE: SELECTED YEARS 1973–1999 (1, 2, 3)

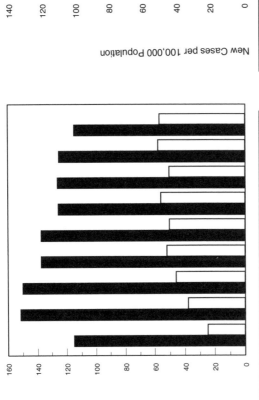

YEAR		1975	1980	1985	1990	1995	1996	1997	1998	1999
White Males	■	89.1	97.6	97.0	96.5	87.6	86.0	84.0	85.1	79.4
White Females	☐	24.8	32.4	40.8	49.0	52.4	52.9	54.6	54.2	52.3

YEAR		1975	1980	1985	1990	1995	1996	1997	1998	1999
Black Males	■	115.1	151.6	150.0	137.5	137.5	125.5	126.1	125.2	115.0
Black Females	☐	24.7	38.1	46.0	52.0	50.3	55.9	50.6	57.9	57.0

New Cases per 100,000 Population

SOURCE: NATIONAL CANCER INSTITUTE: SEER CANCER STATISTICS REVIEW, 1973-1999
Notes:
(1) Rates are per 100,000 and age adjusted by the direct method to the 2000 U.S. standard population.
(2) Data are based on the Surveillance, Epidemiology, and End Results (SEER) Program's population-based registries in Atlanta, Detroit, Seattle-Puget Sound, San Francisco-Oakland, Connecticut, Iowa, Mexico, Utah and Hawaii.
(3) Because these estimates are based on a sample, they may differ from figures that would be obtained from a census of the population. Each data point reported is an estimate of the true population value and subject to sampling variability.

LUNG CANCER HOSPITAL DISCHARGES BY SEX, 1979–2000

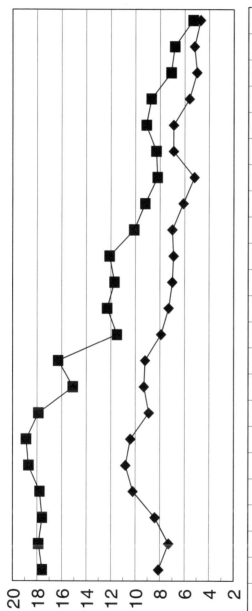

	1979	1980	1981	1982	1983	1984	1985	1986	1987	1988	1989	1990	1991	1992	1993	1994	1995	1996	1997	1998	1999	2000
Male ■	17.6	17.9	17.6	17.8	18.7	18.9	17.9	15.1	16.3	11.5	12.3	11.7	12.1	10.1	9.2	8.2	8.3	9.1	8.7	7.1	6.8	5.3
Female ◆	8.1	7.3	8.4	10.2	10.8	10.4	8.9	9.3	9.2	7.9	7.3	7.0	6.9	7.0	6.1	5.2	6.9	6.9	5.6	5.0	5.2	4.7

Source: National Center for Health Statistics, National Hospital Discharge Survey, 1979-2000

Notes:
(1) Data from 1988-2000 may not be comparable to earlier years due to the redesign of the survey.
(2) Includes malignant neoplasms of the trachea, bronchus and lung.
(3) Because these estimates are based on a sample, they may differ from figures that would be obtained from a census of the population. Each data point reported is an estimate of the true population value and subject to sampling variability.

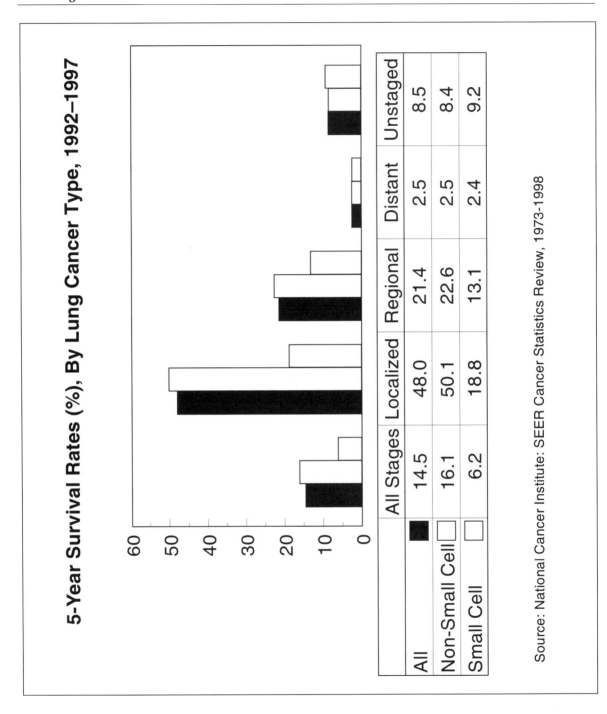

5-Year Survival Rates (%), By Lung Cancer Type, 1992–1997

	All Stages	Localized	Regional	Distant	Unstaged
All	14.5	48.0	21.4	2.5	8.5
Non-Small Cell	16.1	50.1	22.6	2.5	8.4
Small Cell	6.2	18.8	13.1	2.4	9.2

Source: National Cancer Institute: SEER Cancer Statistics Review, 1973-1998

Tables are reprinted with permission © 2001 American Lung Association. For more information, please visit their website at www.lungusa.org or call 1-800-LUNG-USA.

formerly responded. The dose is increased in an attempt to kill more cancerous cells at a time. The side effects of dose-intensity chemotherapy include damage to the bone marrow. New radiation therapies include proton or neuron beam, radiation-activated dyes and photodynamic therapy. In addition, immunotherapy techniques have been designed to boost the immune system, and new drugs are being developed to prevent or reduce the recurrence rate of cancers such as those of the mouth, larynx, and lungs. Retinoids, derived from vitamin A, have been effective against those forms of cancer. The most common chemotherapies are Paraplatin (carboplatin), Platinol (cisplatin), and Taxol (paclitaxel), as well as Gemzar (gemcitabine hydrochloride) and Taxotere (docetaxel), both of which are still in clinical trial stages.

See also APPENDIX III.

lung collapse Atelectasis, or the result of a decrease in intrapulmonic pressure or an increase in intrathoracic pressure. An obstruction in the bronchial tubes, a tumor, an enlarged heart, or pressure placed on the lung by air or fluid in the pleural cavity may cause the change in pressure. When a lung collapses suddenly, the victim also suffers circulatory collapse and has difficulty breathing. A gradual onset may not be indicated by these symptoms. Hypostatic lung collapse refers to lung congestion related to asthenic, or debilitating, diseases, especially when the patient remains inactive and in a recumbent position for prolonged periods of time. Passive lung collapse refers to obstructed blood flow from the lungs to the heart. Treatment may include deep-breathing exercises, changing positions, prevention of congestion, and assisted respiration.

See also ATELECTASIS.

lunger An obsolete term used in the 1800s to describe a person with tuberculosis or a chronic pulmonary disorder.

lung hemorrhage Bleeding that arises from the mouth, larynx, trachea, bronchi, or lungs, usually accompanying an attack of productive coughing up of sputum that contains frothy bright red blood and tastes salty. Lung hemorrhage may also be caused by a parasitic fluke infection of the lungs. Treatment includes cold compresses on the chest, keeping the patient warm, teaching the patient to cough without straining, bedrest with the head slightly elevated, ice packs, sedatives, and tepid fluids. Any hemorrhage requires the attention of a physician.

lung inflammation Another term for pneumonia. See also PNEUMONIA.

lungmotor A device that forces air or a combination of air and oxygen into the lungs.

lung surfactant The substance that regulates the amount of surface tension of the fluid that lines the alveoli, or air sacs. The naturally produced substance has been synthesized and is being used investigationally in cases of infants with respiratory disease syndrome.

lung transplantation The transferal and surgical installation of a lung from a deceased donor into an individual with an imminently life-threatening lung disease. Transplantation of both a single lung and both lungs has become a highly successful surgery and the majority of patients survive.

lungworm Organisms called nematodes that use the lungs of humans and animals as hosts in which to thrive. Nematodes include roundworms and threadworms, certain species of which are parasitic. Infestation requires medical treatment.

lungwort The herb *Pulmonaria officinalis* from which is derived a tonic or remedy for respiratory disorders.

lycoperdonosis A respiratory disease caused by inhaling significant quantities of *Lycoperdon* spores from the mature mushroom commonly known as "puffball." Most puffballs belong to this genus of fungi.

macrophage Important monolytic white blood cell involved in the immune response. Macrophages overtake bacteria and other foreign materials and break them down as an immunological defense. In the respiratory system, alveolar macrophages enter lung tissue and degrade with their enzymes the cell walls of the bacteria or other invader, or transport the bacteria from the lung tissue to the lower airways until they are trapped in mucus and expelled from the respiratory tract via the cilia (also known as the mucociliary transport escalator).

Also, macrophages are capable of transporting bacteria to the lymphatic system, where they are filtered and then destroyed by other cells.

Maimonides, Moses Jewish physician (1135–1204) who wrote *Treatise on Asthma*, among other scientific and philosophical works, which was the first of his medical books available in English translation. In the treatise, Maimonides recommends that attacks of various illnesses, including asthma (which he called shortness of breath), can be made less frequent and less severe if the air is kept clean; if diet, excretions, and spiritual emotions are regulated; and if proper rest and exercise are maintained.

Educated by his father, who was a judge, and by Rabbi ibn Migas, Cordova-born Maimonides also wrote about religion and religious law, logic, astronomy, preventive medicine, drugs, toxins, Galen's teachings, sex, and other topics. He became known as the greatest Jew after Moses and one of the preeminent figures of modern medical ethics along with Hippocrates. Because of religious persecution, Maimonides' family fled to Cairo, where he became a physician. His holistic practice included advocating bathing and massage.

Mantoux test Named for French physician Charles Mantoux (1877–1947), an intracutaneous injection to determine the presence of tuberculosis. One-tenth milliliter of Purified Protein Derivative is injected into the skin, and within 24 to 72 hours the puncture site becomes hard if a person has an active or inactive (exposure to) tubercular infection. The Mantoux test is also known as the tuberculin test.

maple bark disease A form of pneumonitis caused by the inhalation of mold spores *(Cryptostroma corticale)* found in the bark of maple trees.

See also PNEUMONITIS.

marijuana See CANNABIS.

massage An expanded form of the traditional back rub. Various methods of massage are popular, including the Japanese shiatsu, which concentrates on pressure points of the body, and massaging the hands and feet. Essentially, any type of massage induces relaxation and may be particularly useful when stress acts as a trigger for asthma.

See also ACUPRESSURE.

massive collapse of the lung A severe reaction to shock or abdominal or thyroid surgery characterized by chest pain, difficulty breathing, and cyanosis. The collapse is caused by a mucous plug or foreign substance in the main bronchus or by a tension pneumothorax. Treatment includes the administration of carbon dioxide, antibiotics, removal of a foreign body, and oxygen therapy.

See also PNEUMOTHORAX.

mast cells One of the major cells in body tissues responsible for the onset of allergic symptoms. Mast cells contain histamine and other chemically active substances. During a type I, or immediate, allergic reaction, mast cells are activated. There are two types of mast cells, connective tissue mast cells and mucosal mast cells. Each are coated with immunoglobulin E (IgE) antibodies, which bind to receptors on the mast cell's surface. The receptors correlate to individual allergens (substances capable of causing allergy).

One mast cell may have from 5,000 to 500,000 individual IgE antibody receptors on its surface. After exposure to an allergen, the surface antibodies "recognize" their specific allergens, causing the mast cell to release chemical mediators. Chemical mediators are potent biochemicals, including histamine, prostaglandins, and leukotrienes, among others. In an asthmatic patient, the release of the mediators causes a sudden constriction and inflammation of the bronchioles, which results in wheezing and shortness of breath.

The mast cells also produce proteases and cytokines, substances involved in the process of tissue inflammation, growth, and repair.

See also LEUKOTRIENES.

Maxair See PIRBUTEROL.

maximum breathing capacity The largest amount of air, measured in liters per minute, a person can inhale in approximately 30 seconds or other specified time.

maximum expiratory flow rate (MEFR) A measure of a maximal inhalation from a spirometer and a maximal exhalation that yields a calculation of the person's vital capacity, or the total amount of air a person takes in and out. The MEFR is used clinically to approximate the peak expiratory flow rate (PEFR or PEF).

See also PEAK FLOW MEASUREMENTS; SPIROMETRY.

measles, cough accompanying Respiratory symptoms associated with the viral communicable disease known as measles, including coughing that sounds brassy, sneezing, and nasal congestion.

medical alert bracelets and necklaces Engraved metal plates worn like jewelry to identify a chronic medical condition or allergy in the event an individual becomes unable to communicate.

Medihaler-Epi Brand of epinephrine bitartrate, USP.

melanemia Also called melanosis and anthracosis, a black deposit found in the lungs.

See also ANTHROCOSIS; COAL WORKER'S PNEUMOCONIOSIS.

melioidosis A disease resulting from infection by *Pseudomonas pseudomallei* that causes pneumonia. Melioidosis is derived from the Greek word *melis,* meaning a distemper of asses, and *eidos,* meaning form. The causative bacterium thrives in soil and lakes in Asia, Africa, and Australia, but the disease, with pneumonia-like symptoms including high fever, is reportedly nonexistent in the United States and Europe. Similar to glanders, a horse and donkey disease also caused by the inhalation of *P. mallei* but rarely transmitted to humans, melioidosis is potentially fatal. With early detection through pus, sputum, or blood sample analysis, it is curable with antibiotics.

See also PNEUMONIA.

membrane, mucous The soft, pink lining of certain body structures, including the mouth, nose, throat, eyelids, bladder, vagina, and intestinal tract, that secretes mucus, a sticky fluid that keeps the surfaces of these and other organs moist.

meningitis, pneumococcal Inflammation of the membranes of the brain or the spinal cord caused by the pneumococcus, a type of bacterium. Young children are frequently the victims of this disease, which may be life-threatening, but pneumococci may affect any age group. The disease is transmissible through a lung, blood, ear, skull bone, or sinus infection. Individuals who have had their spleen removed or who have a nonfunctioning spleen (the organ that produces antibodies that prevent pneumococcal infection) are particularly at risk should they contract the bacterium. Treatment includes large doses of intravenous or oral antibiotics, usually penicillin. Meningitis caused by viruses is milder and more common than bacterial meningitis, which requires immediate treatment and may be prevented by a pneumococcal vaccine that protects against the most common strains of the bacteria. The vaccine is recommended for people with lung and chronic heart disorders as well as other diseases such as diabetes, sickle cell, Hodgkin's, and HIV.

See also PNEUMOCOCCUS; PNEUMONIA.

meningitis, tuberculous Inflamed cerebral meninges as a result of infection by the tubercle bacillus.

See also TUBERCULOSIS.

mesobronchitis Bronchitis in which the middle layer of the bronchi is inflamed.

See also BRONCHITIS.

mesopneumon The hilus of the lung at which two pleural layers meet.

mesothelioma A rare form of cancer characterized by a malignant tumor that lodges in the mesothelium (lining) of the pleura, pericardium, or peritoneum. Victims of mesothelioma are workers who have inhaled asbestos, a rock made up of silky fireproof fibers used as an effective fire retardant. Asbestos has been used in numerous building materials and products, including hot-water pipe coverings, boilers, furnaces, soundproof tiles, floor coverings, fireproofing and insulation in buildings, trains, and ships, brake and clutch linings in cars and airplanes, plasters, drywall, roof shingles, oven liners, toasters, cements, paints, hair dryers, ironing board covers, joint compounds and tapes, and protective clothing.

When asbestos is inhaled into the lungs and other organs, some of the fibers may remain in the body. Buildings made before 1975 may contain asbestos products, and persons living and working in these buildings risk contracting an asbestos disease, largely because the fibers can be blown into the air through the ventilation system. Asbestos may also be ingested, particularly when tiny fibers

are released into the air during construction work, sanding, cutting, or mixing substances containing asbestos. In addition, workers in industries involving the use of asbestos may contract the disease from bringing home asbestos dust on their clothes. The three most common diseases attributable to prolonged exposure to asbestos are lung cancer, asbestosis, and mesothelioma. Mesothelioma is the only one that may not require a latency period, in which disease develops over long periods of time.

See also ASBESTOSIS; LUNG CANCER.

metal fume fever Also called polymer fume fever, a disease resembling influenza caused by inhaling high concentrations of metallic oxide fumes, including zinc oxide, arsenic, cadmium, cobalt, copper, iron, lead, magnesium, manganese, mercury, nickel, or tin. Symptoms are excessive thirst, diaphoresis (excessive sweating), inflammation of the eyes and respiratory tract, chills, and weakness. Treatment involves leaving the offending environment and getting fresh air. Metal fume fever is considered an occupational disease.

metallic tinkling A ringing, like the sound of metal being tapped, heard through a stethoscope over the chest area in which the lung is collapsed.

See also PNEUMOTHORAX.

metaproterenol A beta-adrenergic agonist, or bronchodilator, drug widely used in the treatment of asthma. Metaproterenol is available as a metered-dose inhaler, tablet, liquid, and solution for nebulizer use.

See also BETA-ADRENERGIC AGONISTS.

methacholine challenge A test to diagnose asthma in individuals with confusing or minimal symptoms by the inhalation of the drug methacholine in gradually increasing quantities. An asthmatic person will have a diminished flow rate during spirometry (pulmonary function study), whereas a normal individual will maintain normal flow rates.

methotrexate A chemotherapeutic agent used in the treatment of cancer, psoriasis, and rheumatoid arthritis. Its effectiveness is being studied as a steroid-sparing, anti-inflammatory drug for severe asthma. Although reports indicate conflicting results, methotrexate is thought to be especially beneficial to corticosteroid-dependent asthmatics. One report recommends that methotrexate be discontinued after 36 months because of the possibility of inducing bronchial hyperreactivity or exacerbation of asthma. Prolonged use and higher doses than those used for the treatment of asthma have been known to cause hepatotoxicity, fibrosis, and cirrhosis; in addition, methotrexate may be lethal to a fetus or cause congenital abnormalities and therefore should not be administered to pregnant women with rheumatoid arthritis, psoriasis, or asthma. Other adverse effects of methotrexate include lung disease, bone-marrow depression, and gastrointestinal disturbances.

methscopolamine nitrate   The generic name for an ingredient in the drugs Dura-Vent DA, Extendryl, Histaspan, Histor-D, Rhinolar, and Dallergy. Methscopolamine nitrate, in conjunction with other agents in these preparations, acts as an antihistaminic decongestant prescribed for relief of respiratory congestion, allergic rhinitis, and allergic skin reactions.

methylprednisolone   The generic name for the adrenal corticosteroid drugs Depo-Medrol and Medrol. An anti-inflammatory glucocorticoid agent, methylprednisolone aids the body in modifying immune responses to various stimuli. It is prescribed for treatment of endocrine, rheumatic, ophthalmic, hematologic, neoplastic, respiratory, and gastrointestinal disorders. In addition, methylprednisolone can control severe allergies, including seasonal allergic rhinitis, contact dermatitis, atopic dermatitis, serum sickness, pemphigus, bullous dermatitis herpetiformis, and bronchial asthma.

See also CORTICOSTEROIDS.

mice allergens   Hair, feces, urine, and other physical aspects of mice, especially in infested buildings or areas, that cause adverse effects, or allergic reactions, in some individuals. Research laboratory workers may experience allergic symptoms and asthma in conjunction with exposure to the urine, skin, and saliva of mice and rats.

See also OCCUPATIONAL ASTHMA.

microlithiasis, pulmonary alveolar   The development of microscopic particles of bone in the lungs.

middle lobe syndrome   See ATELECTASIS.

midge   A small-winged fly of the order Diptera. The larvae of nonbiting midges (chironomids) may cause occupational asthma in those who handle fish foods.

See also OCCUPATIONAL ASTHMA.

miliary tuberculosis   An acute form of tuberculosis characterized by minute tubercles, or small, gray nodules reminiscent of the seeds of millet, in the affected tissue or organ.

military service and asthma   The correlation of armed forces' policies and candidates with asthma. Anyone who has had symptoms of asthma over the age of 12, whether symptoms still occur or not, may be excluded from the military academies. During Operations Desert Shield and Desert Storm, nearly 10 percent of admissions to a fleet hospital in Saudi Arabia were for asthma. Although 12 of the 94 patients did not have asthma, 51 needed to be evacuated from the country. Nearly half of the asthmatics displayed a gas-mask intolerance or phobia. The nerve-gas antidote pyridostigmine increased asthma symptoms in more than 25 percent of asthmatic patients. Desert sand storms triggered asthma in 34 percent of the patients.

mold allergy   Symptoms of allergic rhinitis (hay fever) and asthma caused by the inhalation of indoor and outdoor fungal spores commonly called molds. Wind-borne pollen allergens and dry fungal spores are usually removed from the environmental air during rain. Therefore, allergy symptoms during periods of high humidity are most likely due to high mold spore counts found in clouds and mist. Few individuals are sensitive to fungal allergens alone, but fungal sensitivity is common.

molysmophobia   Morbid fear of contamination or contracting an infection.

mometasone furoate   A topical corticosteroid nasal spray that when used once a day has equal effectiveness of older twice-a-day products. It may prevent allergic nasal symptoms if begun prior to the onset of pollen seasons. The drug has a safety profile that does not differ from that of a placebo.
See also CORTICOSTEROIDS.

Monge's disease   Chronic mountain sickness named for Peruvian pathologist Carlos Monge (1884–1970).
See also ALTITUDE SICKNESS.

monitor, apnea   A device such as an apnea alarm mattress that sets off an alarm when the person, particularly an infant, sleeping on it stops breathing. Apnea monitors are useful in the prevention of sudden infant death syndrome (SIDS) and employed in the care of patients with brain injury, meningitis, heart and kidney diseases, and individuals in a coma.
See also APNEA.

monitoring, respiratory   Also known as respiratory function monitoring, alarm devices and techniques used to alert caregivers when a patient's lung function and breathing require attention. Measuring the amount of oxygen in the blood or carbon dioxide in expired air, pulse oximetry, and use of devices that measure respiratory muscle function and breathing patterns are included.

Montelukast   See SINGULAIR.

mountain fever   See ALTITUDE SICKNESS; BENDS.

mountain sickness, chronic   See ALTITUDE SICKNESS.

movement, respiratory   See RESPIRATORY SYSTEM.

mucormycosis   See ZYGOMYCOSIS.

mucosa   The membrane or layer of tissue that is consistently moistened by mucous secretion, such as in the mouth, nasal passages, throat, and other body cavities and organs.

mucosal tests   Diagnostic tests for bacteria and other harmful microorganisms in mucus.

mucus   See MEMBRANE, MUCOUS.

Müller maneuver   Named after German physician Johannes P. Müller (1801–58), a technique for producing negative intrathoracic pressure. The patient exhales and tries to inhale while the glottis is closed (similar to holding one's breath) to achieve better visualization for the physician during fluoroscopy of the esophagus.

multiple systems organ failure   A highly lethal condition of the body in which two or more of the systems malfunction or become nonfunctional, including the respiratory system.

murmur, bronchial   A vibration that causes a blowing or rasping sound that can be heard in the large bronchi through a stethoscope. A murmur may or may not indicate illness.

murmur, pulmonary   A soft blowing sound heard through a stethoscope when placed over the orifice of the pulmonary artery.
See also MURMUR, BRONCHIAL.

Mycobacterium   From the Greek work meaning little rod, an organism of the Mycobacteriaceae family that causes tuberculosis and leprosy.
See also LEPROSY; TUBERCULOSIS.

mycoderma   Mucous membrane.

Mycoplasma pneumoniae A group of tiny organisms that lack the ability to form cell walls and cause infection of the lungs and upper respiratory tract. The disease is usually treated with tetracycline or erythromycin.

myxasthenia Insufficient production of mucus, which may aggravate respiratory disorders such as asthma.

myxiosis A secretion of mucus.

Nasacort, Nasacort AQ Nasal Spray Brand of the cortisone-like anti-inflammatory drug triamcinolone.

nasal cavity The open space between the cranium floor and the roof of the mouth.

nasal challenge Also called nasal provocation tests, diagnostic allergy tests involving either inhalation or direct mucosal contact with a suspected allergenic substance. The tests are occasionally helpful when allergy skin-test results do not correlate with a person's medical and allergy history. When performing a nasal challenge, the physician must carefully observe the patient for signs of a systemic reaction. The patient should be relatively free of allergic symptoms and must not have taken antihistaminic drugs for the past several days. Positive challenge results are indicated by itching, sneezing, watery discharge from the nose, and swelling of the nasal mucosa. In some cases, the tests fall short because they are time-consuming and because only one allergen at a time can be tested; in addition, if nasal symptoms are already present, the test may not be valid.

nasal congestion Swelling of the nasal passages, which is a symptom of allergic rhinitis (hay fever), vasomotor (nonallergic) rhinitis, upper respiratory infections (colds), and rhinitis medicamentosa (rebound congestion caused by abuse of nasal sprays). Complications of nasal congestion include sinus and ear infection and worsening of asthma. Decongestants are the main treatment of nasal congestions; however, antihistamines and the preventive nasal sprays, cromolyn, and corticosteroids are useful for allergy patients.

Nasalcrom See CROMOLYN SODIUM.

nasal douche See NASAL IRRIGATION.

nasal endoscopy See RHINOSCOPY.

nasal feeding The process of administering liquid food to a patient through a tube that goes into the nose and to the stomach. Nasal feeding is used only when circumstances prevent a patient from taking in nutrients by mouth.

Nasalide A brand of flunisolide, a corticosteroid for topical use as a nasal spray and metered-dose inhaler for prevention of nasal allergy symptoms and asthma.
  See also CORTICOSTEROIDS.

nasal irrigation A procedure that helps rid the nasal passages of excess mucus and bacteria. Saline (salt water) is available from local pharmacies or can be made fresh daily at home with one teaspoon of table salt and a pinch of baking soda in one pint of warm water. Many proprietary brands (Ocean Spray and Salinex are examples) are available as nasal sprays. Saline irrigations should be done before using other medications in the nose. One may inhale or "snuff" the saline solution from the palm of the hand or squirt it into the nose with a rubber ear syringe. When injecting the solution into the nostril, one should keep his mouth open and glottis closed so fluid does not go into the throat and bronchus. Also, no great force should be used.

nasal obstruction Blockage of the nasal passages either uni- or bilaterally. The most common cause of unilateral stuffiness is a deviated septum, which may be a congenital deformity or a result of trauma to the nose. It can be surgically corrected by rhinoplasty ("nose job") if the obstruction is severe. In babies, a frequent cause of obstruction is a foreign body, a tiny object such as a button or a piece of a toy. Unilateral nasal obstruction may also indicate benign or malignant tumors, which should be discovered and treated by the physician.

nasal polyp   See POLYP.

nasal provocation tests   See NASAL CHALLENGE.

nasal reflex   Sneezing, usually caused by an agent that irritates the nasal mucosa.
   See also SNEEZE.

nasal secretions   Mucus discharge from the nose that is characterized by quantity (none, minimal, moderate, or profuse), consistency (none, thin, mucoid, or crusted), and color (colorless, clear, white, or colored). The description aids the diagnosis of allergy, infection, or other anomaly.

nasal septum   The wall separating the two nasal cavities (nostrils).

nasal sinuses   See NOSE.

nasal smear   A screening test used to diagnose nasal symptoms. Nasal secretions are obtained by blowing the nose into waxed paper and transferring the collected material to a glass slide. Hansel's or Wright's stain is applied to the slide, which is examined microscopically for leukocytes, or white blood cells, such as eosinophils or polymorphonuclear leukocytes, or polys. Allergic diseases may be present if eosinophils account for 10 percent or greater of the total white blood cells observed on a nasal smear. A predominance of polys suggests an infection, and absence of a significant number of cells suggests vasomotor, or nonallergic, rhinitis.

nasal spray   Nebulizer or aerosol used to treat excessive nasal discharge and congestion characteristic of hay fever, colds, or other nasal disorders. Nasal sprays include over-the-counter decongestants. However, many individuals quickly develop tolerance, or loss of effectiveness, to these sprays, which leads to a worsening of congestion referred to as rebound. The rebound phenomenon is called rhinitis medicamentosa.

   Saline solution is used to irrigate dry, inflamed nasal passages but has no therapeutic effect to prevent discharge or congestion. The prescription drugs cromolyn sodium and corticosteroids (cortisone derivatives) are effective for long-term prevention of allergy symptoms.
   See also CORTICOSTEROIDS.

nasal spray habituation   See NASAL SPRAY.

nasal turbinates   Four bony structures arising from the nasal septum. The two most important ones are the inferior and middle turbinates. The turbinates are lined with cells similar to those in the tracheobronchial tube and regulate the airflow into the upper respiratory system.
   See also NOSE.

nasitis   Inflammation of the nose.
   See also RHINITIS.

nasopharyngeal airway   Part of the nose that extends to the portion of the throat located above the soft palate or postnasal space.

nasopharyngitis   An inflammation of the nasopharyngeal airway, which may occur in conjunction with postnasal drip and allergic rhinitis.

nasoscope   A medical instrument used for examining the nasal passages.

nasoseptitis   Inflammation of the nasal septum.
   See also NASAL SEPTUM.

nasosinusitis   Inflammation of the nasal accessory sinuses and cavities.
   See also SINUSITIS.

nasotracheal intubation   The insertion of an endotracheal tube, which helps airways remain open, through the nose in patients with clenched teeth or cervical spinal injury, used particularly because the patient's neck does not need to be hyperextended for the insertion of the tube.

nasus   The Latin word for nose.
   See also NOSE.

"natural way" to control asthma   The option of home remedies to treat asthma, or the myth that asthma does not require drugs for treatment.

naturopathy   An alternative healing method that uses natural forces such as air, water, light, and heat and massage instead of drugs and surgery characteristic of allopathic (Western) medicine. Patients with respiratory disorders may seek the advice of a naturopath in conjunction with traditional therapy.

nebulizer   An atomizer or device that produces a fine spray used to deliver allergy and asthma drugs to the nasal passages or lungs.

necropneumonia   Another term for pulmonary gangrene, which refers to death of lung tissue caused by infection, inflammation, degenerative changes, disease, injury, and lack of blood supply to the affected area.

nedocromil sodium (Tilade)   A preventive allergy and asthma anti-inflammatory drug approved for use in the United States in 1993. Although nedocromil has properties similar to those of cromolyn, its effectiveness may be apparent within hours; however, it may take two weeks of regular dosage to realize its full potential. Cromolyn may require several months to realize benefits. Nedocromil may also be needed only twice a day, whereas cromolyn requires use three to four times a day.
   Similar to cromolyn, nedocromil does not interact with other asthma drugs, such as theophylline, and is available as a metered-dose inhaler. This

drug works for children and adults. A solution for aerosol nebulizers, a nasal spray, and eyedrops may also be available. There are no significant side effects of the product, although slightly more than 10 percent of patients complain of an unpleasant taste.
   See also CROMOLYN SODIUM.

Neisseria sicca   A bacterium named for German physician Albert Neisser (1855–1916) that is associated with forms of meningitis and gonorrhea. *Neisseria sicca* is a species of the bacterium that thrives in mucous membrane of the respiratory tract and may cause bacterial endocarditis. *Branhamella (Neisseria) catarrhalis* can be found in the upper respiratory tract and may be mistaken for meningococci.

Neo-Synephrine   Brand name of nosedrops made from phenylephrine hydrochloride, an alpha-adrenergic decongestant drug also used in eyedrops. Phenylephrine hydrochloride is also used in combination with antihistamines for the treatment of hay fever and colds. Tolerance to phenylephrine nasal products often causes a dependency known as rhinitis medicamentosa, which may require treatment with corticosteroids in order to break the cycle and symptoms of dependency.
   See also NASAL SPRAY.

nephrotuberculosis   Condition caused when the *Mycobacterium tuberculosis* affects a kidney.
   See also TUBERCULOSIS.

nerve gas   See BIOTERRORISM; WAR GASSES.

neuraminidase   An enzyme found on the surface of influenza virus particles that allows the particles to detach from cells. When an individual has high levels of antibodies that counteract neuraminidase, he or she may be more resistant to the influenza virus than others.

nicotine gum (Nicorette)   Chewing product containing nicotine that allows smokers to gradually reduce their dependency on the addicting substance in tobacco while avoiding withdrawal symptoms such as irritability and chest pains.

nicotine patches (Habitrol, Nicoderm, Nicotrol, Pro Step) Band-Aid–like adhesive delivery system containing the drug nicotine. The patch is placed on the skin of smokers as a means to stop smoking. Nicotine is the addicting substance in tobacco. The patches contain a varying amount of nicotine, and doses are gradually tapered, usually in two or three steps, to avoid the withdrawal symptoms of nicotine. The adhesive in the patch frequently causes an allergic contact rash.

nicotine poisoning A potentially fatal intoxication of nicotine, a poisonous alkaloid that acts as quickly as cyanide when ingested. Less than 5 milligrams of nicotine per kilogram of body weight may indicate a lethal dose. Death is usually the result of paralysis of the respiratory muscles and respiratory failure. Antidotes include activated charcoal, tannic acid, strong tea and gastric lavage or an emetic substance, oxygen therapy, barbiturates if the victim is having severe convulsions, artificial or mechanically assisted respiration, and maintenance of a patent airway.

nitric acid fuming Vapors or fumes emanating from a concentration of the corrosive toxin nitric acid. If inhaled, the fumes cause choking.

nitrites See INHALANT ABUSE.

nitrogen A gas that constitutes 80 percent of atmospheric volume. Nitrogen is colorless, odorless, tasteless, and a component of all proteins, which makes it essential to plant and animal life.

nitrogen dioxide An environmental pollutant present in the atmosphere that has been associated with an increased incidence of lung disease following prolonged exposure in homes and workplaces.

nitrogen narcosis Euphoria and impaired judgment, motor function, and coordination akin to alcohol intoxication caused by an increased concentration of nitrogen gas in the brain and body tissues. The imbalance of gasses occurs in high altitudes or any situation in which air pressure changes drastically, such as that experienced by divers and submariners.

See also BENDS.

nitrous oxide Also known as laughing gas, a colorless, sweet-tasting, pleasantly aromatic gas used as a light general anesthetic, especially by dentists. In high doses, nitrous oxide may cause asphyxiation. Use of a local anesthetic agent such as lidocaine is probably safer in patients with asthma.

See also INHALANT ABUSE.

N.K.A. An abbreviation for "no known allergies" in medical charts.

Nocardia Named for French veterinary pathologist Edmund I. E. Nocard (1850–1903), a gram-positive bacterium that, when stained on a slide, may be mistaken for *Mycobacterium tuberculosis.* Nocardia causes the disease nocardiosis.

See also NOCARDIOSIS.

nocardiosis A pneumonia-like infection caused by a *Nocardia* bacterium called *Nocardia asteroides,* present in soil dust throughout the world and transmissible by inhalation, skin contact, and ingestion. It may occur in the lungs and spread to the brain, skin, and other parts of the body. It may also be the cause of lower-extremity tumors, particularly a condition known as Madura foot. Nocardiosis may be contracted by individuals with immunodeficiency disorders or other chronic diseases or by those with no preexisting disease. Sometimes nocardiosis is a complication in patients with AIDS. Symptoms include chills, chest pain, shortness of breath, weight loss, loss of appetite, accumulation of fluid in the pleural space, fever, and cough that do not respond to short-term antibiotic therapy and may progress to brain abscess or lung damage. Diagnosis requires analysis of the patient's sputum or body fluid or tissue. Treatment of choice is sulfadiazine, among other drugs, but depending upon the medical condition of the victim and whether or not the infection is contained in the lungs or has already metastasized, nocardiosis may be fatal.

nocturnal asthma   The occurrence of asthma symptoms during the night. Nearly 40 percent of asthmatics experience nightly symptoms; approximately 64 percent have episodes three nights a week, and about 75 percent at least one night per week. Asthma attacks seem to occur most often between 10 P.M. and 7 A.M., peaking at about 4 A.M. When several things simultaneously trigger asthma, results can be severe. The most devastating asthma attacks that lead to respiratory arrest, and possibly death, most often occur between midnight and 6 A.M.

During sleep, mucus secretions accumulate in the bronchial tubes, and the backup, or reflux, of stomach acid may spill over into the lungs, causing irritation and inflammation of lung tissue.

The circadian fall in the body's production of cortisone and adrenaline and the rise of other chemicals, such as histamine, further worsen the situation during the night. In addition, the cell counts of neutrophils and eosinophils (cells that release mediators of inflammation) are higher in patients with nocturnal asthma symptoms. Timing medications to coincide with peak effectiveness and times of greatest need can greatly reduce symptoms and allow patients to sleep through the night.

See also ASTHMA.

nose   One of the chief organs of the respiratory system through which air flows in and out of the body. The external portion of the nose is made of a triangle of cartilage (the top of which constitutes the bridge of the nose, where the two nasal bones are joined) and skin-covered bone lined with mucous membrane. The internal portion contains two chambers divided by a septum. The chambers lead to various sinuses, including accessory nasal sinuses.

The nose is also an olfactory organ that facilitates the sense of smell and warms, moistens, and filters air breathed in. Physicians may observe a patient's nose for its size, shape, color, evidence of injury, discharge, tenderness over sinuses, and interferences with breathing. For example, chronically red nose caused by dilated blood vessels may be a result of alcoholism, acne, boils, or digestive disorders. An offensive discharge may indicate local infection, cavities in the teeth, a cold, or an impacted foreign body. A chronic, clear, watery discharge usually suggests the presence of allergy. Rhinitis refers to inflammation of the nasal mucous membrane; allergic rhinitis refers to seasonal allergy such as hay fever.

nostril reflex   A diminishing of a nostril, or opening at the base of the nose, on the side corresponding to lung disease in which there is a lessened alveolar air capacity in one lung.

notifiable diseases   Highly contagious illnesses that must by law be reported to local authorities, including the board of health. They include tuberculosis, AIDS, chickenpox, rubella, cholera, polio, typhoid fever, typhus, meningococcal meningitis, and syphilis.

obstructive lung disease, chronic   See CHRONIC OBSTRUCTIVE PULMONARY DISEASE.

occupational asthma   Shortness of breath, coughing, wheezing, and other symptoms of asthma from exposure to sensitizing substances found in the workplace. These substances may be allergens, or they may be nonallergic or toxic substances, such as ammonia, chlorine, smoke, or other noxious fumes that inflame the lungs of workers accidentally exposed to them.

History
As early as the second century A.D., miners covered themselves with clothing as protection from dust. In 1713, Bernardino Ramazzini, considered to be the father of industrial or occupational medicine, recommended in his book, *De Morbis Artificum Diatriba,* inquiry into a patient's occupation when he discovered attacks of shortness of breath in sifters and millers exposed to grain dust. Ramazzini described asthma as an occupational hazard in individuals who "are short of breath and cachectic and rarely reach old age." In 1877, the term byssinosis was coined for asthma in cotton workers, and in 1911 platinum salt exposure was recognized as a cause of asthma in photographic workers. More recently British physician Jack Peppys stimulated interest in this problem in the 1960s.

Prevalence
It is estimated that 2 to 15 percent of all asthma cases are caused by occupational or workplace exposure. Up to 44 percent of bakery workers and up to 10 percent of persons exposed to laboratory animals have symptoms. In Japan, an estimated 15 percent of asthma cases in males may be from industrial exposure. In some industries, very few workers develop symptoms, but in others, large numbers are affected. For example, nearly 100 percent of workers exposed to platinum salts for at least five years develop some symptoms.

Causes
More than 200 substances have been reported to cause occupational asthma, and the list continues to grow. To cause an immediate immune response, a substance must have a molecular weight of at least 1,000 daltons, with most weighing more than 20,000. These allergens are proteins or glycoproteins, including animal proteins, biologic enzymes, grain dust, or irritants such as dusts, gases, or fumes that cause early or immediate onset of symptoms and are relatively easy to correlate with exposure.

Lower-molecular-weight allergens (irritants of less than 1,000 daltons), such as anhydrides, diisocyanates, formalin, freon, metals, pharmaceuticals such as penicillin dust, solder fluxes, urea formaldehyde, and wood dust, usually cause late-phase responses; symptoms may not be evident for many hours after exposure.

High-molecular-weight compounds cause a true allergic reaction. The worker inhales the allergen, which stimulates the immune system to produce immunoglobulin E (IgE) antibodies. The antibodies then become attached to structures called receptors on immune cells (mast cells and basophils) in the body tissues. After a person has been sensitized in this manner, subsequent exposures to the same allergen cause a reaction between the allergen and its corresponding antibody that results in the rupturing of these cells and the release of chemicals such as histamine. The released chemicals cause the allergic response or symptoms. Most of the lower-molecular-weight substances fail to elicit such a response, although they do cause similar symptoms to occur via other mechanisms.

Many of the substances responsible for occupational asthma can also be encountered outside the workplace, and materials can be transported outside the original areas of contact on clothing, in the hair, or on the skin of workers. They can also pollute the surrounding environment.

Common fungal and bacterial species may contaminate air-conditioning units and water-cooled machinery, causing an infectious pneumonia such as Legionnaire's disease, or the allergic-type hypersensitivity pneumonitis.

Other occupational exposures include the inhalation of iron particles in dust or fumes, resulting in siderosis, also called arc welder's disease, or hemosiderosis, a pneumonia-like lung disease. Tributyl tin oxide (TBTO) is an organic compound contained in a carpet deodorizer that is a suspected cause of asthma. TBTO is also used in the manufacture of plastics, silicone, and paint products and is an antifungal agent in paper. This substance can also cause an irritant dermatitis.

Talc triggers occupational asthma by acting as an irritant. In the 1970s and 1980s the *Bacillus subtilis* enzyme added to detergents became a major cause of allergic symptoms in workers as well as consumers. Hog trypsin used in the plastics industry is another industrial allergen. Castor bean allergy not only may affect factory workers, but also neighboring inhabitants may become sensitized by exposure to smoke from castor oil factories. Smoking is a complicating factor because of its influence on increasing airway reactivity.

Symptoms

Accompanying the asthma resulting from allergen exposure in the workplace is a latent, or waiting, period between the initial exposure and the onset of symptoms. Often symptoms do not appear for several weeks or take several years to appear. Only about 20 percent of those exposed to occupational allergens develop allergies. Once symptoms occur, they usually become progressively more severe with continued exposure. If exposure is stopped soon enough, symptoms will usually cease unless a person is reexposed. However, if exposure is prolonged, symptoms of asthma may become persis-

tent even after exposure is terminated. Conjunctivitis, or inflammation of the eyes (commonly called "pinkeye"), may be the earliest symptom of allergen or irritant exposure in the workplace. Rhinitis, or runny nose, may also be an early sign. Wheezing, coughing, and shortness of breath can occur within minutes of exposure or not until later in the day or even 24 to 48 hours afterward. The later onset of symptoms often makes diagnosis or proof of cause difficult. A valuable clue to the existence of workplace allergy is that symptoms often improve over the weekend or on holidays; however, it may take weeks, months, or years to improve depending on the length of previous exposure. The asthma caused by a single heavy exposure to toxic fumes may last for years.

Medical-Legal Issues

Documentation of occupational cause of symptoms is often difficult because individuals may have preexisting asthma.This issue may be clarified if other employees have similar symptoms. A survey may be necessary to uncover this. Federal or state public health agencies may be called upon to help affected employees. Patients' symptoms of asthma can be monitored by using objective measuring devices such as a Wright's Peak Flow Meter or much less expensive meters made by various manufacturers such as Access, Mini-Wright, and Vitalograph. These devices can measure the patient's airflow rates both at home and in the workplace every one to two hours for a period of one or two weeks or until a pattern develops.

Individual peak flow should not vary beyond 10 percent of the flow predicted for a normal person throughout the day. A 20 percent or greater decrease in flow rate is considered significant. If peak flow results are inadequate for legal documentation, an inhalation challenge may be necessary to identify the suspected allergen. The challenge carries a risk of a severe attack of asthma and should be performed only by specially trained medical personnel with resuscitation equipment available.

Although it may be difficult, it may be necessary to determine if the patient's symptoms are solely a result of an occupational exposure. The individual with preexisting asthma may have a worsening of symptoms when he or she experiences some trigger such as a dusty environment in a new job or change in working conditions in an existing job. A patient with preexisting but dormant asthma may be exposed to an occupational allergen and then finds it difficult to prove that this is a new occupationally caused asthma. The best objective criterion for diagnosing occupational asthma is the specific bronchoprovocation test, in which the suspected worker is challenged with the implicated substance. In this test, the worker is given the suspected substance by inhalation under carefully controlled conditions. The patient's lung function is studied before and after this challenge.

Unfortunately, this is very difficult to arrange, and less accurate methods of assessment are used instead for practical reasons, including expense and nonavailability of experienced specialists, equipment, or standardized testing materials. The incriminated agent must be standardized so that repeated testing will give the same results (reproducibility) and be specific for the involved materials. An example is the chemical toluene diisocyanate used in plastics and varnishes. When this substance was administered to a control group of known asthmatic patients with no prior exposure to this substance, they did not react to a challenge. However, when previously exposed workers suspected of being sensitized to this substance were given the challenge, they showed a decrease in their lung function tests.

Two main questions must be addressed in these situations: First, is there a disability? Second, can the work environment be improved to allow continued employment? About 70 percent of patients with workplace-induced asthma will continue to have symptoms even years after exposure has stopped. Disability from occupational asthma is often lumped together with that from exposure to silicon and asbestos, a cause of serious lung disease.

Evaluation and Management of Work-Aggravated Asthma and Occupational Asthma Evaluation

Potential for workplace-related symptoms:

- Recognized sensitizers (e.g., isocyanates, plant or animal products)

- Irritants or physical stimuli (e.g., cold/heat, dust, humidity) (NOTE: Material Safety Data may be helpful for identifying respiratory irritants, but many sensitizers are not listed.)

- Coworkers may have similar symptoms

Patterns of symptoms (in relation to work exposures):

- Improvement during vacations or days off (may take a week or more)

- Symptoms may be immediate (<1 hour), delayed (most commonly, 2 to 8 hours after exposure), or nocturnal

- Initial symptoms may occur after high-level exposure (e.g., spill)

Documentation of work relatedness of airflow limitation:

- Serial charting for 2 to 3 weeks (2 weeks at work and up to 1 week off work as needed to identify or exclude work-related changes in peak expiratory flow): Record when symptoms and exposures occur; record when a bronchodilator is used; measure and record peak flow every 2 hours while awake

- Immunologic tests

- Referral for further confirmatory evaluation (e.g., bronchial challenges)

Management

Work-aggravated asthma:

- Work with onsite health care providers or managers/supervisors

- Discuss avoidance, ventilation, respiratory protection, and tobacco smoke-free environment

Occupationally induced asthma:

- Recommend complete cessation of exposure to initiating agent

Control Measures for Environmental Factors That Can Make Asthma Worse

Allergens: Reduce or eliminate exposure to the allergen(s) the patient is sensitive to, including:

- Animal dander: Remove animal from house or, at a minimum, keep animal out of patient's bedroom and seal or cover with filter air ducts that lead to bedroom

- House-dust mites: *(Essential)* Encase mattress in an allergen-impermeable cover; encase pillow in an allergen-impermeable cover or wash it weekly; wash sheets and blankets on the patient's bed in hot water weekly (water temperature of greater than 130 degrees Fahrenheit is necessary for killing mites). *(Desirable)* Reduce indoor humidity to less than 50 percent; remove carpets from the bedroom; avoid sleeping or lying on upholstered furniture; remove carpets that are laid on concrete

- Cockroaches: Use poison bait or traps to control. Do not leave food or garbage exposed

- Pollens (from trees, grass, or weeds) and outdoor molds: To avoid exposure, adults should stay indoors with windows closed during the season in which they have problems with outdoor allergens, especially during the afternoon

- Indoor mold: Fix all leaks and eliminate water sources associated with mold growth; clean moldy surfaces. Consider reducing indoor humidity to less than 50 percent

Tobacco smoke: Advise patients and others in the home who smoke to stop smoking or smoke outside the home. Discuss ways to reduce exposure to other sources of tobacco smoke, such as from day care providers and the workplace.

Indoor/outdoor pollutants and irritants: Discuss ways to reduce exposure to the following:

- Wood-burning stoves or fireplaces
- Unvented stoves or heaters
- Other irritants (e.g., perfumes, cleaning agents, sprays)

Allergens Known to Cause Occupational Asthma

abirukana
acacia
adipic acid
African maple
African zebra wood
Alternaria
aluminum fluoride
aminoethyl ethanolamine
aminophylline

ammonium persulfate
amprolium hydrochloride
animals, laboratory
apple tree mite
aspergillus
azobisformamide
azodicarbonamide
Baby's breath
Bacillus subtilis enzymes
bee moth
bromelain
buckwheat
butterflies
California redwood
carmine
carmine beetle
castor beans
cats
cattle
cedar of Lebanon
Central American walnut
cephalosporins
chromates
chrysanthemum
cibachrome brilliant scarlet
cimetidine
cinnamon
cobalt
cocabolla
cockroaches
coffee beans
colophony (pine resin, or abietic acid)
cotton[1]
crickets
crop storage mites
cyanoacrylate
Daphnia
diastase
dichloramine
diisocyanates
dimethyl ethanolamine
dioazonium salt
dogs
Douglas fir tussock moth
Drimaren brilliant blue and yellow
eastern white cedar
electrocardiography ink
endofluorane anesthetic

ethylenediamine
feathers
flaviastase
flax
fluoride, fluorine
formaldehyde
Freon
fungal amylase
fungal food products
furan base resin
garlic
gentian powder
glue
gluteraldehyde
grain dust[1]
grain dust mite
grain field fungi
grain weevil
guinea pigs
hemp
hexachlorophene
hexahydrophthalic anhydride
hog trypsin
hops
horses
housefly maggots
hoya (sea squirt)
humidifiers
ipecac
iroko
ispaghula
karaya
kejaat
lanau
Levafix brilliant yellow
locusts
lycopodium
magnolia
mahogany
maiko
mayfly
mealworm
methyldopa
methyl methcrylate
Mexican bean weevil
mice
midges
mother of pearl

mulberry
mushroom spores
nickel salts
oak
organophosphate
oyster shells
pancreatic (extract) enzyme
papain
parakeets
paraphenylenediamine
pectinase
penicillins
pepsin
persulfate and henna
phenylene glycine acid chloride
phthalic anhydride
pigeons
piperazine dihydrochloride
platinum salts
Plexiglas dust
polyetheralcohol
polypropylene glycol
polyvinyl chloride
poultry mites
prawns
protease bromelain
psyllium
quillaja ramin
rabbits
rats
salbutamol intermediate
screwworm fly
sheep
silkworm moths and larvae
sky blue
snow crab
South African boxwood
soya bean
spiramycin
sponge
stainless steel
strawberry pollen
styrene
sugar beet
sulfathiazole sulfone chloramide (chloramine T
    and halazone)
sunflower
tamarind

Tanganyika aningre
tannic acid
tea dust
tetrachlorophthalic
tetracycline
tobacco
toluene diisocyanate
tragacanth
triethyl tetramine
trimellitic anhydride
tungsten carbide
urea formaldehyde
vanadium zinc
welding fumes
western red cedar dust (plicatic acid)
wheat flour

[1] Cotton, hemp, and grain dust are irritants and not true allergens.

See also ASBESTOSIS; PNEUMONITIS; SILICOSIS.

oleothorax   The injection of oil into the pleural cavity in the chest, or thorax, as a therapeutic method (oleotherapy) for patients with pulmonary tuberculosis and other respiratory disorders.

olfactory nerves   The first pair of the 12 cranial nerves that facilitate the sense of smell by enervating the mucous membranes of the nose.

oligopnea   The medical term for infrequent, or abnormally shallow or deep, respiration, often as slow as six to 10 respirations per minute, usually as a result of intracranial pressure, hemorrhage of certain parts of the brain, brain tumors, certain forms of meningitis, shock, disease, or drug poisoning. Oligopnea is derived from the Greek words *oligo,* meaning little or few, and *pnoia,* or breath.

Ondine's curse   Named for Undine (French spelling), a mythical water nymph who had a human lover upon whom a curse was cast that he would sleep forever, a reference to primary alveolar hypoventilation, a condition of hypoventilation in the alveoli of the lungs caused by a dysfunction of the respiratory center, such as excessive carbon dioxide, or a lesion in the cervical (neck) portion of the spinal cord. This occurs when the respiratory center does not respond adequately to carbon dioxide. Ondine's curse also refers to a loss of respiratory function as a result of a lesion in the spinal cord.

See also HYPOVENTILATION SYNDROME; PRIMARY PULMONARY HYPERTENSION.

Opticrom   A brand name for cromolyn sodium eyedrops used for allergic disorders.

organic dust toxic syndrome   Abbreviated as ODTS, a respiratory disorder caused by inhaling dust of moldy hay, silage, or similar substances. Symptoms include fever, coughing, and muscle pain. ODTS is a nonallergic and noninfectious illness.

oropharyngeal airway   A tube that can be inserted into the mouth of a patient who is unconscious to prevent obstruction of the air passages by his or her tongue.

orthopnea   From the Greek words *ortho,* meaning straight, and *pnoia,* or breath, a discomfort upon breathing that is relieved by an orthopneic position, i.e., sitting nearly upright in a bed or chair, or standing. Individuals experiencing orthopnea, which may accompany congestive heart failure, bronchial and cardiac asthma, pulmonary edema, emphysema, pneumonia, angina pectoris, and spasmodic coughing, may also be anxious, blue in the face, and using their respiratory muscles forcibly or bracing themselves in order to breathe. Patients usually prop themselves up with several pillows or sit in a chair to sleep in order to avoid feeling as though they are suffocating. A patient may be referred to as having "two-pillow" or "three-pillow" orthopnea, depending on the number of pillows needed to allow him or her to breathe more comfortably.

osmethesia   From the Greek words *osme,* or odor, and *aisthesis,* or sensation, the ability to perceive and distinguish odors.

otolaryngologist Physician who treats diseases of the ears, nose, and throat medically and surgically. Otolaryngologists (also called otorhinolaryngologists) also may perform surgery of the head and neck, and plastic surgery of the face. Otolaryngology is the medical specialty concentrating on diagnoses and treatments of disorders of the ears, nose, and throat.

overventilation See HYPERVENTILATION.

oximeter Photoelectric device for measuring the amount of oxygen in the blood.

oxitriphylline (Choledyl) A derivative of theophylline, a bronchodilating drug used in the treatment of asthma.
See also THEOPHYLLINE.

oxygen An odorless, tasteless, and colorless gas that is essential to life. It is used therapeutically for patients with respiratory distress in diseases such as asthma, emphysema, severe pneumonia, and congestive heart failure. Oxygen content in the body can be determined by measuring arterial blood gases or oximetry.
See also ARTERIAL BLOOD GASES.

oxygenator A mechanism for the purpose of infusing oxygen, such as into the bloodstream during thoracic or open-heart surgery.

oxygen capacity The oxygen measured in cubic centimeters per 100 milliliters of blood. Normal blood contains approximately 20 cubic centimeters of oxygen.

oxygen content The amount of oxygen in the blood.

oxygen debt The deficit of oxygen induced by intense bodily activity (anaerobic exercise) that may be relieved by rest, during which the body has the ability to replenish itself.

oxygen tent An enclosure that surrounds the patient's head and shoulders for the purpose of administering air in which the oxygen content has been increased.
See also OXYGEN THERAPY.

oxygen therapy Treatment of oxygen deficiency by administering oxygen via oxygen mask, tent, or nasal catheter.

oxygen toxicity The inability to ventilate the lungs as a result of pure oxygen breathed for a long period of time. Impaired ventilation causes a lack of oxygen tension in the blood.

oxymetazoline Generic name for the alpha-agonist drug or decongestant nasal sprays or solutions available under the trade names Afrin, Dristan, 4-Way Nasal Spray, NTZ, and Neo-Synephrine. These drugs are noted for their rapid facilitation of nasal decongestion; however, tolerance may develop after only a few days of continuous use. This phenomenon is called rhinitis medicamentosa, or rebound, and is treatable by corticosteroids.

ozone A type of oxygen with a pungent odor and a bluish color, formed by three oxygen atoms and known as the molecule O_3. An environmental pollutant, ozone causes asthma-like hyperreactivity of the bronchioles similar to that in a viral respiratory infection. Inhalation of ozone and other environmental pollutants (including tobacco smoke, nitrogen dioxide, and sulfur dioxide) produces inflammation in the airways. Adverse response to ozone can also be seen in nonasthmatic, or normal, persons. Ozone is formed naturally in the atmosphere by a photochemical reaction. The ozone layer, dubbed in 1929, is located at heights of approximately 20 to 30 miles above Earth.

PA Abbreviation for pulmonary artery.

PA catheter An intravenous catheter (tube) inserted into the pulmonary artery.

pachyderma laryngitis An abnormal thickening and enlargement of the laryngeal mucous membrane, usually a result of chronic laryngitis.
See also LARYNGITIS.

pachypleuritis Inflammation and abnormal thickening of the pleura.
See also RESPIRATORY SYSTEM.

pachyrhinic Referring to a flat, thick nose.

pain, chest Any severe pain in the chest caused by cardiac problems, overexertion, pleurisy (in which there is pain accompanying a deep breath), arthritis, fibrosis, or hiatal or diaphragmatic hernia.

pansinusitis Infection involving all the sinuses.
See also SINUSITIS.

panting Heavy breathing or rapid gasps for breath, usually caused by strenuous physical activity or the onset of fear.

papaverine hydrochloride (Cerespan, Pavabid) Derived from the poppy plant, the salt of an alkaloid from opium that is used as a smooth muscle relaxant for treating bronchial spasm, and stomach and intestinal disturbances.

papilloma, Hopmann's Polyps or epithelial tumors (also warts and condylomas) growing excessively in the nasal mucosa.

para-aminosalicylic acid (PAS) An antituberculosis drug, also known as aminosalicylic acid, often combined with isoniazid and streptomycin. PAS is believed to help delay bacterial resistance to drug therapy.

paracentesis pulmonis The removal of fluid from a lung through puncturing the lung. Patients with excess fluid in a lung may require paracentesis pulmonis, or, in the case of pleural effusion of other abnormal accumulation of fluid in the chest cavity, paracentesis thoracis.
See also ASPIRATION.

paradoxical respiration In the case of collapsed lung, a condition in which the lung inflates on exhalation and deflates on inhalation. Paradoxical respiration also refers to a paralyzed diaphragm that rises during inhalation instead of exhalation.
See also PNEUMOTHORAX.

parainfluenza viruses A variety of microorganisms that cause acute respiratory infections.

paraldehyde poisoning The toxic effect of a liquid polymer of acetaldehyde (trade name Paral), used as a sedative and hypnotic to treat delirium tremens and acute alcoholism. Symptoms include cardiac and respiratory depression. Induced vomiting (if the poisoning is mild), oxygen therapy, artificial ventilation, and tracheostomy are among the treatment options.

paramyxoviruses A subgroup of viruses called myxoviruses that cause parainfluenza, respiratory syncytial viruses, measles, mumps, and Newcastle disease.

paranasal sinuses The frontal, ethmoidal, sphenoidal, and maxillary sinuses that open into the nasal passages.

See also RESPIRATORY SYSTEM.

parapleuritis Inflammation occurring in the chest wall or in the pleura.

parrot fever See PSITTACOSIS.

passive smoking See SMOKING, PASSIVE.

pastille A type of lozenge, or medicated disk, used to soothe or medicate the mouth and throat.

Patanol The brand name of olopatadine hydrochloride, an ophthalmic solution for the treatment of itchy eyes caused by allergic conjunctivitis. Rare adverse reactions include pharyngitis, rhinitis, sinusitis, and cold syndrome.

PBZ Abbreviation for the antihistamine tripelennamine (Pyribenzamine).

peak flow The maximum flow rate that can be generated with the most forcible expiration a person can manage. One of the important indicators of asthma, the peak flow of expired air is measured by a peak flow meter in liters per second. The best of three readings is considered the peak expiratory flow rate (PEFR). The PEFR determines if there is an obstruction in one's airway. This objective measurement is similar to taking a person's blood pressure with a sphygmomanometer. The PEFR provides an accurate way to monitor the response to asthma therapy and exacerbations of asthma, detect asymptomatic deterioration in lung function before it becomes critical, determine the degree of airflow obstruction and detect early stages of obstruction, and indicate when emergency care is required. Because the peak flow measurement tests patency only of the large airways, an individual with mild asthma relating to small airways may be undiagnosed unless spirometry, which measures flow rates at low lung volumes, is employed. An objective measurement of airflow obstruction, such as PEFR, in persons with asthma is desirable because subjective measurements (dyspnea and wheezing, for example) by physicians and patients may be inaccurate. One study demonstrated that only 44 percent of physicians could estimate PEFR with 20 percent of the actual measured PEFR of patients. By the time wheezing can be detected with a stethoscope, the PEFR has already decreased

---

How to Use Your Peak Flow Meter (Patient Handout)

A peak flow meter is a device that measures how well air moves out of your lungs. During an asthma episode, the airways of the lungs usually begin to narrow slowly. The peak flow meter may tell you if there is narrowing in the airways hours—sometimes even days—before you have any asthma symptoms.

By taking your medicine(s) early (before symptoms), you may be able to stop the episode quickly and avoid a severe asthma episode. Peak flow meters are used to check your asthma the way that blood pressure cuffs are used to check high blood pressure.

The peak flow meter also can be used to help you and your doctor:

■ Learn what makes your asthma worse
■ Decide if your treatment plan is working well
■ Decide when to add or stop medicine
■ Decide when to seek emergency care

A peak flow meter is most helpful for patients who must take asthma medicine daily. Patients age 5 and older are usually able to use a peak flow meter. Ask your doctor or nurse to show you how to use a peak flow meter.

How to Use Your Peak Flow Meter

■ Do the following five steps with your peak flow meter:

1. Move the indicator to the bottom of the numbered scale.
2. Stand up.
3. Take a deep breath, filling your lungs completely.
4. Place the mouthpiece in your mouth and close your lips around it. Do not put your tongue inside the hole.
5. Blow out as hard and fast as you can in a single blow.

■ Write down the number you get. But if you cough or make a mistake, don't write down the number. Do it over again.
■ Repeat steps 1 through 5 two more times and write down the best of the three blows in your asthma diary.

Find Your Personal Best Peak Flow Number

Your personal best peak flow number is the highest peak flow number you can achieve over a 2- to 3-week period **when your asthma is under good control.** Good control is when you feel good and do not have any asthma symptoms.

Each patient's asthma is different, and your best peak flow may be higher or lower than the peak flow of someone of your same height, weight, and sex. This means that it is important for you to find your own personal best peak flow number. Your treatment plan needs to be based on your own personal best peak flow number.

To find out your personal best peak flow number, take peak flow readings at least once a day for 2 to 3 weeks. Measure your peak flow at these times:

■ Between noon and 2:00 p.m. each day.
■ Each time you take your short-acting inhaled beta$_2$-agonist to relieve symptoms. (Measure your peak flow *after* you take your medicine.)
■ Any other time your doctor suggests.

The Peak Flow Zone System

Once you know your personal best peak flow number, your doctor will give you the numbers that tell you what to do. The peak flow numbers are put into zones that are set up like a traffic light. This will help you know what to do when your peak flow number changes. For example:

Green Zone (more than ___ L/min [80 percent of your personal best number]) signals *good control*. No asthma symptoms are present. Take your medicines as usual.

Yellow Zone (between ___ L/min and ___ L/min [50 to less than 80 percent of your personal best number]) signals *caution.* You must take a short-acting inhaled beta$_2$-agonist right away. Also, your asthma may not be under good day-to-day control. Ask your doctor if you need to change or increase your daily medicines.

Red Zone (below ___ L/min [50 percent of your personal best number]) signals a *medical alert.* You must take a short-acting inhaled beta$_2$-agonist (quick-relief medicine) right away. Call your doctor or emergency room and ask what to do, or go directly to the hospital emergency room.

Record your personal best peak flow number and peak flow zones in your asthma diary.

Use the Diary To Keep Track of Your Peak Flow

Measure your peak flow when you wake up, before taking medicine. Write down your peak flow number in the diary every day, or as instructed by your doctor.

Actions To Take When Peak Flow Numbers Change

■ PEF goes between ___ L/min and ___ L/min (50 to less than 80 percent of personal best, yellow zone). **ACTION:** Take a short-acting inhaled beta$_2$-agonist (quick-relief medicine) as prescribed by your doctor.
■ PEF increases 20 percent or more when measured before and after taking a short-acting inhaled beta$_2$-agonist (quick-relief medicine)
ACTION: Talk to your doctor about adding more medicine to control your asthma better (for example, an anti-inflammatory medication).

Adapted from *Nurses: Partners in Asthma Care*, National Asthma Education and Prevention Program, National Heart, Lung, and Blood Institute, 1995.

25 percent or more. Patients' symptoms are also an unreliable indicator of airway obstruction. One of the major factors causing delay in treatment of severe asthma and asthma exacerbations is poor perception of the severity on the part of the doctor and the patient.

The accuracy of the PEFR measurement depends on the person's willingness and ability to exhale as hard as he or she can into the peak flow meter.

peak flow meter   A portable device that measures patency of the airways, especially useful in the management of asthma. Various types of peak flow meters are available. The patient takes a deep breath and blows forcibly into the device, after which the flow of air from the lungs can be compared with the normal values predicted for the patient's age, height, and sex. The peak flow meter aids in the diagnosis of asthma and exercise-induced asthma and the detection of an impending asthma attack. It also indicates the severity of an attack and helps to optimize medication dosage.

pearl, Laënnec's   See LAËNNEC'S PEARL.

pectoriloquy   From the Latin words *pectoralis,* or chest, and *loqui,* to speak, words spoken by the patient that can be heard through the chest wall over a particular part of the chest during auscultation, such as over a large bronchus, a pneumothorax, or a pleural effusion.

peenash   An Indian word referring to rhinitis, or inflammation of the nasal passages, caused by insect larvae in the mucous membrane. Certain larvae, such as chironomid larvae (of the red midge, which is a tiny dipteran fly) used as fish food by aquarists have been known to cause an IgE-mediated allergic disease reaction that involved respiratory symptoms, including asthma. Particles of the larvae may be inhaled or cross-react with other allergens, such as mosquitoes, mites, shrimp, and other potentially sensitizing substances. Airborne insect products, insect proteins among them, may result not only in rhinitis

and asthma, but also in conjunctivitis and dermatitis. The deliberate ingestion of insects may cause the life-threatening allergic reaction called anaphylactic shock, and individuals with known or unknown hypersensitivity who eat or inhale insect particles may experience an allergic reaction. For example, mealworm ingestion or inhalation has been reported to cause sensitivity in certain people. Rhinitis, asthma, and rhinoconjunctivitis also can occur in people who fish in rivers and use certain types of live bait, such as the earthworm *Eisenia foetida,* beetle larvae, and marine worms. In addition, a condition called nasal myiasis (infestation of the larvae, or maggots, of Chrysomia flies) exists mostly in the tropics. With atrophic rhinitis as a predisposing factor, the maggots that have reached a body cavity through inhalation or direct contamination can erode the nose, face, and intracranial structures and may cause meningitis and death. A mixture of chloroform and turpentine is among the treatments for killing and removing the maggots. Hypersensitivity treatment includes various medications depending upon the allergen and the specific reaction and condition of the patient.

Nasosinusal myiasis also infects sheep and goats, and dogs can be infected by the *Pneumonyssoides caninum,* or dog nasal mite, irritating and eroding the nasal cavities and frontal sinuses.

See also CORTICOSTEROIDS; HYPERSENSITIVITY; OCCUPATIONAL ASTHMA; RHINITIS.

PEEP   Positive end-respiratory pressure.

penicillins   A group of antibiotics derived from cultures of the mold *Penicillium* or made synthetically and used to kill bacteria, especially cocci, which cause infections. The many derivatives of penicillin include penicillin G, V, ampicillin, amoxicillin, coxicillin, dicloxicillin, carbenicillin, and nafcillin. Penicillins' bactericidal (bacteria-killing) action depends on their ability to interfere with cell wall synthesis of actively multiplying bacteria.

Hypersensitivity reactions, which are common, to the antibacterial drugs of the penicillin family may be of any of the Gell and Coombs allergy types

I through IV. The penicillin molecule, called a hapten, is too small to cause an allergic response, but it is highly chemically reactive: When it combines with a large carrier molecule, usually a protein, it becomes allergenic.

Individuals allergic to one form of penicillin should be considered allergic to all penicillins because they are so chemically similar. The cephalosporin antibiotics are also structurally related to the penicillins. An estimated 5 to 15 percent of penicillin-allergic persons will also react to cephalosporins.

An estimated 13 percent of penicillin-allergic reactions are type I (anaphylactic, immediate, or IgE mediated), and as many as 9 percent, or from 400 to 800, of these prove fatal each year in the United States. Most severe reactions occur when penicillin is administered by injection. Other allergic reactions may result in rashes or serum sickness. Unfortunately, a history of penicillin allergy is often unreliable. In a study by the American Academy of Allergy, only 19 percent of approximately 3,000 persons with a history of penicillin allergy were positive when skin-tested. Seven percent of a group of 1,229 patients with no prior history of penicillin allergy proved positive by skin-test. Furthermore, penicillin can often be detected in individuals who have no knowledge of ever having received it. Exposure is possible from contaminated meat prepared from animals treated with penicillin.

A genus of broomlike molds belonging to the Ascomycetes (sac fungi), *Penicillium* forms the blue molds that grow on fruits, cheese, bread, and other substances. A number of *Penicillium* species are the source of the antibiotic drug penicillin. More than a dozen common types of *Penicillium* are common indoor and outdoor allergens that produce respiratory, external ear, skin, and certain occupational allergies, such as suberosis, caused by the inhalation of *Penicillium frequentans* (a cork-dust mold). Individuals allergic to *Penicillium* mold are not necessarily allergic to penicillin.

Peptostreptococcus An opportunistic bacteria of the Peptococcaceae family that may be normal inhabitants of or cause disease in the respiratory and intestinal tracts of humans.

perennial allergic rhinitis Allergic rhinitis and asthma that are present throughout the year, as opposed to seasonal allergies such as hay fever. Perennial allergens include exposure to animal danders (especially cat and dog), house-dust mites, feathers, and molds.

perfume Alcohol-based liquid (named perfume from the Latin-based French words literally meaning "to smoke thoroughly") made fragrant by adding floral essences or synthetic substances and used cosmetically. It can cause contact skin allergy or trigger asthma by its irritant properties (fumes). Incense was one of the first perfumes in history. Perfumes are eliminated from many products designed to be hypoallergenic.

perfusion Providing an organ or bodily tissue with oxygen and nutrients through the bloodstream.

peribronchial smooth muscle See RESPIRATORY SYSTEM.

peribronchiolitis Inflammation that occurs in the area around the bronchioles. Peribronchitis refers to inflamed areas around the bronchi.

peribronchitis See PERIBRONCHIOLITIS.

peripleuritis Inflammation of the connective tissues between the chest wall and the pleura.

See also RESPIRATORY SYSTEM.

permissible exposure limits The maximum amount of time an individual may be safely exposed to radiation, chemicals, and other physical agents or substances in the environment, particularly the workplace. Workers exposed to hazardous materials or toxic substances may be endangered unless precautions are taken and maximum allowable concentrations of the materials are determined.

pertussis See WHOOPING COUGH.

pertussis vaccine Developed in the 1930s, a preventive substance usually combined with diphtheria and tetanus vaccines for the immunization of infants and children. Pertussis vaccine is not routinely advised after age seven because the infection is rarely serious after this age. Unfortunately, serious adverse effects occur in a small number of infants and the use of this vaccine was severely limited during the 1980s until a government fund was established to deal with liability issues related to the product. Newer vaccine production measures promise to lessen the frequency and severity of reactions.

pharyngalgia Pain in the throat.

pharyngitis, chronic Inflammation of the throat associated with chronic tonsillitis, excessive smoking, dryness caused by mouth-breathing, chronic sinusitis and/or allergic rhinitis, and other ongoing irritation.

pharyngorhinitis Inflammation of the throat and nasal passages.

pharynx The throat, or airway from the nasal cavity to the voice box, or larynx. A musculomembranous tube, the pharynx goes from the base of the skull to the sixth cervical vertebra, and then continues as the esophagus, which leads to the stomach.

See also RESPIRATORY SYSTEM.

phenylephrine hydrochloride (Alconefrin, Neo-Synephrine, Nostril) Alpha-adrenergic, decongestant drug in over-the-counter nasal drops, sprays, and eyedrops. Phenylephrine hydrochloride is also used in combination with antihistamines for the treatment of hay fever and colds. Tolerance to phenylephrine nasal products often causes a dependency known as rhinitis medicamentosa, which may require treatment and corticosteroids in order to break the cycle and symptoms of dependency.

See also RHINITIS MEDICAMENTOSA.

phenylpropanolamine A derivative of the stimulant drug amphetamine used as a decongestant drug for the treatment of nasal allergies and colds. The safety of phenylpropanolamine has been questioned, but in normal decongestant doses it probably does not significantly increase blood pressure. However, the drug is available in higher doses as an over-the-counter appetite suppressant and may be a risk for hypersensitive persons.

phenyltoloxamine An antihistamine usually combined with decongestant drugs for the treatment of hay fever.

See also ANTIHISTAMINE.

phlegm From the Greek word *phlegma,* thick mucus formed in the airways. Also called sputum, phlegm is secreted by cells lining the respiratory tract and capable of causing congestion in upper respiratory passages including the nose and sinuses.

phonasthesia Weakness or hoarseness of the voice attributable to straining the voice.

phosphodiesterase An enzyme that may be involved in causing asthma. Asthma drugs such as theophylline may block this enzyme's action.

photic sneezing Sneezing caused by exposure to bright light or light stimulus.

photodynamic therapy, pulmonary (PDT) A nonsurgical, minimally invasive, localized treatment option for early-stage lung cancer involving a flexible bronchoscope and lasers. In PDT, nonthermal laser light in the visible red to infrared range, or 630 nanometers, activates a light-sensitive drug in order to pinpoint and kill tumor cells. The laser (an acronym meaning light amplification by stimulated emission of radiation) will not burn body tissue, and there is no danger of laser burn because cell destruction occurs through a photochemical reaction.

The patient is given the photosensitive, antineoplastic intravenous drug porfimer sodium (Photofrin), which is absorbed by body tissue and retained only by cancerous and precancerous cells.

When exposed to laser light by way of flexible bronchoscopy 40 to 50 hours after injection of the drug, the drug becomes active and creates a chemical radical known as singlet oxygen. The singlet oxygen targets cell membranes and proteins through oxidation, after which the cancerous cells are destroyed. Twenty-four to 72 hours thereafter, the patient undergoes another bronchoscopy to remove dead cells and, if necessary, for an additional laser treatment. As opposed to chemotherapy and radiation, there are few adverse effects of PDT, which may be repeated as many as three times without damage or abrasion to tissues, pain, or significant risk to the patient. The major side effect is photosensitivity, and patients may need to wear protective clothing and sunglasses when in direct sunlight or bright indoor lighting. Until the porfimer dissipates from the body, patients may also need to limit outdoor activities and take other precautions to minimize exposure to direct sunlight for approximately four to six weeks. Other adverse effects may include localized swelling and inflammation, chest discomfort, nausea, fever, and constipation, but these are easily controlled. A reaction to porfimer specifically may only rarely cause coughing, dysphagia, breathing problems, or hemoptysis.

According to an article in the July 30, 2001, New York–New Jersey edition of *Nursing Spectrum,* "Flexible Scopes and Photodynamic Therapy," "The extent of bronchial invasion and/or nodal extension determines appropriate candidates to PDT. For example, PDT is a local modality only and cannot treat regional lymph nodes. If laser light can't reach the tumor, PDT can't be used. This therapy provides palliative treatment for hemoptysis and shortness of breath secondary to obstructing lung tumors. It is used to treat Stage I lung cancers diagnosed at an early stage as an alternative to surgical resection and as a potentially curative treatment. PDT is also used in combination with chemotherapy and radiation therapy for more comprehensive, localized tumor control. Studies have shown that PDT can produce significant reopening of the bronchial lumen in 70 percent of patients with obstructive bronchial cancers. Clinical trials have found a response rate as high as 89 percent in PDT treatments of patients with early-stage lung tumors. On the other hand, PDT is contraindicated in patients who have tumors that are eroding into a major blood vessel, the trachea, or bronchial tree; a tracheoesophageal or bronchoesophageal fistula; known allergies to porphyrins; or porphyria, a hereditary genetic disorder characterized by a disturbance in porphyrin metabolism. Porphyria causes an abnormal increase in biological pigments (such as the red pigment heme) or coloring (i.e., porphyrins), which are made in the liver, resulting in an abnormal sensitivity to light." Additional information is available at www.cancerlynx.com/photodynamic.html and www.merseyworld.com/lasers.

phrenic avulsion   The condition of one side of the diaphragm that is elevated, and a collapse of the corresponding lung when part of the phrenic nerve is removed, called phrenicectomy or phreniconuerectomy. A motor nerve, the phrenic nerve arises in the cervical plexus and goes into the thorax to the diaphragm.

phrenospasm   A sudden contraction or spasm in the diaphragm.

phthisis   Pulmonary tuberculosis, black lung, and other wasting or atrophic diseases of the lung. Phthistic, from the Greek word *phthisikos,* refers to asthmatic or an asthma sufferer.

Pickwickian syndrome   Also known as hypoventilation syndrome, a state of diminished respiration because of obesity, named for the massively obese character Joe, in *Pickwick Papers,* written by Charles Dickens. The syndrome is characterized by decreased pulmonary function, obesity, and polycythemia.

pigeon breast   Also called chicken breast, a deformity caused by rickets or a childhood respiratory obstruction in which the sternum, or breastbone, projects forward.

pigeon breeder's disease   A pneumonia-like lung disease caused by allergy to pigeon droppings and feathers.

See also HYPERSENSITIVITY; PNEUMONITIS.

pimelorthopnea   Caused by obesity, difficulty in breathing when reclining.

Pins' sign   Named for Austrian physician Emil Pins (1845–1913), the disappearance of pleurisy symptoms in a patient with pericarditis when the patient is in the knee-chest position.

pirbuterol (Maxair)   A beta-adrenergic agonist, or bronchodilating drug, available as a metered-dose inhaler for the treatment of asthma. Maxair opens bronchial tubes to promote easier breathing in individuals with asthma or chronic obstructive pulmonary disease. Nervousness and tremor are the most common side effects, and overuse of Maxair may cause cardiac problems or potentially fatal cardiac complications. This may be seen in patients who are not experiencing significant relief from pirbuterol and who may require further testing or treatment.

Pirquet's test   A skin test for tuberculosis, especially for children. It was named after Austrian pediatrician Clemens P. Pirquet (1874–1929).

plague, pneumonic   A severe type of plague that extensively involves the lungs.
   See also BUBONIC PLAGUE.

plague, white   Another term for tuberculosis.
   See also TUBERCULOSIS.

plastic bronchitis   A type of bronchial inflammation in which fibrin (a protein) exudate sticks to the bronchial tubes like a cast.
   See also BRONCHITIS.

platypnea   Shortness of breath or difficulty breathing that occurs when a patient is standing or sitting.
   See also ORTHOPNEA.

pleura   The moist membrane lining the lungs and the walls of other structures in the thorax and the diaphragm. Because of their serous secretion, both the right and left pleurae help reduce friction between the lungs and other structures during the movements of breathing.

Pleurisy refers to inflammation of a pleura, which often results in painful respiration, coughing, and fever. Pleural fibrosis is a complication of pulmonary tuberculosis in which the pleura thickens and causes crowding in the pleural cavity (space between the layers of the pleurae).

See also RESPIRATORY SYSTEM.

pleural effusion   An abnormal amount of fluid between the visceral and parietal pleura (spaces around the lungs). Effusions, from the Latin word meaning to pour out, may contain serum (hydrothorax), pus (pyothorax), lymph (chylothorax), air (pneumothorax), or combinations of these such as hydropneumothorax and pyopneumothorax. Pleural effusion may result in pain, which may lessen as the fluid builds up due to heart failure, cirrhosis of the liver, pneumonia, or other disorder. Hemothorax, or blood in the pleural space, may be a result of injury or chest trauma, an aortic aneurysm, or impaired blood clotting. Empyema, pus in the pleural space, may be attributable to pneumonia, lung, or abdominal abscess, esophageal rupture, thoracic surgical procedures, and other problems. Lymph, or milky, fluid may be the result of a tumor or injury in the thoracic duct (the main lymphatic duct in the chest. Other causes of pleural effusion include pancreatitis, rheumatoid arthritis, systemic lupus erythematosus, histoplasmosis, blastomycosis, low blood protein levels, coccidiomycosis, tuberculosis, feeding tubes or intravenous catheters that are not properly placed, an abscess under the diaphragm, and certain drugs, such as hydralazine, procainamide, isoniazid, phenytoin, and chlorpromazine, among others.

Treatment for severe pleural effusions may include drainage by way of thoracentesis (aspiration of fluid through a small needle or catheter inserted into the pleural space), or by way of a chest tube. Depending upon the cause of the effusion, corresponding treatment can be administered, such as antibiotics, antitubercular and antitumor drugs, cancer or blood clotting medications, sealing the pleural space, and surgery.

pleurisy   See PLEURA.

pleuroclysis   Washing out the pleural cavity by injecting fluid.

pleurodesis   A treatment for pneumothorax involving the surgical production of adhesions between the parietal and visceral pleura.

pleuropneumonia   The condition of having pneumonia and pleurisy.

pleuroscopy   Examination of the pleural cavity through a surgical incision in the chest.

plombage   Derived from the French word *plomber*, which means to plug, a procedure for a therapeutic deflating of part of a lung in which the parietal pleura is removed from the chest wall and the remaining space is packed with an inert substance such as plastic.

See also DECORTICATION, PULMONARY.

pneodynamics   The mechanism or mechanics of breathing.

See also BREATHING; PNEUMODYNAMICS; RESPIRATORY SYSTEM.

pneopneic reflex   A change in respiratory rate and depth that occurs as a result of inhalation of an irritating vapor. Coughing, shortness of breath, and pulmonary edema may result.

pneumatics   In physics, the study of gases and air.

pneumatocele   A hernia, or protuberance, of lung tissue, usually caused by trauma or a disease process. Pneumatocele also refers to intracranial, extracranial, and scrotal swellings that contain gas. Extracranial pneumatocele refers to gas that collects under the galea aponeurotica (connective tissue of the occipitofrontalis [cranial] muscle), following a fracture in the paranasal sinuses. Intracranial pneumatocele refers to gas pockets in the cranium, brain, or meninges.

pneumatosis   The abnormal presence of air or gas in the body, such as in the peritoneum or in the walls of the intestines, associated with obstructive lung disease caused by pneumatosis coli, or gas in the wall of the colon.

pneumatotherapy   Any treatment of or therapy for the lungs, or a treatment using rarefied or condensed air.

pneumatothorax   An accumulation of air or gas in the pleural cavity.

See also PNEUMOTHORAX.

pneumatype   The moisture that remains on glass from exhaled breath from the nostrils, used to examine the airflow through the nose.

pneumectomy   A surgical removal of a lung or part of a lung, usually as a treatment of malignancies or traumatic injury. The success rate of pneumectomy depends largely on the patient's diagnosis and the presence of aggravating factors, such as concurrent diseases.

pneumoangiography   An X ray of the lung's blood vessels.

pneumocentesis   The surgical aspiration of fluid from the lung.

pneumococcal vaccine polyvalent (Pneumovax, Pnu-Imune)   Immunization for protection against 23 strains of bacteria that cause approximately 90 percent of pneumococcal pneumonia. This type of pneumonia occurs in all age groups but is especially prominent in the elderly. Despite antibiotic therapy, there are still many deaths attributed to this type of pneumonia. Immunization with pneumococcal polysaccharide vaccine is advised for any individual at higher-than-normal risk for serious complications from pneumonia. High-risk persons include anyone older than 65, children older than two, and adults who are immunocompromised, such as those without a spleen or whose spleen is nonfunctional; persons with

Hodgkin's disease, lymphoma, multiple myeloma, chronic renal failure, and nephritic syndrome; persons who have had organ transplantation; and anyone who is HIV positive. Other high-risk patients are those with chronic medical conditions such as heart or lung disease, diabetes mellitus, alcoholism, cirrhosis, and leakage of cerebrospinal fluid.

Protective antibody levels from the pneumococcal vaccine are usually present five years following immunization but then may fall. Revaccination is recommended only for children at extremely high risk of pneumococcal pneumonia, those without a spleen or with nephrotic syndrome.

Adverse effects from pneumococcal vaccine are rare. Most common reactions are cloacal swelling and redness at the injection site or a slight fever. The vaccine should be avoided during an active infection and in children younger than two, and it should not be given during pregnancy unless there is a clear need.

pneumococcus   A gram-positive organism in more than 80 strains that causes pneumonia, meningitis, bronchitis, conjunctivitis, keratitis, mastoiditis, and blood infections.

See also PNEUMONIA.

pneumoconiosis   Lung disorder caused by chronic inhalation of dust and other irritating particles.

See also SILICOSIS.

pneumocystitis carinii pneumonia   See PNEUMONIA.

pneumoderma   Emphysema occurring beneath the skin.

See also EMPHYSEMA.

pneumodynamics   The process of respiration, or the mechanics of breathing involving the exchange of oxygen and carbon dioxide.

See also BREATHING; RESPIRATORY SYSTEM.

pneumoenteritis   Inflammation in the intestinal tract seen in combination with pneumonia.

pneumography   Documentation of the lungs (and also respiratory movements) with a drawing, description, or graph. A pneumograph records frequency and intensity of breathing.

pneumohemorrhagica   Bleeding into the air cells of the lung, also known as apoplexy of the lungs. Hemorrhage, which is abnormal or excessive bleeding, may be caused by certain drugs administered to increase blood volume in patients with pulmonary infections.

pneumohemothorax   More commonly known as hemopneumothorax, the presence of gas, air, and blood in the pleural cavity.

pneumohydrothorax   More commonly known as hydropneumothorax, the presence of gas, air, and fluid in the pleural cavity.

pneumolithiasis   Stone formations, called calculi, in the respiratory tract. Calculus is composed of salts, organic and inorganic acids, and other substances, including cholesterol, and may form in the bronchi, pleura, nose, pharynx, and lungs.

pneumology   A rare term for pulmonology, or the study of diseases of the lungs and airways.

pneumolysis   A surgical procedure performed to loosen a lung that has adhered to the chest wall.

See also PNEUMOTHORAX.

pneumomelanosis   Blackened areas of the lung as seen in pneumoconiosis.

See also PNEUMOCONIOSIS.

pneumometer   See SPIROMETER.

pneumomycosis   A pulmonary disorder caused by a yeast or filamentous fungal infection. Fungi include various forms of mildew, mold, yeasts, and other parasitic life as well as harmless forms that inhabit parts of the body such as the mouth and the intestines. Fungal spores are continually present in the air and in soil. Pathogenic forms of fungi may be inhaled into the respiratory system, especially in individuals who have been on long-term antibiotic therapy for a systemic infection or those who require corticosteroid or immunosuppressive medications. Mycoses, or fungal infections, range from mild to life-threatening, and treatment depends upon the specific fungus and symptoms. Certain fungi cause asthma, allergic rhinitis, and allergic alveolitis, which are not infections but allergic reactions or disorders.

pneumonectasia   Air that causes distention in the lungs.

pneumonia   Inflammation of the lungs characterized by chest pain, fever, cough (often producing bloody or purulent sputum), and other symptoms. The more than 50 causes of various types of pneumonia include bacteria, viruses, and irritating fumes from chemicals. Pneumonia symptoms may be confused with those of hypersensitivity pneumonitis, which is sometimes an allergic reaction to drugs, chemical irritants, plant and animal material, and dust. In addition, allergic alveolitis, or inflammation of the alveoli (air sacs) of the lungs, may produce similar symptoms; the most common causes are inhalation of mold spores, and animal and plant material. Occupational allergies (such as farmer's lung) can simulate pneumonia symptoms.

Pneumonia caused by pneumococci, staphylococci, or bacilli infection is characterized by the sudden onset of high fever, chills, chest pain, cough, and bloody or purulent sputum, and requires immediate treatment with antibiotics. These types of pneumonia are preventable by adhering to rules of hygiene and by immunization.

Bronchial pneumonia refers to infections by mixed bacteria and is often associated with chronic pulmonary conditions including bronchiectasis and emphysema, or as a complication of surgery or anesthesia.

Caseous pneumonia is that associated with tuberculosis involving necrosis (death) of the lung tissue that makes it resemble cheese.

In desquamative interstitial pneumonia, the pulmonary interstitium (tissue surrounding air passages) becomes infiltrated with cells or fibrosis

for unknown reasons. This causes dyspnea, cough, clubbed fingers, and an abnormal diffusion of oxygen and carbon dioxide. Corticosteroids are used to treat this form of pneumonia.

Double pneumonia refers to the illness in both lungs.

Congenital aspiration pneumonia refers to the disease that develops *in utero* or during birth. Intrauterine pneumonia is contracted *in utero.*

Eaton agent pneumonia is caused by the microorganism *Mycobacterium pneumoniae.*

Eosinophilic pneumonia is a lung inflammation caused by roundworms, fungus, and substances including nickel, penicillin, and sulfonamides, and unknown causes.

Hypostatic pneumonia stems from inadequate aeration of the lungs, capillary pooling, and alveolar fluid congestion caused by inactivity, usually in elderly or debilitated patients who stay in the same position for long periods of time. This may be prevented by helping a patient shift positions or ambulate as often as possible.

Pneumocystitis carinii pneumonia occurs when the organism *P. carinii* infects interstitial plasma cells in the lung, trachea, or bronchus, typically in marasmic or debilitated children or in immunocompromised patients. Fever, rapid and/or difficulty breathing, and a nonproductive cough appear as symptoms, and sulfamethoxasole-trimethoprim administered intravenously and inhalation of pentamidine are treatments of choice.

Tuberculous pneumonia is caused by the tubercle bacilli. Varicella and tularemic pneumonias are complications of chickenpox (from the varicella virus) and tularemia (*Francisella tularensis*). Lobar, or central, pneumonia refers to pneumonia, often a result of *Streptococcus pneumoniae,* that affects a lobe or more than one lobe of the lung.

In migratory pneumonia, the infection shifts from one portion of the lung to another, and secondary pneumonia refers to the disease that develops in people with other systemic diseases or conditions such as diphtheria, rheumatic fever, syphilis, typhus, Rocky Mountain fever, typhoid, Q fever, trichiniasis, AIDS, Legionnaire's disease, rickettsial diseases, infectious mononucleosis, brucellosis, psittacosis, tularemia, plague, and acute viral respiratory disease. Embolic pneumonia develops after an embolization of a pulmonary blood vessel. Secondary pneumonia may also be lethal. Microbial causes of pneumonia are adenoviruses, influenza, rhinoviruses, Coxsackie viruses, coronaviruses, respiratory synctitial viruses, mycoplasmas (*Mycoplasma pneumoniae*), cocci (*Pneumococcus, Staphylococcus,* and hemolytic *Streptococcus*), protozoan (*Pneumocystitis carinii*), bacilli (*Haemophilus influenzae, Mycobacterium tuberculosis, Klebsiella pneumoniae,* and gram-negative bacilli), chlamydiae (*Chlamydia trachomatis and C. psittaci*), fungi (*Histoplasma capsulatum, Coccidioides immitis*), and rickettsiae (*Rickettsia rickettsii, R. burnetii*). Pneumonia may also be caused by oil aspiration, radiation, chemicals, vegetable dusts, and silo filler's disease.

See also PNEUMOCOCCAL VACCINE POLYVALENT.

pneumonia, eosinophilic   See PNEUMONIA; PROTEINOSIS; PULMONARY ALVEOLAR.

pneumonic plague   See BUBONIC PLAGUE.

pneumonitis   Also known as pneumonia, an inflammation of the lung. Forms of hypersensitivity (allergic) pneumonitis include bagassosis and other disorders caused by the chronic inhalation of organic dusts. *Mycoplasma pneumonitis* refers to pneumonia (also known as primary atypical pneumonia) that results from infection by mycoplasma organisms. Pneumococcal pneumonitis is pneumonia caused by pneumococci infection.

See also PNEUMONIA.

pneumonocele   Pulmonary hernia, also called pneumatocele.

See also HERNIA, PHRENIC.

pneumopathy   A general term for diseases of the lung.

pneumopleuritis   Inflammation of the lungs and pleura.

pneumopyothorax   The presence of air and pus in the pleural cavity.

See also PNEUMOTHORAX.

pneumorrhagia   Hemorrhage, or abnormal bleeding, in the lung caused by trauma, severe lung infection or disease (including cancer and tuberculosis), blood disease in which there is a coagulation dysfunction, congenital abnormalities, or an adverse effect of certain prescribed medication that increases blood volume for the treatment of respiratory disease. A symptom of lung hemorrhage is red, frothy blood that is coughed up by the patient. Treatment varies and may include surgery.

pneumoserothorax   The presence of air, gas, and serum in the pleural cavity.

See also PNEUMOTHORAX.

pneumosilicosis   See SILICOSIS.

pneumotaxic center   The area in the pons of the brain that rhythmically inhibits inspiration or inhalation.

pneumotherapy   Any treatment of a lung disorder, including one that involves the administration of rarefied or condensed gases.

pneumothorax   Air or gas that collects in the pleural cavity as a result of trauma or the rupture of a lung abscess (such as a tuberculous abscess) or emphysematous bleb. Symptoms include severe sharp pain in the side and difficulty breathing. Treatment may involve the insertion of chest tubes and the administration of oxygen. A spontaneous pneumothorax, characterized by the sudden influx of air into the pleural cavity, may collapse the lung. A tension, or valvular, pneumothorax refers to air that cannot exit the pleural cavity the way it entered, which causes increased pressure in and collapse of the lung. As part of the treatment of pneumonia or pulmonary tuberculosis, a pneumothorax may be artificially induced to give the diseased lung a rest. An artificial pneumothorax is also known as therapeutic pneumothorax.

pneumotomy   A surgical incision made in the lung.

pneumotyphus   Either the development of pneumonia as a complication of typhoid fever, or typhoid with the presence of pneumonia at the onset of disease.

Pneumovax   See PNEUMOCOCCAL VACCINE POLYVALENT.

pneusis   From the Greek word *pnein,* to breathe, breathing, or panting.

Pnu-Imune   See PNEUMOCOCCAL VACCINE POLYVALENT.

pollinosis (hay fever)   Seasonal allergic rhinitis requiring the presence of pollen and capable of eliciting an allergic response in an atopic or allergic subject. The term hay fever is now used regardless of season. Under most circumstances, only anemophilous, or wind-borne pollen present in sufficient quantity can cause hay fever. Huge quantities of pollens are generally required to produce the symptoms of hay fever. Once the symptoms are evident, much smaller amounts of pollen will continue to elicit them. The source of the pollinating plants may be up to hundreds of miles away, being transported by seasonal winds. However, high-pollen–producing trees such as elms, oaks, and others can provoke intense symptoms with exposure to only a single tree.

Pollen release is generally promoted by warm, dry conditions. Ragweed pollen shedding ceases or falls sharply at 10 degrees Celsius (approximately 50 degrees Fahrenheit) or when the relative humidity is above 70 percent. Many flowers store pollen until optimal conditions exist, favoring release during the daytime. Exceptions abound, however, with ragweed and some grasses also releasing pollen at night.

In order to cause hay fever, a plant must meet Thommen's five postulates: (1) the plant must be seed-bearing (spermatophyte); only seed-bearing plants produce pollen; (2) the plant must have wide distribution, or the plant must be close to the human environment; (3) the plant must produce huge quantities of pollen; (4) the pollen must be light enough to be airborne, between 15 and 50 microns (1 micron = 1/25,000 inch) in diameter; (5) the pollen must be allergenic.

A plant species meeting all five rules is considered a primary or index species. Species meeting fewer than five are of little or no significance. Occasionally an individual will seem to have symptoms related to a plant not meeting the criteria, but that is rare, and often the wrong plant is blamed (such as goldenrod, which is blamed for symptoms probably caused by ragweed).

Since pollen is hygroscopic, or able to absorb water vapor from the atmosphere, it becomes too heavy to be wind-borne. Therefore, hay fever-causing plants are rare in humid tropical climates. In these areas, pollination depends upon insects, birds, and bats.

pollutant   Any particle, chemical, irritant, or other substance that contributes to or creates bad air, that is, impure air capable of causing adverse reactions when it flows in and out of the body.

polyblennia   An abnormal secretion of mucus.

polymer fume fever   See METAL FUME FEVER.

polyp, mucous   A soft polyp exhibiting mucoid degeneration.

polyp, nasal   Soft tissue normally found lining the ethmoid sinuses that protrudes into the nasal cavity. Most often nasal polyps occur bilaterally, are usually benign, and cause nasal obstruction. An estimated one to 20 adults per 1,000 population, males by a ratio of from two to four to one, have nasal polyps at some time during their lives. Allergic individuals are no more likely than others to develop polyps. Benign simple polyps are rarely found before age 20, and if present in children before the age of two, a serious defect in the base of the skull may be present. Nasal polyps occur in 8 percent of cystic fibrosis patients, and when seen in children over the age of two, they may be a manifestation of this serious inherited disorder. Polyps are also found in two other rare diseases, Kartagener's syndrome and Young's syndrome. Polyps arising from the maxillary sinuses are called antrocoanal polyps and grow into the postnasal space.

Approximately one-third of patients with nasal polyps are asthmatics, and about 8 percent also have aspirin sensitivity (referred to as a triad, or three-linked disorders). Patients with the triad may develop problems with foods containing the yellow dye tartrazine. Polyps may worsen asthma because the nose's normal warming of the inspired air before it reaches the lungs is blocked, forcing bronchoconstricting cold air to reach the lungs through the mouth because of nasal obstruction.

About half of all cases of nasal polyps respond to corticosteroid nasal sprays. Those not responding will most likely need surgery. Endoscopic resection of polyps is the procedure of choice. Many patients have recurrences.

See also CYSTIC FIBROSIS.

polypnea   Extremely rapid breathing or panting.

polysinusitis   Infection involving more than one of the sinuses.

See also SINUSITIS.

poppers   See INHALANT ABUSE.

porta pulmonis   The point of entry and exit of the bronchi, nerves, and vessels in the lung.

postnasal drip   Sensation of mucus in the back of the throat commonly occurring in persons with nasal allergy, sinusitis, colds, and other upper respiratory infections.

postural drainage   A series of techniques that take advantage of gravity to encourage mucus to move out of the lungs or bronchi. For example, one technique requires the patient to be placed on an incline or over the edge of the bed face down, with his or her head lower than the rest of the body. The health care professional or caregiver then cups his or her hands and gently claps the patient's back over the lung area. The clapping causes productive coughing, that is, expectoration of sputum. Other techniques based on the gravity principle depend upon which part of the lung is affected. Because postural drainage may aggravate a person's asthma or other respiratory disorder, a trained professional should perform the initial therapy and evaluate the patient's tolerance.

potassium chromate poisoning   Toxicity resulting from the inhalation of the chemical potassium chromate, or K_2CrO_4, used in furniture stains, dyes, batteries, photography, and by research laboratories as a tissue preservative. Poisoning and ulcers may also occur when the chemical comes in contact with nasal passages. Treatment includes methods used in cases of toxicity from a strong acid.

potassium iodide   The crystals of the mineral potassium (a salt), having a slight iodine odor, that have been prepared as an expectorant. When used as a mucolytic drug, a potassium iodide solution may help alleviate mucus buildup in the lungs and bronchial passages, but it may also cause acne-like skin lesions and hypothyroidism.

Pott's disease   Named for British surgeon Percivall Pott (1713–88), a tubercular condition of the vertebrae. Not a respiratory disorder, Pott's disease is also known as tuberculous spondylitis, and may result in kyphosis that compresses the spinal cord and nerves.

poultice   From the Latin word *pultes,* a thick paste of hot, moist mustard, linseed, or soap and oil between two pieces of muslin that is applied to the chest or other area to relieve congestion and pain. Also known as a mustard plaster, a poultice counteracts inflammation.

prednisolone   See CORTICOSTEROIDS.

prednisone   The most commonly prescribed corticosteroid drug for the treatment of allergies and asthma.

See also CORTICOSTEROIDS.

pregnancy and rhinitis   Rhinitis, or nasal congestion, that occurs in approximately 35 percent of pregnant women. In one study during pregnancy, the congestion worsened in 34 percent of the women, improved in 15 percent, and was unchanged in the rest. Severe rhinitis can interfere with sleep and aggravate asthma.

As in nonpregnant women, runny and stuffy noses can be caused by allergies or hay fever, or by vasomotor or nonallergic rhinitis, or infections such as colds and sinusitis.

Treatment should be based on the same principles for using any drug during pregnancy. The drug must be necessary and have a long record of use during pregnancy without reported adverse outcomes to the pregnancy, and its use must be monitored by a physician experienced in its use during pregnancy.

preoxygenation   The breathing for two to seven minutes of 100 percent oxygen by a patient before he or she is given anesthesia for surgery. This flushes the nitrogen out of the lungs and replaces it with the oxygen. Preoxygenation is also used to prevent caisson disease, or bends.

See also BENDS.

preparation, heart-lung   The use of devices that take over heart and lung function during open-heart and thoracic surgical procedures.

preventive medicine   Any techniques, modalities, or measures that promote wellness, including methods or regimens followed to stabilize or improve a patient's well-being despite an existing disease. Preventive measures may be considered allopathic, or traditional Western health practices, or alternative, which may involve Eastern medical practices and a variety of other philosophies and modalities. Immunization is also a type of preventive medicine.

See also PNEUMOCOCCAL VACCINE POLYVALENT; VACCINES.

primary pulmonary hypertension   A condition stemming from the insidious onset of respiratory failure in which pressure increases in the blood vessels throughout the lungs. Without proper treatment, the blood vessels become too damaged

to transfer oxygen, thus causing cardiac complications leading to heart failure. Pulmonary hypertension (PH) can also be caused by fibrosis of the lung, sickle cell disease, pulmonary embolic disease, mitral stenosis, atrial septal defects, and chronic hypoxemia in obstructive sleep apnea. Primary pulmonary hypertension (PPH), which also may occur without apparent cause, may possibly be linked to HIV infection, substance abuse (particularly cocaine), appetite suppressant supplements or drugs, and genetic factors.

Treatment for PH includes continuous intravenous epoprostenol (Flolan) and lung transplantation. Flolan, a synthetic substance that performs as the naturally produced prostaglandin does in the body, dilates pulmonary artery vessels, reduces blood clotting, improves cardiac output, and inhibits smooth muscle cell growth. Despite side effects such as headaches and diarrhea, uninterrupted intravenous therapy required for the rest of the patient's life, and administration of a central venous line, Flolan is considered a breakthrough therapy for PH and PPH. If the therapy is interrupted, the patient's symptoms—dyspnea, right-sided heart failure, hepatomegaly, peripheral edema, and angina, among them—may return, and the patient may die. Emotional support is recommended for PH and PPH patients and is available through the Pulmonary Hypertension Association (PHA) at www.phassociation.org or by calling (301) 565-3004.

promethazine (Phenergan)   An antihistaminic, sedative, antimotion-sickness, antinausea, and anticholinergic drug used in the treatment of cough and allergic reactions.

ProStep   See NICOTINE PATCHES.

proteinosis, pulmonary alveolar   A condition in which the alveoli, or air sacs, of the lungs fill with a protein-rich fluid, which prevents the lungs from transferring oxygen to the blood. The cause of this disease that typically affects people between 20 and 60 years old who do not have a history of lung disease is unknown. Some people may be asymptomatic, while others experience shortness of breath or a cough, particularly a productive cough if they smoke. Diagnosed by chest X ray and pulmonary function tests, proteinosis may be treated by antibiotics and bronchopulmonary lavage. If proteinosis is untreated, pulmonary insufficiency may occur and progress into respiratory failure and death. Approximately 25 percent of proteinosis cases clear up spontaneously. The cause of the disease is largely unknown; however, it may be a result of drugs, chemical fumes, or infections by fungi or parasites.

Eosinophils, a type of white blood cell that aids the lungs' immune defenses, may increase by 10 to 15 times the normal number in the event of asthma, allergic reaction, or inflammatory process in the body and contribute to eosinophilic pneumonia, also known as pulmonary eosinophilia syndrome (PIE) and Löffler's syndrome. When eosinophils invade the alveoli, bloodstream, and blood vessel walls, airways may become narrower or, with asthma, plugged with mucus. Diagnostic testing includes microscopic examination of sputum, which would contain clumps of eosinophils, and X ray. Treatment for severe cases of eosinophilic pneumonia may include corticosteroids or other asthma treatment if asthma is present, and drugs corresponding to parasites. Some cases of the disease clear up without treatment.

Proventil   See ALBUTEROL.

pseudocroup   Another name for laryngismus stridulus, or false croup.
   See also LARYNGISMUS STRIDULUS.

pseudoemphysema   Temporary blockage of the bronchi that resembles emphysema.
   See also EMPHYSEMA.

pseudoephedrine   The generic name for Sudafed, Afrinol, and other drugs, including many over-the-counter preparations, used alone or in combination with antihistamines in the treatment of nasal congestion caused by allergies and colds.

pseudotuberculosis   Diseases that have similar characteristics of tuberculosis but are not caused by the same bacillus. Pseudotuberculosis is often caused by the organism *Yersinia pseudotuberculosis.*

psittacosis (parrot fever)   A *Chlamydia pssitaci* infection characterized by headache, nausea, chills, and sometimes pulmonary problems. The disease, rarely fatal, can be transmitted to humans from birds—parrots, pigeons, and fowl are the main carriers—by inhalation of dust contaminated with bird droppings. Approximately 100 cases of psittacosis are reported annually in the United States, though some professionals believe many cases go unreported. Bird or poultry handlers are at the greatest risk of infection. Antibodies specific to the *Chlamydia* species found in human blood confirm the diagnosis. Tetracycline is the treatment of choice. Psittacosis may be confused with asthma or allergy to birds.

ptarmus   Sneezing spasms.

pulmometry   The measurement of the lungs' capacity.

pulmonary arterial webs   Deformities resembling webs that appear in pulmonary angiograms at sites where a patient has had a pulmonary thromboembolism.

pulmonary artery   The major blood vessel that leads from the right ventricle of the heart directly to the lungs. Pulmonary artery wedge pressure refers to the blood pressure in the capillary end of the artery as measured by the insertion of a catheter that inflates a balloon with air. The catheter floats in a "wedged" position until the air in the balloon is deflated and the catheter goes back into the main pulmonary artery. Normal pulmonary artery pressure is 20 to 30 mm Hg (millimeters of mercury) systolic and 8 to 12 mm Hg diastolic. Pulmonary capillary wedged pressure is also measured by the wedge-pressure method.

pulmonary circulation   The process of blood flow from the heart (from the right cardiac vessel) to the lungs. In the lungs, blood becomes oxygenated, and then returns to the heart (left cardiac atrium).

pulmonary edema Edema, or swelling, of the lung.
See also EDEMA, PULMONARY.

pulmonary fibrosis See FIBROSIS, PULMONARY.

pulmonary function tests Procedures used to diagnose and evaluate the severity of asthma and some other lung disorders.
See also PEAK FLOW METER.

pulmonary mucociliary clearance A respiratory tract defense mechanism involving ciliated cells, or cells with fine hairs in the respiratory tract, that have the ability to move mucus, inhaled particles, and other debris up and out of the tracheobronchial tree.

pulmonary stenosis See STENOSIS, PULMONARY.

pulmonary surfactant See RESPIRATORY SYSTEM; SURFACTANT, PULMONARY.

pulmonary valve Located between the right ventricle of the heart and the opening of the pulmonary artery, the membranous structure that separates the ventricle and artery and either closes off or permits the flow of blood.

pulmonary vein The major blood vessel that drains the lungs and brings blood back to the heart's left atrium.
See also RESPIRATORY SYSTEM.

pulmonectomy The surgical excision of all or a portion of lung tissue, also known as pneumonectomy.

pulmonitis Inflammation of the lung.
See also PNEUMONIA.

pulmonologist Physician who specializes in the diagnosis and treatment of lung diseases, including asthma.

pulmotor A device for artificial respiration that forces air or oxygen into the lungs.

pulse, respiratory The pulse corresponding with a person's breathing in and out that may be palpated in the large veins in the neck.

pulse, Riegel's The reduction or diminution of the pulse when a person exhales.

pulsus paradoxus A mercury fall of greater than 10 millimeters in the systolic blood pressure during inspiration that occurs during a severe life-threatening asthma attack.

pump, air (oxygenator) A device that forces air in or suctions air out of a pathway or chamber. A pump-oxygenator not only pumps blood but forces oxygen into it as well.

puna See ALTITUDE SICKNESS.

pursed-lip breathing See BREATHING.

pyohemothorax Blood and pus found in the pleural cavity.

pyothorax Pus found in the pleural cavity.

pyrilamine An antihistaminic drug of the ethylenediamine class used for the treatment of allergic disorders.
See also ANTIHISTAMINE.

Q fever   An infection found throughout the world caused by inhaling dust or other substance contaminated by *Coxiella burnetii (Rickettsia burnetii)*, an organism harbored in farm animals. Ingesting infected raw milk or coming into contact with infected animals' urine, feces, and flesh also transmits the disease. Similar to the symptoms of influenza, Q fever is characterized by fever, severe headache, chills, myalgia, weakness, chest pain, coughing, and pneumonitis. Untreated, Q fever may be fatal. Antibiotic drugs such as tetracyclines are the treatment of choice. A preventive vaccine is available for individuals who may contract the disease through occupations that involve the handling of cows, sheep, goats, and other animals that may be infected.

Q fever has retained its name because its etiology had been previously unknown, and the Q stood for "query." Besides the rickettsial organism that has been identified as a specific cause, all acute infections may include the aforementioned symptoms, and "Q fever" has been used as a generic diagnosis.

quadrangular membrane   Part of the larynx, or vocal cords. The quadrangular membrane is located on the upper portion of the elastic membrane of the larynx.

quanti-Pirquet   A skin test measuring sensitivity to tuberculin developed by Austrian pediatrician Clemens Peter Johann von Pirquet (1874–1929).

quarantine   Derived from the Italian word *quarantina,* meaning 40 days, a designated time during which individuals, groups of people, or animals are not allowed to come into contact with the public, usually because of an infectious disease that may spread to others. The quarantine time begins from the exposure to an infectious disease to the end of its incubation period.

Quibron   See THEOPHYLLINE.

quinolone antibiotics   A unique group of broad-spectrum antibiotics that attack an enzyme, DNA gyrase, essential for the reproduction of infection-causing bacteria. Nalidixic acid, an earlier quinolone drug, had limited usefulness, but derivatives of this drug became available for use in the early 1990s; there are four different clinically important quinolone derivatives now available in the United States: ciprofloxacin (Cipro) and norfloxacin (Noroxin, Floxin, and Maxaquin). Another antibiotic in this category, ofloxacin, was recalled shortly after it was introduced following reports of deaths related to its use.

With the exception of norfloxacin (used primarily for urinary tract infections), these antibiotics are frequently prescribed for patients with respiratory infections. However, since some of the quinolone antibiotics raise theophylline levels, which possibly causes toxicity, they must be used cautiously or avoided in patients who are also taking this asthma drug.

quotient, respiratory   The amount of exhaled carbon dioxide divided by the amount of inhaled oxygen. The typical respiratory quotient is 0.9.

radioallergosorbent tests (RAST) See IMMUNO-GLOBULIN E.

radiofrequency electrophrenic respiration An electronic method of stimulating a patient's breathing when there is respiratory paralysis as a result of spinal cord injury. A radiofrequency transmitter implanted beneath the skin sends electrical stimuli to the phrenic nerves.

radiopulmonography The study of a person's gas flow through the lungs during breathing through the use of radioactive materials.

ragsorters' disease See ANTHRAX.

ragweed Species of the anemophilous (wind-pollinating) genus *Ambrosia* in the plant family Compositae, whose pollen is the most important weed allergen that causes hay fever. Ragweed pollen can be detected as early as late July and usually peaks by early September, when thousands of grains per cubic meter of air afflict an estimated 5 million Americans. The season ends with the first frost about mid-October.

Although ragweed is most abundant in the central plains and eastern rural areas of the United States, approximately 40 species are distributed throughout the warmer regions of the Western Hemisphere. About a dozen species of ragweed are present in sufficient quantity to be important sources of pollen, but the two most prolific are short, common, or dwarf (*Ambrosia artemisifolia*) and giant (*A. trifida*). Short ragweed flourishes in northern Mexico, the Midwest, Ozark plateau, and Gulf states to the Atlantic coast. It is also present to

some extent in the Pacific Northwest. Giant ragweed, whose growth may exceed 15 feet in height, is most abundant along the flood plains of southeastern rivers and the Mississippi delta, as well as over the range of short ragweed (sparing northern Mexico and the Pacific Northwest).

Another important species of ragweed is perennial (*A. psilotachya*), which despite a wide range is significant only in the Great Plains and Great Basin areas, where it grows in dry, sandy soil. Southern, or slender, ragweed (*A. bidentata*) is found from southern Indiana to western Tennessee, Louisiana, Texas, and Nebraska. Perennial slender ragweed (*A. confertiflora*), annual bur ragweed (*A. acanthicarpa*), canyon ragweed (*A. ambrosiodes*), rabbit bush (*A. deltoidea*), and burroweed (*A. dumosa*) are found in dry soils of the West, especially the arid southwestern states. The latter three species are exceptional in that they pollinate in the early spring. Several of these species were called "false ragweed" and classified in the genus *Franseria*. However, they are now recognized as meeting the criteria to be considered true pollinating plants. In the arid Southwest, western, slender, and false ragweed proliferate.

A few species are distributed throughout South America and in the Caribbean, but ragweed-caused hay fever is uncommon in those areas. European ragweed (*A. Maritima*) and an African species (*A. senegalensis*) have a limited range. Short ragweed has appeared in some European countries, with significant hay fever seasons recognized in eastern France, the Balkans, and in the Krasnodar region of the former Soviet Union. Most of Asia, Australia, Africa, and Europe including Great Britain are mainly free from ragweed.

Antigen E, although only 6 percent of the total protein in ragweed extract, is the most reactive allergen, 200 times more potent than the whole extract. Immunotherapy (allergy shots) with standardized ragweed extract is effective for reducing symptoms and medication requirements in most individuals with hay fever sensitive to this pollen.

See also WEED POLLEN ALLERGY.

rale   Any abnormal sound heard through a stethoscope placed on the chest. Produced upon inhalation or exhalation, rales occur when air passes through the bronchi during a spasm, thickening of their walls, or constriction caused by the presence of excess mucus. Moist rales, frequently associated with congestive heart failure, may often be described as crackling sounds in various degrees of severity. Consonating rales are loud and sharp. Dry rales associated with asthma, bronchitis, and early pulmonary tuberculosis may also be described as snoring, whistling, tinkling, low-pitched, or high-pitched. A narrowing of the bronchial tubes caused by a muscular spasm or a thickening of the tubes' mucous lining is responsible for dry rales. The existence of a rale, a French word meaning "rattle," often indicates a pulmonary disease process.

Ramazzini, Bernardino   Italian physician (1633–1714) who suffered from malaria, studied malaria and other epidemiologic problems, and wrote a treatise, *Diseases of Tradesmen,* which addresses 53 trades and illnesses related to them. Ramazzini included graphic descriptions of "pulmonary passages lined with crust" caused by particles of flour in bakers and millers, and intense itching, inflamed and watery eyes, and the obstinate cough of sifters and measurers of grain.

See also BAKERS' ASTHMA; OCCUPATIONAL ASTHMA.

ramus, bronchial   The branches of each main bronchus.

rate, respiration   See RESPIRATORY RATE.

rattle, death   See BREATHING; DEATH RATTLE.

rebreathing   Inhaling gases that have been exhaled.

recompression   Part of treatment for caisson disease (bends), re-exposing a patient to increased atmospheric pressure.

See also BENDS.

reflex, cough   See COUGH.

reflex, lung   Tissue in the lungs that involuntarily dilates when irritated by touch or a sensation of cold.

rehalation   A process of rebreathing sometimes used in anesthesia.

relaxation techniques   Any method that instructs and promotes physiological and emotional calmness and well-being. Meditation, yoga, therapeutic touch, hypnosis, Reiki, massage, and other methods are employed to help control stress. People with hypertension, asthma, and other disorders often benefit from relaxation techniques.

reovirus   An acronym for respiratory enteric orphan virus, one of a group of viruses found in the respiratory and digestive systems of healthy individuals. It has not been determined if reoviruses, formerly classified as ECHO virus, type 10, are pathogenic.

reportable diseases   Communicable diseases, both individual cases and epidemics, that health authorities require physicians to report, as per International Health Regulations and the World Health Organization, including plague, cholera, yellow fever, typhus fever, influenza, relapsing fever, poliomyelitis, and other quarantinable, rarely seen, or previously unrecognized diseases.

reserve air   Additional quantity of air that can be expelled from the lungs after a normal expiration.

residual air   (residual volume)   The quantity of air remaining in the lungs after an individual has exhaled as forcibly as possible.

resistance, airway   The ability to oppose the flow of air into the respiratory tract.

See also RESPIRATORY SYSTEM.

resonance   Sound generated by vibrations. In medicine, resonance of various types is heard through a stethoscope or by percussion over a hollow part of the body, such as the chest. For example, "cracked-pot" resonance, a strange clinking sound, may be heard on percussion of the chest in patients with advanced tuberculosis. Other types of resonance are characteristic of pneumothorax (collapsed lung) and some pulmonary diseases. The lungs also have a normal resonance, that is, a resonance not associated with any abnormality.

Respid   See THEOPHYLLINE.

respiration   See BREATHING; RESPIRATORY SYSTEM.

respirator   A machine or mechanism that produces artificial breathing or supports breathing in patients who cannot breathe normally because of severe lung incapacity. A respirator, or ventilator, promotes pressure into the lungs, which causes the lungs to function without the help of the patient's own breathing reflexes.

respiratory anemometer   A device involving the passage of air through a mask or mouthpiece, which in turn rotates a vane to study pulmonary function.

respiratory arrest   See ARREST, RESPIRATORY.

respiratory center   The area in the medulla oblongata of the brain that regulates the movements—inhalation and exhalation—of breathing. Part of the pons, a fibrous part of the brain, is also responsible for respiratory movements.

See also BREATHING.

respiratory defense function   See RESPIRATORY SYSTEM.

respiratory distress syndrome of premature infants   The leading cause of death of premature infants, a severe breathing dysfunction also known as hyaline membrane disease. It involves atelectasis of the lung, impaired blood supply to the lungs, rapid breathing and heart rate, cyanosis, and other symptoms, as a result of delivery before the infant's enzymatic system can produce adequate pulmonary surfactant. Neonatal intensive care is required.

See also RESPIRATORY SYSTEM.

respiratory failure, acute   A dramatic increase in arterial carbon dioxide concentration and decrease in arterial oxygen concentration that signals a life-threatening situation, possibly caused by an airway obstruction or a disorder resulting in impaired gas exchange.

respiratory failure, chronic   Pulmonary insufficiency caused by any disorder that impairs ventilation and perfusion of the lungs. Among the disorders are asthma, emphysema, chronic bronchitis, sarcoidosis, cystic fibrosis, radiation sickness, and leukemia.

See also RESPIRATORY SYSTEM.

respiratory function monitoring   Techniques used to alert attendants to a patient's change in breathing or lung function, such as pulse oximetry, capnography (for monitoring carbon dioxide content of exhaled air), and other methods to determine breathing patterns and characteristics.

See also APNEA.

respiratory infection, viral (common cold)   A syndrome caused by a virus that includes sneezing, nasal discharge, congestion, sore throat, and coughing, all of which are often confused with or coexist with allergy symptoms. Viral colds can also trigger asthma; shortness of breath and wheezing may persist for a prolonged period following resolution of the viral infection. Some patients have asthma symptoms only when they catch a cold.

respiratory rate   The number of inhalations per minute. The normal respiratory rate is highest in infancy. At six months, the respiratory rate ranges from 22 to 31 breaths per minute while asleep to 58 to 75 breaths per minute while awake. By age six, rates have diminished to 13 to 23 breaths per minute asleep and 15 to 30 awake. Adults inhale at a rate of 15 to 20 breaths per minute.

respiratory syncytial virus (RSV)   A virus that commonly causes a respiratory infection called bronchiolitis in infants. An estimated 35 to 50 percent of children who develop RSV infections will later have bronchial asthma.

See also BRONCHIOLITIS.

respiratory system   The structures of both the upper and lower respiratory tracts in the body, including the nose, nasal cavities, pharynx, larynx (upper respiratory), trachea, bronchi, and lungs (lower respiratory). The upper tract consists of airways that warm, moisten, and conduct air from the environment into the lungs. Airways also provide protection from bacteria and particle contamination and play a role in the sense of smell and the production of speech and sounds.

The nose is made up of three regions beyond the nares (nostrils): a vestibule, an olfactory region, and a respiratory region. Lined with skin and coarse hairs that act as filters for large particles of dust, vestibules conduct air that is inhaled. Lined with olfactory epithelium that has special cells for sensing various smells, the olfactory regions in the roofs of both nasal cavities connect inhaled air with the olfactory nerves in the cranium. In the respiratory regions of the nasal cavities are turbinates, or conchae, bony projections that create channels lined with mucus-secreting epithelial cells, whose cilia (or fine hairs) also serve as a filter for bacteria, dust, and other particles in the air. In the walls of the nasal cavities, too, are openings to the four pairs of paranasal sinuses—frontal, ethmoidal, sphenoidal, and maxillary. Sinuses, or air-filled cavities lined with mucus-secreting epithelium, allow air to vibrate to help in the production of sound. Sinuses that become filled with fluid or are blocked by mucus

that has not drained into the nose may be at risk of infection.

From the oropharynx (the part of the oral cavity, or mouth, that leads to the throat), air breathed in moves down the throat past the larynx and trachea toward the bronchi and lungs. The larynx, also known as the voice box, is a series of cartilages connected by membranes and ligaments; the largest of the cartilages is the thyroid cartilage, which is also called the "Adam's apple." The epiglottis is a flap that opens and closes the opening of the larynx. When a person swallows food or liquid, the larynx is closed off so nothing can get into the airway.

Air goes from the larynx into the trachea, a tube approximately one inch in diameter and five inches long, which begins the lower respiratory tract. The trachea separates into two branches to form the right and left main bronchi, located at the sixth thoracic vertebra. Both bronchi lead to the right and left lungs. The left bronchus, longer and thinner than the right bronchus, passes under the aorta. In the lungs, the bronchi branch out into smaller segments known as bronchopulmonary segments, which then branch into bronchioles (meaning small bronchi and creating the "bronchial tree"). The bronchioles lead to the alveoli, or air sacs, of the lungs. An average lung contains about 300 million alveoli.

Unlike bronchi, bronchioles are not supported by cartilage, but they are lined with a mucus-secreting, ciliated epithelium until the point at which they connect with the alveolar ducts. Oxygen and carbon dioxide are exchanged when each alveolus contacts a network of tiny blood vessels called capillaries.

Situated in the thoracic cavity are the lungs. The right lung has three lobes, or sections, and the left lung has two that are delineated by fissures. Bronchi, blood vessels, and nerves enter the lungs through pedicles located at the root of each lung, and the surface of the lungs are covered by the visceral pleura, a membrane that connects with the parietal pleura lining the rib cage. Between the visceral and parietal pleurae is the pleural space.

Under the lungs and just above the abdomen is the diaphragm, which is a muscle that contracts and relaxes with inspiration and expiration. Like a piston, the diaphragm helps the chest cavity expand during inhalation. In a compartment called the mediastinum between the lungs lie the heart and the major blood vessels leading to and from the heart. Twelve pairs of ribs surround the lungs.

The entire respiratory system supports the process of breathing, that is, the exchange of carbon dioxide from the body for oxygen to the body. External respiration refers to oxygen being taken up by the bloodstream and carbon dioxide being released into the air. Internal respiration refers to the gas exchange that occurs within body tissues, that is, oxygen from the blood passing into cells, and carbon dioxide from the cells passing into the blood for eventual release. The blood vessels involved in pulmonary circulation, characterized by low pressure and low resistance and thinner, more flexible vessel walls than in the systemic circulation, consist of the aorta, pulmonary artery, pulmonary vein, the superior and inferior vena cava, and the ventricles of the heart. The heart pumps blood through both the pulmonary and systemic circulations, although the lungs receive blood from both the pulmonary arteries that carry oxygen-depleted blood to the alveoli and from the bronchial arteries in systemic circulation that carry oxygenated blood to the lungs.

Once in the lung tissue, capillary beds send deoxygenated blood to the alveoli where they are reoxygenated and sent through the pulmonary veins back to the heart. There are two major pulmonary veins from each lung that drain the oxygenated blood into the left side of the heart. From there, the oxygenated blood is pumped through the aorta and into the body's bloodstream. All tissues need a supply of blood for oxygen, nutrients, and to get rid of waste materials. Blood eventually returns from the systemic veins to the inferior and superior vena cava, from which oxygen-depleted blood drains into the right side of the heart.

Respiratory muscles include the peribronchial smooth muscles, located in the bronchial walls, which are innervated by both the sympathetic (or adrenergic) and parasympathetic (or cholinergic) divisions of the autonomic nervous system. The autonomic nervous system regulates unconscious functions such as heart rate, gastrointestinal motility, vascular smooth muscle tone, and peri-

bronchial smooth muscle tone. The adrenergic nervous system stimulates bronchodilation and the reduction of mucus secretion, while the cholinergic system stimulates bronchoconstriction and increased mucus secretion. Medications prescribed for various respiratory disorders are geared to either adrenergic or cholinergic effects. For example, epinephrine (an adrenergic) relaxes peribronchial smooth muscle. Cyclic AMP (cAMP) refers to an intracellular "second messenger" mechanism that also causes peribronchial smooth muscle to relax.

The efficiency of the respiratory system may be evaluated by factors such as ventilation (breathing rate and depth) and perfusion (blood flow into the lungs), and by its two major defense mechanisms: physical and immunologic barriers against "invaders." Physical barriers and autonomic mechanical responses including coughing, sneezing, and expectorating help the body ward off foreign matter that may enter the airways. In the lower airways, immunologic defenses fight off most foreign invaders. They are ingested by alveolar macrophages (originally white blood cells, or monocytes), cells that "eat" undesirable materials such as bacteria. Other white blood cells called lymphocytes and immunoglobulins (large protein molecules) provide defense against pathogenic microorganisms.

Lung function may also be evaluated through technological devices and techniques of measurement, such as the total lung capacity (in a healthy adult, five to six liters, or 5,000 to 60,000 milliliter), tidal volume (the amount of air entering and exiting the body during normal breathing, approximately 400 to 700 milliliter), inspiratory reserve volume (the extra air taken in during inhalation, approximately 2,000 to 3,200 milliliter), expiratory reserve volume (additional air that can be exhaled forcibly, approximately 750 to 1,000 milliliter), residual volume (air remaining in the lungs after a forcible exhalation), functional residual capacity (equal to the expiratory reserve volume and the residual volume), and total lung capacity (equal to the vital capacity and the residual volume).

Pulmonary function tests include spirometry and peak flow measurements.

See also BETA-ADRENERGIC AGONISTS; BETA-AGO-NISTS; BETA-RECEPTORS; BRONCHODILATOR; PEAK FLOW; SPIROMETRY.

respiratory therapy A professional discipline based on methods to improve breathing, preserve the optimal function of the lungs, and treat seriously ill patients with lung disease. Under medical direction, respiratory therapy involves evaluating, diagnosing, treating, controlling, and rehabilitating patients who have asthma, emphysema, and other lung problems (including those associated with air pollution and cigarette smoking) or who are being treated in emergencies such as heart failure, stroke, shock, head injury, drowning, and substance poisoning. For emergency patients, breathing must be restored in three to five minutes to avoid brain damage. If breathing is not restored in nine minutes, the patient may die. Upon orders from the physician, the respiratory therapist administers gas, aerosol, and humidity therapies, intermittent positive-pressure breathing treatments, cardiopulmonary resuscitation, long-term continuous artificial ventilation and other procedures, and may also teach patients breathing exercises and how to use and maintain special respiratory equipment.

respirometer See RESPIRATORY ANEMOMETER.

resuscitation, cardiopulmonary See CARDIOPUL-MONARY RESUSCITATION.

retropharyngitis Inflammation of the tissue behind the pharynx or throat.

review of systems, respiratory The process of taking a thorough patient history as an assessment tool for prevention of illness and diagnosis and treatment of illness. Questions pertaining to the patient's respiratory health may include those concerning exposure to animals, exercise and athletic activity, military service, home environment and circumstances, the health of family members, criminal record, travel, occupation, medical history, smoking and tobacco use, substance abuse, exposure to individuals with contagious respiratory diseases, and current symptoms involving the nose, mouth, and pulmonary function.

Reye's syndrome Named for Australian pathologist R. D. K. Reye (1912–77), an anomaly characterized by acute encephalopathy and fatty infiltration of the liver (and possibly affecting other organs including the heart, kidney, spleen, pancreas, and lymph nodes) that begins with a viral upper respiratory infection. A syndrome usually seen in children younger than 15 years, Reye's appears to be associated with aspirin used to reduce fever as a result of the virus. Caregivers are advised not to administer aspirin to children suffering from chickenpox or influenza. Reye's syndrome may be life-threatening.

rhinalgia Painful nose.

rhinitis Inflammation of the mucous membrane lining the nasal passages. Rhinitis caused by allergies is called allergic rhinitis, or hay fever. Rhinitis can also be caused by respiratory infections; and if the cause is unknown, it is referred to as vasomotor rhinitis.

rhinitis medicamentosa Severe nasal congestion with swelling of the mucous lining of the nasal passages from overuse of over-the-counter decongestant nasal sprays. Abuse of these nasal sprays results in rebound phenomenon, in which nasal congestion initially improves but the spray loses its effectiveness and is required with increased frequency until the individual is using the spray or drops constantly. Use of these products should be limited to three to five days. Corticosteroids are frequently needed to improve the condition. Oral drugs, such as the reserpine used to treat high blood pressure, can also cause rhinitis medicamentosa. Symptoms of rhinitis medicamentosa are often confused with allergies, and the condition should be considered before a person is evaluated for allergy.

rhinoanemometer A mechanism that measures the air flow through the nose to determine if there is obstruction in the nasal passages.

rhinoantritis Inflammation of nasal cavities and the maxillary antra, cavities in the maxillary bone.

rhinocleisis A nasal obstruction.

Rhinocort Nasal Spray Brand of cortisone-like anti-inflammatory drug budesonide.
See also CORTICOSTEROIDS.

rhinodynia Pain in the nose.

rhinolaryngitis Inflammation of the nasal passages and larynx, or voice box.

rhinolithiasis The formation of stones, or calculi, in the nasal passages.

rhinomycosis The presence of fungus in mucous membranes of the nose and nasal secretions.

rhinopharyngitis Inflammation of the nasal passages and the pharynx, or throat, usually caused by the inhalation of allergenic substances or infectious spores and other organisms.
See also PHARYNGITIS; RHINITIS.

rhinophycomycosis An infection by the fungus *Entomophthora coronata* that affects the nasal and paranasal sinuses. Occurring in both humans and animals, the infection may spread to the brain. Treatment includes antifungal drugs.
See also PNEUMOMYCOSIS.

rhinopneumonitis Inflammation of the mucous membranes of the lungs and nose.
See also PNEUMONIA; RHINITIS.

rhinorrhagia A severe nosebleed.
See also EPISTAXIS.

rhinorrhea A thin watery discharge from the nose. Conditions causing rhinorrhea include allergies, the common cold, and cluster headaches. A watery discharge following a serious head injury may indicate the leakage of cerebrospinal fluid.

rhinoscleroma A disease caused by the bacillus *Klebsiella rhinoscleromatis* that results in extremely hard, nodular growths in the nose and respiratory tract. Treatment includes surgery and streptomycin therapy.

rhinoscopy A diagnostic procedure in which an instrument, a rhinoscope (rigid or flexible fiberoptic), is introduced into the nostrils to view the nasal passages. With the fiberoptic rhinoscope, the observer can also see openings to the sinuses and eustachian tube, and the oropharynx and trachea. The procedure is useful for determining the cause of nasal symptoms such as allergic rhinitis, sinus infections, or obstructions such as a deviated septum or tumor.

rhinosporidiasis Also known as rhinosporidiosis, a fungal infection contracted from cattle and caused by *Rhinosporidium seeberi* in which a chronic granulomatous disease produces polyps that form on mucous membranes of the nose, larynx, eyes, penis, vagina, and skin. Rhinosporidiasis may be seen in India, Sri Lanka, and other locations. Antifungal drugs are among the treatments.

rhinostenosis Obstruction or constriction of the nasal passages.

rhinotracheitis Inflammation of the nasal passages and the windpipe, or trachea.

rhinovirus A species of picornavirus that causes the common cold. It is estimated there are more than 100 rhinoviruses that occur throughout the world.

rhonchus Snoring, or any rattling in the windpipe or chest.

rifampin Also known by the trade names Rimactane and Rifadin, an antibiotic used to treat tuberculosis caused by the *Mycobacterium tuberculosis* and to treat carriers of *Neisseria meningitidis*.
See also TUBERCULOSIS.

rima respiratoria   The space located behind the arytenoid cartilages.

Robitussin   The trade name for guaifenesin, an expectorant.

room, dust-free   An area or chamber designated for individuals with allergies or sensitivity to airborne microorganisms and particles that may be harmful if inhaled. Devices may be installed that filter or purify the air in the room, thus reducing the number of offending particles or allergens.

rose fever (rose cold)   Another name for hay fever occurring in the spring pollen season. Rose pollen is transferred by insects and is not an important allergen. Persons who have hay fever symptoms in the spring are allergic to tree and/or grass pollens.

See also RHINITIS, ALLERGIC.

Rotacaps   Capsules containing the dry, powdered bronchodilating asthma drug albuterol (Ventolin). The capsules are placed in a device called a Rotahaler, which is activated by puncturing the capsule and releasing the powder into a small chamber. The powder is then inhaled through the mouth into the airways. This Rotahaler method of inhalation is useful for patients lacking the coordination necessary to activate a metered-dose inhaler.

See also ALBUTEROL.

S

sac, alveolar   Air sacs found in the lungs.
See also ALVEOLUS; LUNG.

St. Joseph's Cough Syrup for Children   A brand of dextromethorphan hydrobromide, a derivative of a synthetic morphine used to treat coughing. It reportedly does not cause dependence, although as an antitussive, it is not as effective as codeine.
See also ANTITUSSIVE.

salbutamol   See ALBUTEROL.

saline solution   A combination of salt and water. A saline nasal spray contains the concentration of tears (.09 percent) and is used as a spray to irrigate the nasal passages.

salmeterol (Serevent)   A bronchodilating drug of the beta-adrenergic agonist type for the treatment of asthma. Salmeterol is also available as a metered-dose inhaler. Its effects last for 12 hours or longer without tolerance or loss of effectiveness. Studies also indicate that continued use does not result in worsening asthma symptoms.
See also BETA-ADRENERGIC AGONISTS.

salpingopharyngeal   Pertaining to the pharynx, or throat, and the eustachian tube of the ear.

salt   The chemical sodium chloride (the same as table salt), an inorganic, mineral constituent of the body that is vital to cell function and life. English researchers have reported that excessive intake of dietary salt may increase asthma mortality.

Salter, Henry H.   British physician (1823–71) who practiced in London and was associated with R. B. Todd at King's College. Salter, an asthmatic, published a respected work entitled *On Asthma: Its Pathology and Treatment,* in which he pointed out the dangers and questioned the effectiveness of the use of opium in treating asthma. He saw in opium a tendency to cause involuntary muscular action and induce spasms. He attributed its prescription by physicians of his day to their unthinking acceptance of its routine use and their failure to monitor closely their own patients' responses.

Salter also wrote articles on the pancreas and tongue for Todd's *Cyclopedia.* In 1854, he became a lecturer in physiology and in medicine at Charing Cross Hospital in London.

salts, smelling   Aromatized ammonium carbonate, used to revive a person who has fainted.

saltwater sprays   See SALINE SOLUTION.

Samuelsson, Bengt I.   Swedish physician and scientist, born in 1934, who shared the Nobel Prize for physiology or medicine in 1982 with Sune Bergstrom and John Vane. Samuelsson identified and described leukotrienes and their role in asthma, allergy, and inflammation. At the Karolinska Institute in Stockholm, Sweden, since 1972, he has served as professor of medical and physiologic chemistry, chairman of the Department of Chemistry, dean of the medical faculty, and rector.
See also LEUKOTRIENES.

sanatorium   A facility, also called a sanatarium, dedicated to the prevention and treatment of chronic illness, particularly tuberculosis, and the promotion of health.

sandfly fever   A tropical and subtropical viral disease caused by arboviruses carried by the sandfly *Phlebotomus papatasi.* Sandfly (or pappataci or phlebotomus) fever resembles influenza but does not include respiratory distress. Sandflies of the order Diptera and the genus *Phlebotomus,* however, may transmit sandfly fever, Oroya fever, and forms of leishmaniasis.

See also LEISHMANIASIS.

sanitizer   Any substance or agent that disinfects an area or reduces bacteria to make the materials or area that is sanitized safe according to standards for public health.

sarcoidosis   A chronic, often asymptomatic, disease that can affect the skin, lungs, lymph nodes, spleen, eyes, and the small bones of the hands and feet. Although the cause of sarcoid (formerly known as Boeck's sarcoid) is unknown, it is characterized by granulomatous lesions in body tissue. A routine chest X ray often reveals the presence of the disease, but symptoms may occur and include fever, fatigue, malaise, arthritis, cough, shortness of breath on minimal exertion, nervous system disturbances, painful red bumps on the shins, abnormal heart rhythm, and elevated blood calcium. Steroids are the treatment of choice, although in some patients, the disease resolves spontaneously.

saturation, oxygen   The ratio of the amount of oxygen in a certain amount of blood to the amount of oxygen the blood could optimally carry.

scaleniotomy   Referring to the three scalenus muscles on each side of the neck, a surgical incision into one of the muscles to check expansion of the lung's apex in patients with tuberculosis.

scarlatina anginosa   A type of scarlet fever (an acute, contagious disease caused by more than 40 strains of streptococci) that involves ulceration and severe necrosis of the throat and abscess of the tonsils and surrounding areas.

schneiderian membrane   The nasal mucosa, named after the German anatomist Conrad Viktor Schneider (1614–80) who identified it.

scleroderma   A chronic disease of unknown etiology that causes sclerosis or hardening of skin and other organs, including the lungs. Scleroderma is not considered a respiratory disorder per se because it affects several major organs after the skin becomes tough and leathery, a primary manifestation. There is no special therapy, but various drugs are prescribed according to pathological changes.

scoliosis, empyemic   A lateral curvature of the spine as a result of empyema (pus in a body cavity, usually the lungs) and retraction of one side of the chest.

screening   Diagnostic testing, including chest X ray and tuberculin tests, to identify either risk factors or the presence of disease in large groups of people. Screening plays an important role in public health and prevention of disease.

scrofula   A type of tuberculosis adenitis, considered a complication of a pulmonary lesion that has spread to the cervical lymph nodes. Treatment involves antituberculosis drug therapy.

scuba   See SELF-CONTAINED UNDERWATER BREATHING APPARATUS.

seal, velopharyngeal   The closed area between the mouth, nose, and throat cavities.

seasonal allergy (seasonal hay fever)   Nasal and eye allergies and asthma that occur in the spring and fall upon exposure to pollinating trees, grasses, and weeds in susceptible persons. Many who suffer from perennial, or year-round, allergies also have seasonal allergies and tend to suffer more in the spring and fall.

See also ALLERGIC RHINITIS; ASTHMA; HAY FEVER; POLLINOSIS.

segment, bronchopulmonary A subdivision of the lobes of the lung, usually a small section.

Seldane A brand name for terfenadine, a second-generation or nonsedating antihistaminic drug used to treat allergic rhinitis and urticaria. There have been rare but life-threatening cardiac arrhythmias (irregular heartbeat) associated with the use of terfenadine given simultaneously with other drugs, including the antibiotic erythromycin, the antifungal drug ketoconazole, and with grapefruit juice. A risk is also associated with the use of this drug in persons with liver disorders.

self-contained underwater breathing apparatus (SCUBA) A watertight device connected to a tank of compressed air worn by swimmers and divers.
See also BENDS.

self-treatment risks The danger of underestimating the severity of asthma or allergic reactions until they become more difficult to treat, cause serious irreparable damage to the lungs, or provoke a life-threatening situation. A person with asthma may have gradually become accustomed to his or her shortness of breath and have an unrealistic perception of its severity.
See also ASTHMA.

Semprex-D (Prolert) A brand name for acrivistine, a nonsedating antihistamine. In clinical trials subjects did not develop tolerance (loss of effectiveness of a drug with continued use) after several weeks of use. Onset of the drug effect starts within one to two hours of the first dose, but the drug must be taken three or four times a day.
See also ANTIHISTAMINE.

sense of smell, loss (anosmia) Inability to detect odors, either permanently by destruction of the olfactory (or first) cranial nerve, or temporarily by nasal obstruction or allergies.

sensitivity A person's level of susceptibility to allergens, also known as antigens, which may produce a varied number of symptoms. Sensitogens are all the allergens of the body that can possibly produce an allergic reaction. Sensitogens include anaphylactogen and sensibilisinogen.

septicemia, bronchopulmonary A potentially life-threatening condition characterized by pathogenic bacteria that have entered the bronchi and lungs through the blood. An abscess, a preexisting disease such as cancer, diabetes mellitus or an immunodeficiency disorder, or an infection such as pneumonia may contribute to the onset of septicemia. Symptoms of septicemia, or blood poisoning, include chills, fever, rapid respirations, and shock. If treated with antibiotic drugs, usually administered by intravenous infusion, septicemia can be arrested before septic shock or damage to lung and other tissue occurs. Oxygen therapy may be employed, and surgery may be required to remove the site of the infection.

septotomy A surgical incision made in the nasal septum.

septum, nasal See NASAL SEPTUM.

sequestration, pulmonary A nonfunctioning part of the lung that is supplied with blood from systemic circulation.

Serevent See SALMETEROL.

sexual activity and asthma The physical exertion of intercourse that in asthmatic persons may result in wheezing or shortness of breath and should be treated as exercise-induced asthma.
See also ASTHMA.

Shen-Nung The legendary founder of Chinese medicine and agriculture and the "Fire Emperor" of China from 2838 to 2698 B.C. who devised the *Pen-Ts'ao*, or the *Divine Husbandman's Materia Medica*. This reference described how drugs and plants could be used to treat diseases. Shen-Nung's work was continued by other investigators long after his death. His original reference to Ma-Huang, the plant source of the drug epinephrine, has been studied pharmacologically up through today. According to Shen-Nung, Ma-Huang, or ephedra, redirects a reversed flow of *ch'i* (in Eastern medicine, *ch'i* refers to the air, or essential spirit, of the human body), which causes coughing and difficulty in breathing. Today, ephedrine is an effective drug in the treatment of hay fever and asthma.

See also EPHEDRINE.

shock A set of symptoms indicating great physical and/or emotional trauma, including inadequate peripheral blood flow to the heart, infection, hemorrhage, trauma, myocardial infarction (heart attack), poisoning, dehydration, excess or lack of insulin, allergic reaction, anesthetic overdose, acidosis, electric current, toxins from gram-negative bacteria, insufficient amount of blood in the circulatory system, mental or psychic trauma, protein administered parenterally, injection of certain serum, adverse surgical effects, and other causes.

Shock is considered a medical emergency and requires immediate treatment, depending upon type and severity.

sick building syndrome (tight building syndrome)
Symptoms suggestive of allergy occurring in groups of office workers. Since the energy crisis of the 1970s, changes in construction were designed to improve heating and air-conditioning efficiency. These changes frequently resulted in poor ventilation, which leads to respiratory irritation and the possible retention of allergens in the air.

Symptoms range from itching and burning of the mucous membranes of the respiratory system to rashes and central nervous system complaints. In more than 450 evaluations made by the National Institute of Occupational Safety and Health (NIOSH), there have rarely been severe or permanent illnesses as a result of these symptoms. The exceptions have been cases of hypersensitivity pneumonitis, an allergic lung disease caused by repeated exposure to organic dusts or other offending agents, or infectious pneumonias such as Legionnaire's disease.

See also LEGIONNAIRE'S DISEASE; PNEUMONITIS.

sickness, mountain See ALTITUDE SICKNESS.

siderosis A chronic, pneumonia-like lung disease, also known as arc welder's disease or hemosiderosis, caused by the inhalation of iron particles in dust or fumes.

sigh A deep breath and exhalation that may be accompanied by a sound.

signs, vital Temperature, respiration rate, blood pressure, and pulse rate monitored regularly as functions that are essential to life.

silicosiderosis See SIDEROSIS.

silicosis A chronic, pneumonia-like lung disease caused by the chronic occupational inhalation of quartz dust, or silica, stone dust, sand dust, or flint dust that contains silicon dioxide. Silicosis is also called grinder's disease, or pneumoconiosis.

See also GRINDER'S DISEASE; PNEUMOCONIOSIS.

silicotuberculosis Pulmonary tuberculosis concurrent with silicosis.

See also SILICOSIS; TUBERCULOSIS.

silo filler's disease An occupational, lung-damaging irritation of nitrogen oxide (NO_2), a poisonous gas produced by fermenting material in silos. Silo workers may experience eye and throat irritation, but the condition may be as severe as to cause unconsciousness and injury to the lungs. Among preventive measures are forbidding entrance to the silo for seven to 10 days after it has been filled, adequate ventilation above the silo's base for that seven- to 10-day period, a blower fan installed in the silo that can be turned on upon entering, and constructing a fence around the area of the silo to prevent children and animals from possible toxicity exposure.

Singulair Brand name of montelukast.

singultation From the Latin word *singultus*, a hiccup.

sinobronchitis Bronchitis occurring simultaneously with paranasal sinusitis.

See also BRONCHITIS; SINUSITIS.

sinopulmonary infections and immunoglobulin A (IgA) deficiency A higher incidence of respiratory infections in the sinuses and lungs in persons with a deficiency in antibodies of the IgA class.

See also IMMUNE COMPLEX DISORDERS.

sinuses, accessory nasal Hollow air-filled cavities in the bones of the skull located over the eyes (frontal), behind the eyes (ethmoidal), behind the nose (sphenoid), and behind the cheeks (maxillary). The frontal sinus is not present at birth and usually develops fully by the late teens (or it may never develop in some persons). The function of the sinuses is unknown; however, infection in one or more of the sinus cavities is a source of frequent disability that can be severe.

See also SINUSITIS.

sinuses, pleural Open regions or spaces in the pleural sac located in the lower and inferior portions of the lung.

sinuses, sphenoidal See SINUSES, ACCESSORY NASAL.

sinusitis An inflammation of the mucous membrane lining in one or more of the sinus cavities in the head, caused by inadequate drainage characteristic of allergy, infection, or physical obstruction. Sinusitis may be acute, lasting for a few days to weeks, or chronic, lasting for many months to years. It has a tendency to recur.

During an attack of sinusitis, tiny hairs that keep the sinuses clear lose their effectiveness, and the sinus cavities become blocked. The blockage results in the symptoms of pressure or pain characteristic of sinusitis. Headache and facial pain caused by migraine, trigeminal neuralgia, or from a dental problem are often erroneously called "sinus headache" but must be distinguished from sinusitis. Fever and a thick yellow-green mucus discharge are often associated with sinus infection.

The diagnosis of a sinus condition is usually suggested by a history of the typical symptoms described above. However, the diagnosis may be unclear at times. As many as 10 percent of sinus infections are related to dental problems. Diagnostic procedures to confirm the presence of sinusitis include transillumination of the frontal and maxillary sinuses in a completely darkened room. A bright light source is placed over the orbital area of the face, and the hard palate is observed for the absence of transmission of light indicative of sinusitis. The light source is then placed against the hard palate to observe light transmission over the cheekbones behind which the maxillary sinuses are located. Transillumination is of lesser value for the frontal sinuses and of no use to diagnose disease in the ethmoid and sphenoid sinuses.

Ultrasound is a technique in which inaudible sound waves in the frequency of approximately 20,000 to 10 billion cycles per second are passed through body tissues. Differences in the velocity with which sound passes through various tissues are used to outline their shape and aid in the diagnosis of disorders. Despite early promises of being a safe, noninvasive means to diagnose sinus conditions, unfortunately it lacks the sensitivity to be a reliable diagnostic method.

X rays are the mainstay for accurate diagnosis of sinus disease. Plain films are useful for detecting thickness suggestive of chronic sinus disease or air-fluid levels correlating with acute infection. However, X rays have limited ability to view the deeper ethmoid and sphenoid sinuses. Computerized tomography (CT or CAT scan) is the most sensitive means for the diagnosis of sinus disorders. Magnetic resonance imaging (MRI) is capable of detecting minute changes in tissues, but it is two or three times more expensive than a CT scan.

Allergies are probably the most common cause of sinus symptoms, and skin and blood tests are helpful in making that diagnosis. Although bacterial infections frequently complicate sinusitis, cultures of material obtained from nasal secretions are unreliable in determining the cause. *Streptococcus pneumoniae* and *Haemophilus influenzae* are responsible for approximately 50 percent of proven sinus infection, but *Branhamella catarrhalis* (formerly called *Neisseria catarrhalis*) and other bacteria are important causes of infected sinuses. Less frequently, fungal infections occur in the sinuses. Many sinus infections are preceded by viral upper respiratory infections or colds.

Most sinus conditions respond to decongestant drugs, antihistamines for allergic individuals, and antibiotics. Antibiotics should be taken for a minimum of 10 to 14 days but may be needed for up to six weeks in persistent cases. Anti-inflammatory, corticosteroid nasal sprays may be helpful in controlling sinus symptoms and preventing recurrences. Sinus irrigation, the mainstay of treatment prior to the introduction of antibiotics, is still useful in stubborn cases. If adequate antibiotic therapy and sinus drainage are unsuccessful, surgical procedures by otolaryngologists (ENT doctors) skilled in various procedures may be necessary. Unfortunately, sinus surgery has a high rate of failure in preventing recurrences of sinusitis.

skier's nose   Also known as cold-induced rhinorrhea, a runny nose that occurs upon exposure to cold air. It is not an allergy and does not respond to antihistamines, but it may be prevented by using a mixture of atropine sulfate and saline solution as a nasal spray.

Skoda's rales   Named for Austrian physician Josef Skoda (1805–81), crackling noises heard on auscultation in the bronchial tubes of pneumonia patients.

See also SKODA'S RESONANCE.

Skoda's resonance   Sounds heard above the presence of fluid in the case of pleuritic effusion or pneumonia.

sleep apnea   See APNEA.

Slo-Bid   See THEOPHYLLINE.

Slo-Phyllin   See THEOPHYLLINE.

slow-reacting substance of anaphylaxis (SRS-A)
Also known as slow-releasing substance (SRS), leukotriene C and D, a potent biochemical substance produced and released by mast cells of the immune system during anaphylaxis (severe allergic reaction). SRS causes smooth-muscle contraction especially in the bronchial tubes and increased permeability of blood vessels.

See also LEUKOTRIENES.

smog   A type of air pollution caused by a combination of smoke and fog.

smoke inhalation   See SMOKE POISONING.

smokeless tobacco   See TOBACCO.

smoke poisoning   Deleterious effects of inhaling gases, usually carbon monoxide, and smoke that is the result of burning. Affected most is the respiratory system, namely injured mucosa, which may lead to pulmonary edema, shock, and death. Therapy includes oxygen, corticosteroids, and other measures specific to pulmonary edema.

smoker's cancer   See LUNG CANCER.

smoking   See LUNG CANCER.

smoking, passive   The exposure of nonsmokers to the same gases and particulate matter as smokers except to a somewhat lesser degree. Cigarette smoke contains slightly different compositions from each end of the cigarette. Smoke from the lighted end produces "sidestream" smoke; the smoker's end is called "mainstream" smoke. Sidestream smoke constitutes about 85 percent of the smoke in a smoke-filled room and contains a much greater concentration of potential carcinogens; therefore, it is a great risk to nonsmokers present in any smoking environment. Healthy children exposed to passive smoke, especially during the first year of life, suffer from an increased number of upper respiratory infections, including ear infections and tonsillitis, and lower respiratory infections, such as bronchitis, bronchiolitis, and pneumonia. There is also diminished resistance to viral infections and a small but statistically significant decrease in lung function or breathing capacity in otherwise healthy children. In allergic and asthmatic children and adults, there is also a worsening of their usual symptoms. However, there is no evidence that exposure to passive smoking increases allergic tendencies in newborn or older children. Passive smoking was the most important environmental factor occurring in 62 percent of children younger than three, hospitalized for asthma in a New York inner-city hospital.

sneeze From the Anglo-Saxon word *fneosan*, meaning to pant, a forcible expulsion of air through the nose and/or mouth caused by a spasm in the expiratory muscles or an irritant to nasal membranes. Also known as sternutation, a sneeze may have many or unknown causes, the presence of allergens or infection among them.

sneeze reflex, solar A sneeze of unknown mechanism occurring upon exposure to bright sunlight, which may be normal or associated with rhinitis.

sniffing See INHALANT ABUSE.

snore See STERTOR.

snoring rale A low-pitched, sonorous rale, similar to the sound of snoring.

snuff Pulverized tobacco that can be inhaled, chewed, or put next to the gums. The word is derived from the Dutch word *snuftabak*. Snuff is also a medicinal powder that can be inhaled through the nose. Anatomical snuffbox refers to the dorsal base of the thumb on which a small quantity of snuff could be placed and inhaled through the nose.

snuffles The condition of nasal discharge and obstructed breathing, usually seen in infants as a result of the mother's congenital syphilis.

S.O.B. The medical abbreviation for short (or shortness) of breath.

sob Crying that involves heaving or convulsive moving of the chest due to sudden inspiration of air and the subsequent glottal spasm.

sonorous rale A sound produced in a bronchus that is low-pitched and dry, indicating the presence of mucous secretion.

soot A black substance that produces fine particles on combustion. The particles create a carbon powder that sticks to pipes, chimneys, smoke, and other substances. Considered a major pollutant, soot in the air has been linked with illness that causes thousands of premature deaths each year, according to the Environmental Protection Agency (EPA).

In an April 21, 2001, article in the *New York Times*, the EPA's study on fine soot and its effects noted that in 1999, "the latest year with comprehensive data, New York City, Los Angeles, Atlanta, Chicago, and several other cities had annual average levels of 2.5 micron particles that would—if seen for three years in a row—violate the proposed rule" to cut levels of soot and other smog ingredients produced mainly by power plants and vehicles. Before her appointment to the Bush administration as EPA administrator, former New Jersey governor Christie Whitman endorsed a Clinton administration ruling that would "sharply curtail emissions of soot and other emissions from diesel engines."

Soot particles, composed of metals, carbons, and other ingredients, have the ability to be breathed into the lungs and go easily into the bloodstream, putting people susceptible to or already suffering from respiratory problems at risk. The Harvard School of Public Health and the American Cancer Society reported that they found that high levels of small particles in the air corresponded with a rise in death rates. Other studies indicate that more than 50,000 people die prematurely each year from illness resulting from inhaling fine soot, and that sooty air corresponded with a rise in hospital admissions of children having asthma attacks. A 632-page research review was posted on the EPA website, www.epa.gov/ncea/. A paper recommending how to interpret information from the studies and cut the level of fine soot is currently being drafted by the EPA's Clean Air Science Advisory Committee. Industry representatives are questioning the validity of the studies and the EPA's proposed course of action, which is basically that a standard would be established to limit the concentrations of soot particles smaller than 2.5 microns to an average of 15 micrograms per cubic meter measured over three consecutive years.

sore throat   Pain accompanying an inflammation of the pharynx (throat), tonsils, or larynx. The inflammation may be the result of an infection, such as in streptococcal, quinsy, diphtheritic or septic sore throat.

soroche   A type of mountain sickness that is prevalent in the Andes.

See also MOUNTAIN SICKNESS.

sounds, breath   See SOUNDS, RESPIRATORY.

sounds, respiratory   Any sound arising from the trachea, larynx, bronchi, or lungs that can be heard with or without the use of a stethoscope. Various sounds, such as rales or rhonchi, may indicate the presence of infection or obstruction in the airways or respiratory structures. Bronchial sound may indicate pulmonary disease involving infiltration and solidification of the lung. Cracked pot sound can be heard over the pulmonary cavities. When two inflamed mucous surfaces rub together, they produce a friction sound. Breath sounds heard through a stethoscope over a normal chest are categorized as vesicular, tracheal, and bronchovesicular. Vesicular sound is that produced by the lung during inhalation, which causes the alveoli to expand. Bronchovesicular refers to the sound made by both the bronchi and lungs. Normal tracheal sounds are heard over both the trachea (windpipe) and larynx (voice box). Tubular sounds may be heard over the large bronchi or the trachea.

space, retropharyngeal   The region located behind the pharynx (throat) that can serve as a pathway for an infection to spread from the mouth to organs of the trunk of the body.

See also RETROPHARYNGITIS.

spacer   A drug-delivery device in various shapes and sizes for metered-dose inhalers that affords the user, including small children or poorly coordinated individuals, the full benefits of an aerosol asthma medication. Spacers allow small particles of active medication to enter the airways, and trap large inactive particles that could irritate the mouth and throat. The spacer is especially helpful with the corticosteroid metered-dose inhalers and lessens the likelihood of oral yeast infections.

spasm, bronchial   A sudden contraction of the bronchial tube muscles that occurs during an asthma attack.

See also ASTHMA.

spasmatic asthma   Symptoms of asthma triggered by spasm in the bronchioles.

See also ASTHMA.

spasmatic croup   Another term for laryngismus stridulus, or spasm of the larynx.

See also LARYNGITIS STRIDULUS; LARYNX.

speech   The act of speaking, making words, or sounds that range from the simplest expressions to a highly complex pattern of communication. The physical ability to speak involves the coordination of the mouth, lips, larynx, chest, and abdominal muscles and the manipulation of air flowing in and out of the body. Speech abnormalities may occur in conjunction with certain respiratory disorders.

Spinhaler   A drug-delivery device formerly used with cromolyn sodium (Intal) capsules. The powder-containing capsules were placed inside a whistlelike plastic tube and activated by twisting the device and inhaling the released drug. The Spinhaler has been replaced by the metered-dose inhaler.

See also AEROSOLS; INHALER.

spirit of glyceryl trinitrate   An alcoholic liquid once used as a relaxant for the treatment of asthma and angina pectoris (chest pain related to heart disease).

spirogram   A printout made by a spirometer that records breathing function.
  See also SPIROMETER.

spirometer   An instrument that measures the air capacity of the lungs. It is used to make treatment decisions for patients with asthma and other lung disorders. It is also used to determine the severity of lung disease and to help determine disability or if a specific job should be precluded. Spirometry equipment must meet rigid specifications as recommended by the American Thoracic Society in an official policy statement published in the *American Review of Respiratory Diseases* in 1987.

spore   Derived from the Greek word meaning seed, a reproductive cell of certain plants, especially fungi and protozoans (the simplest, mostly unicellular, animal form). Spores are usually asexual (able to reproduce by fission), but certain sexual forms are associated with molds, such as oospores, zygospores, and ascospores. Fungal or mold spores are a significant source of allergic symptoms.

sputum   A combination of mucus, pus, blood, cellular debris, infectious microorganisms, and caseous material expelled by individuals with pneumonia and other pulmonary diseases when they cough or clear their throats. Types of sputum vary according to the diagnosis. In bronchial asthma, sputum is often purulent (containing pus), grayish, and possibly frothy and contains Charcot-Leyden crystals (hard formations from salts and other substances). In bronchitis, sputum contains thick mucus and pus that is greenish yellow. In bronchopneumonia, mucus may look like prune juice in color and can be frothy, thin, mucoid, purulent, and bloody.

squatting in asthmatic children   The crouching position assumed by some children with asthma, heart disease, or other disorders affecting normal breathing during play or physically strenuous activity. This characteristic squatting helps relieve chronic oxygen deprivation, especially after exertion, by facilitating use of accessory muscles of respiration and thus making breathing easier.

staircase breaths   A technique involving the administration of several small breaths as opposed to a single large-volume breath during cardiopulmonary resuscitation.
  See also CARDIOPULMONARY RESUSCITATION.

staphylitis   Inflammation of the uvula.
  See also RESPIRATORY SYSTEM.

status asthmaticus   The condition of intractable asthma, a diagnosis that indicates that a patient is so debilitated that emergency management in a hospital is required.

steam tent   An enclosure devised to facilitate the inhalation of steam or vapors to relieve respiratory distress. Although benzoin, menthol, camphor, and other ingredients may be added to the boiling water, the real therapeutic value is the water vapor itself.

stenosis, pulmonary   From the Greek word *stenos*, meaning narrow, a narrowing of the opening into the pulmonary artery from the right ventricle of the heart.

stenothorax   The condition of having an unusually narrow chest cavity.

sternutation   The medical term for sneezing. A sternutator refers to any agent that causes sneezing, and convulsive sternutation refers to paroxysmal or spasmodic sneezing accompanied by extremely watery eyes.
  See also SNEEZE.

steroid   Any substance in a large group of sterol-related chemicals, including compounds containing a 17-carbon, 4-ring system (the perhydrocyclopentanophenanthrene ring).

See also CORTICOSTEROIDS.

stertor   The medical term for snoring. Stertorous breathing also refers to loud breathing that sometimes sounds like a hen's clucking. Hen cluck stertor is often found in patients with postpharyngeal abscess. Stertorous breathing may also occur in persons with asthma or respiratory allergy symptoms. Snoring is actually the vibrating sound made by inhaled air passing through the mouth and then the soft tissues in the throat, including the roof of the mouth, tonsils, adenoids, and uvula. As the body ages, the soft tissues stretch and further restrict the passage of inhaled air. Overweight men over 40 are most likely to snore and experience sleep apnea, and women who are pregnant or postmenopausal may also snore because they produce less progesterone, a hormone that, among other properties, helps stabilize respiratory muscles. The use of alcohol and tranquilizers and sleeping on one's back may also contribute to snoring. (Sewing golf balls or marbles on pajamas has been suggested as a way to prevent sleeping on one's back.) The FDA has approved nasal strips designed to be worn across the bridge of the nose to help keep nasal passages open for optimal breathing through the nose during sleep. Another breathing device is the Continuous Positive Airway Pressure mask, which pushes air through the nose, down the throat, and into the lungs. Surgical procedures, such as tonsillectomy and/or adenoidectomy, and radio frequency ablation that uses microwaves to adjust soft tissues in the throat, may be effective in treating severe snoring and breathing problems.

stethoscope   An instrument consisting of two rubber tubes connected to a bell at one end and ear pieces at the other. It is used to listen to respiratory, cardiac, pleural, arterial, venous, uterine, fetal, intestinal, and other body sounds for diagnostic purposes.

stillicidium lacrimarum   The medical term for watery eyes.

stillicidium narium   The medical term for watery mucus discharged from the nose and associated with allergies or the common cold.

stimulant, respiratory   Any substance that increases breathing function.

stonecutter's phthisis   A wasting form of bronchopneumonia as a result of irritation of the lung by inhaled stone dust.

See also PHTHISIS.

stramonium   An antispasmodic drug derived from the dried leaves of *Datura stramonium* and related to the drug atropine. Atropine blocks the constricting action of the vagus nerve on the bronchial tubes. Stramonium was the active ingredient in Asthmador cigarettes, inhaled by asthma patients to relax smooth muscles in the bronchial tubes in a now-obsolete treatment of asthma. Adverse effects of this treatment, including irritation from the cigarette smoke, eventually outweighed any possible benefit. Atropine-like drugs, however, are now prescribed mainly for the treatment of chronic bronchitis and occasionally asthma.

See also ATROPINE.

Streptococcus pneumoniae   A species of gram-positive, nonmotile bacteria that causes lobar and other types of pneumonia and is associated with infections including endocarditis, septicemia, meningitis, and conjunctivitis.

See also PNEUMONIA.

stress   Physical or emotional tension that may be well-tolerated by the body for efficient function or ill-tolerated, which often results in some form of debilitation. Negative stress, or distress, is considered a trigger for asthma.

stridor   A shrill or harsh sound, like wind whistling through pipes, created during respiration by individuals with severe asthma or acute obstruction of the larynx.

subcrepitant   A rale that makes a partially crackling or crepitant sound.

suction, post-tussive   The sucking sound heard through a stethoscope over the lung after a patient has coughed.

suffocation   The state of being smothered, choked, gassed, drowned, or otherwise having one's breathing impaired to the point of unconsciousness or death.

sulfating agents   Food additives used to prevent discoloration of food and to inhibit growth of certain microorganisms in the fermentation process during the manufacture of wine. Sulfur dioxide gas, or powdered or liquid potassium metabisulfite, and other sulfating agents have been used for hundreds of years and are the most important additives that can cause serious adverse reactions. Ingestion of sulfites has no apparent effects on normal persons, but approximately 5 percent of asthmatic individuals are sulfite-sensitive, with symptoms ranging from mild wheezing to death. The average diet in the United States contains about 2 to 3 milligrams of sulfites daily. Each ounce of beer or wine contains 5 to 10 milligrams. Prior to a Food and Drug Administration ban in 1986 on the use of sulfites in restaurants, a meal contained from 25 to 200 milligrams of sulfites. As little as 5 milligrams of ingested sulfite can provoke an asthmatic response in susceptible persons, and there are at least 12 documented asthma deaths from sulfating agents. Allergic symptoms including urticaria (hives), angioedema (tissue swelling), and anaphylaxis (allergic shock) may be caused by sulfites, but only a few individuals who react to these additives have positive skin tests to them. The cause of sulfite reactions may be related to a deficiency of the enzyme sulfite oxidase, which is required to inactivate sulfite in the body.

Highest levels of sulfites are found in dried fruits, potatoes, seafoods, and wine. Sulfite use is prohibited in any food served fresh in restaurants. Since January 1988, packaged foods and bottled wines must be labeled if they contain more than 10 parts per million of sulfur dioxide (SO_2). Some medications used as solutions in the emergency treatment of asthma contain sulfites. Isoetharine (Bronkosol) solution contains sodium bisulfite as a preservative, and isoproterenol (Isuprel) contains sodium metabisulfite, also as a preservative. Although these medications are rarely used since the introduction of albuterol and metaproterenol, asthma patients and their physicians should be aware that these solutions for aerosol treatment of asthma may actually worsen asthma in some individuals.

The most common foods that may contain sulfites are processed potatoes (chips, fries, dehydrated); dried and packaged fruits and beverages; shrimp and other seafood; beer and wine; salads and all ingredients in salad bars in countries outside the United States (sulfite use is banned in restaurant salad bars in the United States); precut fruit outside the United States; avocado, guacamole, and other dips; cider and wine vinegars; pickled vegetables; white grapes; Maraschino cherries; fresh mushrooms; beet sugar; wet-milled corn; and conditioned dough.

supplemental air   See RESERVE AIR.

surfactant, pulmonary   A natural, fatty substance that lubricates the lungs and prevents them from collapsing during expiration, and reduces or controls surface tension of air-liquid emulsion found in the lungs. In cases of pulmonary edema, prematurity, and hyaline membrane disease, the surfactant is inadequate or abnormal.

surgery, related to allergic and asthmatic persons   Individuals with asthma and/or allergies to drugs including anesthesia need to consider certain factors when they require an elective surgical procedure. (1) Do not schedule surgery when a viral infection or exacerbation of asthma is present. (2) Have the physician evaluate breathing status, blood oxygenation, and lung function one or two days before the surgery. (3) Review all medications and blood levels of medications with the physician and surgical team before the surgery. (4) Use local anesthesia, which does not interfere with breathing mechanisms, if possible. (5) Avoid nitrous oxide (laughing gas) as dental anesthesia; a local anesthetic and a mild tranquilizer are recommended. (6) Ensure that the patient will be assisted in bringing up mucus and secretions after the surgery, if necessary.

In the event of emergency surgery and the use of general anesthesia, most often there is minimal increased risk for the allergic or asthmatic patient in light of available medications and adequate monitoring.

Sus-Phrine   The brand name for epinephrine hydrochloride.

See also EPINEPHRINE.

suspiration   From the Latin word *suspirare*, sighing, or a sigh. The word suspirious also refers to sighing, or breathing with emphasis or effort.

sweat chloride test   A diagnostic test used to determine the presence of cystic fibrosis. The test, which measures the salt content in the sweat, is performed on children who are wheezing or who have a family history of cystic fibrosis, failure to thrive, recurrent pneumonia, or other pulmonary disorder that involves gastrointestinal disturbances.

See also CYSTIC FIBROSIS.

sympathomimetic drugs   See AGONIST.

symptoms of allergy   From the Greek word meaning occurrence, a symptom is a change or ill effect experienced by an individual and potentially indicating a disease process. Specific symptoms of allergy include sneezing, itching, wheezing, runny nose, nasal congestion, shortness of breath, tightness in the chest, rashes, swelling of body tissues, discharge from the eyes, and other discomforts.

See also RHINITIS.

Syngamus laryngeus   A species of parasitic worm that thrives in the respiratory tract of birds, mammals, and sometimes humans.

system, respiratory   See RESPIRATORY SYSTEM.

tabacosis Tobacco poisoning, especially from the inhalation of tobacco dust by tobacco handlers. Exposure to tobacco dust is a cause of occupational asthma.

See also OCCUPATIONAL ASTHMA.

tachypnea Abnormally rapid breathing.

See also BREATHING.

talcosis A condition resulting from the inhalation or implantation of talc, powdered soapstone, or hydrous magnesium silicate, in the body. Talc, also called talcum, is commonly used as a dusting powder, as a counterirritant for prickly heat, diaper rash, and other skin eruptions, and for industrial products. It is also an irritant that can trigger asthma.

See also OCCUPATIONAL ASTHMA; PNEUMOCONIOSIS.

tampon, nasal A nostril plug made of a rubber bulb inflated with compressed air that is designed to stop nasal hemorrhaging.

Tapia syndrome Named for Spanish physician Antonio Garcia Tapia (1875–1950), a lesion affecting the vagus and hypoglossal cranial nerves and resulting in pharyngeal (throat) and laryngeal (voice box) paralysis on one side and atrophy of the tongue on the other side.

Tavist A brand of clemastine fumarate, an antihistamine drug.

technician, respiratory therapy An individual trained to treat noncritical respiratory care patients.

A technician may also respond to emergency calls for respiratory care.

tent, oxygen See OXYGEN TENT.

terbutaline sulfate (Brethaire, Brethine, Bricanyl) A selective beta$_2$ bronchodilating drug used to treat asthma. As an oral or inhaled medication, its effectiveness and safety are similar to those of albuterol. It can be administered by subcutaneous injection for asthma emergencies and has an action similar to that of epinephrine, but it takes up to 15 minutes to become effective (epinephrine usually works within one minute).

See also BETA-ADRENERGIC AGONISTS.

terfenadine (Seldane) A second-generation of nonsedating antihistaminic drug used to treat allergic rhinitis (hay fever) and urticaria (hives). There have been rare but life-threatening cardiac arrythmias (irregular heartbeat) associated with the use of terfenadine given simultaneously with certain other drugs, including the antibiotic erythromycin, the antifungal drug ketaconazole, and with grapefruit juice. A risk is also associated with the use of terfenadine in persons with liver disorders.

terpin hydrate An over-the-counter expectorant, which helps rid the body of excess bronchial secretions.

test, tuberculin See MANTOUX TEST.

tetracyclines A group of broad-spectrum antibiotics first discovered as a result of systemic screening of soil samples collected from around the world in a search for microorganisms that could produce antibiotics. The first of these drugs produced was chlortetracycline in 1948. Since then three other naturally occurring antibiotics have been produced from species of the bacteria *Streptomyces*, tetracycline (Achromycin, Sumycin, Panmycin, Robitet), oxytetracycline (Terramycin), and demeclocycline (Declomycin). Methacycline (Rondomycin), doxycycline (Vibramycin, Doryx), and minocycline (Minocin) are semisynthetically derived by manipulation of the natural tetracyclines.

The antibiotic affect of tetracyclines is due to their ability to interfere with protein synthesis in bacteria. However, by some other mechanism, the drugs are effective against *Rickettsia* and *Chlamydia* infections. Although tetracyclines are frequently used for the treatment of respiratory infections such as sinusitis, bronchitis, and pneumonia in patients with asthma or allergic rhinitis, many microorganisms have developed a resistance to them. Adverse effects of the tetracyclines include rare cases of anaphylaxis, and all drugs in this class should be avoided in persons with a history of serious allergic reaction to any of them. More commonly, rashes occur, especially with sun exposure. Demeclocycline causes the most severe and frequent photosensitivity reactions; doxycycline reactions are less severe. Most of the photosensitivity rashes resemble severe sunburn and occur on exposed skin areas. Paresthesias (tingling of the hands, feet, and nose) may be the first sign of adverse reactions to tetracyclines and the sun.

Tetracyclines also cause numerous other adverse effects, most often gastrointestinal upset, which are usually mild and self-limiting. Rarely, neurologic disturbances are exhibited, such as pseudotumor cerebri (increased pressure in the brain that gives symptoms suggestive of a brain tumor).

Tetracyclines are absorbed by bones and teeth and depress bone growth and tooth development. Therefore they should probably not be given to pregnant women or to children before the age of eight or nine. In rare instances with life-threatening infections such as Rocky Mountain spotted fever, their use may be necessary.

theophylline   Derived from the Latin word *thea*, or tea, and the Greek word *phyllon*, or plant, a spas-molytic drug that relaxes smooth muscle in the respiratory system. Theophylline, a white crystalline powder with action like caffeine and theobromine, is used to treat bronchial asthma, bronchospasm that accompanies chronic obstructive lung disease (COLD), and chronic bronchitis. Trade names include Accurbron, Aerolate Slo-Phyllin, Aquaphyllin, Bronkodyl, Elixomin, Slo-Phyllin, Respbid, Theophylline Oral, Theospan-SR, Theovent, T-Phyls and Uniphyl.

Theophylline was first isolated from tea leaves in 1888. At first, it was used as a diuretic for cases of congestive heart failure, and for a brief period in the 1950s it was used to treat angina. A modified version of the drug, aminophylline, became popular in the 1940s to treat asthma, but it was not until the late 1970s and 1980s that its popularity peaked with the introduction of long-acting formulas.

The basis of theophylline's activity has not been well defined but is thought to be complex. Theophylline is known to block the action of adenosine, which causes constriction of the bronchioles in asthma. The drug strengthens the contractability of the diaphragmatic muscle and diminishes fatigue. Theophylline seems to stimulate the respiratory center; in patients with both chronic bronchitis or emphysema and heart failure (cor pulmonale), theophylline strengthens cardiac output. The drug also may inhibit the release of inflammatory mediators.

There is considerable disagreement among physicians about the role of theophylline in the treatment of asthma. Some researchers feel theophylline is more effective than beta$_2$-agonists and should be a primary drug, whereas others have relegated theophylline to a backup role to be added to a regimen of other asthma drugs.

Despite its reputation for causing many side effects, the only major drawback of theophylline is overdose, which can be avoided by monitoring serum levels. Tachyphylaxis (tolerance) does not occur, and it is the only bronchodilator drug for which there is a fixed dose that is independent of the severity of the disease.

The use of theophylline in children is also controversial. The drug has been blamed for causing both learning disabilities and hyperactivity. Studies have demonstrated normal school performance in students with asthma taking theophylline on a daily basis when compared with nonasthmatic children.

Guidelines for the safe use of theophylline are

1. Serum levels from 15 to 20 micrograms/ml were considered optimal until recently. Now levels from 5 to 15 are considered adequate and safer for most patients.
2. During pregnancy, and in chronic bronchitis or emphysema, levels from 8 to 12 are advised.
3. Doses should be taken at regular intervals and in the same relationship to meals.
4. Various brand-name products and generic formulations are not interchangeable, and levels may vary greatly when switching from one formulation to another.
5. If another illness occurs while on theophylline, especially heart failure, liver disease, or upper respiratory infections (including the common cold), theophylline doses may need to be adjusted downward. If unable to reach your doctor, you should skip a dose and lower subsequent doses until the physician can be consulted.
6. Many drugs affect the theophylline level by diminishing its excretion from the body, thus raising levels to a possible toxic degree. Cimetidine (Tagamet), mexiletine, ciprofloxacin, and other quinolone antibiotics, erythromycin, allopurinol, propanolol, and oral contraceptives may increase levels. Influenza vaccine also raises theophylline levels for a short time. The anticonvulsant medications phenytoin, phenobarbital, and carbamazepine, the antibiotic rifampin, and cigarette smoking may lower theophylline levels.
7. The following patient types should probably avoid theophylline except in very carefully monitored settings: (a) elderly frail patients with multiple medical problems; (b) patients susceptible to nausea and vomiting; (c) premature babies and infants under one year; (d) patients known to have sudden changes in their heart rhythm (arrhythmias); and (e) any patient who might misuse medications.

therapist, respiratory   An individual trained in the techniques and use of equipment for patients with acute and chronic respiratory disorders.

thoracentesis   A diagnostic surgical procedure involving the aspiration of fluid from the thoracic cavity, or chest, with a large-bore needle. Also known as pleurocentesis, thoracentesis is usually preceded and followed by chest X rays.

thoracic cavity   The area of the chest and the organs it contains, including the lungs, heart, thoracic aorta, pulmonary artery and veins, vena cava, thymus gland, lymph nodes, trachea, bronchi, esophagus, and thoracic duct. The thorax is enclosed by thoracic walls and is located above the diaphragm. The thoracic cage is the skeletal component of the chest that consists of 12 pairs of ribs, the thoracic vertebrae, and the sternum or breastbone.

thoracic outlet compression syndrome   Symptoms caused by nerves or vessels becoming compressed in the neck and axilla that may be confused with cervical disk lesions, lung cancer, bursitis, and angina.

thoracic squeeze   A divers' phenomenon, particularly when divers hold their breath and go approximately 80 to 100 feet in depth, in which the lungs become so compressed that alveolar capillaries rupture. Divers suffering from thoracic squeeze must be removed from the water immediately and given artificial respiration and oxygen therapy.

thoracograph   A device that records on paper the shape of the thorax and its movements during a patient's respirations.

thoracopneumoplasty   Plastic surgery procedures that involve the thorax and lung.

thoracostenosis   Also known as "wasp waist," a narrowing of the chest, or thorax, due to wasting or atrophy of the muscles.

thorax   The medical term for the chest cavity, organs, and other structures.

throat   The pharynx and fauces of the respiratory system, which extends from the arch of the palate to the glottis and superior opening of the esophagus. Essentially, the throat is an airway.

tidal air The air inhaled and exhaled in normal breathing.

Tilade inhaler An aerosol medication of nedocromil sodium used to treat severe perennial bronchial asthma and to prevent exercise-induced or environmental pollutant bronchospasm.

tobacco The dried leaves of the Nicotiana tabacum and other plant species that are used to make cigarettes, cigars, pipe tobacco, snuff, and chewing tobacco, all of which have ill effect on the lungs and respiratory passages. When lit and smoked, the tobacco's nicotine is released and widely known to cause addiction and respiratory disease.

See also LUNG CANCER; SMOKING.

tonsil From the Latin word *tonsilla*, meaning almond-shaped, lymphatic tissue masses in the mucous membrane of the fauces and pharynx that help form white blood cells in the event of infection and to help filter harmful bacteria from the body. Nasal tonsils are located in the lymphoid tissue on the nasal septum. Pharyngeal tonsils, also called Luschka's tonsils, are on the roof of the back of the throat. The lingual tonsil lies at the root of the tongue, and palatine tonsils are located on either side of the oral pharynx.

toxic-allergic syndrome A lung disorder caused by the ingestion of grapeseed oil tainted with aniline and containing acetanilide. Symptoms include respiratory distress, fever, headache, nausea, muscle and abdominal pain, rash, enlarged spleen and liver, and eosinophilia. Treatment may involve corticosteroid drugs and mechanically assisted respiration.

trachea A cartilaginous, membranous tube known commonly as the windpipe, the main airway between the mouth and the lungs. The inside of the trachea looks like about 20 horseshoes piled up flat against each other. These cartilage "horseshoes" maintain the tube's shape, thus keeping it open for airflow. The trachea, part of the throat, extends from the larynx (vocal cords) to the bronchi branching into the lungs. An inflammation of the trachea, or tracheitis, may be associated with bronchitis and laryngitis.

See also TRACHEITIS.

tracheitis An inflammation of the trachea, or windpipe, which may be acute or chronic. Tracheitis is usually caused by a viral respiratory infection and may also involve the larynx and bronchioles. When the trachea becomes obstructed, a surgical procedure called a tracheostomy, or tracheotomy, may be necessary: An incision is made into the skin over the throat, and a hollow tube is inserted so that patient can breathe through it.

See also TRACHEA.

tracheobronchomegaly Congenital abnormal enlargement of the trachea and bronchi.

tracheocele A herniated mucous membrane protruding through the wall of the trachea, or windpipe.

tracheostomy Also called tracheotomy, the surgical creation of an opening in the trachea, or windpipe, to allow air into the body in the event that an individual's other airways are obstructed. In emergencies, an endotracheal tube is inserted in the opening to keep the airway patent. Tracheostomy care involves suctioning excess secretions that may impede the flow of air.

trachitis Inflammation of the trachea.

See also TRACHEITIS.

tract, respiratory See RESPIRATORY SYSTEM.

transpiration, pulmonary The release of water vapor from the bloodstream to the air in the lungs.

transplantation, lung See LUNG.

tree, bronchial   See BRONCHI.

tree pollen allergy   Seasonal hay fever and/or asthma caused by the inhalation of the pollen of wind-pollinating, or anemophilous, trees. Insect-pollinating, or entomophilus, trees and wind-pollinating conifers, whose pollen has a thick outer covering, have a very low potential for causing allergic symptoms. Each tree genus has pollen that is distinct from any other. An individual may exhibit allergy to one or many of the trees in his or her region. Pollinating seasons are brief, often intense, and usually occur before, during, or shortly after leaves develop in deciduous trees, especially in the spring.

TREES THAT ARE A CAUSE OF HAY FEVER IN THE UNITED STATES AND CANADA

Common Name	Technical Name	Plant Family	Distribution	Pollination Season
Acacia	*Acacia decurrens*	Leguminosae	Cultivated ornamental (subtropical)	Mar.–May
Acacia, Bailey's	*A. baileyana*	Leguminosae	Cultivated ornamental (subtropical)	Mar.–May
Acacia, longleaf	*A. longifolia*	Leguminosae	Cultivated ornamental (subtropical)	Mar.–May
Alder, red (Oregon)	*Alnus rubra*	Betulaceae	Pacific coast from S.W. Y.T. to So. CA, rarely more than 50 mi. from salt or over 2,500 A. elev.	Mar.–Apr.
Alder, Sitka[1]	*A. sinuata (A. sitchensis)*	Betulaceae	AK So. to Olympic Mts., Cascade Mts., No. CA, E. WA, N.E. OR, Rocky Mts.	May–July
Alder, slender[1]	*A. tenuifolia*	Betulaceae	N.E. MN, ND to B.C., So. to NM	Mar.–May
Alder, tag (speckled)[1]	*A. incana (A. rugosa)*	Betulaceae	Nfld. to N.W.T. and B.C. So. to MD., No. to IN and MN, MT, ID, WA	Mar.–May
Alder, white	*A. rhombifolia*	Betulaceae	No. ID to E. slope Cascades, to So. OR, W. slope of Sierra Nevada, So. to Coast Range in CA	Jan.–Apr.
Arborvitae, Chinese	*Thuja orientalis*	Cupressaceae	Cultivated ornamental	Apr.–May
Arborvitae, western (white cedar)	*T. occidentalis*	Cupressaceae	P.Q. and N.S. to Hudson Bay, So. to NJ, OH, No. IN and IL, WI, MN, Mts. NC and TN	Apr.–May
Ash (Arizona velvet)	*Fraxinus velutina*	Oleaceae	CA, AZ, So. NM, E. TX. Cultivated in these areas	Mar.–Apr.
Ash, black	*F. nigra*	Oleaceae	Nfld. and P.Q. to Man., So. to DE, KY, IA	Spring
Ash, green (ash, red)	*F. pennsylvanica*	Oleaceae	P.Q. to Man., So. to FL and TX	Spring
Ash, Mexican	*F. uhdei*	Oleaceae	Cultivated ornamental	Winter
Ash, Oregon	*F. oregona*	Oleaceae	C. CA, No. to B.C.	Mar.–May
Ash, white	*F. americana*	Oleaceae	N.S. to MN, So. to FL and TX	Spring
Aspen	*Populus tremuloides*	Salicaeae	Lab. to AK, So. to NJ, VA, TN, MO, Rocky Mts., Sierra Nevada, Cascades	Spring
Beech, American	*Fagus grandifolia*	Fagaceae	N.S. to MN, So. to FL and TX	Spring
Beefwood (Austral. pine)	*Casuarina equisetifolia*	Casuarinaceae	Cultivated ornamental (subtropical)	Jan.–Mar.

TREES THAT ARE A CAUSE OF HAY FEVER IN THE UNITED STATES AND CANADA (continued)

Common Name	Technical Name	Plant Family	Distribution	Pollination Season
Birch, cherry (black)	*Bettila lenta*	Betulaceae	IA, So. ME and So. W. P.Q. to DE and KY, along Appalachians to GA	Mar.–May
Birch, European (white)	*B. pendula alba*	Betulaceae	Cultivated ornamental	Mar.–May
Birch, paperback	*B. papyrifera*	Betulaceae	Lab. to AK, So. to NJ, WV, No. IN, N. E. IA, W. to MT, WA	Mar.–May
Birch, river (red)	*B. nigra*	Betulaceae	NH to FL, W. to So. OH, So. MI, S.E. MN, E. KS, and TX	Feb.–June
Birch, spring	*B. fontinalis*	Betulaceae	AK to CA, E. to Sask., ND, SD, Rocky Mt. States	Feb.–June
Birch, yellow	*B. lutea*	Betulaceae	Nfld. to Man., So. to DE, PA, No. OH	Spring
Bottlebrush	*Calistemon species*	Myrtaceae	Cultivated ornamental (subtropical)	All seasons
Box elder, ash–leaved (maple)	*Acer negundo*	Aceraceae	So. Canada, VT to FL, W. nearly to pacific coast Man.	Mar.–May
Butternut (white walnut)	*Juglans cinerea*	Juglandaceae	Cultivated ornamental and native tree, N.B. to Ont., No. MI, ND, So. to VA, CA, AR, KS	Apr.–May
Carob	*Ceratonia silitlua*	Leguminoseae	Cultivated ornamental	Late winter, early spring
Cedar, Atlantic	*Cedrus atlantica*	Pinaceae	Cultivated ornamental	Winter
Cedar, deodar	*C. deodara*	Pinaceae	Cultivated ornamental	Winter
Cedar, giant (canoe)	*Thuja plicata*	Cupressaceae	AK to C. CA, W. MT	Apr.–May
Cedar, incense	*Libocedrus decurrens*	Cupressaceae	CA to No. OR, W. to NV	Apr.–May
Cedar, Japanese	*Cryptomeria japonica*	Taxodiaceae	Cultivated ornamental	Spring
Cedar, Salt	*Tamarix gallica*	Tamaricaceae	Introduced, common in alkali western soils, along watercourses	Mar.–Aug.
Cherry	*Prunus cerasus*	Rosaceae	Cultivated crop and ornamental	Mar.–May
Chestnut, American	*Castanea dentata*	Fagaceae	Appalachia; rare; nearly exterminated by blight	Spring
Chestnut, horse	*Aesctilus hippocastanum*	Hippocastanaceae	Cultivated ornamental	May–June
Cottonwood, black	*Populus trichocarpa*	Salicaceae	So. CA to AK, IN, NV	Feb.–Apr.
Cottonwood (Carolina poplar)	*P. deltoides (includes P. sargentii)*	Salicaceae	P.Q. and New England to So. Man., MN, to eastern Rocky Mts., So. to FL and TX	Mar.–Apr.
Cottonwood, Fremont	*P. fremontii*	Salicaceae	C. and So. CA to NV, AZ	Mar.–Apr.

TREES THAT ARE A CAUSE OF HAY FEVER IN THE UNITED STATES AND CANADA *(continued)*

Common Name	Technical Name	Plant Family	Distribution	Pollination Season
Cypress, Arizona	*Cupressus arizonica*	Cuppressaceae	Native to AZ and E. NM; cultivated in CO and S.W.	Mar.–Apr.
Cypress, bald	*Taxodium distichum*	Taxodiaceae	DE to FL, W. to IL, MO, AR, and TX	Spring
Cypress, Italian	*Cupressus sempervirens*	Cupressaceae	Cultivated ornamental	Feb.–Mar.
Cypress, Monterey	*C. macrocapa*	Cupressaceae	Monterey peninsula	Spring
Elderberry	*Sambuctis glauca*	Sambucaceae	So. CA. to B.C., Alta., ID	June–Sept.
Elm, American (white elm)	*Ulnitis americana*	Ulmaceae	Nfld. to Man., So. to FL and TX, also cultivated	Feb.–Apr.
Elm, Chinese	*U. irvifolia*	Ulmaceae	Cultivated ornamental	Aug.–Sept.
Elm, fall-blooming (cedar elm)	*U. crassifolia*	Ulmaceae	MS to AR and TX	July–Oct.
Elm, Siberian (Chinese)	*Ulmus pumila*	Ulmaceae	Cultivated ornamental	Mar.–Apr.
Elm, slippery (red elm)	*U. fulva*	Ulmaceae	P.Q. and ME to ND, So. to FL and TX	Mar.–Apr.
Fir, Douglas	*Pseudotsuga menziesii*	Pinaceae	S.W. B.C. to C. CA, E. to S.W., Alta., MT, WY, CO, W. TX	Apr.–May
Fir, noble (red)	*Ables nobilis*	Pinaceae	Cascade Mts., WA, OR, CA	June–July
Fir, white	*A. concolor*	Pinaceae	W. WY, So. ID to NM, AZ, CA	May–June
Gum, blue	*Eucalyptus globulus*	Myrtaceae	Cultivated ornamental	Dec.–May
Gum, sweet	*Liquidambar styraciflua*	Altingiaceae	CT to So. OH, So. IL, OK, So. to FL, TX, cultivated ornamental	May
Hackberry	*Ceitis occidentalis*	Ulmaceae	P.Q. to Man., So. to NC, TN, AR	Spring
Hazelnut, America	*Corylus americana*	Corylaceaeto	ME to Sask., So. CA and OK	Jan.–Apr.
Hazelnut, beaked	*C. cornuta*	Corylaceae	Nfld. to B.C., So. to No. NJ, PA, OH, MO, No. CA, W. to No. CA, OR, WA	Jan.–Apr.
Hemlock, Canada (eastern)	*Tsuga canadensis*	Pinaceae	N.B. to Ont. and No. MN, So. to DE, WV, E. OH, C. MI, WI	May–June
Hemlock, western	*T. heterophylla*	Pinaceae	AK, to No. CA, to S.E. B.C., No. ID, to N.W. MT	May–June
Hickory, shagbark	*Carya ovata*	Juglandaceae	P.Q. and ME to MI and S.E. MN, S. FL and TX	May–June
Hickory, shellbark	*C. laciniosa*	Juglandaceae	NY. to So. Ont. to IA, So. to NC, MS, OK	May–June

TREES THAT ARE A CAUSE OF HAY FEVER IN THE UNITED STATES AND CANADA (continued)

Common Name	Technical Name	Plant Family	Distribution	Pollination Season
Hickory, white (mockernut)	C. tomentosa	Juglandaceae	MA. to Ont., MI, IA, So. to FL and TX	May–June
Hornbeam, American	Carpinus carolineana	Carpinaceae	N.S. to MN, So. to FL and TX	Mar.–May
Hornbeam, hop (ironwood)	Ostrya virginiana	Carpinaceae	N.S. to Man., So. to FL and TX	Mar.–Apr.
Juniper, California	Juniperus californica	Cupressaceae	C. and So. CA	Jan.–Mar.
Juniper, Chinese	J. chinensis	Cupressaceae	Cultivated ornamental	Winter–spring
Juniper, mountain	J. sabinoides	Cupressaceae	W. and So. TX into Mexico	Winter
Juniper, one-seed	J. monosperma	Cupressaceae	N.W. OK, W. TX to UT, NV, S.E. AZ, and NM	Spring
Juniper, Pinchot	J. pinchotii	Cupressaceae	C. TX. to S.E. NM, W. OK	Spring
Juniper, Rocky Mountain	J. scopulorum	Cupressaceae	So. B.C. to MT, ND, SD, Rocky Mt. states	May–June
Juniper, Utah	J. utahensis	Cupressaceae	CA. to S.W. ID, S.W. WY, W. NM	Spring
Juniper, Virginia (red cedar)	J. virginiana	Cupressaceae	So. P.Q. and ME to ND, So. to AL, TX	Mar.–Apr.
Juniper, western	J. occidentalis	Cupressaceae	Mountain slopes and higher. Prairies of E. WA, W. ID, So. in mt. ranges to So. CA	May–June
Larch (tamarack)	Larix occidentalis	Pinaceae	So. B.C., So. to E. Cascades to OR, E. to N.W. MT, N. ID	May–June
Linden American	Tilia americana	Tiliaceae	P.Q. to ND, So. to VA, NC, KY, MO	June–July
Locust, black	Robinia pseudoacacia	Leguminosae	PA to So. IN and OK, So. to GA, LA, cultivated ornamental	June
Maple, bigleaf (canyon, coast)	Acer macrophyllum	Aceraceae	CA to AK	Apr.–May
Maple, red	A. rubrum	Aceraceae	P.Q. to MN, So. to FL and TX	Mar.–Apr.
Maple, silver (soft map)	A. saccharinum	Aceraceae	N.B., P.Q. to MN, SD, So. to FL, TN, OK, cultivated ornamental	Mar.–Apr.
Maple, sugar	A. saccharum	Aceraceae	P.Q. and NJ to Man., ND, So. to NJ, GA, AL, TX	Apr.–May
Mesquite	Prosopis juliflora	Leguminosae	C. and So. CA to Gulf of Mexico	Apr.–June
Mock orange (syringa)	Philadelphus species	Philadelphaceae	Cultivated ornamentals and widespread native shrubs	May–June
Mulberry, black	Morus tatarica	Moraceae	Cultivated ornamental	Spring
Mulberry, paper	Broussonetia papyrifera	Moraceae	Cultivated ornamental	Winter–spring
Mulberry, red	Morus rubra	Moraceae	Cultivated ornamental	spring

TREES THAT ARE A CAUSE OF HAY FEVER IN THE UNITED STATES AND CANADA *(continued)*

Common Name	Technical Name	Plant Family	Distribution	Pollination Season
Mulberry, white	*M. alba*	Moraceae	Cultivated ornamental	Spring
Oak, Ariz. Scrub (canyon oak)	*Quercus chrysolepsis*	Fagaceae	So. CA to OR, NM	Apr.–May
Oak, Arizona (white)	*Q. arizonica*	Fagaceae	W. TX to AZ	Apr.–May
Oak, black	*Q.velutina*	Fagaceae	So. ME. to MI, MN, So. to FL and TX	Spring
Oak, black jack	*Q. marilandica*	Fagaceae	So. NY. to So. MI, IA, So. to FL and TX	Spring
Oak, Blue	*Q. douglasii*	Fagaceae	CA	Apr.–May
Oak, Bur	*Q. macrocarpa*	Fagaceae	N.B., P.Q. to Ont. and So. Man., So. to VA, AL, AR, TX. Shrub in W. MN and IA to Canada	Spring
Oak, California (Black)	*Q. kelloggii*	Fagaceae	So. CA to OR	Apr.–May
Oak, California scrub	*Q. dumosa*	Fagaceae	CA	Mar.–May
Oak, chestnut	*Q. prinus*	Fagaceae	Appalachian Mts., ME to No. CA to Atlantic coast as far as So. VA, W. to So. IN	Spring
Oak, coast live (Encina)[1]	*Q. agrifolia*	Fagaceae	C. and So. CA	Mar.–Apr.
Oak, Emory	*Q. emoryi*	Fagaceae	TX to AZ	Spring
Oak, Engelmann	*Q. engelmannii*	Fagaceae	So. CA	Apr.–May
Oak, Gambel	*Q. gambelii*	Fagaceae	So. W. TX to CO, WY, So. to AZ, abundant on dry slopes of Rockies	Spring
Oak, Garry1	*Q. garryana*	Fagaceae	No. CA, W. OR, WA	Spring
Oak, holly	*Q. ilex*	Fagaceae	Cultivated ornamental	Spring
Oak, interior live	*Q. wislizenii*	Fagaceae	C. and No. CA	Mar.–May
Oak, Palmer	*Q. palmeri*	Fagaceae	So. CA, AZ	Apr.–May
Oak, pin	*Q. palustris*	Fagaceae	MA to MI, IA, E. KS, So. to NC, TN, OK	Spring
Oak, post	*Q. stellata*	Fagaceae	S.E. MA, So. NY to IN, IA, So. to FL and TX	Spring
Oak, red (northern red oak)	*Q. rubra (Q. borealis)*	Fagaceae	N.S. to No. MI and MN, So. to VA, AL, MS, AR	Spring
Oak, Spanish (southern red oak)	*Q. falcata*	Fagaceae	NJ, PA to FL and TX, along coastal plain and No. in interior to OH, IN, MD	Spring
Oak valley (Roble)	*Q. lobata*	Fagaceae	C. and So. CA	Mar.–Apr.
Oak, Virginia live	*Q. virginiana*	Fagaceae	Coastal plain, S.E. VA to FL and TX	Spring

TREES THAT ARE A CAUSE OF HAY FEVER IN THE UNITED STATES AND CANADA *(continued)*

Common Name	Technical Name	Plant Family	Distribution	Pollination Season
Oak, water	*Q. nigra*	Fagaceae	Coastal plain, DE to FL and S.E. TX, No. in interior to S.E. MO	spring
Oak, white	*Q. alba*	Fagaceae	ME to MI and MN, So. to FL and TX	Spring
Olive	*Olea europaea*	Oleaceae	Cultivated crop and ornamental	Spring
Orange, Osage	*Maclura pomifera*	Moraceae	Cultivated hedge and native tree, AR, OK, TX	Apr.–May
Palm, Canary Island date	*Phoenix canariensis*	Palmae	Cultivated ornamental	Spring
Palm, date	*P. dactylifera*	Palmae	Cultivated crop and ornamental	Spring
Palm, dwarf	*Chamaerops humilus*	Palmae	Cultivated ornamental	Spring
Palm, queen	*Cocos plumosa*	Palmae	Cultivated ornamental	Spring
Palo Verde	*Cercidium torreyana*	Leguminosae	So. CA, AZ	Mar.–May
Peach	*Prunus persica*	Rosaceae	Cultivated crop and ornamental	Mar.–May
Pear	*Pyrus communis*	Rosaceae	Cultivated crop	Mar.–May
Pecan	*Carya pecan*	Juglandaceae	Cultivated crop and ornamental, S.W. OH to IA, So. to AL, TX	Spring
Peppertree, Brazilian	*Schinus terebinthifolius*	Anacardiaceae	Cultivated ornamental naturalized in So. FL	Jan.–Dec.
Peppertree, Peruvian	*So. molle*	Anacardiaceae	Cultivated ornamental	Winter
Pine, Australian (beefwood)	*Casuarina equisetifolia*	Causuarinaceae	Cultivated ornamental	Spring
Pine, bull (digger)	*Pinus sabiniana*	Pinaceae	C. and So. CA	Apr.–May
Pine, Canary Island	*P. canariensis*	Pinaceae	Cultivated ornamental	Spring
Pine, eastern white	*P. strobus*	Pinaceae	Nfld. to Man., So. to DE, GA, KY, IA	Spring
Pine, Japanese (black)	*P. thunbergii*	Pinaceae	Cultivated ornamental	Spring
Pine, loblolly	*P. taeda*	Pinaceae	NJ to FL, TX, No. in interior to AR and TN	Spring
Pine, lodgepole	*P. contorta*	Pinaceae	CA, AK, Rocky Mts.	June–July
Pine, longleaf	*P. palustris (P. australis)*	Pinaceae	Coastal plain, S.E. VA to FL and TX	Spring
Pine, Monterey	*P. radiata*	Pinaceae	Monterey peninsula and adjacent coastal counties	April
Pine, Pinyon	*P. edulis*	Pinaceae	So. CA to WY, TX, AZ	Spring

TREES THAT ARE A CAUSE OF HAY FEVER IN THE UNITED STATES AND CANADA *(continued)*

Common Name	Technical Name	Plant Family	Distribution	Pollination Season
Pine, ponderosa (west. yellow)	*P. ponderosa*	Pinaceae	So. CA to B.C., Rocky Mts.	May–June
Pine, red (Norway)	*P. resinosa*	Pinaceae	NS. to Man., So. MA, PA, MI, MN, in mts. to WV	Spring
Pine, short-leaf (yellow)	*P. echinata*	Pinaceae	So. NY to WV, So. IL, S.E. KS, So. to FL and TX	Spring
Pine, single-leaf (one-leaved)	*P. monophylla*	Pinaceae	C. and E. CA to UT, AZ	May
Pine, Virginia scrub (Jersey)	*P. virginiana*	Pinaceae	So. NY to So. IN, So. to GA, AL	Spring
Pine, western white	*P. monticola*	Pinaceae	So. B.C. to CA, W. NV, E. to ID, S.W. AK, W. MT	May–June
Plum	*Prunus domestica*	Rosaceae	Cultivated crop and ornamental	Mar.–May
Poplar, balsam	*Populus balsamifera*	Saliaceae	Lab. to AK, So. to CT, No. PA, No. IN, IA, N.B., OR	Mar.–Apr.
Poplar, black	*P. nigra*	Saliaceae	Cultivated ornamental	Mar.–Apr.
Poplar, Lombardy	*P. nigra italica*	Saliaceae	Cultivated ornamental	Mar.–Apr.
Poplar, white (silver)	*P. alba*	Saliaceae	Cultivated ornamental	Mar.–Apr.
Privet, California	*Ligustrum ovalifolium*	Oleaceae	Cultivated ornamental	Spring
Privet, common	*L. vulgare*	Oleaceae	Cultivated ornamental	Spring–summer
Privet, southern	*L. lucidum*	Oleaceae	Cultivated ornamental	Spring
Redwood	*Sequoia sempervirens*	Taxodiaceae	C. CA. to S.W. OR	Mar.
Silk tassel bush	*Garrya eliptica*	Garryaceae	C. CA to OR	Jan.–Mar.
Spiraea (bridal wreath)	*Spiraea species*	Rosaceae	Cultivated ornamentals and widespread native shrubs	Spring–summer
Spruce, Colorado blue	*Picea pungens*	Pinaceae	Cultivated ornamentals, native to C. CO	June–July
Spruce, red	*P. rubens*	Pinaceae	P.Q. and Ont. to PA, NJ, So. in mts. to NC and TN	Spring–summer
Spruce, Sitka	*P. sitchensis*	Pinaceae	AK to C. CA in coastal mts.	May
Sweet gale	*Myrica gale*	Myricaceae	Circumboreal, in North America, So. to NY, PA, NC, MI, MN, WA	Apr.–June
Sycamore (London Plane)	*Platanus orientalis*	Platanaceae	Cultivated ornamental	Spring
Sycamore, eastern (buttonwood)	*P. occidentalis*	Platanaceae	S.W. ME to So. MI and S.E. MN, So. to FL, TX	Spring

TREES THAT ARE A CAUSE OF HAY FEVER IN THE UNITED STATES AND CANADA (continued)

Common Name	Technical Name	Plant Family	Distribution	Pollination Season
Sycamore, mapleleaf	P. acerifolia	Platanaceae	Cultivated ornamental	Spring
Sycamore, western	P. racemosa	Platanaceae	C. and So. CA	Feb.–Apr.
Tree of heaven	Ailanthus altissima	Simaroubaceae	Cultivated ornamentals and urban weed	June
Viburnum	Viburnum	Caprifoliaceae	Cultivated ornamental, widespread native shrubs	May–July
Walnut, Arizona	Juglans rupestris	Juglandaceae	W. OK, TX to S.E. NM, AZ	Spring
Walnut, black	J. nigra	Juglandaceae	Cultivated crop, ornamental native W. New England to MI, MN, N.B., So. to FL, TX	Apr.–May
Walnut, California	J. californica	Juglandaceae	So. CA	Apr.–May
Walnut, English	J. regia	Juglandaceae	Cultivated crop	Apr.–May
Walnut, Hinds black	J. hindsii	Juglandaceae	C. and No. CA	Apr.–May
Walnut, Japanese	J. sieboldiana	Juglandaceae	Cultivated ornamental	Apr.–May
Willow, Arroyo	Salix lasiolepis	Salicaeae	CA to WA, ID, NM	Feb.–Apr.
Willow, black	So. nigra	Salicaeae	So. N.B. to C. MN, So. to FL, TX	Spring
Willow, pussy	So. discolor	Salicaeae	Cultivated ornamental, native shrub, Nfld. to B.C., So. to DE, KY, MO, SD, MT	Spring
Willow, red	So. laevigata	Salicaeae	CA, UT, AZ	Mar.–May
Willow, yellow	So. lasiandra	Salicaeae	CA to AK, ID	Mar.–May

[1]Pollen is a major source of hay fever.
Adapted from *Pollen Guide for Allergy,* Hollister-Stier.

trepopnea   Breathing that is easier when a person is in a certain position.

triage   A process usually during war, disaster, or other emergency in which patients are assessed for the severity of their illness or injury in order to save the most lives. The first priority treatment is given to patients whose airways are not functioning. The second priority is given to those who are bleeding and in shock, and third priority has been established for patients with possible nerve damage and injured bones and tissues.

triamcinolone (Aristocort, Azmacort, Kenacort)   A corticosteroid drug frequently used in the treatment of allergies and asthma.
   See also CORTICOSTEROIDS.

trigeminal cough   A reflex cough caused by irritation of the trigeminal nerve endings in the upper respiratory passages.

trigger, asthma   Any agent, substance, or condition that brings on asthma symptoms or an asthma attack.
   See also ASTHMA.

tripelennamine (Pyribenzamine or PBZ)   An antihistaminic drug of the ethylenediamine class. This drug is especially useful for the treatment of allergic disorders during pregnancy because of its long history of safe use. It has a mild sedative effect, but it may cause some gastrointestinal distress that can be minimized by taking the drug with food. Tripelennamine is available as a topical cream for the relief of itching, but it can be a cause of allergic rashes in some individuals, worsening the skin condition for which it is prescribed. Because of this adverse effect, it is rarely prescribed.

triprolidine (Actidil)   An antihistamine of the alkylamine class with mildly sedating properties. It is usually combined with pseudoephedrine in the proprietary product Actifed. This combination drug is widely used for the treatment of the nasal congestion of colds and hay fever.

troche   From the Greek word meaning a small wheel, a type of mildly medicated throat lozenge.

tube, endobronchial   Used in anesthesia, a tube with a double lumen. One lumen is inserted into a part of one lung for the purpose of aeration, while the other lumen is constricted so the other lung or part of it can deflate.

tube, endotracheal   See TRACHEOSTOMY.

tuberculin   From the Latin word *tuberculum,* meaning little swelling, a preparation of cells from the tubercle bacillus used in diagnostic testing to determine the presence of the disease tuberculosis. A solution called new tuberculin has been replaced by Tuberculin, USP. Old tuberculin refers to Koch's cultures of *Mycobacterium tuberculosis.* Purified Protein Derivative tuberculin is a preparation like old tuberculin but for a synthetic broth in which the *Mycobacterium tuberculosis* is cultured.
See also KOCH, ROBERT.

tuberculin tine test   A test in which the skin is pierced by an instrument with multiple sharp points, or tines, to which tuberculin has been applied. Redness or sign of inflammation occurring at the puncture site within two or three days after the skin is penetrated indicates the possible presence of tuberculosis in the individual.

tuberculofibrosis   Another term for interstitial pneumonia, a chronic lung inflammation from which fibrous tissue forms.
See also PNEUMONIA.

tuberculosis   A highly infectious, often life-threatening disease caused most frequently by the *Mycobacterium tuberculosis,* an airborne bacterium that has a history of causing illness from ancient times to epidemics in the recent past. However, tuberculosis (TB) has been and can be controlled or cured by antibiotics, including isoniazid (INH), pyrazinamide (PZA), rifampin (RMP), streptomycin, and ethambutol, and combinations of two or more of these. Depending upon the severity of the disease, surgery may be necessary to drain accumulated pus from the lungs or other infection site or to repair a spinal deformity that was caused by the disease. TB is characterized by pulmonary lesions, inflammation, tubercle formation, abscesses, fibrosis, calcification, and other processes that manifest as respiratory symptoms, particularly productive coughing. Sputum streaked with blood, difficulty breathing, a feeling of being unwell or fatigued, and cold night sweats may also appear.

TB is considered a threat to public health because it is extremely contagious and, more recently, because antibiotics that have long been used to treat the disease have become less effective due to the resistance of some tuberculosis-causing strains of bacteria. In 1995, nearly 23,000 cases of TB were reported in the United States, with 28 percent involving people age 65 and older. Others at high risk of contracting TB include persons of lower socioeconomic groups, immunosuppressed individuals (particularly those with AIDS), persons with chronic renal failure, diabetes mellitus, malignancies, silicosis, gastrectomy, and jejunoileal bypass, and infants who weigh 10 percent or more below the ideal weight. On May 6, 2001, *The New York Times* reported a serious tuberculosis epidemic in Russia, with one in every 1,000 Russians suffering from the disease. That is triple the rate of 10 years ago and approximately 15 times the rate in America.

"The threat is heightened by the size of Russia's prison population—at 963,000, one of the world's largest and a major incubator of the disease. In some prisons, as many as one-fifth of all TB cases are multidrug resistant," the article says.

TB may be contracted by inhaling indoor air containing tuberculosis bacteria. The bacteria may also be coughed or sneezed into the air by an infected person. An infant may be exposed through breathing infected droplets, and a fetus may breathe in or swallow infected amniotic fluid. People who live in crowded conditions or underdeveloped countries may also be at higher risk of contamination. Active tubercular infection typically begins in the lungs, but it may spread into the bloodstream and to other parts of the body (extrapulmonary tuberculosis). Often a person who is exposed to the TB bacterium will be able to ward off the disease through his or her immune system, which accounts for approximately 90 to 95 percent of all TB infections healing without causing active symptoms of the disease. Also, other diseases caused by mycobacteria similar to *Mycobacterium tuberculosis* can mimic tuberculosis, including lung and lymph node infections, and a persistent cough may be attributed erroneously to smoking or a bout with influenza.

Methods of diagnosis include a tuberculin skin test and a follow-up chest X ray if the skin test is positive. An abnormal chest X ray, which may be confused with other infections or the presence of cancer, may be followed by a laboratory sputum, chest fluid or tissue (biopsy) analysis to determine the presence of the tuberculosis bacterium, and a bronchoscopy to examine the bronchial tubes and obtain mucus samples. Spinal cord fluid may also be analyzed to diagnose tuberculous meningitis, which affects the brain and spinal cord. A polymerase chain reaction (PCR) test can reveal tuberculosis meningitis as well as tuberculosis in the kidneys. Samples of uterine, liver, and lymph node tissue and bone marrow may also be tested.

Preventive measures against TB include the prophylactic prescription of isoniazid, the use of a ger-micidal ultraviolet light in communal areas, tuberculin skin testing, and the BCG vaccine used in high-risk, developing countries.

See also MILIARY TUBERCULOSIS; TEST, TUBERCULIN.

tularemia Also called rabbit or deer fly fever, a bacterial infection caused by the organism *Francisella tularensis*. There are four types of tularemia: ulceroglandular, the most common and one that causes ulcers to form on the hands; oculoglandular, which affects the eyes; glandular, causing swelling of lymph nodes; and typhoidal, characterized by fever, abdominal pain, and exhaustion, and can lead to pneumonia. Although people become infected with tularemia from eating or touching infected animals or being bitten by ticks and insects infected by the animals, a June 6, 2001, article in the *Journal of the American Medical Association* cited the *F. tularensis* organism as one that can be inhaled and therefore used as a biological weapon. Person-to-person transmission does not occur, but the bacterium is highly infectious and has the potential to cause illness and death through environmental exposure. Treatment, usually with expectations of full recovery and subsequent immunity, includes antibiotics either injected or taken orally, and dressings and compresses for topical therapy. In cases involving severe headaches, analgesics may be prescribed.

See also BIOTERRORISM.

turkey raiser's disease Continuous exposure to an allergen in turkey droppings that may cause hypersensitivity pneumonitis, an allergic pneumonia-like lung disorder.

See also PNEUMONITIS.

turpentine poisoning The toxic effect of inhaling turpentine, characterized by symptoms including a burning sensation in the esophagus, vomiting, diarrhea, weak pulse and respiration, and urinary and neurological disturbances. Gastric lavage, increased fluid intake, and other measures may be necessary for treatment.

tussiculation A brief, dry cough.

Tussi-Organidin Mucolytic expectorant containing a mixture of several iodinated compounds formed by the reaction of iodine and glycerin. This prescription drug, also known as Iodur, Iotuss, Organidin, and Par-Glycerol, is frequently combined with the cough suppressants dextromethorphan or codeine. Iodine-containing preparations should be avoided during pregnancy, in nursing mothers, or in the newborn. These products should be avoided or used with caution in those individuals with thyroid disorders or who have experienced an adverse reaction to these or other iodine-containing foods or drugs in the past. Allergic or other adverse reactions include rashes, enlarged thyroid glands, and swelling of the parotid glands (acute parotitis).

tussis The medical term for cough. Tussis convulsiva refers to whooping cough, and tussis stomachalis is a reflex cough that results from an irritation of the mucosal stomach lining.

tylophora asthmatica An herb reported to have anti-inflammatory properties and long-term benefits in controlling asthma, particularly because it is thought to reduce congestion and mucus production.

typhoid fever, respiratory symptoms in Rapid respiratory rate, cough, and bronchial rales associated with typhoid fever and acute infectious disease. Typhoid fever is not considered a respiratory disorder per se, but certain symptoms resembling respiratory disease are present.

unconsciousness Insensibility characterized by the inability to swallow, nonreactive eyes, and generally a sleeplike state, possibly caused by lack of oxygen, alcohol or drug intoxication, carbon monoxide poisoning, brain tumor, cerebral hemorrhage or thrombosis, cardiac decompensation, meningitis, pneumonia, uremia, subdural hematoma, diabetes, epilepsy, fear, fright, heat stroke, and a number of other problems. Also known as twilight sleep, coma, shock, stroke, stupor, asphyxia, and apoplexy, unconsciousness may be treated by artificial respiration or cardiopulmonary resuscitation.

See also CARDIOPULMONARY RESUSCITATION.

upper airway obstruction A blockage in the main bronchus, larynx, mouth, or nose that prevents breathing.

upper respiratory infection An invasion of disease-causing microorganisms in the nose, throat, and bronchi.

uvulopalatopharyngoplasty A surgical procedure in which the soft palate, uvula, pillars, fauces, and a certain portion of pharyngeal mucosa are removed in order to prevent intractable snoring, sleep apnea, and other sleep disorders.

vaccine Inoculation with bacteria, bacterial products, or viral products in order to immunize, or protect, an individual against a certain disease.

vacuum cleaners for allergic patients Dust- and dirt-collecting devices with double bags, which offer protection to allergic persons. The ordinary-type vacuum cleaners allow small suspended particles containing most collected allergens to pass through the collection bag back into the surrounding air. An allergic person should avoid a recently vacuumed room for an hour or two following vacuuming. If possible, have a nonallergic person do the vacuuming. An alternative is for the allergic individual to wear a mask capable of trapping small particles.

Vacuum cleaners with elaborate special HEPA, or water-filtering, devices may not be more efficient than ordinary vacuums. However, vacuums with double bags may be the most effective. When possible, such as when planning a new home, install a central vacuum system with motor and collection bag in the garage.

valley fever See COCCIDIOMYCOSIS.

valve, pulmonary A membrane that separates the pulmonary artery and the right ventricle of the heart.

Vanceril inhaler See BECLOMETHASONE.

vaporizers See HUMIDIFIERS.

vasoconstrictor Any substance that can cause constriction, or narrowing, of blood vessels.

vasodilator Any substance that dilates or increases the circumference of blood vessels.

vasomotor rhinitis Nasal congestion that cannot be attributed to any other cause, such as allergic rhinitis (hay fever) or upper respiratory infections (colds, sinusitis). Vasomotor rhinitis is thought to be caused by excessive stimulation of certain nerve endings in the nose for unknown reasons.

Nasal congestion, often accompanied by large amounts of clear watery mucus, does not respond to antihistamines or allergy nasal sprays containing the drugs cromolyn or corticosteroids. Alpha-agonist (decongestant) drugs, such as pseudoephedrine (Sudafed) orally or topical nasal sprays, are sometimes helpful. Abuse of over-the-counter nasal sprays may cause a rebound effect. The worsening of nasal congestion caused by the overuse of drugs is called rhinitis medicamentosa. Treatment with oral or topical (nasal sprays or drops) decongestant drugs and anticholinergic drugs such as atropine and ipratropium may be effective. However, antihistamines are not effective, and anti-inflammatory corticosteroid nasal sprays are occasionally helpful.

vent, alveolar Opening between adjacent alveoli, or air sacs, in the lungs.

ventilation From the Latin word *ventilare*, meaning to air, the air circulation in a room, the amount of air inhaled on a daily basis, and the oxygenation of the bloodstream. Ventilation is the act of drawing air into and expressing air out of the body through the respiratory system in order to oxygenate the blood. It also refers to heating and cooling systems in buildings. Artificial ventilation is another term for respirator. Pulmonary ventilation refers to the inhalation and exhalation of air from the lungs. Continuous positive-pressure ventilation refers to a mechanical device that administers oxygen or air to the lungs with continuous pressure; intermittent positive-pressure ventilation is a mechanical method that assists pulmonary ventilation by inflating the lungs under positive pressure. High frequency jet ventilation provides respiration in the case of respiratory failure. This continuous ventilation is administered at 100 to 150 breathing cycles per minute.

A ventilation coefficient refers to the amount of air that must be taken in for every liter of oxygen to be absorbed into the blood.

ventilation rate   The amount of air breathed during the course of one minute.

ventilator   A device that provides artificial respiration either by hand or machine.

Ventolin   See ALBUTEROL.

ventricle of larynx   Space between the true and the false vocal cords.

Venturi mask   Named after Giovanni Battista Venturi, an Italian scientist (1746–1822), a device placed over the nose and mouth that administers a controlled dose of oxygen to an individual.

vestibule of nose, mouth, and larynx   The front part of the nostrils, the part of the mouth between the lips, cheeks, gums and teeth, and the part of the larynx above the vocal cords. A vestibule is a tiny space at the front or the beginning of a structure.

vicarious respiration   The increase of activity in a lung that makes an effort to compensate for the other lung that may be injured or diseased.

viruses   From the Latin word for poison, organisms that can produce disease in the host in which they thrive. There are hundreds of viruses (300 or more isolated from animals). Although some appear to be harmless to people, many viruses cause diseases including influenza, AIDS, the common cold, smallpox, yellow fever, certain lymphomas, leukemias and other forms of cancer, poliomyelitis, communicable childhood diseases such as chickenpox, and most upper respiratory infections. The respiratory syncytial virus causes many of the lower respiratory diseases in infants and young children. Some antiviral drugs have been developed, and certain viruses are susceptible to preventive vaccines.

See also BIOTERRORISM.

vital capacity   The volume of air that can be exhaled following a full inspiration. The timed vital capacity is the volume of air that can be forcibly exhaled in a given time. In asthma patients this important value is often expressed as the forced expiratory volume in one second, or FEV_1. The FEV_1 is considered by most physicians to be the most important guide to the severity of an asthma attack.

See also SPIROMETRY.

vital signs   Body temperature, pulse, and number of respirations as measured or counted per minute.

vocal cords   The pair of thin membranes in the larynx that vibrate when air passes between them. This creates our ability to make sounds, speak, and sing.

Vollmax   Brand of sustained-release albuterol.
See also ALBUTEROL.

volume, expiratory reserve   The largest amount of air that can be forced out of the lungs after normal breathing out, or exhaling.

volume, inspiratory reserve   The largest amount of air that can be forced out of the lungs after normal breathing in.

volume, residual   The amount of air remaining in the lungs after exhalation.

volume, tidal The amount of air inhaled and exhaled in a normal breathing cycle.

vomer From the Latin word for plowshare, the bone reminiscent of a plow at the lower back of the nasal septum. The vomer connects with the two palate bones, the ethmoid, sphenoid, and two upper maxillary bones.

von Pirquet's test See QUANTI-PIRQUET.

war gases Any type of chemical substance used deliberately to inflict irritation or to poison.

See also BIOTERRORISM.

weed pollen allergy Hay fever caused by exposure to the windblown, or anemophilous, pollen of plants that grow wild. Weeds often grow in areas despite minimal nutrition and water and tend to choke out more attractive plants. Most weeds are considered of little or no value and a nuisance. However, notable exceptions include the crops alfalfa, beets, castor bean, hemp, hops, sunflower, and ornamental plants such as roses and tulips. Various species of ragweed are the most important producers of allergy-causing weed pollen.

See also RAGWEED.

WEEDS THAT ARE A CAUSE OF HAY FEVER IN THE UNITED STATES AND CANADA

Common Name	Technical Name	Plant Family	Distribution	Pollination Season
Alfalfa	*Medicago sativa*	Leguminosae	Cultivated crop	May–Oct.
Allscale[1]	*Atriplex polycarps*	Chenopodiaceae	Colorado and Mojave Desert, alkali flats of C. CA, So. NV, UT and AZ	July–Oct.
Aster	*Aster* species	Compositae	Cultivated ornamentals and native weeds	Fall
Balsamroot	*Balsamorrhiza sagittata*	Compositae	So. B.C. to So. CA, E. to MT, SD, CO	Apr.–July
Bassia	*Bassia hyssopifolia*	Chenopodiaceae	B.C. to CA, E. to MT, ID, NV, spreading elsewhere	July–Oct.
Beachbur	*Franseria bipinnatifidia*	Compositae	Coastal beaches and dunes B.C. to So. CA	Mar.–Sept.
Beachbur, San Francisco	*F. chamissonis*	Compositae	Coastal beaches and dunes B.C. to So. CA	July–Sept.
Beet	*Beta vulgaris*	Chenopodiaceae	Cultivated crop (sugar and red) established locally in So. U.S.	July–Oct.
Bractscale[1]	*Atriplex bracteosa*	Chenopodiaceae	C. and So. CA, E. to NM, TX	July–Nov.
Brewers scale[1]	*A. breweri*	Chenopodiaceae	C. and So. CA	July–Oct.
Brittle bush (incienso)	*Encelia farinosa*	Compositae	C. and So. CA, to S.W. UT, AZ	Mar.–May
Broom, Scotch	*Cystisus scoparius*	Leguminosae	Naturalized, CA, No. to WA, B.C.	Apr.–June

WEEDS THAT ARE A CAUSE OF HAY FEVER IN THE UNITED STATES AND CANADA (*continued*)

Common Name	Technical Name	Plant Family	Distribution	Pollination Season
Broomweed	*Gutierrezia dracunculoides*	Compositae	C. TX and OK	July–Oct.
Bulrush	*Scirpus microcorpus*	Cyperaceae	So. CA, No. to AK, Rocky Mts., NM	May–Aug.
Burrobrush[1]	*Hymenoclea monogyra*	Compositae	So. CO E. to TX	Aug.–Nov.
Burrobrush[1]	*H. salsola*	Compositae	So. CA, NV, S. UT, AZ	Mar.–June
Canaigre (wild rhubarb)	*Rumex hymenosepalus*	Polygonaceae	C. and So. CA, WY, W. TX	Jan.–May
Carelessweed[1]	*Amaranthus palmeri*	Amaranthaceae	So. CA, E. to C. U.S.	Aug.–Nov.
Castor bean[1]	*Ricinus communis*	Euphorbiaceae	Cultivated ornamental, established in So. U.S.	Jan.–Dec.
Cattail, broad-leaf	*Typha latifolia*	Typhaceae	Widespread weed	June–Aug.
Cattail, narrow-leaf	*T. angtistifolia*	Typhaceae	Widespread weed	June–Aug.
Chamise (greasewood)	*Adenostoma fasciculatum*	Rosaceae	Common component of California chaparral	May–June
Clover, red	*Trifolium pratense*	Leguminosae	Cultivated hay crop	June–Aug.
Clover, sweet	*Melilotus* species	Leguminosae	Cultivated hay crop, widespread weed	May–Nov.
Clover, white	*Trifolium repens*	Leguminosae	Cultivated lawn plant	Apr.–Sept.
Cocklebur, common[1]	*Xanthium strumarium*	Compositae	Widespread weed	Aug.–Oct.
Cocklebur, spiny	*X. spinosum*	Compositae	Widespread weed in warm and temperate regions	July–Oct.
Daisy, ox-eye	*Chrysanthemum leucantheum*	Compositae	Widespread weed, cultivated as Shasta daisy	June–Aug.
Dandelion officinale	*Taraxacum*	Compositae	Widespread weed	Jan.–Dec.
Dock, bitter[1]	*Rumex obtrusifolis*	Polygonaceae	Widespread weed	June–Dec.
Dock, green[1]	*R. conglomeratus*	Polygonaceae	Widespread weed	Apr.–Oct.
Dock, white[1]	*R. mexicanus*	Polygonaceae	Widespread weed	June–Sept.
Dock, yellow (curly dock)[1]	*R. crispis*	Polygonaceae	Widespread weed	May–Oct.
Dog fennel (mayweed)	*Anthemis cotula*	Compositae	Widespread weed	June–Oct.
Fern, bracken	*Pterdium aquilinum*	Dennstaedtiaceae	Widespread weed	June–Aug.
Fern, royal	*Osmunda regalis*	Osmundaceae	Widespread weed	Summer

WEEDS THAT ARE A CAUSE OF HAY FEVER IN THE UNITED STATES AND CANADA *(continued)*

Common Name	Technical Name	Plant Family	Distribution	Pollination Season
Fern, sword Christmas fern	*Polystichum munitum*	Polypodiaceae	AK to So. CA, to ID and MT	Summer
Firebush, Mex. (smr. cypress)[1]	*Kochia scoparia*	Chenopodiaceae	Widespread weed	Aug.–Oct.
Fireweed	*Epilobrium angustifolium*	Onagraceae	Widespread weed	July–Sept.
Goldenrod	*Solidago* species	Compositae	Widespread weed	May–Oct.
Goosefoot, Lamb's-quarter[1]	*Chenopodium album*	Chenopodiaceae	Widespread weed	June–Oct.
Goosefoot, nettle-leaf	*Chenopodium murale*	Chenopodiaceae	Widespread weed	Most of year, esp. spring
Greasewood	*Sarcobatus vermiculatus*	Chenopodiaceae	So. CO to E. WA, Alta., ND, TX	May–Aug.
Hemp	*Cannabis sativa*	Cannabidaceae	Cultivated crop and widespread weed, diminishing	July–Sept.
Hops, cultivated	*Humulus lupulus*	Cannabidaceae	Cultivated crop	Summer
Hop-sage	*Grayia spinosa*	Chenopodiaceae	CA to E. WA, WY, AZ	Mar.–June
Iodine bush	*Allenrolfea occidentalis*	Chenopodiaceae	CA to OR, UT	June–Aug.
Jerusalem oak	*Chenopodium botrys*	Chenopodiaceae	Widespread weed	June–Oct.
Lenscale[1]	*Atriplex lentiformis*	Chenopodiaceae	So. and C. CA, to UT	Aug.–Oct.
Marshelder, August	*Iva augustifolia*	Compositae	AR, OK, TX, LA	Late summer–fall
Marshelder, rough (poverty weed)[1]	*I. ciliata*	Compositae	IL to LA, W. to N.B., NM	Late spring–summer
Mugwort[1]	*Artemisia douglasiana*	Compositae	CA E. to W. NV, to WA, ID	June–Oct.
Mugwort[1]	*A. heterophylla*	Compositae	CA. E. to W. NV, to WA, ID	June–Oct.
Mustard (Black)	*Brassica nigra*	Cruciferae	Widespread weed	Apr.–July
Mustard	*B. campestris*	Cruciferae	Widespread weed, esp. in CA	Jan.–May
Nettle	*Urtica dioica*	Urticaceae	Widespread weed	July–Sept.
Pea, sweet	*Lathyrus odoratus*	Leguminosae	Cultivated ornamental	Jan.–Dec.
Phlox	*Phlox* species	Polemoniaceae	Cultivated ornamental	Spring–summer
Pickleweed (glasswort)	*Salicornia ambigua*	Chenopodiaceae	Atlantic and Pacific coastal, salt marshes and adjacent salt flats	Aug.–Nov.
Pigweed, green	*Amaranthus hybridus*	Amaranthaceae	Widespread weed	June–Nov.

WEEDS THAT ARE A CAUSE OF HAY FEVER IN THE UNITED STATES AND CANADA *(continued)*

Common Name	Technical Name	Plant Family	Distribution	Pollination Season
Pigweed, redroot[1]	A. retroflex	Amaranthaceae	Widespread weed	June–Nov.
Pigweed, spiny	A. spinosus	Amaranthaceae	Advancing weed	June–Sept.
Pigweed, spreading	A. blitoides	Amaranthaceae	Widespread weed	July–Nov.
Plantain, common	*Plantago major*	Plantaginaceae	Widespread weed	Jan.–Dec.
Plantain, English (buck-horn)[1]	*P. lanceolata*	Plantaginaceae	Widespread weed	June–Sept.
Poppy, California	*Escholzia californica*	Papaveraceae	CA, cultivated ornamental elsewhere	Feb.–Sept.
Povertyweed, giant	*Iva xanthifolia*	Compositae	P.Q. to Alta., So. to DC, OH, MD, TX, NM, AZ	July–Sept.
Povertyweed, small	*I. axilaris*	Compositae	CA to No.B., Canada	May–Sept.
Rabbitbrush	*Chrysothamnus nauseosus*	Compositae	E. CA, No. to B.C., E. to Sask., TX	July–Oct.
Rabbitbrush[1]	*Franseria deltoides*	Compositae	So. AZ and Mexico	Spring
Ragweed, canyon[1]	*F. ambrosiodes*	Compositae	So. CA, So. AZ	Mar.–June
Ragweed, desert (burroweed)[1]	*F. dumosa*	Compositae	So. CA, S.W. UT, AZ	Mar.–May
Ragweed, false (Sandbur)[1]	*F. acanthicarpa*	Compositae	C. and So. CA to WA, Sask., TX, advancing eastward	Aug.–Nov.
Ragweed, giant (crownweed)[1]	*Ambrosia trifida*	Compositae	So. Canada and U.S. to Rocky Mts.	July–Sept.
Ragweed, short[1]	*A. artemisifolia*	Compositae	So. Canada and U.S., except W. and S.W. U.S.	Aug.–Oct.
Ragweed, silver[1]	*Dicoria canescens*	Compositae	So. CA, S.W. AZ, NV, S.W. UT	Sept.–Jan.
Ragweed, slender[1]	*Franseria tenuifolia*	Compositae	C. and So. CA, to KS, TX	May–Nov.
Ragweed, southern[1]	*Ambrosia bidentata*	Compositae	So. IL, to LA, W. to N.B. and TX	Aug.–Sept.
Ragweed, western[1]	*A. psilostachya*	Compositae	CA to WA, Sask., IL	July–Nov.
Redscale	*Atriplex rosea*	Chenopodiaceae	CA to WA, Atlantic coast	July–Oct.
Rose	*Rosa species*	Rosaceae	Cultivated ornamentals and native shrubs	Jan.–Dec.
Sagebrush, annual	*Artemisia annua*	Compositae	Widespread weed	July–Sept.

WEEDS THAT ARE A CAUSE OF HAY FEVER IN THE UNITED STATES AND CANADA (continued)

Common Name	Technical Name	Plant Family	Distribution	Pollination Season
Sagebrush, biennial	A. biennis	Compositae	Widespread weed	Aug.–Sept.
Sagebrush, California[1]	A. californica	Compositae	Coastal C., and So. CA	Aug.–Dec.
Sagebrush, carpet (pasture)[1]	A. frigida	Compositae	Some forms cultivated annuals	July–Sept.
Sagebrush, common (giant)[1]	A. tridentata	Compositae	So. CA to B.C., Rocky Mts.	Aug.–Oct.
Sagebrush, prairie[1]	A. ludoviciana	Compositae	CA to WA, Alta., Ont., AR, NM	July–Sept.
Sagebrush, sand dune	A. ludoviciana	Compositae	Coastal C. CA, and OR	June–Aug.
Sagebrush, Sukasdorf	A. pycnocephala	Compositae	Coastal N. CA to Vancouver Island	May–Aug.
Saltbush, annual	A. suksdorfii	Chenopodiaceae	So. AZ and So. NM	July–Sept.
Sea blite (seepweed)	Suaeda moquini	Chenopodiaceae	So. CA to Alta.	July–Oct.
Sea blite (seepweed)	S. californica	Chenopodiaceae	Coastal salt marsh, San Francisco Bay to So. CA	July–Oct.
Sea blite (seepweed)	S. suffrutescens	Chenopodiaceae	C. CA to WA, Rocky Mts.	July–Sept.
Sedge	Carex species	Cyperaceae	Widespread, largest genus of flowering plants in North America	Spring–summer
Shadscale (sheep fat)	Atriplex conifertifolia	Chenopodiaceae	So. CA to E. OR, ND	Apr.–July
Sheep sorrel[1]	Romex acetosella	Polygonaceae	Widespread weed	Mar.–Aug.
Silverscale	Atriplex argentea	Chenopodiaceae	So. CA to B.C., ND, NM	June–Sept.
Snapdragon	Antirrhinum majus	Scrophulariaceae	Cultivated crop	Jan.–Dec.
Spearscale	Atriplex patula	Chenopodiaceae	Widespread weed	June–Nov.
Sunflower	Helianthus species	Compositae	Cultivated crop, ornamental, native So. Canada to Mexican border	Feb.–Oct.
Tansy	Tanacetum vulgare	Compositae	Cultivated ornamental, naturalized weed	July–Sept.
Tarragon (green sagebrush)	Artemisia dracunculus	Compositae	C. and So. CA, N. to B.C., WI, TX, cultivated form sterile	Aug.–Oct.
Tarweed	Hemizonia species	Compositae	30 species, all in CA	Apr.–Nov.
Tea, Mexican (wormseed)	Chenopdium ambrosiodes	Chenopodiaceae	Widespread weed	June–Dec.
Thistle, Russian[1]	Salsola kali	Chenopodiaceae	Widespread weed	July–Oct.
Tulip	Tulipa species	Liliaceae	Cultivated ornamentals	Spring

WEEDS THAT ARE A CAUSE OF HAY FEVER IN THE UNITED STATES AND CANADA *(continued)*

Common Name	Technical Name	Plant Family	Distribution	Pollination Season
Water hemp[1]	*Acnida tamariscina*	Amaranthaceae	E. TX, No. to So. OK, E. to IN	Aug.–Sept.
Wingscale, (shadescale)[1]	*Atriplex canescens*	Chenopodiaceae	C. and So. CA to E. WA, SD, KS, TX	June–Aug.
Winter fat	*Eurotia lanata*	Chenopodiaceae	C. and So. CO, WA, Rocky Mts., TX	Mar.–June
Wormwood	*Artemisia absinthium*	Compositae	Cultivated ornamental, naturalized weed	July–Sept.

[1]Pollen is a major source of hay fever.
Adopted from *Pollen Guide for Allergy*, Hollister-Stier.

wheeze A breathing difficulty characterized by a high-pitched whistling or moaning sound produced when a lumen, or the space, of a respiratory passage narrows, such as in the case of asthma, hay fever, croup, or pleural effusion. Wheezing may be caused by a bronchial spasm, tumor, obstruction by a foreign body, edema, obstructive emphysema, or tuberculosis. Wheezing may be offensively loud or audible only through a stethoscope in the case of asthma, bronchitis, pulmonary edema, a foreign object inhaled into an airway, and other respiratory disorders.

whiff A brief inhalation or exhalation, or puff of air that may carry a particular odor, such as that of tobacco smoke.

whooping cough A respiratory infection caused by *Bordetella pertussis* that is characterized by coughing spasms that end with a high-pitched whooping sound. Also known as pertussis, whooping cough is extremely contagious and is considered a major disease in the world, although in the United States, where there had been epidemics, there is now a routine, combined immunization called DTP, or diphtheria-tetanus-pertussis, for infants and children.

Pertussis is spread through droplets of moisture from an infected person's cough. Symptoms start approximately seven to 10 days after exposure, when the bacteria attack the throat lining, trachea, and other airways and increase the production of mucus. The three stages of whooping cough, which usually lasts six weeks, are the catarrhal stage, with mild symptoms similar to a cold; the paroxysmal stage, with severe coughing; and the convalescent stage, when the patient begins to recover. It may be easy to confuse the catarrhal stage of whooping cough with symptoms of bronchitis, influenza, and other viral infections, or the onset of tuberculosis. A nose and throat culture determines the presence of the pertussis bacteria most of the time. If a child develops pneumonia secondary to a pertussis infection, pneumothorax (collapse of the lung), difficulty breathing or apnea, and other complications may be fatal. Other complications of pertussis include vomiting, choking spells, otitis media, bleeding or swelling of the brain, paralysis, rectal prolapse, convulsions, and certain neurological problems.

Whooping cough is often transmitted to young children by infected older children and adults with only mild symptoms. Treatment may consist of oxygen therapy, suctioning of mucus from the throat, intravenous fluids, and antibiotic therapy, particularly erythromycin.

Wilson-Mikity syndrome Named for American pediatrician Miriam G. Wilson (b. 1922) and American radiologist Victor G. Mikity (b. 1919), a pulmonary syndrome seen in premature babies. Symptoms include difficulty breathing, rapid breathing, and cyanosis during the infant's first month of life. Known as a dysmaturity syndrome, Wilson-Mikity is also characterized by evidence of emphysema, pulmonary insufficiency, and heart failure, and approximately 25 percent of the victims die from the disease.

windpipe A layman's term for the trachea, a tube through which inhaled air goes from the larynx (voice box or vocal cords) into the lungs. The end of the trachea branches into two bronchi, each one connected to a lung. Trachealgia refers to pain in the windpipe. Tracheitis is an inflammation of the trachea that may be a symptom of bronchitis or laryngitis. A tracheostomy is the surgical creation of an opening into the trachea to relieve airway obstruction.

A tracheal tickle refers to a technique to induce a reflex cough. Tracheal tugging means a pulling down of the trachea or laryngeal pulsation associated with thoracic aneurysm.

wood- and coal-burning stoves Home heating alternatives that may be excellent sources of inexpensive fuel. More than 11 million wood-burning stoves are in use in the United States since the energy crisis of the 1970s caused a significant increase in home heating costs. Wood stoves should have a catalytic converter to burn off smoke produced by burning wood. Do not store wood in the home. Always keep the doors to stoves or fireplaces closed. Once the fire has been started, use only hard wood. Soft pine, poplars, twigs, or unseasoned wood should be avoided. Coal stoves may be safe but only if they are airtight. Poorly ventilated coal stoves may result in unsafe levels of carbon monoxide, nitrogen and sulfur dioxides, formaldehyde, and benzopyrene in the home. Kerosene heaters produce unpleasant fumes that can trigger asthma.

woolsorter's disease A type of anthrax, caused by *Bacillus anthracis,* that affects the lungs of indi-viduals who handle contaminated wool and wool products. A highly contagious disease, anthrax may be life-threatening. Woolsorter's anthrax usually is the result of inhaling spores of the bacterium, which multiply in lymph nodes and spread to the lungs. When lymph nodes begin to deteriorate and bleed, the bacterium travels throughout the thorax, creating flulike symptoms, breathing difficulty, shock, coma, meningoencephalitis, and death.

Anyone who works in textile mills that process wool, veterinarians, laboratory technicians, animal workers, certain military personnel, and others at high risk of contracting pulmonary anthrax should be vaccinated. Treatment for the infection includes intravenous penicillin, antibiotics, and corticosteroids. In the 1950s, an anthrax vaccine was developed for humans and licensed by the FDA in the 1970s.

According to the U.S. Department of Defense Anthrax Vaccine Immunization Program, the vaccine manufactured by the BioPort Corporation, of Lansing, Michigan, is safely and routinely administered to people at risk, but it is not available to the general public and the supply is limited. Developed over a four-year period from 1951 to 1955, the vaccine helps the immune system prevent the anthrax bacteria from growing and leading to complications and death from anthrax. Dr. G. G. Wright and associates of the U.S. Army Chemical Corps, of Fort Detrick, Maryland, reported on the development of the vaccine that was produced by growth of the R1-NP (a non-encapsulated, nonproteolytic mutant of a Vollum strain of *B. anthracis*).

The original study showed 92.5 percent fewer cutaneous and inhaled anthrax cases among vaccinated people compared to unvaccinated people.

For more information on the vaccine, you may log on to www.anthrax.osd.mil, or call the U.S. Department of Defense Anthrax Vaccine Immunization Agency at 1-877-GETVACC.

See also ANTHRAX.

xeromycteria From the Greek words *xero,* or dry, and *mycter,* or nose, the medical term for dry nasal passages.

X ray, chest A diagnostic test using a high-energy electromagnetic wave, or X ray, to determine the health or disease of the thoracic cavity and the organs therein. Chest X rays are commonly performed when lung cancer or various forms of pneumonia and tuberculosis are suspected.

yawn The involuntary opening of the mouth followed by a deep breath, ordinarily a sign of fatigue or boredom. Observing a person who yawns may induce yawning, also known as oscitation.

yoga The Hindu philosophy embracing various methods of mental and physical exercise that renders one capable of lowering blood pressure and heart rate and suppressing other bodily functions in order to achieve a state of total relaxation. Yoga techniques, including meditation, stretching, and breathing, may have a positive outcome for asthmatics, according to P. K. Vedanthan, M.D., a Fort Collins, Colorado, allergist. Vedanthan conducted a 12-week study of patients with mild asthma whose lung function, exercise tolerance, relaxation levels, and attitude improved significantly with the practice of yoga three times a week. The patients also required less asthma medication, especially adrenergic inhalers, whereas other similar patients who did not practice yoga required the same or increased medication.

Z

Zafirlukast (Accolate) Leukotriene-receptor antagonist, or drug that blocks the effects of leukotriene D_4, a substance produced in certain cells of the immune system. Leukotrienes contribute to inflammation and obstruction in the airways of asthma patients.

See also LEUKOTRIENE.

Ziehl-Neelsen method Named for Franz Ziehl, a German bacteriologist (1857–1926), and German pathologist Friedrich Karl Adolf Neelsen (1854–94), a microbiological test to determine the presence of *Mycobacterium tuberculosis*. The two scientists used carbolfuchsin, a solution that stays on the organism after it is rinsed with acid alcohol, to stain the organism in order to identify it.

Zileuton (Zyflo) Leukotriene inhibitor—a drug that prevents the action of 5-lipoxygenase, an enzyme that causes inflammation in the airways of asthmatic patients. Although Zyflo is not effective for acute attacks of asthma, it may add to the beneficial effects of inhaled corticosteroids in the prevention of asthma symptoms. Another leukotriene inhibitor, Zileutron (Leutrol), may cause changes in liver functioning and periodic liver function tests are advised. In addition, individuals with liver disease, alcohol abuse problems, or those who are taking theophylline, warfarin, or terfenadine increase their risk of complications when taking Zileutron, which is metabolized in the liver.

See also LEUKOTRIENES.

Zileutron (Leutrol) See ZILEUTON.

Zithromax Brand of azithromycin, an antibacterial drug used to treat mild to moderate infections of the upper and lower respiratory tracts caused by the influenza, pneumonia, and other microorganisms.

zygomycosis Another term for mucormycosis, a disease caused by the family of fungi known as Mucoraceae (class Zygomycetes) that usually causes thrombosis and infarction of blood vessels. Persons with diabetes mellitus who contract the disease may suffer paranasal sinus infections that may be mistaken initially for an allergic condition. The pulmonary form of this rare disease, characterized by lung infarctions, is the result of inhaling the fungus. Treatment includes prevention of diabetic acidosis, amphotericin B, and surgical repair.

Zyrtec Brand name for the antihistamine cetirizine, which is used to treat allergic rhinitis and other allergy symptoms. Cetirizine is an H_1-histamine antagonist.

APPENDIXES

APPENDIX I

PROGRESS REPORT OF THE AMERICAN LUNG ASSOCIATION, 2000

In 1996, The American Lung Association's Board of Directors voted to fund three National Asthma Research Centers, as the first step in an intensive search for the causes of asthma and ultimately for a means of prevention and cure. This joint effort of the ALA and the American Thoracic Society was named Asthmattack!, reflecting the urgent need to turn around the alarming increase in asthma's prevalence and the rising number of deaths for which it is responsible. Since the inception of Asthmattack!, the three research centers have focussed on putting the essential building blocks of knowledge in place that will lead to better ways of treating asthma, and one day to a cure.

"Basic research in the laboratory is the first step on the road to overcoming asthma," says Spencer Koerner, M.D., an ALA board member and former chairman of the Research Coordinating Committee. "Sometimes it's difficult to grasp just how scientists studying cells in test tubes are going to lead us to new asthma treatments, but in every area of medicine it's been proven time and again that basic research is the only route to success at the patient's bedside."

Scientific research is a painstaking process of linking together many studies and experiments, not a single, amazing discovery made in a vacuum. The journey to a cure is a long one, requiring collaboration among many different kinds of specialists to arrive at the final destination. "The history of medical advances abounds with examples of how basic research leads to the knowledge that allows clinicians to heal patients, sometimes by what may seem to be an indirect route," Dr. Koerner points out.

Asthma is no exception, and this year, Asthmattack! has begun a new phase, with the establishment of Asthma Clinical Research Centers around the country to conduct clinical research on large groups of patients.

Meanwhile, work continues, thanks to the wisdom and commitment of those who recognize that steady progress is leading us to the day when asthma will no longer take its toll on millions of Americans of all ages.

The first two Asthma Research Centers were initially funded in the summer of 1996. One is based at The National Jewish Medical and Research Center in Denver, Colorado, with Dr. Richard J. Martin as Principal Investigator. Dr. Martin is head of the Pulmonary Division at his institution, as well as Vice Chair of the Department of Medicine. The second center is located at The Human Molecular Biology and Genetics Institute at the University of Utah in Salt Lake City. Dr. Thomas McIntyre, Principal Investigator, is a professor of internal medicine and pathology at the University of Utah, where he has been a faculty member since 1983. The third center was funded as of January 1, 1997 and is located at the University of New Mexico in Albuquerque, with Dr. Mary Lipscomb as Principal Investigator. Dr. Lipscomb is a professor and chair of the Department of Pathology at the University of New Mexico School of Medicine.

While these three locations serve as home bases, the centers are not bound by bricks and mortar. Instead, they are far-flung organizations in a constantly expanding network of connections among specialists in many different fields at their base locations, at other institutions and private enterprise in this country, and at similar organizations around the world. "Our projects involve pulmonologists, immunologists, allergists and basic researchers in the areas of inflammation, corticosteroid receptors, and physiology," comments Dr. Martin. "This year, we are joined by a leader in pulmonary epidemiology at Harvard. We also have brought prominent experts in other fields into asthma research, some for the first time. As our projects succeed, we are continually developing more national and international collaborative research. All of these investigators have an impact on our ongoing research."

Some of these scientists are as far away as Australia, while others are located in premier institutions in the United States, such as Johns Hopkins Medical School in Baltimore, and Brigham and Women's Hospital in Boston. In New Mexico, a strong research relationship has been developed between researchers at the ALA Asthma Research Center and the Lovelace Respiratory Research Institute in Albuquerque. Scientists at the Asthma Research Center in Utah have worked with a prominent asthma center in London. Since they were initially funded, the three centers have continued to reap the benefits of collaboration on local, national and global levels.

DENVER 2000 ASTHMA RESEARCH CENTER PROGRESS REPORT

At the Asthma Research Center in Denver, Dr. Richard Martin and colleagues continue to expand and clarify the concept that infection plays a key role in the origin of chronic asthma, at least in some people. During the past four years, they have firmly established that mycoplasma and chlamydia, two classes of bacteria which are very common and often cause pneumonia, are present in the airways of a large subset of asthmatics. When such individuals are treated with antibiotics to suppress the bacteria, their lung function improves and their asthma symptoms lessen.

"We have found mycoplasma or chlamydia to be present in over fifty percent of the asthmatics in the studies we have conducted," comments Dr. Martin. "We are now confident that these bacteria are involved in the development of asthma in a significant number of people."

In the past year, an epidemiologic study has been launched and is currently investigating a group of children who had pneumonia caused by mycoplasma or chlamydia between seven and nine years ago. Another group of children who had pneumonia that was not caused by bacteria will serve as a control group. At this writing, the researchers have found that 75 percent of the children who had mycoplasma pneumonia now have asthma. "This is a very high percentage, since the incidence of asthma in the general populations is only six percent," Dr. Martin explains. While this is a relatively small study which will eventually include 45 children in the study group and 45 controls, it will provide the preliminary data that is needed to decide whether to embark on a larger one.

The results of the discovery that certain microbes play a role in the development of asthma will in due course have an impact on how physicians treat asthma all over the country, and indeed all over the world. "We're beginning to publish our findings, and as they are disseminated others will try this approach and further evaluate it," Dr. Martin explains. "We are already receiving queries from physicians throughout the United States about the relationship between chronic infection and chronic asthma and how that impacts on treatment. And we are getting feedback from them that corroborates our findings. While we are researchers, you might say we're getting closer and closer to the bedside."

The Denver center has also developed a laboratory animal model of mycoplasma. These animals provide a means for studying the relationship between the presence of mycoplasma infection and the development of bronchial hyperresponsiveness that is a hallmark of asthma.

Another major focus in this center is to gain a greater understanding of the cellular and immunologic mechanisms by which mycoplasma contributes to chronic asthma. These investigations have revealed that the tiny bacteria has the capacity to act as either an antigen or a superantigen. An antigen is a substance that causes an allergic reaction by inducing the immune system to produce antibodies. Antigens require memory recall from the body's cells: a familiar example is poison ivy infection, which does not occur the first time a person is exposed to the plant. But when exposed for a second time, cellular memory kicks in and the unpleasant symptoms appear. A superantigen, however, can induce a reaction upon initial exposure. "It's intriguing that this organism can affect the immune system in two different manners," Dr. Martin says. "It's also important, because someone with an initial exposure can develop bronchial hyperresponsiveness. Then if they are reexposed to mycoplasma, the memory recall aspect may also come into play, and the combination of the two may worsen the situation." Studies to further elucidate the precise events and interactions that take place at the cellular level will continue in the coming year.

The Denver center also undertakes several pilot projects annually, consisting of innovative studies that are related to its major areas of investigation. One such project has investigated the role of surfactant proteins and how they interact with mycoplasma. Surfactants perform a variety of functions in the body, but their involvement in defending against invaders that are inhaled has not previously been well studied. "We began looking at surfactants several years ago, and the results were so promising that we have continued and expanded this pilot project," says Dr. Martin. In 1999, it was found that mycoplasma can bind to two surfactants called SP-A and SP-D, and that this may cause an inflammatory response in the lungs. During the coming year, this pilot project will examine the biochemistry and cell biology of the interaction of SP-A and SP-D with mycoplasma, hoping to determine whether the surfactants inhibit or enhance infection with mycoplasma.

Another pilot project that will be continued in the coming year has the goal of developing a non-invasive method for diagnosing mycoplasma and chlamydia in asthmatics. This is currently done by performing a bronchoscopy, which involves inserting a tube through the throat, a costly and uncomfortable procedure. Collecting a sample of induced sputum for laboratory analysis would be cost effective, less stressful and less risky. In the first year of this project, investigators found that the induced sputum technique is not as sensitive to the presence of mycoplasma and chlamydia as bronchoscopy. Their current efforts are aimed at increasing its sensitivity, as well as studying the inflammatory mediators that are present in the sputum of patients with mycoplasma and chlamydia, and those found in the sputum of individuals who do not harbor the bacteria.

A new pilot project will take basic research into the clinical arena by investigating patients to see whether surfactant proteins differ in those who have mycoplasma and chlamydia, and in patients who do not. Another new project will examine the ways in which mycoplasma alters the tight junction between the epithelial cells that line the airways, allowing inflammatory mediators and edema fluid to move through these junctions.

UTAH 2000 ASTHMA RESEARCH CENTER PROGRESS REPORT

The Asthma Research Center at the University of Utah, under the leadership of Principal Investigator Thomas Mc. McIntyre, Ph.D., is taking a reductionist approach to understanding the complex chain of events that occurs when asthma develops. "We know that a person's genetic susceptibility to asthma depends on a fairly large number of genes, perhaps as many as twenty or thirty," explains Dr. McIntyre. "They interact with each other, and because of their genetic background people with certain combinations of genes are more susceptible to developing asthma when they meet up with a trigger. There are many, many asthma triggers, making it even more complicated to understand precisely why some people have asthma and others do not."

By studying asthma in the laboratory, these researchers have been able to isolate and clarify certain key steps in its development. "We have shown that when one particular genetic defect is present, which we have found to produce a modest increase in susceptibility to asthma, the incidence of asthma can be further modified by a second gene mutation that by itself has little or no effect on asthma susceptibility," Dr. McIntyre says. "Our studies are now focussed on substantiating the idea that asthma involves interactions among many genes, each of which has a small part to play, but that together appear to have a synergistic effect."

The symptoms of asthma wax and wane as inflammatory changes take place in the branching network of tubes that conducts air into the lungs. These changes occur when inflammatory cells enter the airway tubes, causing fluid to be retained in the lining of the airways. Fluid retention narrows the airways, while other inflammatory events trigger contractions of smooth muscle cells that also reduce the size of the airways. Over time, these inflammatory exacerbations lead to tissue remodeling and eventually to structural changes that chronically decrease the size of the airways.

"Our goal is to understand the genesis of this process. We want to know how and why inflammatory cells enter the airways," Dr. McIntyre comments. Understanding such early changes will provide tools and guidance for alleviating the symptoms of asthma, and perhaps for a means of preventing it altogether.

A major difficulty for researchers studying asthma is that in humans the disease is well established before any symptoms appear. Nonetheless, scientists at this center have been able to explore in the laboratory a genetic defect in certain people that leads to an increased incidence of severe asthma. These studies have allowed them to begin unraveling the genetic basis of the disease.

In 1998, they found that individuals who lack an enzyme called PAF acetylhydrolase, which stops the activity of an inflammation-inducing agent called PAF (platelet-activating factor), are missing the enzyme due to a very specific single mutation in the gene that codes for it, a change that leads to a loss of the enzyme's activity. A person who lacks PAF-acetylhydrolase is at a small but detectable increased risk of developing severe asthma. During the past year, the researchers have identified a second mutation in humans that modifies the effect of the PAF-acetylhydrolase gene mutation, further increasing the incidence of asthma. This observation is important because it describes a common but "silent" mutation that may be present in a large number of people and thus have significant impli-

cations regarding who may be at risk for asthma.

Another milestone in the past year involves defining, at a molecular level, the changes in inflammatory cells that occur in response to their environment. This type of signaling from the outside to the inside of the cell has been shown to induce a new receptor in inflammatory cells that makes them more sensitive to chemicals that had previously been invisible to them. "Some of these chemicals mimic the inflammatory mediator PAF, while others act on an intracellular receptor, and so we now know a new way that cells become sensitive to external inflammatory signals and become activated," Dr. McIntyre comments. This finding provides another clue to how the inflammatory process is turned on, leading to the airway inflammation that is characteristic of asthma.

The genetic difference between mice that lack a specific class of inflammatory cells called mast cells is also being explored as a means of understanding the genetic basis for airway sensitivity to asthma triggers. Mast cells are thought to be the sentries that rapidly react to the presence of antigens, or foreign invaders, triggering an acute asthma episode. Significant differences involving dozens of genes were identified when genes from mice lacking mast cells, who tend not to develop asthma, were compared with genes from normal animals. In the past year, genes from mast cell–deficient mice have been studied and found to code for certain proteins that may be responsible for the loss of mast cells. This information can eventually lead to identification of genes that may be involved in asthma in humans.

In other studies of mice with defective inflammatory cells, a gene that controls the processing of certain destructive enzymes has been defined. Currently, the investigators are attempting to "knock out" or remove this gene to determine whether mice who lack it are less susceptible to developing asthmatic lung complications. "Once we are able to create mice that lack this enzyme and that pass this trait on to the next generation, we hope to find that they develop less severe symptoms of asthma, especially when exposed to airborne triggers," according to Dr. McIntyre. A mutation in humans has been found with this exact condition, but it is so rare that it cannot be studied, highlighting the importance of examining asthma in a laboratory model, such as genetically engineered mice.

When will the knowledge and understanding that is being acquired in this basic research pay off with clinical applications? "Science is a slow process," says Dr. McIntyre. "It's been a challenge for me in my role as President of the American Lung Association of Utah to explain why this is so, and why we need to support this lengthy effort. All research takes time, because systems are complicated, and with asthma that's especially true because it's so complex. Even a disease caused by a single genetic event is complicated, and many genes are involved in asthma, as well as many triggers. What we and the other Asthma Research Centers are working on now is the basic knowledge we have to have before we can start designing new therapies. We need to know who all the players are to be able to influence the process, and each year we are getting closer to our goal."

NEW MEXICO 2000 ASTHMA RESEARCH CENTER

The centerpiece of the Asthma Research Center at the University of New Mexico is its Pilot Project Program, designed to foster new ideas in asthma research and to bring scientists from other disciplines to the study of asthma. In the first four years of the program, scientists from many different areas of interest and perspectives have become involved, including basic researchers, clinicians, and even anthropologists. The Pilot Project Program has also succeeded in developing significant collaborative efforts between junior and senior scientists. A total of 18 research awards have been made, many to junior faculty members and promising post-doctoral research fellows. The investigations begun thanks to this funding have resulted in a number of papers published in respected scientific journals, and in additional funding from other sources.

Pilot project grantees are also integrated into other research activities that target asthma, which are largely supported by a Specialized Center of Research (SCOR) grant from the National Heart, Lung and Blood Institute of the National Institutes of Health (NIH). This synergy has created a climate in which asthma research can grow exponentially.

As one example of this process, former pilot project grantees have made important contributions to this year's SCOR grant renewal application. "Their asthma-related research, which was initially funded by the ALA Asthma Research Center, provided key data and new insights that were important in the growth and refinement of the SCOR research program," comments Mary F. Lipscomb, M.D., the Center's Principal Investigator, as well as the Principal Investigator of the SCOR grant. "If our SCOR grant is renewed, certainly the ALA's support has helped make that possible."

In addition, a number of former and current Pilot Project awardees are active in the National Institute of Environmental Health Sciences (NIEHS) Developmental Center, which is directed by Pope Mosely, M.D., who is also director of the Asthma Research Center's Pilot Project Program. The NIEHS Center, now in its second year of funding, focuses on asthma and lung cancer among Native American populations within New Mexico. "One key reason for this center's success is the environment created by the combined asthma research efforts of the ALA center and the SCOR grant," Dr. Lipscomb explains. "Each entity supports the other two, and the whole is greater than the sum of the parts."

Members of all three centers meet weekly for a discussion group or journal club, which serves as a forum for new work on asthma and related fields. They also participate in "work-in-progress" sessions where fellow investigators present their work and receive feedback from colleagues who are active in different scientific disciplines, bringing new viewpoints to bear on each project. Presentations are also made by senior members of the SCOR and NIEHS centers, who report their own research progress.

Of the pilot projects funded in 1999, two were designed to develop animal models for studying asthma, and both accomplished their goals. Another project succeeded in casting new light on how antibodies could be used to suppress the activity of mast cells and basophils, two types of cells that are triggered in the lungs of people with asthma and play an important role in causing the airways to narrow. "The information this investigator developed has resulted in three papers published in scientific journals, and has given the researcher enough preliminary data to apply for an NIH grant that would provide major funding," Dr. Lipscomb comments. Another 1999 project studied eosinophils, cells that are significantly involved in both acute asthma episodes and the long-term chronic effects of asthma. This investigator made important observations about how eosinophils are selectively recruited into the lungs of asthmatics, findings that are contributing to a new grant proposal for a project in the asthma SCOR program.

In January of 2000, new pilot project grants were awarded to four talented young scientists who are committed to careers in pulmonary diseases with a focus on asthma. One of these projects concerns the increased risk of developing asthma among infants whose mothers have asthma. The investigator hypothesizes that the antibodies in a pregnant woman that are responsible for her asthma may cross the placenta and play a role in the development of childhood asthma in the baby. Using a laboratory animal model, the role of the mother's response to a particular allergen in the development of an allergic response in her offspring is being studied.

A second project, headed by a cardiovascular and endocrine physiologist who was attracted by the rich asthma research climate at the University of New Mexico, is concerned with airway smooth muscle. This investigator has developed a new approach to determining the factors that contribute to the propensity of the smooth muscle that surrounds the airways to constrict during asthma episodes.

Another project is investigating immunoglobin E (IgE), a type of antibody that can bind to inhaled allergens, and its role in enhancing the function of dendritic cells in the lungs of people who have asthma. Dendritic cells are essential components of the immune response that occurs in asthma. Their role is to present the allergen to a type of white blood cell called T-lymphocytes, which then help to orchestrate the immune system-mediated inflammation that is characteristic of asthma. It is already known that IgE plays a role in causing mast cells to release their contents in asthmatic airways and contribute to the inflammatory process, but this project proposes new ways in which IgE antibodies participate in the development of asthma episodes.

The fourth pilot project is studying the role of the respiratory syncytial virus (RSV), a common childhood infection, in the subsequent development of asthma. "We know children infected with RSV in early childhood are at increased risk for asthma, but the reason why is unclear," Dr. Lipscomb says. "This scientist is investigating a protein from the Clara cells that line the airways, which may help us understand why children infected with RSV tend to develop asthma." Known as Clara cell secretory protein or CCSP, it dampens inflammatory responses in the lungs by decreasing inappropriate and excessive inflammation in lung tissue. "Asthmatics may not make enough CCSP when they need it," speculates Dr. Lipscomb. "If a child who is genetically predisposed to asthma is infected with RSV, and is unable to make enough CCSP, the result would be prolonged inflammation, and that could set the stage for developing asthma." This study, using genetically manipulated laboratory animals, may provide important insight into the relationship between CCSP levels, RSV infection, and asthma. Eventually, the information developed in studies like this could lead to new treatments for asthma.

Much has been accomplished by the Asthma Research Centers during the past four years, and much work still lies ahead. This ambitious enterprise has been fruitful in producing new and valuable information, and in encouraging more scientists to become involved in asthma research. Their long-term efforts will pay off many times over in alleviating suffering, reducing health care costs, and improving the productivity of the national economy. The painstaking work of basic research, however, requires time, patience and perseverance as one building block after another is cemented into place. Only through the commitment of programs like the Asthma Research Centers can these scientists reach their final goal: a better life for the millions of people who are adversely affected by asthma.

For more information about the American Lung Association's research program, contact Ray M. Vento, Assistant Vice President, Scientific Programs Administration, American Lung Association, 1740 Broadway, New York, NY 10019-4374.

Reprinted by permission of the
American Lung Association

APPENDIX II

THE ESTIMATED PREVALENCE AND INCIDENCE OF LUNG DISEASE BY LUNG ASSOCIATION TERRITORY

EXECUTIVE SUMMARY

The Best Practices and Program Services Division has compiled this issue of *The Estimated Prevalence and Incidence of Lung Disease by Lung Association Territory* to provide lung associations with lung disease morbidity data pertinent to the areas they serve. This document depicts prevalence estimates of chronic conditions and the incidence of lung cancer at the state, county, constituent, and affiliate levels. The data are based upon the 1998 National Health Interview Survey and the 1997 Surveillance, Epidemiology, and End Results (SEER) program.

In previous years this document included incidence estimates of acute lung diseases such as the common cold, acute bronchitis, pneumonia, and influenza. However, the National Health Interview Survey (NHIS), a scientifically designed population sample survey that serves as the principal source of magnitude data on chronic and acute lung disease, redesigned its questionnaire in 1997. Originally, questions on these acute lung diseases were included in the survey, however the National Center for Health Statistics staff eliminated acute lung disease because of difficulties in compiling accurate data. Therefore, the most recent year of data for acute lung diseases is for 1996. *The latest acute lung disease estimates by lung association are in the April 2000 Estimated Prevalence and Incidence of Lung Disease by Lung Association Territory.*

In addition, the NHIS questions on chronic lung disease questions were revised as well. All questions now ask for a medical diagnosis instead of self-report. This change in definition of disease has made it impossible to compare the estimates in this year's estimates with those of the past.

Preceding the data is a statistical methodology section, which defines the procedures used to compute local lung disease prevalence and incidence estimates. This section also delineates the limitations of these data.

Please note that these numbers reflect the *estimated* prevalence and incidence of lung disease within each lung association area, and not the *actual number*. That is, the estimate is derived from national data and adjusted for the age-specific population of each area. Many other factors may affect *actual* prevalence. When releasing this information to the public or press, please be careful to ensure that the nature and derivation of these estimates are understood.

April 2001

STATISTICAL METHODOLOGY

Introduction

Presently, state and county-specific measurements of the number of persons with chronic lung disease are not available. In order to assess the magnitude of lung disease at the state and county levels, we have utilized a synthetic estimation technique originally developed by the U.S. Bureau of the Census. This method uses age-specific national estimates of diagnosed lung disease to project the prevalence and incidence of lung disease within the counties served by lung association constituents and affiliates. Table 1 summarizes these prevalence and incidence estimates.

Prevalence Estimates: Chronic Bronchitis, Emphysema, and Asthma

With the revision of the National Health Interview Survey (NHIS) questionnaire, chronic disease estimates have changed dramatically. Questions now ask for a medical diagnosis instead of self-report, making it impossible to compare this year's estimates with those of the past.

Revisions to the chronic obstructive pulmonary disease (COPD) questions include a change in prevalence time frames (stopping the use of overall COPD estimates) and the elimination of childhood estimates. Prior to 1997 survey respondents were asked "Have you or someone in your family had chronic bronchitis or emphysema in the past year?" After 1997, the chronic bronchitis question states, "Have you been diagnosed with chronic bronchitis by a health professional in the past year?" while the emphysema question asks respondents, "Have you been diagnosed with emphysema by a health professional during your lifetime?"

In addition to the change seen with chronic bronchitis and emphysema, questions asked on asthma were revised. Previously, survey respondents were asked "Have you or someone in your family had asthma?" After 1997, this question was replaced with two new asthma questions. The first measures lifetime prevalence (as in the case of emphysema): "Have you been diagnosed with asthma by a health professional within your lifetime?" The second measures point prevalence (as in the case of chronic bronchitis): "If diagnosed with asthma in your lifetime, have you had an asthma attack or episode in the past year?" For the purposes of this publication we will use data from the latter question to obtain county estimates. Information on pediatric asthma is still collected.

In 1998, the NHIS estimated that 8.9 million Americans reported a physician diagnosis of chronic bronchitis within the year and that an estimated 3 million Americans had been diagnosed with emphysema sometime in their life. The NHIS estimates that 10.6 million diagnosed people (3.8 million under 18) had an asthma attack in 1998.

Previous results from the NHIS showed that an estimated 16 million people (14.2 million chronic bronchitis and 1.8 million emphysema) had self-reported COPD in the past year. During that same year an estimated 14.6 million people (4.4 million children under age 18) said they had asthma.

Local area prevalence of chronic bronchitis, emphysema, and asthma are estimated by applying age-specific national prevalence rates from the 1998 NHIS to age-specific county-level resident populations. Prevalence estimates for chronic bronchitis, emphysema, and adult asthma are calculated for those 18 to 44, 45 to 64, and 65+. The prevalence estimate for pediatric asthma is calculated for those under age 18.

The procedure for determining local prevalence estimates is as follows. First, the age-specific county-level resident population for July 1, 1998, is obtained from the U.S. Bureau of the Census website. The age-specific national prevalence rate for each chronic lung disease is applied to the age-specific county-level population of each county. Thereafter, the age-specific prevalence estimates for each county within a lung association area are summed to determine its overall prevalence.

An individual respondent to the NHIS can report the presence of more than one chronic lung disease, i.e., chronic bronchitis and emphysema. For this reason and the fact that prevalence estimates are over different time frames (chronic bronchitis prevalence over a year vs. emphysema over a lifetime), adding these estimates to calculate COPD prevalence should not be performed, as it would *overestimate* the prevalence in your community.

Incidence Estimates: Lung Cancer

The Surveillance, Epidemiology, and End Results (SEER) program of the National Cancer Institute derives nationwide lung cancer incidence estimates. The SEER program was initiated in 1973 to collect cancer incidence data and includes nine population-based cancer registries, covering about 10 percent of the U.S. population.

Unlike the estimates for chronic lung diseases, lung cancer estimates are for the year 1997. Data for 1998 has not been released by the time of printing. Based on the lack of current information on age- and state-specific national incidence rates derived from SEER (the most recent year for which these data are available is 1989) the following modified methodology to obtain county estimates was employed. The Data Evaluation and Publication Committee, a standing committee of the North American Association of the Central Cancer Registries (NAACR), recommended dividing the national incidence rate by the national mortality rate published by the SEER program to estimate county-level lung cancer incidence (in 1997 - 54.4/41.7 = 1.30). This number was then applied to county-level mortality data derived from CDC Wonder to generate county-level lung cancer incidence estimates. The rationale behind this methodology stems from measured lung cancer survival rates, which relates closely to the mortality rate of lung cancer.

Limitations of Estimates

The National Health Interview Survey (NHIS), the principal source of magnitude data on chronic and acute lung disease, redesigned its questionnaire in 1997. Unfortunately, acute lung disease questions were excluded and chronic lung disease questions were edited, obliterating all trends. This has made it impossible to compare this year's estimates with those in past publications.

Since the statistics presented by the NHIS are based on a sample, they will differ (due to random sampling variability) from figures that would be derived from a complete census, or case registry of people in the United States with these diseases. The results are also subject to reporting, non-response, and processing errors. These types of errors are kept to a minimum by methods built into the survey.

Additionally, a major limitation of the survey is that the information represents physician-diagnosed data so estimates are certainly low. However, the NHIS is the best available source that depicts the magnitude of acute and chronic lung disease on the national level.

Local estimates of chronic and acute lung diseases are scaled in direct proportion to the base population of the county and its age distribution. No adjustments are made for other factors that may affect local prevalence (e.g., race, socioeconomic status, income, local prevalence of cigarette smokers, or occupational exposures) since the health surveys that obtain such data are rarely conducted on the county level.

REFERENCES

1. Irwin, R. Guide to Local Area Populations U.S. Bureau of the Census Technical Paper Number 39 (1972).
2. National Center for Health Statistics. Raw Data from the National Health Interview Survey, U.S., 1998 (Analysis by the American Lung Association Best Practices Division, Using SPSS and SUDAAN software).
3. Population Estimates Branch, U.S. Bureau of the Census. County Resident Population Estimates, by Age: July 1, 1998.
4. Population Estimates Branch, U.S. Bureau of the Census. Estimates of Population of Minor Civil Divisions: Annual Time Series, July 1, 1998.
5. National Institutes of Health, National Cancer Institute (NCI). SEER Cancer Statistics Review, 1973–1997.
6. CDC Wonder. Unpublished Mortality Data, 1997.

TABLE 1 ESTIMATED PREVALENCE AND INCIDENCE OF LUNG DISEASE BY COUNTY, STATE, AND LUNG ASSOCIATION, 1998

Association	Population	Lung Cancer[1]	CHRONIC LUNG DISEASES			
			Emphysema	Chronic Bronchitis	Adult Asthma	Pediatric Asthma
ALABAMA CONSTITUENT: ALA OF ALABAMA	4,313,456	3,713	48,723	147,797	112,064	56,564
Autauga County	42,193	40	457	1,386	1,051	623
Baldwin County	132,857	121	1,503	4,559	3,457	1,735
Barbour County	26,936	26	297	901	683	379
Bibb County	18,987	13	206	626	474	278
Blount County	46,292	48	524	1,589	1,205	603
Bullock County	11,325	3	122	370	281	169
Butler County	21,658	16	232	705	534	328
Calhoun County	117,083	116	1,339	4,062	3,080	1,477

TABLE 1 ESTIMATED PREVALENCE AND INCIDENCE OF LUNG DISEASE BY COUNTY,
STATE, AND LUNG ASSOCIATION, 1998 *(continued)*

Association	Population	Lung Cancer[1]	CHRONIC LUNG DISEASES			
			Emphysema	Chronic Bronchitis	Adult Asthma	Pediatric Asthma
ALA OF ALABAMA (cont.)						
Chambers County	36,706	43	415	1,258	954	481
Cherokee County	21,827	21	254	770	584	261
Chilton County	36,926	30	411	1,248	946	505
Choctaw County	15,829	20	173	524	397	229
Clarke County	28,531	13	308	934	708	425
Clay County	13,966	17	160	486	368	175
Cleburne County	14,283	9	161	488	370	188
Coffee County	42,222	43	482	1,461	1,108	536
Colbert County	52,924	55	614	1,862	1,412	637
Conecuh County	13,863	9	153	464	352	195
Coosa County	11,637	14	133	405	307	146
Covington County	37,461	49	427	1,296	982	477
Crenshaw County	13,626	17	153	463	351	183
Cullman County	74,944	69	854	2,590	1,964	957
Dale County	48,916	35	541	1,641	1,244	682
Dallas County	46,803	49	496	1,504	1,140	730
De KalbCounty	58,274	35	662	2,009	1,523	750
Elmore County	61,985	46	697	2,115	1,604	823
Escambia County	36,732	35	415	1,259	955	481
Etowah County	103,923	133	1,196	3,627	2,750	1,286
Fayette County	18,096	14	205	623	472	234
Franklin County	29,684	26	340	1,032	782	372
Geneva County	24,875	25	284	862	654	315
Greene County	9,843	13	103	311	236	160
Hale County	16,750	13	176	534	405	267
Henry County	15,798	20	178	541	410	208
Houston County	85,613	75	945	2,867	2,174	1,200
Jackson County	51,339	66	584	1,772	1,343	658
Jefferson County	660,039	560	7,591	23,026	17,460	8,176
Lamar County	16,012	16	183	555	421	203
Lauderdale County	84,206	78	978	2,967	2,250	1,008
Lawrence County	33,447	17	375	1,138	862	449
Lee County	100,481	43	1,184	3,592	2,723	1,144
Limestone County	62,247	17	712	2,159	1,637	786
Lowndes County	12,984	3	131	397	301	226
Macon County	23,207	21	263	799	606	300
Madison County	278,008	187	3,212	9,742	7,387	3,393
Marengo County	23,375	23	251	761	577	353
Marion County	30,857	36	355	1,078	817	381
Marshall County	80,192	82	921	2,795	2,119	997
Mobile County	398,886	426	4,375	13,269	10,061	5,695
Monroe County	24,005	17	256	778	590	367
Montgomery County	217,392	170	2,423	7,350	5,573	2,966
Morgan County	109,218	77	1,237	3,752	2,845	1,421
Perry County	12,682	14	133	405	307	201
Pickens County	21,019	20	230	698	530	301
Pike County	28,648	27	326	987	749	369
Randolph County	20,025	14	227	687	521	261
Russell County	50,368	51	567	1,721	1,305	666
Saint ClairCounty	62,018	55	694	2,105	1,596	836
Shelby County	140,853	68	1,560	4,731	3,587	1,958
Sumter County	15,765	12	167	507	384	246
Talladega County	77,025	72	853	2,588	1,963	1,069
Tallapoosa County	40,360	18	459	1,391	1,055	519
Tuscaloosa County	160,761	129	1,861	5,644	4,280	1,949

Association	Population	Lung Cancer[1]	CHRONIC LUNG DISEASES			
			Emphysema	Chronic Bronchitis	Adult Asthma	Pediatric Asthma
Walker County	71,006	66	808	2,452	1,859	909
Washington County	17,663	17	191	579	439	262
Wilcox County	13,451	16	137	415	314	230
Winston County	24,130	32	278	843	639	298
ALASKA						
CONSTITUENT:	615,205	251	6,324	19,185	14,547	10,281
ALA OF ALASKA						
Aleutians East Borough	2,221	1	25	75	57	31
Aleutians West						
Census Area	3,941	2	48	146	111	39
Anchorage Borough	255,618	104	2,734	8,294	6,289	3,894
Bethel Census Area	16,005	7	137	417	316	363
Bristol Bay Borough	1,090	0	10	32	24	21
Denali Borough	1,938	1	22	66	50	26
Dillingham Census						
Area	4,488	2	40	120	91	98
Fairbanks North Star						
Borough	84,253	34	869	2,636	1,999	1,398
Haines Borough	2,321	1	25	77	58	34
Juneau Borough	30,143	13	321	973	738	465
Kenai Peninsula Borough	48,321	20	496	1,505	1,141	810
Ketchikan Gateway						
Borough	14,228	6	151	457	347	222
Kodiak Island Borough	14,479	6	146	444	337	250
Lake and Peninsula						
Borough	1,736	1	15	47	35	38
Matanuska-Susitna						
Borough	55,793	22	547	1,659	1,258	1,027
Nome Census Area	9,004	4	79	239	181	200
North Slope Borough	7,017	3	62	188	142	154
Northwest Arctic						
Borough	6,764	0	53	162	123	170
Prince of Wales-Outer						
Ketchikan Ce	6,863	3	67	205	155	126
Sitka Borough	8,305	4	86	261	198	136
Skagway-Hoonah-Angoon						
Census Area	3,655	2	35	108	82	69
Southeast Fairbanks						
Census Area	5,984	2	58	176	133	112
Valdez-Cordova Census						
Area	10,256	4	109	329	250	160
Wade Hampton Census						
Area	6,868	3	53	160	121	178
Wrangell-Petersburg						
Census Area	6,813	3	71	214	162	112
Yakutat Borough	790	0	8	24	19	13
Yukon-Koyukuk Census						
Area	6,311	3	57	171	130	135
ARIZONA/NEW MEXICO						
CONSTITUENT:	6,400,812	4,053	69,149	209,750	159,042	95,094
ALA OF ARIZONA/						
NEW MEXICO						
ARIZONA	4,667,277	3,137	50,641	153,609	116,475	68,563
Apache County	68,734	9	611	1,855	1,406	1,485
Cochise County	112,404	91	1,204	3,652	2,769	1,707
Coconino County	114,087	29	1,169	3,545	2,688	1,921

TABLE 1   ESTIMATED PREVALENCE AND INCIDENCE OF LUNG DISEASE BY COUNTY,
STATE, AND LUNG ASSOCIATION, 1998 *(continued)*

Association	Population	Lung Cancer[1]	CHRONIC LUNG DISEASES			
			Emphysema	Chronic Bronchitis	Adult Asthma	Pediatric Asthma
ALA OF ARIZONA/						
NEW MEXICO (cont.)						
Gila County	48,839	52	538	1,632	1,237	689
Graham County	31,711	14	314	952	722	573
Greenlee County	9,323	4	90	274	208	175
La Paz County	14,830	N/A	168	510	387	192
Maricopa County	2,783,779	1,772	30,306	91,929	69,705	40,534
Mohave County	130,647	212	1,517	4,601	3,489	1,568
Navajo County	96,838	34	902	2,735	2,074	1,950
Pima County	790,333	529	8,788	26,656	20,212	10,858
Pinal County	146,947	117	1,550	4,700	3,564	2,317
Santa Cruz County	38,155	12	370	1,123	852	715
Yavapai County	148,748	152	1,741	5,281	4,004	1,735
Yuma County	131,902	110	1,373	4,164	3,158	2,144
NEW MEXICO	1,733,535	916	18,508	56,141	42,567	26,531
Bernalillo County	524,686	272	5,866	17,795	13,493	7,093
Catron County	2,812	0	32	96	73	37
Chaves County	62,618	49	655	1,988	1,507	1,005
Cibola County	26,506	N/A	273	828	628	441
Colfax County	13,586	12	147	447	339	200
Curry County	44,873	34	469	1,424	1,080	721
DeBaca County	2,362	3	27	81	61	31
Dona Ana County	168,967	86	1,775	5,385	4,083	2,688
Eddy County	53,446	43	562	1,705	1,293	848
Grant County	31,628	22	337	1,023	776	485
Guadalupe County	4,041	1	43	130	99	63
Harding County	904	3	10	30	23	12
Hidalgo County	6,174	4	63	190	144	106
Lea County	56,442	55	575	1,744	1,322	962
Lincoln County	16,432	17	187	566	429	212
Los Alamos County	18,273	6	209	634	480	231
Luna County	23,985	13	253	767	582	378
McKinley County	67,332	13	626	1,898	1,439	1,360
Mora County	4,830	3	52	157	119	73
Otero County	54,315	29	575	1,745	1,323	847
Quay County	10,010	14	111	337	255	138
Rio Arriba County	37,839	14	387	1,173	889	640
Roosevelt County	17,824	14	192	583	442	266
Sandoval County	88,037	29	904	2,742	2,079	1,475
San Juan County	106,169	38	1,031	3,127	2,371	1,989
San Miguel County	28,714	12	302	916	694	456
Santa Fe County	122,826	48	1,378	4,179	3,169	1,645
Sierra County	10,988	16	132	402	304	115
Socorro County	16,343	14	172	522	396	258
Taos County	26,759	13	289	877	665	398
Torrance County	16,021	4	166	503	382	263
Union County	3,986	1	44	132	100	58
Valencia County	63,807	34	664	2,015	1,528	1,037
ARKANSAS						
CONSTITUENT:	2,538,202	2,597	28,166	85,425	64,771	35,088
ALA OF ARKANSAS						
Arkansas County	20,657	23	227	687	521	295
Ashley County	24,337	35	264	801	607	358
Baxter County	36,319	65	439	1,330	1,009	376

Association	Population	Lung Cancer[1]	CHRONIC LUNG DISEASES			
			Emphysema	Chronic Bronchitis	Adult Asthma	Pediatric Asthma
Benton County	133,875	114	1,497	4,542	3,444	1,808
Boone County	31,797	35	360	1,092	828	414
Bradley County	11,408	10	127	386	292	156
Calhoun County	5,684	9	63	190	144	80
Carroll County	22,438	20	255	772	586	290
Chicot County	15,021	20	158	478	362	240
Clark County	21,586	22	251	762	577	257
Clay County	17,122	34	199	603	457	206
Cleburne County	22,890	20	271	821	623	257
Cleveland County	8,421	13	94	285	216	115
Columbia County	25,109	23	281	852	646	339
Conway County	19,828	20	221	669	507	272
Craighead County	77,199	65	873	2,647	2,007	1,010
Crawford County	50,267	36	535	1,623	1,231	775
Crittenden County	49,794	47	515	1,562	1,184	821
Cross County	19,414	30	204	620	470	307
Dallas County	9,051	9	101	306	232	124
Desha County	15,075	12	157	475	360	246
Drew County	17,475	17	190	575	436	257
Faulkner County	78,238	53	869	2,635	1,998	1,079
Franklin County	16,825	10	185	560	425	240
Fulton County	10,946	12	127	386	293	130
Garland County	83,661	124	991	3,006	2,279	934
Grant County	15,843	14	175	530	402	223
Greene County	36,010	35	405	1,227	931	480
Hempstead County	22,035	26	240	728	552	320
Hot Spring County	28,874	31	322	978	742	392
Howard County	13,682	22	149	452	343	199
Independence County	32,908	32	366	1,109	841	453
Izard County	13,108	18	154	468	355	149
Jackson County	17,720	20	202	612	464	227
Jefferson County	81,588	81	890	2,699	2,047	1,182
Johnson County	21,456	25	241	732	555	285
Lafayette County	8,942	12	98	297	225	128
Lawrence County	17,207	30	195	593	449	222
Lee County	12,912	14	136	414	314	203
Lincoln County	14,326	8	164	499	378	179
Little River County	13,154	14	144	437	331	189
Logan County	21,099	25	232	703	533	300
Lonoke County	50,004	39	530	1,608	1,219	779
Madison County	13,242	12	145	441	335	188
Marion County	14,860	23	174	527	400	174
Miller County	39,526	31	427	1,294	981	589
Mississippi County	50,515	57	522	1,583	1,200	835
Monroe County	10,125	12	108	327	248	156
Montgomery County	8,648	6	100	304	231	104
Nevada County	9,981	20	109	331	251	144
Newton County	8,163	12	89	269	204	119
Ouachita County	27,779	34	309	939	712	380
Perry County	9,629	5	108	327	248	130
Phillips County	27,302	35	271	823	624	490
Pike County	10,546	16	117	356	270	145
Poinsett County	24,634	36	272	825	625	346
Polk County	19,653	27	218	663	502	270
Pope County	52,041	49	574	1,741	1,320	732
Prairie County	9,344	5	105	318	241	125
Pulaski County	348,813	274	3,882	11,776	8,929	4,779
Randolph County	17,788	21	200	606	460	237
St. Francis County	28,127	43	286	866	657	483

TABLE 1 ESTIMATED PREVALENCE AND INCIDENCE OF LUNG DISEASE BY COUNTY,
STATE, AND LUNG ASSOCIATION, 1998 *(continued)*

Association	Population	Lung Cancer[1]	CHRONIC LUNG DISEASES			
			Emphysema	Chronic Bronchitis	Adult Asthma	Pediatric Asthma
ALA OF ARKANSAS						
(cont.)						
Saline County	77,156	72	847	2,568	1,947	1,100
Scott County	10,585	12	119	360	273	142
Searcy County	7,735	6	88	268	203	98
Sebastian County	105,898	90	1,171	3,553	2,694	1,477
Sevier County	14,608	29	161	487	369	207
Sharp County	16,904	17	197	597	453	200
Stone County	11,092	17	128	387	293	137
Union County	45,228	55	496	1,505	1,141	646
Van Buren County	15,533	25	182	552	418	181
Washington County	144,989	114	1,630	4,945	3,749	1,928
White County	64,629	77	727	2,205	1,672	859
Woodruff County	8,837	12	95	288	218	133
Yell County	18,987	29	212	643	488	258
CALIFORNIA						
CONSTITUENT:	32,682,794	17,963	356,489	1,081,351	819,926	473,486
ALA OF CALIFORNIA						
Alameda County	1,397,050	762	15,763	47,816	36,256	18,381
Alpine County	1,192	3	13	41	31	16
Amador County	33,415	40	402	1,219	924	352
Butte County	194,347	212	2,178	6,606	5,009	2,611
Calaveras County	39,642	46	445	1,350	1,023	530
Colusa County	18,596	8	188	571	433	321
Contra Costa County	917,970	559	10,246	31,078	23,565	12,475
Del Norte County	27,006	36	294	892	677	393
El Dorado County	158,322	121	1,733	5,258	3,987	2,271
Fresno County	755,051	399	7,611	23,086	17,505	13,151
Glenn County	26,176	20	266	808	613	447
Humboldt County	122,163	107	1,348	4,087	3,099	1,717
Imperial County	143,735	74	1,436	4,356	3,303	2,548
Inyo County	18,071	20	205	621	471	234
Kern County	631,615	356	6,405	19,430	14,732	10,864
Kings County	118,667	60	1,223	3,709	2,812	1,973
Lake County	55,076	83	617	1,871	1,419	741
Lassen County	33,281	14	384	1,166	884	406
Los Angeles County	9,223,807	4,324	100,540	304,970	231,241	133,874
Madera County	114,523	57	1,201	3,642	2,762	1,830
Marin County	236,377	169	2,869	8,704	6,600	2,394
Mariposa County	15,786	16	182	553	419	193
Mendocino County	83,754	82	904	2,743	2,080	1,247
Merced County	197,261	108	1,892	5,740	4,352	3,776
Modoc County	9,338	9	101	307	233	138
Mono County	10,307	5	115	350	265	139
Monterey County	366,631	157	3,897	11,821	8,963	5,673
Napa County	119,540	120	1,360	4,124	3,127	1,534
Nevada County	91,114	72	1,030	3,123	2,368	1,193
Orange County	2,723,782	1,330	30,324	91,984	69,746	37,285
Placer County	229,216	156	2,511	7,618	5,776	3,281
Plumas County	20,362	23	227	687	521	279
Riverside County	1,480,708	932	15,511	47,050	35,676	23,716
Sacramento County	1,166,699	809	12,702	38,529	29,214	16,987
San Benito County	48,984	18	494	1,497	1,135	854
San Bernardino County	1,635,967	800	16,562	50,238	38,092	28,241
San Diego County	2,766,123	1,565	30,697	93,116	70,604	38,212

Association	Population	Lung Cancer[1]	CHRONIC LUNG DISEASES			
			Emphysema	Chronic Bronchitis	Adult Asthma	Pediatric Asthma
San Francisco County	745,756	502	9,289	28,175	21,364	6,718
San Joaquin County	549,684	333	5,670	17,198	13,040	9,118
San Luis Obispo County	234,074	152	2,700	8,190	6,210	2,872
San Mateo County	701,080	398	8,135	24,675	18,710	8,431
Santa Barbara County	389,472	218	4,396	13,335	10,111	5,119
Santa Clara County	1,641,848	706	18,506	56,134	42,563	21,672
Santa Cruz County	243,200	114	2,715	8,235	6,244	3,303
Shasta County	164,156	153	1,768	5,363	4,066	2,458
Sierra County	3,376	3	37	112	85	48
Siskiyou County	44,024	42	481	1,460	1,107	634
Solano County	376,748	265	3,989	12,101	9,176	5,883
Sonoma County	433,777	341	4,828	14,645	11,105	5,942
Stanislaus County	426,872	256	4,333	13,144	9,967	7,327
Sutter County	77,069	44	814	2,469	1,872	1,211
Tehama County	54,016	42	579	1,755	1,331	820
Trinity County	13,043	14	144	437	331	182
Tulare County	354,527	185	3,449	10,461	7,932	6,617
Tuolumne County	53,029	51	616	1,868	1,416	636
Ventura County	732,143	329	7,861	23,846	18,081	11,048
Yolo County	153,293	91	1,703	5,167	3,918	2,110
Yuba County	59,953	52	600	1,820	1,380	1,060
AFFILIATES:						
ALA OF CENTRAL CA						
Fresno County	755,051	399	7,611	23,086	17,505	13,151
Kings County	118,667	60	1,223	3,709	2,812	1,973
Madera County	114,523	57	1,201	3,642	2,762	1,830
Mariposa County	15,786	16	182	553	419	193
Merced County	197,261	108	1,892	5,740	4,352	3,776
Tulare County	354,527	185	3,449	10,461	7,932	6,617
ALA OF CENTRAL COAST						
Monterey County	366,631	157	3,897	11,821	8,963	5,673
San Luis Obispo County	234,074	152	2,700	8,190	6,210	2,872
Santa Cruz County	243,200	114	2,715	8,235	6,244	3,303
ALA OF EAST BAY						
Alameda County	1,397,050	762	15,763	47,816	36,256	18,381
Contra Costa County	917,970	559	10,246	31,078	23,565	12,475
Solano County	376,748	265	3,989	12,101	9,176	5,883
ALA OF INLAND COUNTIES						
Inyo County	18,071	20	205	621	471	234
Mono County	10,307	5	115	350	265	139
Riverside County	1,480,708	932	15,511	47,050	35,676	23,716
San Bernardino County	1,635,967	800	16,562	50,238	38,092	28,241
ALA OF LOS ANGELES COUNTY						
Los Angeles County	9,223,807	4,324	100,540	304,970	231,241	133,874
Orange County	2,723,782	1,330	30,324	91,984	69,746	37,285
ALA OF SACRAMENTO- EMIGRANT TRAILS						
Alpine County	1,192	3	13	41	31	16
Amador County	33,415	40	402	1,219	924	352
Colusa County	18,596	8	188	571	433	321
El Dorado County	158,322	121	1,733	5,258	3,987	2,271

TABLE 1 ESTIMATED PREVALENCE AND INCIDENCE OF LUNG DISEASE BY COUNTY, STATE, AND LUNG ASSOCIATION, 1998 (continued)

Association	Population	Lung Cancer[1]	CHRONIC LUNG DISEASES			
			Emphysema	Chronic Bronchitis	Adult Asthma	Pediatric Asthma
ALA OF SACRAMENTO-EMIGRANT TRAILS (cont.)						
Nevada County	91,114	72	1,030	3,123	2,368	1,193
Placer County	229,216	156	2,511	7,618	5,776	3,281
Sacramento County	1,166,699	809	12,702	38,529	29,214	16,987
Sierra County	3,376	3	37	112	85	48
Yolo County	153,293	91	1,703	5,167	3,918	2,110
ALA OF SAN DIEGO & IMPERIAL COUNTIES						
Imperial County	143,735	74	1,436	4,356	3,303	2,548
San Diego County	2,766,123	1,565	30,697	93,116	70,604	38,212
ALA OF SAN FRANCISCO & SAN MATEO COUNTIES						
San Francisco County	745,756	502	9,289	28,175	21,364	6,718
San Mateo County	701,080	398	8,135	24,675	18,710	8,431
ALA OF SANTA BARBARA & VENTURA COUNTIES						
Santa Barbara County	389,472	218	4,396	13,335	10,111	5,119
Ventura County	732,143	329	7,861	23,846	18,081	11,048
ALA OF SANTA CLARA-SAN BENITO						
San Benito County	48,984	18	494	1,497	1,135	854
Santa Clara County	1,641,848	706	18,506	56,134	42,563	21,672
COLORADO CONSTITUENT: *ALA OF COLORADO*	3,968,967	1,722	43,851	133,011	100,857	55,524
Adams County	323,427	135	3,423	10,385	7,874	5,055
Alamosa County	14,543	5	152	460	349	235
Arapahoe County	472,579	165	5,209	15,800	11,980	6,654
Archuleta County	9,154	5	97	295	223	142
Baca County	4,327	6	50	150	114	54
Bent County	5,798	4	64	196	148	80
Boulder County	266,671	69	3,074	9,323	7,069	3,279
Chaffee County	15,174	10	177	537	408	178
Cheyenne County	2,322	0	24	73	55	38
Clear Creek County	9,017	5	101	306	232	122
Conejos County	7,983	4	79	238	181	146
Costilla County	3,642	0	39	117	89	56
Crowley County	4,313	5	50	152	115	52
Custer County	3,438	0	38	115	88	48
Delta County	26,633	14	302	915	694	347
Denver County	498,402	290	5,725	17,365	13,167	6,200
Dolores County	1,821	3	20	61	46	26
Douglas County	141,449	36	1,469	4,457	3,379	2,310
Eagle County	33,709	3	370	1,124	852	479
Elbert County	18,612	3	193	585	444	305
El Paso County	490,044	192	5,327	16,159	12,252	7,163
Fremont County	44,225	30	522	1,583	1,201	501
Garfield County	39,377	13	427	1,294	981	581

Association	Population	Lung Cancer[1]	CHRONIC LUNG DISEASES			
			Emphysema	Chronic Bronchitis	Adult Asthma	Pediatric Asthma
Gilpin County	4,184	1	47	144	109	54
Grand County	10,099	0	113	343	260	136
Gunnison County	12,425	3	146	444	337	141
Hinsdale County	736	0	9	28	21	7
Huerfano County	6,789	6	75	227	172	95
Jackson County	1,521	1	17	52	40	20
Jefferson County	500,802	220	5,596	16,975	12,871	6,782
Kiowa County	1,647	1	18	53	40	25
Kit Carson County	7,312	3	78	237	179	112
Lake County	6,351	4	68	206	156	96
La Plata County	40,519	20	451	1,367	1,037	556
Larimer County	231,104	91	2,581	7,829	5,937	3,135
Las Animas County	14,547	10	161	488	370	203
Lincoln County	5,686	1	66	202	153	67
Logan County	17,897	8	199	603	457	247
Mesa County	112,899	90	1,246	3,780	2,866	1,583
Mineral County	703	1	9	26	20	7
Moffat County	12,564	4	129	392	297	210
Montezuma County	22,365	18	235	712	540	357
Montrose County	30,790	16	337	1,022	775	443
Morgan County	25,088	9	262	793	602	406
Otero County	20,665	14	219	664	504	322
Ouray County	3,318	3	38	115	87	42
Park County	13,403	3	147	446	338	191
Phillips County	4,301	4	48	145	110	59
Pitkin County	13,345	0	167	508	385	116
Prowers County	13,704	13	141	428	325	228
Pueblo County	134,919	81	1,483	4,497	3,410	1,916
Rio Blanco County	6,263	3	67	203	154	96
Rio Grande County	11,473	8	119	362	275	187
Routt County	17,490	6	196	593	450	237
Saguache County	6,050	3	61	184	139	107
San Juan County	526	0	5	17	13	9
San Miguel County	5,448	1	63	191	145	66
Sedgwick County	2,553	4	29	89	68	31
Summit County	18,781	1	222	674	511	211
Teller County	20,553	3	221	670	508	310
Washington County	4,550	3	51	153	116	63
Weld County	159,501	64	1,698	5,152	3,906	2,457
Yuma County	9,436	4	101	307	233	143
CONNECTICUT CONSTITUENT: ALA OF CONNECTICUT	3,272,563	2,437	36,976	112,157	85,042	42,883
Fairfield County	837,476	594	9,515	28,862	21,884	10,787
Hartford County	827,706	646	9,382	28,458	21,578	10,740
Litchfield County	181,311	131	2,032	6,164	4,674	2,434
Middlesex County	150,015	117	1,714	5,198	3,942	1,899
New Haven County	792,879	593	8,961	27,182	20,610	10,380
New London County	246,959	199	2,757	8,362	6,340	3,355
Tolland County	131,360	84	1,486	4,506	3,417	1,717
Windham County	104,857	73	1,129	3,425	2,597	1,571
DELAWARE CONSTITUENT: ALA OF DELAWARE	744,066	634	8,461	25,666	19,460	9,557
Kent County	124,311	92	1,365	4,140	3,139	1,769
New Castle County	482,562	365	5,515	16,729	12,684	6,101
Sussex County	137,193	177	1,581	4,797	3,637	1,687

TABLE 1 ESTIMATED PREVALENCE AND INCIDENCE OF LUNG DISEASE BY COUNTY,
STATE, AND LUNG ASSOCIATION, 1998 *(continued)*

| Association | Population | Lung Cancer[1] | CHRONIC LUNG DISEASES | | | |
			Emphysema	Chronic Bronchitis	Adult Asthma	Pediatric Asthma
DISTRICT OF COLUMBIA CONSTITUENT: *ALA OF THE DISTRICT OF COLUMBIA*	521,426	452	6,340	19,232	14,582	5,244
District of Columbia	521,426	452	6,340	19,232	14,582	5,244
FLORIDA CONSTITUENT: *ALA OF FLORIDA*	14,908,230	15,048	170,709	517,823	392,634	187,314
Alachua County	198,221	148	2,271	6,888	5,223	2,487
Baker County	21,049	17	214	650	493	359
Bay County	146,730	157	1,610	4,883	3,703	2,092
Bradford County	24,836	32	279	848	643	330
Brevard County	464,818	580	5,393	16,360	12,404	5,590
Broward County	1,507,770	1,381	17,450	52,932	40,135	18,290
Calhoun County	12,409	17	135	411	311	180
Charlotte County	134,763	229	1,683	5,104	3,870	1,200
Citrus County	113,640	220	1,385	4,202	3,186	1,130
Clay County	137,581	95	1,440	4,369	3,313	2,207
Collier County	199,775	202	2,362	7,164	5,432	2,248
Columbia County	52,914	64	568	1,722	1,306	800
DeSoto County	24,708	26	277	839	636	333
Dixie County	12,869	18	144	436	330	175
Duval County	734,664	554	7,949	24,110	18,282	10,873
Escambia County	284,098	292	3,143	9,534	7,229	3,960
Flagler County	47,043	72	571	1,733	1,314	475
Franklin County	10,100	20	114	347	263	132
Gadsden County	44,007	30	459	1,393	1,056	711
Gilchrist County	13,819	13	152	461	350	195
Glades County	8,586	14	98	298	226	108
Gulf County	13,490	23	155	469	356	169
Hamilton County	12,680	10	134	408	309	198
Hardee County	21,041	18	221	671	509	334
Hendry County	29,392	20	297	901	683	510
Hernando County	126,590	214	1,531	4,645	3,522	1,301
Highlands County	74,918	138	906	2,749	2,084	770
Hillsborough County	925,413	774	10,278	31,177	23,640	12,755
Holmes County	18,623	22	206	624	473	261
Indian River County	99,112	157	1,186	3,597	2,727	1,065
Jackson County	44,498	36	495	1,500	1,138	612
Jefferson County	13,196	16	142	430	326	199
Lafayette County	6,318	6	71	217	164	83
Lake County	202,115	277	2,392	7,256	5,502	2,265
Lee County	392,909	525	4,661	14,139	10,721	4,363
Leon County	215,116	98	2,439	7,398	5,609	2,789
Levy County	31,685	49	355	1,077	817	425
Liberty County	6,732	14	76	231	175	88
Madison County	17,740	17	191	579	439	267
Manatee County	239,629	304	2,826	8,573	6,501	2,719
Marion County	241,269	316	2,794	8,476	6,427	2,919
Martin County	115,949	181	1,416	4,294	3,256	1,145
Miami-Dade County	2,150,877	1,208	24,221	73,471	55,708	28,469
Monroe County	80,853	81	989	2,999	2,274	793
Nassau County	55,405	49	600	1,821	1,380	817

Association	Population	Lung Cancer[1]	CHRONIC LUNG DISEASES			
			Emphysema	Chronic Bronchitis	Adult Asthma	Pediatric Asthma
Okaloosa County	168,532	162	1,840	5,580	4,231	2,436
Okeechobee County	31,971	47	336	1,020	773	507
Orange County	804,489	616	8,935	27,103	20,551	11,088
Osceola County	145,744	101	1,589	4,819	3,654	2,116
PalmBeach County	1,032,872	1,206	12,220	37,068	28,107	11,586
Pasco County	325,129	563	3,862	11,716	8,884	3,591
Pinellas County	877,273	1,078	10,559	32,030	24,287	9,203
Polk County	452,649	506	5,053	15,326	11,621	6,150
Putnam County	70,305	95	774	2,347	1,780	994
St. Johns County	116,065	114	1,330	4,035	3,059	1,454
St. Lucie County	179,360	231	2,044	6,200	4,701	2,288
Santa Rosa County	117,678	103	1,263	3,830	2,904	1,779
Sarasota County	303,341	473	3,784	11,478	8,703	2,712
Seminole County	350,489	242	3,848	11,673	8,851	4,988
Sumter County	41,524	57	480	1,456	1,104	505
Suwannee County	32,496	42	352	1,067	809	480
Taylor County	18,873	17	204	618	469	281
Union County	12,548	14	141	429	325	166
Volusia County	420,668	551	4,970	15,076	11,431	4,743
Wakulla County	18,613	20	197	598	453	291
Walton County	37,422	47	423	1,284	973	489
Washington County	20,239	29	226	684	519	276
AFFILIATES:						
ALA OF CENTRAL FLORIDA						
Lake County	202,115	277	2,392	7,256	5,502	2,265
Marion County	241,269	316	2,794	8,476	6,427	2,919
Orange County	804,489	616	8,935	27,103	20,551	11,088
Osceola County	145,744	101	1,589	4,819	3,654	2,116
Seminole County	350,489	242	3,848	11,673	8,851	4,988
Sumter County	41,524	57	480	1,456	1,104	505
ALA OF GULF COAST FLORIDA						
Charlotte County	134,763	229	1,683	5,104	3,870	1,200
Citrus County	113,640	220	1,385	4,202	3,186	1,130
Collier County	199,775	202	2,362	7,164	5,432	2,248
DeSoto County	24,708	26	277	839	636	333
Hardee County	21,041	18	221	671	509	334
Hernando County	126,590	214	1,531	4,645	3,522	1,301
Highlands County	74,918	138	906	2,749	2,084	770
Hillsborough County	925,413	774	10,278	31,177	23,640	12,755
Lee County	392,909	525	4,661	14,139	10,721	4,363
Levy County	31,685	49	355	1,077	817	425
Manatee County	239,629	304	2,826	8,573	6,501	2,719
Pasco County	325,129	563	3,862	11,716	8,884	3,591
Pinellas County	877,273	1,078	10,559	32,030	24,287	9,203
Polk County	452,649	506	5,053	15,326	11,621	6,150
Sarasota County	303,341	473	3,784	11,478	8,703	2,712
ALA OF SOUTH FLORIDA						
Broward County	1,507,770	1,381	17,450	52,932	40,135	18,290
Glades County	8,586	14	98	298	226	108
Hendry County	29,392	20	297	901	683	510
Miami-Dade County	2,150,877	1,208	24,221	73,471	55,708	28,469
Monroe County	80,853	81	989	2,999	2,274	793

TABLE 1 ESTIMATED PREVALENCE AND INCIDENCE OF LUNG DISEASE BY COUNTY,
STATE, AND LUNG ASSOCIATION, 1998 *(continued)*

Association	Population	Lung Cancer[1]	CHRONIC LUNG DISEASES			
			Emphysema	Chronic Bronchitis	Adult Asthma	Pediatric Asthma
ALA OF SOUTHEAST						
FLORIDA						
Indian River County	99,112	157	1,186	3,597	2,727	1,065
Martin County	115,949	181	1,416	4,294	3,256	1,145
Okeechobee County	31,971	47	336	1,020	773	507
PalmBeach County	1,032,872	1,206	12,220	37,068	28,107	11,586
St. Lucie County	179,360	231	2,044	6,200	4,701	2,288
GEORGIA						
CONSTITUENT:	7,636,522	5,091	84,156	255,274	193,563	107,578
ALA OF GEORGIA						
Appling County	16,547	20	177	536	407	253
Atkinson County	7,158	12	74	226	171	116
Bacon County	10,364	8	109	330	251	165
Baker County	3,627	1	39	117	89	55
Baldwin County	41,883	31	484	1,468	1,113	510
Banks County	12,821	10	142	430	326	179
Barrow County	40,438	29	435	1,319	1,000	608
Bartow County	71,937	48	785	2,381	1,805	1,041
Ben Hill County	17,471	9	182	552	419	283
Berrien County	16,317	21	177	537	407	240
Bibb County	155,946	140	1,728	5,241	3,974	2,165
Bleckley County	11,157	8	124	376	285	154
Brantley County	13,528	17	143	434	329	212
Brooks County	15,914	17	167	507	384	253
Bryan County	23,395	17	238	723	548	399
Bulloch County	50,554	22	578	1,753	1,329	639
Burke County	22,825	10	229	694	527	402
Butts County	17,822	12	198	602	456	244
Calhoun County	5,002	1	53	161	122	77
Camden County	47,322	18	493	1,495	1,133	768
Candler County	9,099	9	99	299	227	134
Carroll County	82,904	51	911	2,764	2,096	1,176
Catoosa County	50,709	46	568	1,723	1,307	682
Charlton County	9,433	12	98	297	225	154
Chatham County	225,297	203	2,495	7,567	5,738	3,132
Chattahoochee County	16,408	3	175	531	403	252
Chattooga County	22,748	39	256	777	589	301
Cherokee County	134,352	56	1,452	4,404	3,339	1,995
Clarke County	90,516	48	1,074	3,258	2,470	1,005
Clay County	3,493	3	38	114	86	53
Clayton County	208,997	116	2,266	6,873	5,212	3,076
Clinch County	6,649	3	70	212	161	106
Cobb County	566,060	259	6,369	19,318	14,648	7,513
Coffee County	34,230	27	360	1,091	827	545
Colquitt County	40,229	34	429	1,302	987	617
Columbia County	90,854	58	963	2,921	2,215	1,416
Cook County	14,988	14	160	486	369	228
Coweta County	85,118	42	913	2,769	2,099	1,289
Crawford County	10,655	3	115	349	265	158
Crisp County	20,693	30	218	661	501	327
Dade County	15,057	10	169	514	389	200
Dawson County	14,898	5	163	493	374	215
Decatur County	27,021	17	285	863	654	428
DeKalb County	592,870	290	6,771	20,539	15,574	7,511
Dodge County	18,120	22	202	613	464	247

Association	Population	Lung Cancer[1]	CHRONIC LUNG DISEASES			
			Emphysema	Chronic Bronchitis	Adult Asthma	Pediatric Asthma
Dooly County	10,409	6	109	330	250	167
Dougherty County	95,019	87	1,004	3,045	2,309	1,492
Douglas County	89,398	42	967	2,934	2,225	1,323
Early County	12,171	10	128	388	294	194
Echols County	2,361	4	25	75	57	38
Effingham County	36,565	26	380	1,154	875	595
Elbert County	19,322	23	214	648	491	270
Emanuel County	21,017	25	220	667	506	337
Evans County	9,923	8	105	319	242	154
Fannin County	18,575	22	217	658	499	218
Fayette County	88,733	40	960	2,913	2,208	1,313
Floyd County	85,138	78	975	2,956	2,242	1,071
Forsyth County	86,409	34	960	2,913	2,209	1,189
Franklin County	19,061	20	219	666	505	235
Fulton County	737,222	445	8,370	25,390	19,252	9,515
Gilmer County	18,747	17	213	647	491	240
Glascock County	2,514	0	29	88	67	31
Glynn County	67,187	57	752	2,282	1,730	904
Gordon County	41,078	27	453	1,373	1,041	579
Grady County	21,416	16	231	701	532	319
Greene County	13,663	5	143	433	328	220
Gwinnett County	522,666	164	5,670	17,199	13,041	7,682
Habersham County	31,734	26	365	1,109	841	391
Hall County	119,334	74	1,325	4,020	3,048	1,645
Hancock County	9,139	6	96	291	220	146
Haralson County	24,590	34	272	825	626	343
Harris County	22,297	18	251	763	578	294
Hart County	21,793	20	247	750	568	282
Heard County	10,088	9	108	329	249	152
Henry County	104,925	55	1,144	3,470	2,631	1,521
Houston County	105,638	75	1,148	3,483	2,641	1,545
Irwin County	9,048	9	97	294	223	138
Jackson County	37,711	36	416	1,263	958	528
Jasper County	10,166	9	110	334	253	150
Jeff Davis County	12,707	17	138	418	317	187
Jefferson County	17,829	16	188	569	432	282
Jenkins County	8,446	9	90	274	208	129
Johnson County	8,293	9	88	268	203	127
Jones County	22,997	14	251	762	578	332
Lamar County	14,700	14	164	497	376	201
Lanier County	6,988	9	74	224	170	110
Laurens County	43,687	46	472	1,431	1,085	650
Lee County	22,767	10	232	702	532	389
Liberty County	59,081	17	603	1,828	1,386	1,004
Lincoln County	8,226	6	91	277	210	114
Long County	8,576	10	88	268	203	142
Lowndes County	85,049	56	917	2,780	2,108	1,272
Lumpkin County	19,003	13	215	651	494	249
McDuffie County	21,697	22	232	703	533	332
McIntosh County	10,018	6	109	330	251	146
Macon County	13,207	8	137	414	314	218
Madison County	24,426	22	270	820	622	340
Marion County	6,703	4	72	217	165	102
Meriwether County	23,078	26	247	749	568	352
Miller County	6,360	5	69	211	160	92
Mitchell County	21,198	26	218	661	501	354
Monroe County	19,625	16	217	658	499	274
Montgomery County	7,725	1	85	259	196	108
Morgan County	15,092	12	165	499	379	218

TABLE 1 ESTIMATED PREVALENCE AND INCIDENCE OF LUNG DISEASE BY COUNTY,
STATE, AND LUNG ASSOCIATION, 1998 *(continued)*

Association	Population	Lung Cancer[1]	CHRONIC LUNG DISEASES			
			Emphysema	Chronic Bronchitis	Adult Asthma	Pediatric Asthma
ALA OF GEORGIA (cont.)						
Murray County	32,714	26	352	1,068	810	490
Muscogee County	182,414	125	2,006	6,085	4,614	2,584
Newton County	57,862	38	626	1,899	1,440	856
Oconee County	23,707	16	255	774	587	355
Oglethorpe County	11,437	9	127	385	292	158
Paulding County	73,888	35	781	2,369	1,796	1,159
Peach County	24,475	23	269	816	619	347
Pickens County	19,733	13	223	675	512	260
Pierce County	15,763	12	171	518	393	233
Pike County	12,667	12	139	423	321	179
Polk County	36,280	43	401	1,217	923	506
Pulaski County	8,412	3	93	281	213	119
Putnam County	17,561	18	197	599	454	234
Quitman County	2,488	3	28	84	64	34
Rabun County	13,380	14	158	480	364	150
Randolph County	7,954	6	84	255	194	124
Richmond County	191,374	161	2,111	6,404	4,856	2,688
Rockdale County	68,278	49	743	2,254	1,709	995
Schley County	3,953	3	42	127	97	61
Screven County	14,451	13	155	469	356	220
Seminole County	9,762	9	107	326	247	138
Spalding County	57,603	34	623	1,891	1,434	852
Stephens County	25,358	25	291	884	670	315
Stewart County	5,410	6	59	180	137	77
Sumter County	31,288	23	332	1,008	765	485
Talbot County	6,977	8	77	234	177	97
Taliaferro County	1,917	0	21	63	48	28
Tattnall County	19,039	23	215	652	494	250
Taylor County	8,228	8	89	271	205	121
Telfair County	11,537	12	125	378	286	172
Terrell County	11,142	18	118	357	271	175
Thomas County	42,891	36	461	1,399	1,061	645
Tift County	36,787	31	393	1,192	904	562
Toombs County	25,822	17	271	823	624	410
Towns County	8,477	6	107	324	245	72
Treutlen County	5,966	9	64	195	148	90
Troup County	58,574	60	634	1,924	1,459	865
Turner County	9,188	8	95	288	218	152
Twiggs County	10,116	5	107	325	246	158
Union County	16,506	14	195	591	448	186
Upson County	27,061	17	304	921	698	362
Walker County	62,690	79	705	2,137	1,621	835
Walton County	54,629	34	593	1,798	1,364	802
Ware County	35,414	32	392	1,189	901	493
Warren County	6,070	5	66	200	152	88
Washington County	20,055	21	214	650	493	306
Wayne County	25,360	29	272	824	625	385
Webster County	2,200	1	24	74	56	31
Wheeler County	4,900	5	52	159	120	75
White County	17,485	13	204	618	469	207
Whitfield County	82,042	58	908	2,754	2,088	1,143
Wilcox County	7,361	13	79	240	182	110
Wilkes County	10,606	12	118	359	272	144
Wilkinson County	10,863	6	116	351	266	168
Worth County	22,446	20	235	713	541	359

Association	Population	Lung Cancer[1]	CHRONIC LUNG DISEASES			
			Emphysema	Chronic Bronchitis	Adult Asthma	Pediatric Asthma
HAWAII CONSTITUENT: ALA OF HAWAII	1,190,472	631	13,424	40,717	30,873	15,696
Hawaii County	141,805	98	1,529	4,638	3,517	2,117
Honolulu County	871,768	452	9,956	30,199	22,898	11,048
Kalawao County	67	N/A	1	2	2	1
Kauai County	56,208	26	613	1,859	1,409	815
Maui County	120,624	55	1,325	4,019	3,047	1,715
IDAHO/NEVADA CONSTITUENT: ALA OF IDAHO/ NEVADA	2,974,695	2,012	32,321	98,030	74,330	43,550
IDAHO	1,230,923	667	13,185	39,988	30,321	18,693
Ada County	275,623	114	3,037	9,211	6,984	3,886
Adams County	3,785	0	42	128	97	52
Bannock County	74,272	40	779	2,364	1,792	1,185
Bear Lake County	6,511	6	64	193	147	120
Benewah County	9,088	9	99	300	228	132
Bingham County	41,825	14	400	1,213	920	805
Blaine County	17,203	6	195	591	448	224
Boise County	5,121	3	57	172	130	72
Bonner County	35,338	29	389	1,181	895	499
Bonneville County	80,699	32	819	2,483	1,883	1,387
Boundary County	9,820	9	103	314	238	156
Butte County	3,041	1	31	93	71	53
Camas County	841	0	9	27	20	13
Canyon County	120,385	66	1,262	3,828	2,902	1,926
Caribou County	7,403	4	73	220	167	136
Cassia County	21,324	10	209	634	481	393
Clark County	889	0	10	29	22	13
Clearwater County	9,347	5	108	327	248	115
Custer County	4,091	1	45	135	102	60
Elmore County	25,359	14	267	810	614	401
Franklin County	11,113	1	104	315	239	222
Fremont County	11,933	3	117	354	268	220
Gem County	14,849	9	164	496	376	209
Gooding County	13,658	5	146	443	336	208
Idaho County	15,007	12	167	508	385	204
Jefferson County	19,534	9	181	550	417	395
Jerome County	17,957	6	186	564	428	295
Kootenai County	101,305	99	1,137	3,449	2,615	1,355
Latah County	32,667	9	386	1,172	889	367
Lemhi County	8,041	1	89	271	206	111
Lewis County	3,995	3	44	134	102	55
Lincoln County	3,778	0	40	121	92	60
Madison County	25,125	3	268	813	617	385
Minidoka County	20,205	6	202	612	464	358
Nez Perce County	36,842	38	429	1,301	986	438
Oneida County	4,030	1	39	120	91	74
Owyhee County	10,254	8	105	317	241	174
Payette County	20,450	22	217	658	499	317
Power County	8,412	4	84	254	192	151
Shoshone County	13,863	20	158	480	364	176
Teton County	5,490	0	55	168	128	95
Twin Falls County	62,222	35	669	2,029	1,538	936
Valley County	8,010	4	90	272	206	108
Washington County	10,218	6	110	334	253	152

TABLE 1 ESTIMATED PREVALENCE AND INCIDENCE OF LUNG DISEASE BY COUNTY,
STATE, AND LUNG ASSOCIATION, 1998 (continued)

			CHRONIC LUNG DISEASES			
Association	Population	Lung Cancer[1]	Emphysema	Chronic Bronchitis	Adult Asthma	Pediatric Asthma
NEVADA	1,743,772	1,345	19,136	58,042	44,009	24,857
Churchill County	23,147	13	241	730	554	377
Clark County	1,161,259	910	12,764	38,717	29,357	16,479
Douglas County	36,815	31	407	1,234	935	515
Elko County	46,021	14	444	1,346	1,021	873
Esmeralda County	1,150	0	13	39	30	15
Eureka County	1,990	1	21	64	49	31
Humboldt County	18,083	6	179	544	412	326
Lander County	6,972	3	66	200	151	137
Lincoln County	4,178	4	41	124	94	77
Lyon County	30,131	30	320	970	735	468
Mineral County	5,332	3	57	172	131	82
Nye County	28,657	42	327	991	751	365
Pershing County	4,834	1	48	146	110	87
Storey County	2,951	5	33	100	76	39
Washoe County	313,008	237	3,503	10,626	8,057	4,220
White Pine County	10,081	5	109	330	250	150
Carson City[2]	49,163	40	563	1,709	1,296	616
ILLINOIS CONSTITUENTS:	12,069,774	8,691	133,349	404,487	306,704	168,852
ALA OF METROPOLITAN CHICAGO						
Cook County	5,192,396	3,689	57,647	174,862	132,587	71,647
ALA OF ILLINOIS						
Adams County	67,324	69	749	2,273	1,724	922
Alexander County	10,057	14	107	326	247	154
Bond County	17,287	8	201	609	461	208
Boone County	38,748	16	416	1,263	958	583
Brown County	6,882	10	83	251	190	72
Bureau County	35,477	26	391	1,187	900	498
Calhoun County	4,903	3	56	169	128	63
Carroll County	16,897	17	190	576	437	225
Cass County	13,270	18	148	447	339	182
Champaign County	169,835	98	1,980	6,006	4,554	2,009
Christian County	35,800	36	405	1,230	932	466
Clark County	16,516	18	186	564	428	219
Clay County	14,479	14	161	490	371	197
Clinton County	35,674	30	393	1,192	904	503
Coles County	51,960	42	616	1,870	1,418	577
Crawford County	20,950	16	239	726	551	265
Cumberland County	11,118	9	120	363	276	166
DeKalb County	85,896	42	1,004	3,045	2,309	1,007
De Witt County	16,737	16	186	565	428	229
Douglas County	19,885	13	215	651	494	296
DuPage County	880,996	406	9,729	29,513	22,378	12,339
Edgar County	19,780	27	221	669	508	269
Edwards County	6,950	5	79	239	181	91
Effingham County	33,536	20	352	1,068	810	534
Fayette County	22,125	20	249	755	572	294
Ford County	14,068	13	156	474	360	193
Franklin County	40,456	53	459	1,391	1,055	525
Fulton County	38,712	43	441	1,339	1,015	493
Gallatin County	6,627	9	76	230	175	83

Association	Population	Lung Cancer[1]	CHRONIC LUNG DISEASES			
			Emphysema	Chronic Bronchitis	Adult Asthma	Pediatric Asthma
Greene County	15,735	9	173	526	399	222
Grundy County	36,748	31	398	1,206	915	544
Hamilton County	8,616	13	98	296	225	112
Hancock County	21,153	23	236	715	543	288
Hardin County	4,932	10	57	172	131	61
Henderson County	8,621	8	96	292	221	117
Henry County	51,542	48	566	1,717	1,302	733
Iroquois County	31,274	35	348	1,056	801	428
Jackson County	60,851	36	732	2,219	1,683	641
Jasper County	10,635	6	114	345	261	163
Jefferson County	39,040	47	433	1,313	996	541
Jersey County	21,515	20	236	716	543	306
Jo Daviess County	21,502	20	240	729	553	291
Johnson County	13,546	10	164	497	377	139
Kane County	391,686	194	4,063	12,325	9,345	6,415
Kankakee County	102,318	87	1,094	3,320	2,517	1,559
Kendall County	51,793	27	546	1,655	1,255	818
Knox County	55,606	46	638	1,936	1,468	693
Lake County	608,348	303	6,582	19,964	15,138	9,004
La Salle County	110,193	108	1,229	3,727	2,826	1,502
Lawrence County	15,325	23	174	529	401	196
Lee County	35,973	29	401	1,215	922	492
Livingston County	39,641	25	443	1,344	1,019	536
Logan County	31,892	25	370	1,122	850	385
McDonough County	35,480	29	434	1,315	997	349
McHenry County	241,046	133	2,555	7,750	5,876	3,756
McLean County	143,366	87	1,637	4,966	3,765	1,817
Macon County	113,675	134	1,268	3,845	2,916	1,549
Macoupin County	48,753	43	541	1,641	1,244	674
Madison County	259,185	265	2,891	8,768	6,648	3,530
Marion County	41,932	55	461	1,397	1,059	596
Marshall County	12,895	8	145	440	334	171
Mason County	16,833	14	187	566	429	233
Massac County	15,528	18	176	535	406	200
Menard County	12,525	6	136	412	313	184
Mercer County	17,622	9	194	589	446	249
Monroe County	26,640	14	293	889	674	378
Montgomery County	31,440	31	353	1,071	812	419
Morgan County	35,412	48	404	1,226	929	450
Moultrie County	14,455	8	159	482	366	205
Ogle County	50,522	34	549	1,664	1,262	741
Peoria County	181,505	139	2,009	6,094	4,621	2,526
Perry County	21,261	22	236	717	544	292
Piatt County	16,430	16	184	558	423	221
Pike County	17,278	20	194	588	446	231
Pope County	4,777	4	55	166	126	59
Pulaski County	7,286	13	77	233	177	115
Putnam County	5,804	8	65	196	149	79
Randolph County	33,675	40	382	1,159	879	436
Richland County	16,782	14	186	565	428	232
Rock Island County	147,920	143	1,651	5,008	3,798	2,010
St. Clair County	261,792	182	2,795	8,480	6,430	4,005
Saline County	26,184	40	297	900	682	341
Sangamon County	191,487	155	2,135	6,476	4,910	2,610
Schuyler County	7,569	9	85	258	196	101
Scott County	5,616	10	62	188	142	79
Shelby County	22,686	10	252	764	579	313
Stark County	6,315	5	71	214	163	85
Stephenson County	48,868	31	544	1,651	1,252	668

**TABLE 1 ESTIMATED PREVALENCE AND INCIDENCE OF LUNG DISEASE BY COUNTY,
STATE, AND LUNG ASSOCIATION, 1998 (continued)**

Association	Population	Lung Cancer[1]	CHRONIC LUNG DISEASES			
			Emphysema	Chronic Bronchitis	Adult Asthma	Pediatric Asthma
ALA OF ILLINOIS (cont.)						
Tazewell County	129,324	105	1,444	4,381	3,321	1,755
Union County	18,003	20	206	625	474	227
Vermilion County	84,469	100	940	2,852	2,162	1,157
Wabash County	12,567	12	140	425	322	172
Warren County	18,919	16	211	641	486	256
Washington County	15,301	18	168	511	388	216
Wayne County	16,958	13	192	582	441	221
White County	15,603	17	179	543	412	195
Whiteside County	59,829	65	658	1,995	1,513	848
Will County	460,225	248	4,830	14,650	11,108	7,341
Williamson County	61,348	62	699	2,121	1,608	783
Winnebago County	267,665	212	2,956	8,968	6,800	3,748
Woodford County	35,193	23	377	1,143	867	534
INDIANA CONSTITUENT:	5,907,617	4,861	65,818	199,648	151,379	80,699
ALA OF INDIANA						
Adams County	33,019	9	340	1,032	783	548
Allen County	314,422	235	3,436	10,423	7,903	4,532
Bartholomew County	69,432	43	781	2,368	1,796	923
Benton County	9,756	10	106	321	243	144
Blackford County	13,946	6	158	478	363	182
Boone County	43,851	36	482	1,463	1,109	621
Brown County	15,948	12	182	552	419	202
Carroll County	20,004	20	222	674	511	276
Cass County	38,830	31	432	1,311	994	532
Clark County	93,991	101	1,059	3,213	2,436	1,242
Clay County	26,725	30	297	899	682	369
Clinton County	33,192	30	362	1,098	832	481
Crawford County	10,589	14	116	352	267	151
Daviess County	28,945	30	310	939	712	441
Dearborn County	47,169	29	509	1,543	1,170	704
Decatur County	25,558	16	275	833	632	385
De Kalb County	39,308	32	422	1,280	970	594
Delaware County	116,334	98	1,371	4,158	3,152	1,325
Dubois County	39,651	25	431	1,308	992	579
Elkhart County	172,718	95	1,869	5,670	4,299	2,555
Fayette County	26,025	22	290	880	667	355
Floyd County	71,819	75	798	2,422	1,837	987
Fountain County	18,328	27	205	623	472	246
Franklin County	21,819	21	233	708	537	333
Fulton County	20,665	16	229	693	526	288
Gibson County	32,161	25	362	1,097	832	428
Grant County	72,652	81	835	2,532	1,920	903
Greene County	33,328	20	375	1,137	862	443
Hamilton County	162,772	64	1,755	5,322	4,035	2,432
Hancock County	54,495	47	602	1,826	1,385	763
Harrison County	34,618	21	377	1,143	866	505
Hendricks County	95,533	69	1,052	3,191	2,420	1,349
Henry County	48,690	51	557	1,689	1,281	614
Howard County	83,410	91	931	2,824	2,141	1,133
Huntington County	37,291	32	407	1,236	937	538

Association	Population	Lung Cancer[1]	CHRONIC LUNG DISEASES Emphysema	Chronic Bronchitis	Adult Asthma	Pediatric Asthma
Jackson County	41,044	31	452	1,372	1,041	578
Jasper County	29,070	22	312	948	719	437
Jay County	21,715	23	242	733	556	297
Jefferson County	31,452	23	356	1,080	819	410
Jennings County	27,754	23	305	925	701	394
Johnson County	109,390	74	1,209	3,666	2,780	1,530
Knox County	39,261	52	454	1,377	1,044	478
Kosciusko County	71,151	57	769	2,332	1,768	1,057
Lagrange County	33,393	12	330	1,000	758	606
Lake County	480,969	410	5,246	15,912	12,065	6,970
La Porte County	109,844	78	1,243	3,772	2,860	1,431
Lawrence County	45,695	49	515	1,563	1,185	602
Madison County	131,236	146	1,498	4,545	3,446	1,665
Marion County	812,662	731	9,119	27,660	20,973	10,872
Marshall County	45,568	31	493	1,495	1,134	674
Martin County	10,470	12	116	352	267	145
Miami County	33,510	32	363	1,103	836	493
Monroe County	116,569	64	1,427	4,329	3,282	1,138
Montgomery County	36,464	31	412	1,249	947	479
Morgan County	65,560	61	719	2,180	1,653	937
Newton County	14,798	12	158	480	364	226
Noble County	42,607	31	454	1,378	1,045	655
Ohio County	5,447	12	61	185	140	73
Orange County	19,592	23	216	656	498	274
Owen County	20,431	29	227	687	521	283
Parke County	16,852	16	192	583	442	214
Perry County	19,308	13	216	657	498	259
Pike County	12,899	9	147	447	339	163
Porter County	146,253	95	1,609	4,881	3,701	2,070
Posey County	26,454	20	289	876	664	382
Pulaski County	13,431	9	145	440	334	200
Putnam County	34,551	26	398	1,208	916	425
Randolph County	27,503	25	308	935	709	369
Ripley County	27,251	26	294	890	675	408
Rush County	18,238	22	199	603	457	265
St. Joseph County	258,185	203	2,907	8,818	6,686	3,419
Scott County	23,055	21	252	763	578	334
Shelby County	43,329	32	477	1,447	1,097	612
Spencer County	21,017	18	230	699	530	300
Starke County	23,935	23	260	789	598	350
Steuben County	31,447	13	350	1,061	805	431
Sullivan County	21,354	26	246	747	566	262
Switzerland County	8,838	6	97	294	223	126
Tippecanoe County	141,274	83	1,677	5,086	3,856	1,567
Tipton County	16,654	12	187	566	429	224
Union County	7,236	12	79	240	182	104
Vanderburgh County	167,736	155	1,936	5,872	4,452	2,054
Vermillion County	16,946	21	191	581	440	222
Vigo County	104,963	113	1,214	3,684	2,793	1,275
Wabash County	34,572	9	387	1,173	889	467
Warren County	8,336	8	93	282	214	113
Warrick County	51,556	48	561	1,703	1,291	750
Washington County	27,800	20	303	920	698	402
Wayne County	71,462	70	809	2,453	1,860	931
Wells County	26,849	29	292	885	671	393
White County	25,329	27	279	847	642	357
Whitley County	30,358	18	330	1,001	759	444

TABLE 1 ESTIMATED PREVALENCE AND INCIDENCE OF LUNG DISEASE BY COUNTY,
STATE, AND LUNG ASSOCIATION, 1998 *(continued)*

Association	Population	Lung Cancer[1]	CHRONIC LUNG DISEASES			
			Emphysema	Chronic Bronchitis	Adult Asthma	Pediatric Asthma
IOWA						
CONSTITUENT:	2,861,025	2,249	32,082	97,300	73,776	38,367
ALA OF IOWA						
Adair County	8,103	9	92	278	210	106
Adams County	4,386	3	50	153	116	55
Allamakee County	14,052	0	155	470	357	197
Appanoose County	13,568	9	153	463	351	180
Audubon County	6,806	6	77	234	178	88
Benton County	25,399	26	277	839	636	370
Black Hawk County	120,918	116	1,367	4,146	3,144	1,582
Boone County	26,113	23	297	899	682	337
Bremer County	23,343	10	265	805	611	300
Buchanan County	21,152	14	222	673	510	338
Buena Vista County	19,412	6	218	662	502	258
Butler County	15,631	10	175	530	402	212
Calhoun County	11,373	14	130	393	298	145
Carroll County	21,616	21	231	700	531	330
Cass County	14,642	6	165	501	380	193
Cedar County	17,957	12	200	606	459	246
Cerro Gordo County	46,073	62	526	1,597	1,211	583
Cherokee County	13,190	10	147	445	338	181
Chickasaw County	13,425	8	146	443	336	196
Clarke County	8,303	6	93	282	213	112
Clay County	17,474	17	193	586	445	243
Clayton County	18,711	12	204	620	470	270
Clinton County	49,924	40	555	1,685	1,278	685
Crawford County	16,462	12	181	548	415	235
Dallas County	36,865	22	400	1,214	920	541
Davis County	8,462	1	93	282	213	121
Decatur County	8,241	10	96	290	220	99
Delaware County	18,541	9	196	594	450	291
Des Moines County	42,069	32	475	1,440	1,092	554
Dickinson County	16,209	10	188	570	432	196
Dubuque County	87,879	69	975	2,958	2,243	1,214
Emmet County	10,850	12	121	368	279	147
Fayette County	21,794	26	243	737	559	297
Floyd County	16,369	18	184	558	423	218
Franklin County	10,865	4	122	371	281	144
Fremont County	7,771	10	87	263	199	106
Greene County	10,075	10	115	348	264	128
Grundy County	12,234	5	138	418	317	162
Guthrie County	11,506	10	131	396	300	149
Hamilton County	16,010	18	181	548	415	211
Hancock County	12,044	8	131	398	302	175
Hardin County	18,350	23	209	633	480	236
Harrison County	15,336	18	169	512	388	217
Henry County	20,038	20	227	688	521	261
Howard County	9,680	6	107	324	245	136
Humboldt County	10,327	14	117	354	268	136
Ida County	7,917	1	87	263	200	113
Iowa County	15,513	9	174	527	400	208
Jackson County	20,139	26	221	669	507	288
Jasper County	36,541	36	416	1,261	956	469
Jefferson County	17,043	13	194	589	447	217
Johnson County	102,556	36	1,231	3,735	2,832	1,087
Jones County	20,138	9	226	687	521	268

Association	Population	Lung Cancer[1]	CHRONIC LUNG DISEASES			
			Emphysema	Chronic Bronchitis	Adult Asthma	Pediatric Asthma
Keokuk County	11,469	9	128	389	295	155
Kossuth County	17,721	12	194	588	446	255
Lee County	38,488	44	432	1,311	994	513
Linn County	182,779	136	2,071	6,283	4,764	2,373
Louisa County	11,935	12	131	397	301	170
Lucas County	9,098	3	104	316	239	115
Lyon County	12,036	10	128	387	294	187
Madison County	13,888	13	151	458	347	203
Mahaska County	21,899	21	243	738	560	301
Marion County	31,327	18	351	1,063	806	422
Marshall County	38,740	53	439	1,330	1,009	504
Mills County	14,481	9	158	479	363	210
Mitchell County	11,033	13	123	374	284	149
Monona County	10,068	12	115	349	264	128
Monroe County	8,033	13	90	274	207	107
Montgomery County	11,850	13	134	408	309	154
Muscatine County	40,991	26	445	1,349	1,023	602
O'Brien County	14,887	12	165	502	380	205
Osceola County	6,956	4	77	233	176	98
Page County	17,271	25	199	602	457	214
Palo Alto County	10,059	8	112	340	258	138
Plymouth County	24,609	18	263	799	606	375
Pocahontas County	8,815	20	99	301	228	117
Polk County	359,713	255	4,066	12,332	9,351	4,709
Pottawattamie County	86,190	84	951	2,885	2,188	1,210
Poweshiek County	18,759	16	215	651	494	236
Ringgold County	5,358	3	62	188	143	65
Sac County	11,893	9	132	401	304	164
Scott County	158,333	110	1,727	5,239	3,972	2,294
Shelby County	12,934	5	144	436	330	178
Sioux County	31,425	13	337	1,022	775	476
Story County	74,875	31	901	2,734	2,073	785
Tama County	17,766	14	199	603	457	240
Taylor County	7,149	5	80	242	184	97
Union County	12,522	10	140	424	322	170
Van Buren County	7,862	1	88	266	202	106
Wapello County	35,387	21	406	1,232	934	441
Warren County	40,209	26	440	1,334	1,012	578
Washington County	20,938	8	232	702	533	292
Wayne County	6,677	9	77	233	176	83
Webster County	38,975	44	438	1,330	1,008	517
Winnebago County	11,942	6	135	410	310	156
Winneshiek County	20,962	14	240	729	553	262
Woodbury County	101,547	99	1,099	3,332	2,527	1,503
Worth County	7,742	5	88	266	202	101
Wright County	14,039	20	160	486	369	178
KANSAS CONSTITUENT: *ALA OF KANSAS*	2,638,667	2,001	29,116	88,318	66,968	37,044
Allen County	14,532	21	159	483	366	208
Anderson County	8,046	6	89	269	204	113
Atchison County	16,858	22	184	557	423	245
Barber County	5,336	4	59	179	136	74
Barton County	28,936	25	320	971	736	404
Bourbon County	15,160	8	169	512	388	208
Brown County	11,040	8	120	364	276	161
Butler County	61,883	46	667	2,024	1,535	924
Chase County	2,941	4	33	100	76	40

TABLE 1 ESTIMATED PREVALENCE AND INCIDENCE OF LUNG DISEASE BY COUNTY,
STATE, AND LUNG ASSOCIATION, 1998 *(continued)*

Association	Population	Lung Cancer[1]	CHRONIC LUNG DISEASES			
			Emphysema	Chronic Bronchitis	Adult Asthma	Pediatric Asthma
ALA OF KANSAS (cont.)						
Chautauqua County	4,343	8	50	152	115	54
Cherokee County	22,499	27	248	752	570	317
Cheyenne County	3,160	5	36	109	83	40
Clark County	2,353	0	26	80	61	31
Clay County	9,086	10	101	307	233	124
Cloud County	10,062	10	117	355	269	120
Coffey County	8,680	8	94	286	217	127
Comanche County	2,002	3	23	69	53	25
Cowley County	37,092	32	411	1,246	945	515
Crawford County	36,360	46	418	1,267	961	452
Decatur County	3,446	3	39	118	89	45
Dickinson County	19,602	21	218	662	502	268
Doniphan County	7,872	3	88	267	203	106
Douglas County	96,554	29	1,149	3,486	2,643	1,059
Edwards County	3,287	8	37	112	85	43
Elk County	3,386	5	39	120	91	40
Ellis County	26,585	16	299	906	687	354
Ellsworth County	6,277	6	73	221	167	76
Finney County	36,621	16	359	1,088	825	675
Ford County	29,461	16	310	941	713	466
Franklin County	24,853	21	268	813	616	371
Geary County	25,226	18	273	827	627	374
Gove County	3,045	6	34	103	78	42
Graham County	3,189	6	36	109	83	42
Grant County	7,996	4	78	238	180	147
Gray County	5,575	3	57	173	131	94
Greeley County	1,694	3	18	54	41	27
Greenwood County	8,101	18	92	279	212	105
Hamilton County	2,369	5	27	81	61	32
Harper County	6,411	9	73	220	167	83
Harvey County	34,148	22	380	1,153	874	467
Haskell County	3,962	4	40	122	93	68
Hodgeman County	2,215	0	24	73	55	32
Jackson County	12,111	13	131	398	302	179
Jefferson County	18,175	17	199	603	457	262
Jewell County	3,873	4	45	135	102	48
Johnson County	429,649	230	4,760	14,438	10,948	5,964
Kearny County	4,138	1	42	126	96	73
Kingman County	8,559	5	93	284	215	124
Kiowa County	3,420	1	38	116	88	46
Labette County	23,050	13	255	773	586	321
Lane County	2,245	0	25	75	57	32
Leavenworth County	71,178	56	783	2,376	1,802	1,006
Lincoln County	3,331	1	38	115	87	43
Linn County	9,166	6	102	309	234	127
Logan County	2,990	1	33	101	77	41
Lyon County	33,785	25	370	1,121	850	485
McPherson County	28,549	10	319	967	733	388
Marion County	13,609	16	157	475	360	168
Marshall County	10,994	10	122	369	280	153
Meade County	4,431	1	48	146	111	64
Miami County	26,456	17	287	872	661	388
Mitchell County	6,950	3	77	233	177	97
Montgomery County	37,046	39	415	1,258	954	500
Morris County	6,155	9	69	210	159	82

Association	Population	Lung Cancer[1]	CHRONIC LUNG DISEASES			
			Emphysema	Chronic Bronchitis	Adult Asthma	Pediatric Asthma
Morton County	3,428	1	36	109	83	55
Nemaha County	10,205	9	110	333	253	153
Neosho County	16,706	26	187	566	429	227
Ness County	3,628	8	41	123	93	49
Norton County	5,735	4	67	204	154	67
Osage County	17,158	8	187	568	431	248
Osborne County	4,680	1	53	162	123	60
Ottawa County	5,881	0	65	198	150	81
Pawnee County	7,245	13	82	247	188	96
Phillips County	6,036	4	68	207	157	79
Pottawatomie County	18,638	22	197	598	453	292
Pratt County	9,682	10	108	328	249	131
Rawlins County	3,130	4	35	107	81	42
Reno County	63,241	44	712	2,160	1,637	838
Republic County	6,098	6	70	214	162	74
Rice County	10,427	8	116	352	267	143
Riley County	63,940	20	751	2,278	1,727	737
Rooks County	5,688	3	63	191	144	80
Rush County	3,405	10	40	121	92	39
Russell County	7,535	4	88	266	202	89
Saline County	51,399	46	571	1,732	1,314	707
Scott County	5,023	5	52	159	120	82
Sedgwick County	447,819	318	4,868	14,767	11,197	6,546
Seward County	20,072	21	204	619	470	343
Shawnee County	170,349	148	1,904	5,776	4,380	2,305
Sheridan County	2,721	3	30	90	68	40
Sherman County	6,556	1	73	221	167	90
Smith County	4,594	4	54	163	124	54
Stafford County	5,049	5	56	170	129	70
Stanton County	2,244	0	23	70	53	38
Stevens County	5,415	5	56	170	129	89
Sumner County	27,197	22	289	878	666	419
Thomas County	8,030	3	87	263	200	119
Trego County	3,293	8	37	111	84	45
Wabaunsee County	6,613	5	73	221	167	93
Wallace County	1,812	3	19	59	45	27
Washington County	6,512	9	73	223	169	86
Wichita County	2,646	1	27	83	63	44
Wilson County	10,266	20	114	347	263	140
Woodson County	3,946	6	45	136	103	51
Wyandotte County	152,521	150	1,642	4,980	3,776	2,287
KENTUCKY CONSTITUENT: ALA OF KENTUCKY	3,934,310	4,019	44,392	134,655	102,097	51,766
Adair County	16,451	20	189	572	434	206
Allen County	16,567	25	185	561	425	225
Anderson County	18,501	18	206	626	475	252
Ballard County	8,489	14	99	299	227	102
Barren County	36,971	35	422	1,281	972	468
Bath County	10,586	8	120	365	277	136
Bell County	29,155	46	324	984	746	400
Boone County	79,761	51	861	2,611	1,980	1,188
Bourbon County	19,337	14	218	660	500	257
Boyd County	49,514	69	580	1,759	1,334	576
Boyle County	27,102	30	313	949	719	332
Bracken County	8,419	14	94	286	217	113
Breathitt County	15,728	38	171	519	393	230
Breckinridge County	17,455	25	196	596	452	232

TABLE 1 ESTIMATED PREVALENCE AND INCIDENCE OF LUNG DISEASE BY COUNTY,
STATE, AND LUNG ASSOCIATION, 1998 *(continued)*

Association	Population	Lung Cancer[1]	CHRONIC LUNG DISEASES			
			Emphysema	Chronic Bronchitis	Adult Asthma	Pediatric Asthma
ALA OF KENTUCKY						
(cont.)						
Bullitt County	59,344	40	643	1,951	1,479	874
Butler County	11,932	21	133	405	307	161
Caldwell County	13,335	12	154	469	355	161
Calloway County	33,422	43	406	1,231	933	338
Campbell County	87,301	78	972	2,950	2,237	1,193
Carlisle County	5,337	6	62	187	141	66
Carroll County	9,624	12	107	324	245	133
Carter County	26,900	25	301	912	691	364
Casey County	14,788	25	166	503	382	198
Christian County	72,436	60	805	2,441	1,851	997
Clark County	31,941	35	362	1,098	833	414
Clay County	22,760	25	242	733	556	353
Clinton County	9,347	12	107	325	246	117
Crittenden County	9,587	13	109	331	251	123
Cumberland County	6,848	13	80	241	183	82
Daviess County	90,973	101	1,014	3,077	2,333	1,240
Edmonson County	11,347	6	128	388	294	150
Elliott County	6,593	12	71	216	164	98
Estill County	15,581	9	174	529	401	210
Fayette County	241,697	185	2,844	8,627	6,542	2,766
Fleming County	13,478	12	153	463	351	175
Floyd County	43,324	49	470	1,425	1,081	637
Franklin County	46,501	39	539	1,635	1,239	562
Fulton County	7,548	9	86	260	197	98
Gallatin County	7,182	10	78	237	180	105
Garrard County	13,920	9	160	486	368	172
Grant County	20,314	16	219	666	505	302
Graves County	35,966	46	413	1,253	950	447
Grayson County	23,736	23	267	809	613	316
Green County	10,565	10	123	375	284	124
Greenup County	36,970	49	423	1,284	974	464
Hancock County	8,963	10	97	293	222	134
Hardin County	90,576	74	989	3,001	2,275	1,308
Harlan County	34,820	43	379	1,149	871	508
Harrison County	17,542	22	195	593	449	240
Hart County	16,723	20	188	570	432	223
Henderson County	44,482	30	499	1,513	1,147	596
Henry County	14,774	12	167	507	384	193
Hickman County	5,197	6	60	183	139	62
Hopkins County	46,380	55	523	1,586	1,203	612
Jackson County	12,931	10	140	424	322	191
Jefferson County	671,595	719	7,743	23,487	17,809	8,252
Jessamine County	36,577	22	405	1,229	932	508
Johnson County	23,986	17	266	808	613	331
Kenton County	146,731	140	1,615	4,899	3,715	2,074
Knott County	17,948	23	194	588	446	267
Knox County	31,890	53	347	1,051	797	467
Larue County	13,067	14	149	452	343	166
Laurel County	50,847	38	561	1,700	1,289	715
Lawrence County	15,606	14	170	517	392	225
Lee County	8,029	12	90	273	207	108
Leslie County	13,589	22	145	440	334	208
Letcher County	26,237	29	286	867	657	382
Lewis County	13,513	5	149	451	342	191

Association	Population	Lung Cancer[1]	CHRONIC LUNG DISEASES			
			Emphysema	Chronic Bronchitis	Adult Asthma	Pediatric Asthma
Lincoln County	22,403	36	250	758	575	305
Livingston County	9,440	10	111	337	255	108
Logan County	26,195	29	294	891	676	351
Lyon County	8,009	8	102	308	234	66
McCracken County	64,405	87	742	2,250	1,706	794
McCreary County	16,634	29	176	535	406	259
McLean County	9,841	18	112	341	258	125
Madison County	66,454	55	780	2,365	1,794	768
Magoffin County	13,846	8	146	442	335	220
Marion County	17,038	13	188	571	433	238
Marshall County	30,174	51	354	1,073	814	350
Martin County	12,083	9	127	384	291	193
Mason County	16,913	21	191	579	439	222
Meade County	28,732	13	292	887	672	491
Menifee County	5,774	4	64	193	146	81
Mercer County	20,664	22	237	720	546	257
Metcalfe County	9,573	8	110	333	252	120
Monroe County	11,143	13	128	388	294	139
Montgomery County	21,006	30	236	716	543	280
Morgan County	13,575	12	154	466	353	177
Muhlenberg County	32,060	52	363	1,101	835	417
Nelson County	35,929	36	388	1,176	892	535
Nicholas County	7,007	8	80	241	183	90
Ohio County	22,013	46	244	741	562	304
Oldham County	44,436	22	485	1,470	1,114	644
Owen County	10,350	16	115	349	264	143
Owsley County	5,398	8	60	182	138	74
Pendleton County	13,735	9	148	449	341	205
Perry County	30,995	35	338	1,026	778	448
Pike County	72,020	88	796	2,415	1,831	1,006
Powell County	12,913	10	137	417	316	199
Pulaski County	56,313	46	648	1,966	1,491	696
Robertson County	2,206	3	25	77	58	27
Rockcastle County	15,923	14	178	539	409	216
Rowan County	22,118	16	265	804	610	236
Russell County	16,182	13	188	571	433	193
Scott County	30,782	26	340	1,033	783	429
Shelby County	29,640	21	336	1,020	773	384
Simpson County	16,467	12	183	556	422	225
Spencer County	9,665	3	107	325	246	134
Taylor County	22,981	25	264	801	607	286
Todd County	11,263	9	126	381	289	153
Henderson County	44,482	30	499	1,513	1,147	596
Trigg County	12,409	20	146	442	335	144
Trimble County	7,685	4	86	260	197	105
Union County	16,546	21	180	546	414	242
Warren County	87,310	56	1,007	3,055	2,316	1,071
Washington County	10,892	17	121	368	279	149
Wayne County	19,056	23	212	643	487	262
Webster County	13,537	25	152	460	349	181
Whitley County	35,827	30	398	1,207	915	494
Wolfe County	7,383	14	80	242	183	110
Woodford County	22,731	13	256	775	588	302
LOUISIANA CONSTITUENT: ALA OF LOUISIANA	4,362,758	3,657	47,449	143,928	109,136	63,692
Acadia Parish	57,814	46	605	1,836	1,392	928
Allen Parish	24,204	23	273	829	629	317

TABLE 1 ESTIMATED PREVALENCE AND INCIDENCE OF LUNG DISEASE BY COUNTY,
STATE, AND LUNG ASSOCIATION, 1998 *(continued)*

Association	Population	Lung Cancer[1]	CHRONIC LUNG DISEASES			
			Emphysema	Chronic Bronchitis	Adult Asthma	Pediatric Asthma
ALA OF LOUISIANA						
(cont.)						
Ascension Parish	71,679	46	746	2,262	1,715	1,167
Assumption Parish	23,023	17	242	733	556	368
Avoyelles Parish	40,786	36	444	1,347	1,021	594
Beauregard Parish	31,977	25	348	1,056	800	466
Bienville Parish	15,799	9	174	527	400	224
Bossier Parish	92,334	68	1,006	3,053	2,315	1,340
Caddo Parish	242,484	213	2,659	8,066	6,116	3,463
Calcasieu Parish	180,111	153	1,961	5,948	4,510	2,622
Caldwell Parish	10,377	20	113	342	260	151
Cameron Parish	9,034	10	97	294	223	137
Catahoula Parish	11,050	10	118	359	272	168
Claiborne Parish	17,027	17	195	590	448	215
Concordia Parish	20,752	20	222	674	511	316
De Soto Parish	24,984	25	269	816	619	374
East Baton Rouge Parish	393,656	238	4,374	13,267	10,060	5,420
East Carroll Parish	8,866	9	88	266	202	160
East Feliciana Parish	20,964	16	227	690	523	308
Evangeline Parish	34,167	39	359	1,088	825	544
Franklin Parish	22,094	22	235	712	540	342
Grant Parish	18,951	20	203	615	467	288
Iberia Parish	72,946	70	759	2,303	1,746	1,186
Iberville Parish	31,457	30	342	1,038	787	459
Jackson Parish	15,497	12	171	517	392	219
Jefferson Parish	449,708	386	5,049	15,314	11,612	6,007
Jefferson Davis Parish	31,571	38	335	1,016	771	490
Lafayette Parish	186,150	130	2,026	6,146	4,660	2,712
Lafourche Parish	89,010	65	960	2,913	2,209	1,327
La Salle Parish	13,681	25	151	459	348	190
Lincoln Parish	41,140	25	477	1,447	1,097	495
Livingston Parish	88,274	72	930	2,822	2,139	1,395
Madison Parish	12,934	14	131	398	302	222
Morehouse Parish	31,467	31	334	1,014	769	487
Natchitoches Parish	37,040	42	396	1,202	911	564
Orleans Parish	464,578	439	5,131	15,563	11,801	6,507
Ouachita Parish	146,830	124	1,584	4,803	3,642	2,191
Plaquemines Parish	26,177	14	277	841	638	408
Pointe Coupee Parish	23,527	12	252	764	580	357
Rapides Parish	126,475	101	1,377	4,178	3,168	1,840
Red River Parish	9,606	5	101	307	233	152
Richland Parish	21,040	13	222	673	510	332
Sabine Parish	23,804	30	260	790	599	342
St. Bernard Parish	65,847	83	740	2,244	1,701	878
St. Charles Parish	48,164	35	508	1,540	1,168	761
St. Helena Parish	9,572	8	101	306	232	151
St. James Parish	21,033	23	222	674	511	330
St. John the Baptist Parish	42,195	36	431	1,307	991	716
St. Landry Parish	83,781	69	880	2,670	2,024	1,333
St. Martin Parish	47,448	31	494	1,500	1,137	769
St. Mary Parish	57,232	43	598	1,814	1,375	923
St. Tammany Parish	188,727	138	2,028	6,150	4,663	2,844
Tangipahoa Parish	96,943	81	1,030	3,123	2,368	1,503
Tensas Parish	6,599	6	68	206	156	110

Association	Population	Lung Cancer[1]	CHRONIC LUNG DISEASES			
			Emphysema	Chronic Bronchitis	Adult Asthma	Pediatric Asthma
Terrebonne Parish	104,725	91	1,095	3,322	2,519	1,684
Union Parish	22,037	26	242	735	557	313
Vermilion Parish	52,056	56	554	1,680	1,274	804
Vernon Parish	51,380	27	570	1,730	1,312	709
Washington Parish	43,127	46	472	1,430	1,085	621
Webster Parish	42,724	40	475	1,442	1,094	585
West Baton Rouge Parish	20,617	17	222	674	511	308
West Carroll Parish	12,152	14	132	401	304	177
West Feliciana Parish	13,661	9	165	499	379	143
Winn Parish	17,693	18	199	603	457	236
MAINE CONSTITUENT: ALA OF MAINE	1,247,554	1,122	14,327	43,458	32,953	15,527
Androscoggin County	101,266	105	1,154	3,500	2,654	1,293
Aroostook County	76,648	58	881	2,671	2,026	952
Cumberland County	254,429	195	2,977	9,032	6,848	2,970
Franklin County	28,852	27	327	992	752	374
Hancock County	49,840	55	580	1,761	1,335	592
Kennebec County	115,115	96	1,321	4,006	3,037	1,438
Knox County	37,985	32	441	1,336	1,013	458
Lincoln County	31,760	29	367	1,114	845	386
Oxford County	53,845	64	610	1,851	1,404	698
Penobscot County	144,431	117	1,672	5,071	3,845	1,751
Piscataquis County	18,191	21	207	627	476	234
Sagadahoc County	35,651	29	403	1,223	927	466
Somerset County	52,420	51	584	1,771	1,343	716
Waldo County	36,529	27	409	1,240	940	492
Washington County	35,573	40	406	1,233	935	451
York County	175,019	176	1,988	6,030	4,573	2,256
MARYLAND CONSTITUENT: ALA OF MARYLAND	5,130,072	3,709	57,572	174,642	132,420	68,593
Allegany County	72,130	94	836	2,535	1,922	872
Anne Arundel County	474,682	347	5,314	16,120	12,223	6,393
Baltimore County	721,556	630	8,408	25,504	19,338	8,550
Calvert County	71,757	46	763	2,315	1,755	1,108
Caroline County	29,519	26	322	976	740	429
Carroll County	149,690	90	1,633	4,954	3,756	2,167
Cecil County	82,348	72	884	2,683	2,034	1,242
Charles County	118,060	78	1,235	3,747	2,841	1,896
Dorchester County	29,584	30	337	1,023	776	377
Frederick County	186,621	108	2,034	6,171	4,679	2,708
Garrett County	29,275	22	318	964	731	430
Harford County	214,569	127	2,326	7,056	5,350	3,159
Howard County	235,118	90	2,593	7,867	5,965	3,304
Kent County	19,002	20	224	679	515	217
Montgomery County	839,158	373	9,547	28,960	21,959	10,762
Prince George's County	776,907	395	8,701	26,394	20,013	10,451
Queen Anne's County	39,692	43	445	1,350	1,023	532
St. Mary's County	87,645	51	924	2,802	2,124	1,384
Somerset County	24,252	30	290	880	668	260
Talbot County	33,154	23	390	1,183	897	379
Washington County	127,477	92	1,462	4,436	3,364	1,592
Wicomico County	79,441	116	886	2,688	2,038	1,081
Worcester County	42,771	51	497	1,507	1,143	512
Baltimore City[2]	645,664	755	7,203	21,848	16,566	8,788

TABLE 1 ESTIMATED PREVALENCE AND INCIDENCE OF LUNG DISEASE BY COUNTY, STATE, AND LUNG ASSOCIATION, 1998 (continued)

Association	Population	Lung Cancer[1]	CHRONIC LUNG DISEASES			
			Emphysema	Chronic Bronchitis	Adult Asthma	Pediatric Asthma
MASSACHUSETTS CONSTITUENT: ALA OF MASSACHUSETTS	6,144,407	4,717	70,330	213,337	161,759	77,300
Barnstable County	208,477	229	2,462	7,467	5,662	2,356
Berkshire County	132,839	122	1,531	4,643	3,521	1,635
Bristol County	516,975	387	5,790	17,563	13,317	6,955
Dukes County	13,852	13	159	483	366	172
Essex County	700,370	551	7,899	23,962	18,169	9,226
Franklin County	70,626	56	790	2,396	1,816	955
Hampden County	439,336	387	4,849	14,709	11,153	6,163
Hampshire County	150,344	96	1,794	5,442	4,126	1,633
Middlesex County	1,422,465	962	16,704	50,669	38,419	16,400
Nantucket County	7,891	6	93	281	213	91
Norfolk County	642,089	524	7,551	22,906	17,368	7,363
Plymouth County	467,041	361	5,108	15,495	11,749	6,717
Suffolk County	641,333	477	7,443	22,578	17,119	7,706
Worcester County	730,769	546	8,157	24,743	18,761	9,928
Middlesex County [1]	1,293,020	875	15,183	46,011	34,659	15,024
ALA OF GREATER NORFOLK COUNTY						
Norfolk County	642,089	524	7,551	22,906	17,368	7,363
Holliston Town	13,578	9	116	432	542	197
Natick Town	31,526	21	366	1,133	870	333
Newton City	80,200	54	994	2,951	2,241	789
Sherborn Town	4,141	3	44	142	107	57
ALA OF WESTERN COUNTY						
Berkshire County	132,839	122	1,531	4,643	3,521	1,635
Franklin County	70,626	56	790	2,396	1,816	955
Hampden County	439,336	387	4,849	14,709	11,153	6,163
Hampshire County	150,344	96	1,794	5,442	4,126	1,633
MICHIGAN CONSTITUENT: ALA OF MICHIGAN	9,820,231	7,263	109,072	330,853	250,863	135,345
Alcona County	11,061	18	132	399	302	122
Alger County	9,984	12	115	348	264	124
Allegan County	101,680	64	1,072	3,252	2,466	1,604
Alpena County	30,475	30	339	1,030	781	417
Antrim County	21,473	14	240	727	551	292
Arenac County	16,405	20	182	551	418	228
Baraga County	8,602	12	97	296	224	112
Barry County	54,465	44	595	1,805	1,369	785
Bay County	109,980	105	1,226	3,720	2,821	1,498
Benzie County	14,743	9	169	513	389	184
Berrien County	159,831	142	1,762	5,345	4,053	2,249
Branch County	43,702	46	479	1,453	1,102	624
Calhoun County	140,806	133	1,558	4,727	3,584	1,961
Cass County	49,975	60	553	1,679	1,273	695
Charlevoix County	24,496	29	271	821	622	343
Cheboygan County	23,813	29	267	809	613	320
Chippewa County	37,906	32	439	1,331	1,009	460

Association	Population	Lung Cancer[1]	CHRONIC LUNG DISEASES			
			Emphysema	Chronic Bronchitis	Adult Asthma	Pediatric Asthma
Clare County	29,514	46	327	992	752	410
Clinton County	63,407	39	685	2,078	1,576	942
Crawford County	14,128	23	157	477	362	194
Delta County	38,936	55	431	1,308	992	541
Dickinson County	27,062	17	302	916	694	368
Eaton County	101,022	48	1,109	3,364	2,550	1,439
Emmet County	28,633	18	317	962	729	398
Genesee County	435,691	368	4,750	14,409	10,926	6,319
Gladwin County	25,341	36	283	858	650	344
Gogebic County	17,243	20	202	613	465	200
Grand Traverse County	74,224	64	818	2,480	1,881	1,047
Gratiot County	40,145	20	442	1,340	1,016	568
Hillsdale County	46,572	32	506	1,535	1,164	682
Houghton County	35,617	14	411	1,247	946	436
Huron County	35,273	40	390	1,182	896	494
Ingham County	285,874	117	3,245	9,844	7,464	3,691
Ionia County	66,710	42	738	2,237	1,696	931
Iosco County	25,715	34	289	877	665	342
Iron County	12,882	23	151	459	348	148
Isabella County	58,394	43	673	2,041	1,548	719
Jackson County	156,130	129	1,748	5,302	4,020	2,103
Kalamazoo County	229,627	122	2,615	7,932	6,015	2,936
Kalkaska County	15,554	26	165	501	380	241
Kent County	544,781	298	5,875	17,819	13,511	8,132
Keweenaw County	2,099	1	25	74	56	25
Lake County	10,424	13	116	352	267	142
Lapeer County	88,229	61	942	2,858	2,167	1,350
Leelanau County	19,142	9	216	654	496	253
Lenawee County	98,609	83	1,072	3,252	2,465	1,442
Livingston County	146,317	66	1,583	4,803	3,641	2,165
Luce County	6,791	4	78	236	179	85
Mackinac County	11,041	10	124	377	286	146
Macomb County	786,866	662	9,085	27,558	20,896	9,621
Manistee County	23,485	22	271	823	624	287
Marquette County	62,585	42	703	2,133	1,617	834
Mason County	27,896	22	310	941	714	383
Mecosta County	40,156	30	461	1,400	1,061	499
Menominee County	24,393	27	271	823	624	335
Midland County	81,562	46	901	2,734	2,073	1,140
Missaukee County	13,887	12	147	446	338	217
Monroe County	143,365	127	1,550	4,701	3,564	2,127
Montcalm County	60,602	51	652	1,979	1,500	909
Montmorency County	9,999	14	115	350	265	123
Muskegon County	166,849	129	1,811	5,492	4,165	2,450
Newaygo County	45,769	43	485	1,470	1,115	715
Oakland County	1,175,057	734	13,370	40,557	30,752	15,065
Oceana County	24,745	17	263	796	604	384
Ogemaw County	21,085	35	234	710	538	292
Ontonagon County	7,842	14	91	275	209	95
Osceola County	22,138	22	235	713	541	343
Oscoda County	8,890	8	102	310	235	111
Otsego County	22,232	14	240	728	552	331
Ottawa County	225,407	92	2,406	7,298	5,533	3,453
Presque Isle County	14,535	12	165	502	381	186
Roscommon County	23,355	42	278	842	638	258
Saginaw County	210,032	146	2,288	6,939	5,262	3,054
St. Clair County	159,465	142	1,738	5,273	3,998	2,314
St. Joseph County	61,141	62	657	1,994	1,512	919

TABLE 1 ESTIMATED PREVALENCE AND INCIDENCE OF LUNG DISEASE BY COUNTY, STATE, AND LUNG ASSOCIATION, 1998 (continued)

Association	Population	Lung Cancer[1]	CHRONIC LUNG DISEASES Emphysema	Chronic Bronchitis	Adult Asthma	Pediatric Asthma
ALA OF MICHIGAN						
(cont.)						
Sanilac County	43,051	32	465	1,409	1,068	642
Schoolcraft County	8,782	17	100	303	229	113
Shiawassee County	72,489	48	785	2,380	1,805	1,072
Tuscola County	57,965	40	627	1,901	1,441	860
Van Buren County	75,637	55	807	2,449	1,857	1,159
Washtenaw County	302,787	134	3,566	10,816	8,201	3,455
Wayne County	2,116,540	1,628	23,298	70,671	53,585	29,913
Wexford County	29,118	22	314	952	722	435
MINNESOTA						
CONSTITUENT:	4,726,411	2,769	51,958	157,604	119,505	67,048
ALA OF MINNESOTA						
Aitkin County	14,182	20	163	494	375	177
Anoka County	292,324	140	3,103	9,413	7,137	4,538
Becker County	29,495	22	315	955	724	452
Beltrami County	38,664	25	405	1,228	931	620
Benton County	34,114	18	357	1,084	822	546
Big Stone County	5,652	4	63	192	146	76
Blue Earth County	53,727	25	622	1,888	1,432	649
Brown County	27,069	22	299	906	687	380
Carlton County	31,303	25	342	1,037	786	452
Carver County	64,821	23	679	2,061	1,563	1,037
Cass County	26,310	30	287	872	661	380
Chippewa County	13,052	16	143	434	329	187
Chisago County	40,950	30	424	1,286	975	673
Clay County	51,522	18	579	1,757	1,332	686
Clearwater County	8,241	13	87	265	201	128
Cook County	4,751	0	55	166	126	59
Cottonwood County	12,031	12	134	408	309	163
Crow Wing County	51,741	48	570	1,728	1,310	731
Dakota County	342,059	121	3,624	10,993	8,335	5,334
Dodge County	17,169	8	177	536	406	286
Douglas County	31,077	18	342	1,037	787	440
Faribault County	16,260	13	181	549	416	222
Fillmore County	20,763	16	226	686	520	302
Freeborn County	31,560	29	355	1,077	817	419
Goodhue County	43,130	27	467	1,417	1,074	637
Grant County	6,108	6	68	207	157	83
Hennepin County	1,058,943	601	12,169	36,912	27,988	13,152
Houston County	19,267	22	207	629	477	289
Hubbard County	16,909	18	186	563	427	240
Isanti County	30,036	12	310	941	714	497
Itasca County	43,919	43	477	1,448	1,098	642
Jackson County	11,496	10	126	383	290	164
Kanabec County	14,161	14	149	451	342	226
Kandiyohi County	40,887	25	438	1,329	1,008	620
Kittson County	5,301	6	60	180	137	71
Koochiching County	15,068	12	170	515	391	199
Lac qui Parle County	7,995	12	89	270	205	109
Lake County	10,664	14	123	374	284	130
Lake of the Woods County	4,562	5	50	151	115	66
Le Sueur County	25,319	12	270	818	620	390
Lincoln County	6,486	1	72	219	166	89

Association	Population	Lung Cancer[1]	CHRONIC LUNG DISEASES			
			Emphysema	Chronic Bronchitis	Adult Asthma	Pediatric Asthma
Lyon County	24,398	16	266	807	612	354
Mc Leod County	34,142	12	365	1,108	840	520
Mahnomen County	5,051	1	52	157	119	85
Marshall County	10,280	9	111	335	254	155
Martin County	22,000	12	244	740	561	305
Meeker County	21,739	8	231	701	531	337
Mille Lacs County	21,067	23	225	683	518	321
Morrison County	30,518	18	316	959	727	502
Mower County	37,104	21	417	1,265	959	494
Murray County	9,531	5	105	318	241	135
Nicollet County	29,482	8	325	985	747	417
Nobles County	19,275	8	214	649	492	266
Norman County	7,539	4	83	251	190	108
Olmsted County	116,931	58	1,277	3,874	2,937	1,688
Otter Tail County	54,794	44	607	1,841	1,396	762
Pennington County	13,541	6	148	449	341	194
Pine County	24,096	30	260	787	597	361
Pipestone County	10,057	5	109	329	250	150
Polk County	31,081	29	335	1,018	772	463
Pope County	10,913	9	119	361	274	158
Ramsey County	485,709	282	5,466	16,579	12,571	6,443
Red Lake County	4,237	1	45	136	103	67
Redwood County	16,504	10	179	542	411	244
Renville County	16,931	16	184	559	424	247
Rice County	54,198	34	602	1,825	1,384	748
Rock County	9,723	13	105	320	243	143
Roseau County	16,086	12	165	502	380	269
St. Louis County	193,463	168	2,196	6,661	5,051	2,499
Scott County	79,114	29	819	2,484	1,884	1,302
Sherburne County	60,339	35	616	1,869	1,417	1,022
Sibley County	14,641	9	158	478	363	219
Stearns County	128,736	51	1,394	4,230	3,207	1,900
Steele County	31,723	10	340	1,031	782	481
Stevens County	10,036	4	116	350	266	124
Swift County	11,495	17	130	395	299	150
Todd County	24,035	18	251	760	577	389
Traverse County	4,248	10	47	144	109	57
Wabasha County	20,891	18	224	680	516	316
Wadena County	13,114	5	143	433	328	191
Waseca County	18,534	10	199	604	458	279
Washington County	196,675	68	2,069	6,277	4,759	3,118
Watonwan County	11,519	16	126	381	289	167
Wilkin County	7,372	4	80	241	183	110
Winona County	48,022	26	545	1,652	1,252	622
Wright County	85,022	31	862	2,615	1,983	1,463
Yellow Medicine County	11,417	10	125	380	288	162
MISSISSIPPI CONSTITUENT: ALA OF MISSISSIPPI	2,751,335	2,400	29,917	90,763	68,822	40,174
Adams County	34,141	47	375	1,139	863	484
Alcorn County	32,755	40	372	1,128	856	422
Amite County	13,852	13	150	455	345	205
Attala County	18,325	20	203	617	468	253
Benton County	8,086	1	87	264	201	121
Bolivar County	40,185	40	410	1,245	944	681
Calhoun County	14,891	14	167	507	385	199
Carroll County	9,989	9	110	332	252	143
Chickasaw County	18,039	20	194	588	446	271

TABLE 1 ESTIMATED PREVALENCE AND INCIDENCE OF LUNG DISEASE BY COUNTY,
STATE, AND LUNG ASSOCIATION, 1998 (continued)

			CHRONIC LUNG DISEASES			
Association	Population	Lung Cancer[1]	Emphysema	Chronic Bronchitis	Adult Asthma	Pediatric Asthma
ALA OF MISSISSIPPI (cont.)						
Choctaw County	9,401	3	100	304	231	144
Claiborne County	11,513	6	125	380	288	168
Clarke County	18,239	13	199	604	458	264
Clay County	21,622	8	229	696	528	336
Coahoma County	31,277	30	316	957	726	543
Copiah County	28,827	38	310	942	714	432
Covington County	17,723	13	188	569	431	277
DeSoto County	97,110	73	1,058	3,210	2,434	1,411
Forrest County	74,484	73	838	2,542	1,927	989
Franklin County	8,287	5	89	270	205	125
George County	19,600	20	208	632	479	303
Greene County	12,745	9	142	432	327	173
Grenada County	22,408	29	244	739	561	327
Hancock County	40,271	55	447	1,355	1,027	557
Harrison County	177,194	199	1,948	5,909	4,480	2,513
Hinds County	247,262	237	2,739	8,309	6,300	3,433
Holmes County	21,513	10	216	656	498	377
Humphreys County	11,318	17	112	341	258	203
Issaquena County	1,636	3	17	51	39	27
Itawamba County	21,093	10	241	732	555	265
Jackson County	130,799	107	1,416	4,296	3,257	1,932
Jasper County	17,666	10	188	571	433	272
Jefferson County	8,451	9	85	259	197	146
Jefferson Davis County	13,815	13	146	444	336	216
Jones County	63,616	74	706	2,141	1,623	879
Kemper County	10,573	8	115	349	264	154
Lafayette County	34,756	20	414	1,256	952	380
Lamar County	37,041	26	395	1,198	909	569
Lauderdale County	76,107	73	839	2,545	1,930	1,071
Lawrence County	12,999	8	140	424	322	195
Leake County	19,437	21	212	644	488	281
Lee County	74,621	72	817	2,478	1,879	1,071
Leflore County	37,241	26	392	1,188	901	591
Lincoln County	31,859	30	349	1,060	804	455
Lowndes County	61,045	38	658	1,997	1,514	911
Madison County	72,879	30	784	2,379	1,804	1,094
Marion County	26,404	25	281	853	647	407
Marshall County	32,170	23	346	1,050	796	482
Monroe County	38,105	31	415	1,257	953	556
Montgomery County	12,402	14	136	412	313	178
Neshoba County	27,502	13	293	888	673	425
Newton County	21,597	21	238	723	548	303
Noxubee County	12,413	9	127	385	292	210
Oktibbeha County	39,635	17	464	1,409	1,068	461
Panola County	33,326	29	347	1,052	798	542
Pearl River County	46,833	36	509	1,544	1,171	685
Perry County	11,858	9	125	378	287	188
Pike County	37,835	43	405	1,229	932	575
Pontotoc County	25,307	23	279	847	642	356
Prentiss County	24,356	25	277	840	637	312
Quitman County	9,858	16	101	305	231	167
Rankin County	109,600	52	1,220	3,701	2,806	1,501
Scott County	25,015	12	268	814	617	378
Sharkey County	6,602	3	65	196	149	122

| Association | Population | Lung Cancer[1] | CHRONIC LUNG DISEASES | | | |
			Emphysema	Chronic Bronchitis	Adult Asthma	Pediatric Asthma
Simpson County	25,295	17	273	827	627	378
Smith County	15,268	16	167	505	383	221
Stone County	13,225	3	143	435	330	195
Sunflower County	33,537	26	361	1,095	830	503
Tallahatchie County	14,787	10	152	460	349	248
Tate County	23,973	27	259	786	596	355
Tippah County	21,016	18	233	708	537	290
Tishomingo County	18,660	27	217	657	498	224
Tunica County	8,041	9	77	235	178	153
Union County	23,861	25	267	809	613	323
Walthall County	14,391	13	151	458	347	229
Warren County	49,357	32	529	1,606	1,218	747
Washington County	65,173	44	663	2,013	1,526	1,112
Wayne County	20,297	16	213	647	491	323
Webster County	10,585	14	118	357	271	146
Wilkinson County	9,158	9	98	298	226	138
Winston County	19,286	16	209	634	481	284
Yalobusha County	12,416	18	137	414	314	176
Yazoo County	25,500	39	264	802	608	418
MISSOURI CONSTITUENTS: ALA OF EASTERN MISSOURI	5,437,562	4,805	60,541	183,616	139,221	74,452
Adair County	24,241	10	290	879	667	261
Audrain County	23,555	35	261	791	600	328
Bollinger County	11,552	5	127	385	292	164
Boone County	128,963	58	1,487	4,511	3,420	1,584
Butler County	40,434	62	451	1,367	1,036	552
Callaway County	37,499	29	416	1,262	957	519
Cape Girardeau County	66,229	42	756	2,293	1,739	841
Carter County	6,382	8	69	210	159	94
Clark County	7,449	6	81	247	187	107
Cole County	69,227	48	781	2,369	1,797	911
Crawford County	22,295	23	244	739	560	321
Dent County	14,134	23	156	472	358	199
Dunklin County	32,707	53	359	1,088	825	467
Franklin County	91,852	68	987	2,993	2,270	1,384
Gasconade County	14,824	17	167	507	384	196
Howell County	35,748	40	396	1,201	910	497
Iron County	10,909	14	119	362	274	157
Jefferson County	195,472	179	2,073	6,287	4,767	3,043
Knox County	4,360	3	50	151	114	55
Lewis County	10,194	6	117	355	269	127
Lincoln County	36,610	34	385	1,169	886	580
Macon County	15,329	14	172	523	396	204
Madison County	11,550	23	129	390	296	158
Maries County	8,433	3	94	284	215	116
Marion County	27,864	26	303	920	697	406
Mississippi County	13,473	6	143	433	328	210
Monroe County	9,039	8	98	297	225	133
Montgomery County	12,065	18	133	403	305	171
New Madrid County	20,357	23	215	651	494	321
Oregon County	10,175	8	116	352	267	130
Osage County	12,465	6	135	409	310	185
Pemiscot County	21,448	23	219	663	503	365
Perry County	17,497	8	188	569	432	265
Phelps County	38,555	27	441	1,337	1,014	487
Pike County	16,395	16	179	543	412	236

**TABLE 1 ESTIMATED PREVALENCE AND INCIDENCE OF LUNG DISEASE BY COUNTY,
STATE, AND LUNG ASSOCIATION, 1998 *(continued)***

			CHRONIC LUNG DISEASES			
Association	Population	Lung Cancer[1]	Emphysema	Chronic Bronchitis	Adult Asthma	Pediatric Asthma
ALA OF EASTERN MISSOURI (cont.)						
Pulaski County	39,331	27	417	1,264	958	614
Ralls County	8,876	13	98	296	224	126
Randolph County	23,912	16	270	818	620	315
Reynolds County	6,648	3	74	223	169	93
Ripley County	14,050	22	154	466	353	202
St. Charles County	272,101	142	2,884	8,748	6,633	4,240
St. Francois County	55,355	52	620	1,881	1,426	745
St. Louis County	997,347	840	11,343	34,407	26,089	12,805
Ste. Genevieve County	17,357	10	189	573	434	253
Schuyler County	4,454	8	50	151	114	61
Scotland County	4,821	4	54	163	123	66
Scott County	40,288	48	431	1,308	992	613
Shannon County	8,299	8	91	277	210	118
Shelby County	6,749	5	74	226	171	95
Stoddard County	29,681	34	335	1,015	769	392
Texas County	22,373	20	247	748	567	315
Warren County	24,512	18	265	803	609	364
Washington County	23,042	30	245	742	562	358
Wayne County	13,061	26	150	455	345	162
St. Louis City[2]	338,946	378	3,723	11,294	8,564	4,817
ALA OF WESTERN MISSOURI						
Andrew County	15,551	6	171	518	392	222
Atchison County	7,035	6	82	249	188	83
Barry County	33,179	31	369	1,120	849	455
Barton County	12,071	13	132	400	303	174
Bates County	15,826	18	175	531	402	221
Benton County	16,955	23	200	607	460	192
Buchanan County	81,799	109	908	2,756	2,090	1,127
Caldwell County	8,812	10	97	294	223	125
Camden County	33,936	32	401	1,215	922	384
Carroll County	10,201	9	113	342	259	143
Cass County	80,572	55	863	2,619	1,986	1,222
Cedar County	13,195	14	151	458	348	166
Chariton County	8,654	4	96	292	221	119
Christian County	48,982	34	527	1,598	1,212	736
Clay County	176,428	162	1,976	5,992	4,544	2,375
Clinton County	19,050	18	206	624	473	283
Cooper County	16,041	16	182	552	419	207
Dade County	7,840	6	88	266	202	105
Dallas County	15,314	13	167	505	383	224
Daviess County	7,901	12	86	261	198	115
DeKalb County	11,210	23	134	406	308	121
Douglas County	12,443	9	138	417	317	174
Gentry County	6,923	6	78	236	179	92
Greene County	226,574	188	2,623	7,957	6,034	2,745
Grundy County	10,189	14	117	354	268	128
Harrison County	8,466	14	98	296	224	104
Henry County	21,256	22	240	729	553	278
Hickory County	8,603	17	104	315	239	90
Holt County	5,539	6	62	187	142	76
Howard County	9,731	9	109	331	251	130
Jackson County	655,055	520	7,299	22,139	16,787	8,946

Association	Population	Lung Cancer[1]	CHRONIC LUNG DISEASES			
			Emphysema	Chronic Bronchitis	Adult Asthma	Pediatric Asthma
Jasper County	99,620	92	1,112	3,372	2,557	1,355
Johnson County	47,685	22	536	1,627	1,234	633
Laclede County	30,974	34	340	1,030	781	443
Lafayette County	32,670	32	360	1,092	828	460
Lawrence County	33,124	40	362	1,100	834	476
Linn County	13,796	14	155	469	356	185
Livingston County	14,140	17	160	485	368	185
McDonald County	20,010	12	216	656	497	297
Mercer County	3,982	1	46	139	105	49
Miller County	22,465	23	245	743	563	326
Moniteau County	13,256	6	143	435	330	196
Morgan County	18,427	34	213	645	489	226
Newton County	49,210	47	543	1,648	1,249	690
Nodaway County	20,712	18	241	731	554	247
Ozark County	9,913	21	114	347	263	121
Pettis County	37,086	42	411	1,246	945	516
Platte County	69,994	35	780	2,367	1,795	954
Polk County	25,557	25	288	875	663	336
Putnam County	4,898	4	57	172	131	59
Ray County	23,661	20	254	770	584	357
St. Clair County	9,070	16	104	316	240	112
Saline County	22,668	23	254	770	584	305
Stone County	26,841	30	315	955	724	310
Sullivan County	6,998	9	80	244	185	87
Taney County	34,457	40	405	1,229	932	396
Vernon County	19,488	10	215	652	495	274
Webster County	29,176	21	313	949	719	442
Worth County	2,289	0	26	78	59	30
Wright County	19,580	22	210	638	484	295
NEBRASKA CONSTITUENT: *ALA OF NEBRASKA*	1,660,772	1,140	18,248	55,348	41,970	23,598
Adams County	29,414	23	334	1,014	769	379
Antelope County	7,288	4	77	233	177	115
Arthur County	426	0	5	15	11	6
Banner County	876	0	9	29	22	13
Blaine County	578	1	6	19	14	9
Boone County	6,376	3	69	209	158	95
Box Butte County	12,764	6	130	395	299	217
Boyd County	2,563	3	28	86	65	36
Brown County	3,532	1	39	119	90	48
Buffalo County	40,335	23	450	1,364	1,035	549
Burt County	7,922	6	88	266	202	110
Butler County	8,679	4	94	286	217	128
Cass County	24,485	16	263	798	605	369
Cedar County	9,631	6	102	308	234	152
Chase County	4,266	4	46	140	106	64
Cherry County	6,292	6	69	208	158	91
Cheyenne County	9,481	6	104	315	238	136
Clay County	7,135	8	78	238	181	101
Colfax County	10,657	6	120	363	275	143
Cuming County	9,989	10	109	330	251	145
Custer County	11,957	10	131	398	302	170
Dakota County	18,779	6	196	594	450	305
Dawes County	8,872	6	101	305	231	115
Dawson County	23,157	12	250	757	574	346
Deuel County	2,021	1	22	68	52	28
Dixon County	6,312	4	68	207	157	94

TABLE 1 ESTIMATED PREVALENCE AND INCIDENCE OF LUNG DISEASE BY COUNTY, STATE, AND LUNG ASSOCIATION, 1998 (continued)

Association	Population	Lung Cancer[1]	CHRONIC LUNG DISEASES			
			Emphysema	Chronic Bronchitis	Adult Asthma	Pediatric Asthma
ALA OF NEBRASKA						
(cont.)						
Dodge County	35,304	36	396	1,201	911	473
Douglas County	443,370	328	4,888	14,826	11,242	6,240
Dundy County	2,281	3	26	78	59	30
Fillmore County	6,940	5	76	231	175	99
Franklin County	3,716	4	43	130	98	46
Frontier County	3,107	1	34	102	78	46
Furnas County	5,430	6	62	188	142	69
Gage County	22,791	13	260	788	598	290
Garden County	2,129	5	25	76	57	25
Garfield County	2,045	1	23	70	53	27
Gosper County	2,325	0	27	81	62	29
Grant County	745	1	8	25	19	11
Greeley County	2,861	3	30	92	70	45
Hall County	51,730	36	557	1,689	1,281	775
Hamilton County	9,454	6	102	308	234	142
Harlan County	3,701	9	42	128	97	47
Hayes County	1,059	3	12	35	27	15
Hitchcock County	3,440	4	37	113	86	50
Holt County	12,018	12	128	389	295	185
Hooker County	697	0	8	24	18	9
Howard County	6,498	4	70	213	162	96
Jefferson County	8,348	8	95	287	218	108
Johnson County	4,572	10	52	157	119	60
Kearney County	6,849	3	75	228	173	98
Keith County	8,680	6	95	288	218	125
Keya Paha County	973	0	11	33	25	13
Kimball County	4,074	5	45	138	104	56
Knox County	9,186	8	103	312	236	124
Lancaster County	235,537	118	2,698	8,183	6,205	2,957
Lincoln County	33,477	23	358	1,087	824	509
Logan County	882	0	9	27	21	15
Loup County	672	3	7	22	17	9
Mc Pherson County	554	0	6	18	14	8
Madison County	34,567	21	374	1,133	859	513
Merrick County	8,063	10	88	266	202	117
Morrill County	5,423	4	58	177	134	82
Nance County	4,101	8	44	134	102	61
Nemaha County	7,674	9	87	264	201	99
Nuckolls County	5,204	8	59	178	135	68
Otoe County	14,720	12	164	497	377	202
Pawnee County	3,129	5	36	110	84	37
Perkins County	3,191	5	34	103	78	50
Phelps County	9,898	6	109	330	250	140
Pierce County	7,963	4	85	257	195	123
Platte County	30,680	20	316	959	727	510
Polk County	5,616	1	62	187	142	80
Red Willow County	11,242	12	125	379	287	155
Richardson County	9,435	6	107	324	245	123
Rock County	1,730	4	19	57	44	25
Saline County	12,960	12	146	443	336	171
Sarpy County	120,329	46	1,245	3,775	2,863	1,983
Saunders County	19,231	18	208	631	478	285
Scotts Bluff County	36,016	30	387	1,174	890	543
Seward County	16,384	9	183	555	421	222

Association	Population	Lung Cancer[1]	CHRONIC LUNG DISEASES			
			Emphysema	Chronic Bronchitis	Adult Asthma	Pediatric Asthma
Sheridan County	6,447	5	70	213	161	94
Sherman County	3,452	0	38	114	87	50
Sioux County	1,479	1	16	50	38	20
Stanton County	6,238	0	63	193	146	107
Thayer County	6,261	5	71	216	164	81
Thomas County	797	0	8	25	19	13
Thurston County	7,172	4	69	210	159	136
Valley County	4,632	6	52	159	120	61
Washington County	18,674	13	205	623	472	265
Wayne County	9,329	3	108	326	247	115
Webster County	4,019	4	46	139	105	52
Wheeler County	930	0	10	29	22	15
York County	14,554	10	160	487	369	205
NEW HAMPSHIRE CONSTITUENT: ALA OF NEW HAMPSHIRE	1,185,823	849	13,285	40,298	30,554	15,939
Belknap County	52,932	36	591	1,792	1,358	720
Carroll County	39,382	46	450	1,366	1,036	497
Cheshire County	72,021	47	815	2,473	1,875	938
Coos County	32,865	25	372	1,128	855	429
Grafton County	78,237	61	902	2,735	2,074	963
Hillsborough County	362,477	226	4,027	12,217	9,263	4,990
Merrimack County	127,894	99	1,427	4,330	3,283	1,738
Rockingham County	270,643	183	3,006	9,117	6,913	3,731
Strafford County	109,498	83	1,249	3,788	2,872	1,393
Sullivan County	39,874	43	446	1,352	1,025	540
NEW JERSEY CONSTITUENT: ALA OF NEW JERSEY	8,095,542	6,141	91,513	277,593	210,480	105,914
Atlantic County	237,988	200	2,691	8,164	6,190	3,110
Bergen County	854,428	655	10,066	30,534	23,152	9,736
Burlington County	421,283	299	4,689	14,223	10,784	5,772
Camden County	504,268	436	5,433	16,479	12,495	7,545
Cape May County	98,001	117	1,123	3,405	2,582	1,230
Cumberland County	140,389	125	1,523	4,621	3,504	2,062
Essex County	748,322	543	8,356	25,346	19,218	10,156
Gloucester County	248,012	200	2,673	8,109	6,149	3,705
Hudson County	553,030	374	6,327	19,192	14,552	6,968
Hunterdon County	122,389	69	1,377	4,178	3,168	1,623
Mercer County	331,474	252	3,783	11,474	8,700	4,211
Middlesex County	712,638	552	8,244	25,007	18,961	8,657
Monmouth County	603,214	458	6,721	20,386	15,458	8,240
Morris County	459,012	308	5,255	15,940	12,086	5,771
Ocean County	490,104	598	5,574	16,909	12,821	6,291
Passaic County	483,050	296	5,342	16,205	12,287	6,738
Salem County	64,935	52	714	2,166	1,643	920
Somerset County	282,274	152	3,257	9,879	7,490	3,460
Sussex County	143,139	96	1,523	4,620	3,503	2,209
Union County	498,893	312	5,749	17,440	13,223	6,139
Warren County	98,699	47	1,093	3,316	2,514	1,371
NEW YORK CONSTITUENTS: ALA OF BROOKLYN	18,159,175	12,377	205,358	622,916	472,322	237,291
Kings County	2,266,242	1,221	24,671	74,835	56,743	33,002

TABLE 1 ESTIMATED PREVALENCE AND INCIDENCE OF LUNG DISEASE BY COUNTY,
STATE, AND LUNG ASSOCIATION, 1998 (continued)

Association	Population	Lung Cancer[1]	CHRONIC LUNG DISEASES			
			Emphysema	Chronic Bronchitis	Adult Asthma	Pediatric Asthma
ALA OF NEW YORK						
Bronx County	1,191,319	556	12,593	38,199	28,964	18,680
New York County	1,546,508	774	18,952	57,488	43,590	15,029
Richmond County	406,899	289	4,536	13,759	10,433	5,549
ALA OF QUEENS						
Queens County	1,993,172	1,153	23,226	70,451	53,419	23,619
ALA OF NEW YORK STATE						
Albany County	293,025	250	3,419	10,371	7,864	3,456
Allegany County	50,567	46	556	1,688	1,280	716
Broome County	196,531	200	2,263	6,865	5,205	2,425
Cattaraugus County	84,940	70	912	2,766	2,098	1,282
Cayuga County	82,164	69	901	2,733	2,073	1,173
Chautauqua County	138,310	107	1,535	4,656	3,530	1,911
Chemung County	92,207	120	1,025	3,109	2,357	1,268
Chenango County	50,985	47	549	1,666	1,263	764
Clinton County	79,780	57	891	2,702	2,049	1,083
Columbia County	63,102	64	709	2,152	1,632	839
Cortland County	48,215	43	537	1,630	1,236	658
Delaware County	46,388	47	521	1,579	1,197	620
Dutchess County	265,413	194	3,008	9,123	6,917	3,447
Erie County	933,702	923	10,666	32,353	24,531	11,823
Essex County	37,557	36	427	1,294	981	484
Franklin County	48,669	43	544	1,651	1,252	657
Fulton County	53,084	56	582	1,767	1,340	757
Genesee County	60,689	58	663	2,012	1,526	875
Greene County	48,145	48	552	1,673	1,269	604
Hamilton County	5,187	1	62	187	141	58
Herkimer County	64,021	57	707	2,144	1,626	897
Jefferson County	111,014	100	1,199	3,637	2,758	1,651
Lewis County	27,424	18	284	861	653	452
Livingston County	65,640	48	740	2,245	1,702	865
Madison County	70,915	61	787	2,388	1,811	978
Monroe County	714,936	512	8,001	24,271	18,403	9,638
Montgomery County	50,777	43	565	1,713	1,299	697
Nassau County	1,300,995	930	15,151	45,958	34,847	15,448
Niagara County	217,788	211	2,436	7,388	5,602	2,943
Oneida County	230,704	190	2,609	7,913	6,000	3,015
Onondaga County	457,916	359	5,145	15,606	11,833	6,103
Ontario County	99,526	100	1,108	3,361	2,548	1,363
Orange County	329,795	214	3,524	10,689	8,105	5,037
Orleans County	44,911	27	491	1,490	1,130	645
Oswego County	123,818	88	1,321	4,006	3,037	1,900
Otsego County	60,570	53	690	2,092	1,586	775
Putnam County	93,350	49	1,036	3,144	2,384	1,288
Rensselaer County	152,203	139	1,721	5,220	3,958	1,990
Rockland County	280,968	169	3,106	9,420	7,143	3,926
St. Lawrence County	113,147	98	1,265	3,836	2,909	1,531
Saratoga County	197,436	157	2,189	6,639	5,034	2,736
Schenectady County	145,112	133	1,663	5,044	3,825	1,819
Schoharie County	32,075	30	360	1,091	827	430
Schuyler County	19,194	14	210	636	482	277
Seneca County	31,939	38	351	1,065	808	453
Steuben County	97,966	81	1,062	3,221	2,443	1,442
Suffolk County	1,370,549	907	15,353	46,571	35,312	18,427

Association	Population	Lung Cancer[1]	CHRONIC LUNG DISEASES			
			Emphysema	Chronic Bronchitis	Adult Asthma	Pediatric Asthma
Sullivan County	69,393	56	772	2,342	1,776	952
Tioga County	52,428	35	562	1,706	1,293	793
Tompkins County	97,239	35	1,162	3,526	2,673	1,049
Ulster County	166,826	133	1,909	5,792	4,391	2,100
Warren County	61,258	61	684	2,076	1,574	830
Washington County	60,170	49	664	2,015	1,528	843
Wayne County	95,096	46	1,019	3,092	2,345	1,441
Westchester County	900,861	620	10,462	31,734	24,062	10,801
Wyoming County	44,151	23	485	1,472	1,116	626
Yates County	24,264	21	265	803	609	351
AFFILIATES:						
ALA OF CENTRAL						
NEW YORK						
Cortland County	48,215	43	537	1,630	1,236	658
Franklin County	48,669	43	544	1,651	1,252	657
Jefferson County	111,014	100	1,199	3,637	2,758	1,651
Lewis County	27,424	18	284	861	653	452
Onondaga County	457,916	359	5,145	15,606	11,833	6,103
Oswego County	123,818	88	1,321	4,006	3,037	1,900
Saint Lawrence County	113,147	98	1,265	3,836	2,909	1,531
Tompkins County	97,239	35	1,162	3,526	2,673	1,049
ALA OF FINGER LAKES						
REGION						
Cayuga County	82,164	69	901	2,733	2,073	1,173
Chemung County	92,207	120	1,025	3,109	2,357	1,268
Livingston County	65,640	48	740	2,245	1,702	865
Monroe County	714,936	512	8,001	24,271	18,403	9,638
Ontario County	99,526	100	1,108	3,361	2,548	1,363
Orleans County	44,911	27	491	1,490	1,130	645
Schuyler County	19,194	14	210	636	482	277
Seneca County	31,939	38	351	1,065	808	453
Steuben County	97,966	81	1,062	3,221	2,443	1,442
Wayne County	95,096	46	1,019	3,092	2,345	1,441
Yates County	24,264	21	265	803	609	351
ALA OF HUDSON						
VALLEY						
Greene County	48,145	48	552	1,673	1,269	604
Orange County	329,795	214	3,524	10,689	8,105	5,037
Putnam County	93,350	49	1,036	3,144	2,384	1,288
Rockland County	280,968	169	3,106	9,420	7,143	3,926
Sullivan County	69,393	56	772	2,342	1,776	952
Ulster County	166,826	133	1,909	5,792	4,391	2,100
Westchester County	900,861	620	10,462	31,734	24,062	10,801
ALA OF NASSAU						
SUFFOLK						
Nassau County	1,300,995	930	15,151	45,958	34,847	15,448
Suffolk County	1,370,549	907	15,353	46,571	35,312	18,427
ALA OF WESTERN						
NEW YORK						
Allegany County	50,567	46	556	1,688	1,280	716
Cattaraugus County	84,940	70	912	2,766	2,098	1,282
Chautauqua County	138,310	107	1,535	4,656	3,530	1,911
Erie County	933,702	923	10,666	32,353	24,531	11,823
Genesee County	60,689	58	663	2,012	1,526	875

TABLE 1   ESTIMATED PREVALENCE AND INCIDENCE OF LUNG DISEASE BY COUNTY,
STATE, AND LUNG ASSOCIATION, 1998 *(continued)*

Association	Population	Lung Cancer[1]	CHRONIC LUNG DISEASES			
			Emphysema	Chronic Bronchitis	Adult Asthma	Pediatric Asthma
ALA OF WESTERN NEW YORK (cont.)						
Niagara County	217,788	211	2,436	7,388	5,602	2,943
Wyoming County	44,151	23	485	1,472	1,116	626
NORTH CAROLINA CONSTITUENT:	7,545,828	6,035	84,513	256,350	194,374	101,517
ALA OF NORTH CAROLINA						
Alamance County	119,657	109	1,384	4,197	3,182	1,456
Alexander County	31,291	16	349	1,057	802	428
Alleghany County	9,808	4	115	349	265	113
Anson County	24,390	16	269	817	619	342
Ashe County	24,042	22	280	851	645	284
Avery County	15,711	16	180	546	414	197
Beaufort County	44,518	62	491	1,489	1,129	626
Bertie County	20,405	25	217	658	499	315
Bladen County	30,822	22	337	1,023	776	442
Brunswick County	68,445	75	782	2,372	1,799	866
Buncombe County	194,456	155	2,232	6,770	5,134	2,424
Burke County	82,357	78	928	2,815	2,134	1,088
Cabarrus County	120,319	91	1,343	4,073	3,088	1,636
Caldwell County	75,911	75	859	2,606	1,976	989
Camden County	6,812	9	77	233	177	90
Carteret County	59,803	62	690	2,092	1,586	734
Caswell County	22,254	23	256	776	588	276
Catawba County	132,400	125	1,489	4,518	3,426	1,758
Chatham County	45,581	30	525	1,594	1,209	560
Cherokee County	22,745	22	260	788	598	288
Chowan County	14,207	21	156	473	359	202
Clay County	8,570	6	98	297	225	108
Cleveland County	93,064	75	1,041	3,157	2,394	1,257
Columbus County	52,739	57	571	1,733	1,314	778
Craven County	88,814	74	964	2,926	2,218	1,302
Cumberland County	284,224	166	2,994	9,082	6,886	4,494
Currituck County	17,789	21	194	589	447	257
Dare County	28,812	25	332	1,006	763	356
Davidson County	141,132	152	1,587	4,813	3,649	1,878
Davie County	31,998	32	362	1,099	833	416
Duplin County	43,126	53	470	1,425	1,081	627
Durham County	202,311	142	2,304	6,989	5,300	2,586
Edgecombe County	55,010	58	586	1,777	1,347	847
Forsyth County	287,689	235	3,307	10,031	7,606	3,570
Franklin County	44,577	42	496	1,505	1,141	611
Gaston County	183,856	192	2,029	6,155	4,667	2,579
Gates County	10,150	12	112	339	257	143
Graham County	7,596	8	85	259	197	101
Granville County	43,802	30	494	1,499	1,137	576
Greene County	18,384	14	203	617	468	257
Guilford County	387,633	306	4,456	13,516	10,249	4,809
Halifax County	56,313	65	609	1,848	1,401	833
Harnett County	82,414	53	896	2,717	2,060	1,206
Haywood County	51,494	58	607	1,842	1,396	585
Henderson County	81,205	90	949	2,878	2,182	954
Hertford County	21,989	30	239	725	550	322
Hoke County	30,348	17	307	933	707	523

Association	Population	Lung Cancer[1]	CHRONIC LUNG DISEASES			
			Emphysema	Chronic Bronchitis	Adult Asthma	Pediatric Asthma
Hyde County	5,854	5	66	201	153	76
Iredell County	113,522	86	1,272	3,859	2,926	1,524
Jackson County	29,967	25	353	1,070	811	343
Johnston County	106,559	81	1,175	3,565	2,703	1,497
Jones County	9,363	10	103	311	236	134
Lee County	49,199	48	538	1,632	1,238	708
Lenoir County	58,877	51	648	1,964	1,490	834
Lincoln County	58,046	48	646	1,959	1,485	796
Mc Dowell County	40,058	29	454	1,376	1,044	521
Macon County	28,281	43	336	1,018	772	314
Madison County	18,776	18	216	656	497	232
Martin County	26,157	22	286	867	658	377
Mecklenburg County	630,813	333	7,045	21,370	16,203	8,557
Mitchell County	14,794	21	172	522	396	177
Montgomery County	24,124	25	265	803	609	344
Moore County	71,349	73	821	2,491	1,889	882
Nash County	90,879	68	1,012	3,070	2,328	1,243
New Hanover County	149,837	135	1,714	5,198	3,941	1,890
Northampton County	21,330	31	239	725	550	286
Onslow County	143,376	82	1,565	4,746	3,599	2,074
Orange County	109,905	57	1,303	3,953	2,997	1,223
Pamlico County	12,310	16	141	427	323	156
Pasquotank County	35,589	31	388	1,176	892	517
Pender County	39,367	34	442	1,340	1,016	526
Perquimans County	11,194	12	126	383	290	148
Person County	33,609	34	375	1,137	862	458
Pitt County	126,630	110	1,407	4,269	3,237	1,742
Polk County	16,731	18	200	606	459	181
Randolph County	121,375	116	1,361	4,127	3,129	1,628
Richmond County	45,985	35	498	1,511	1,146	678
Robeson County	115,675	86	1,189	3,606	2,734	1,934
Rockingham County	90,056	83	1,017	3,084	2,338	1,183
Rowan County	125,057	120	1,404	4,259	3,229	1,671
Rutherford County	60,917	73	680	2,064	1,565	826
Sampson County	52,367	52	570	1,731	1,312	761
Scotland County	35,712	27	373	1,132	859	575
Stanly County	55,836	44	621	1,883	1,428	767
Stokes County	43,275	34	483	1,465	1,111	589
Surry County	67,251	64	767	2,325	1,763	857
Swain County	12,265	14	135	410	311	173
Transylvania County	28,453	27	331	1,005	762	338
Tyrrell County	4,005	4	44	133	101	57
Union County	110,188	60	1,177	3,569	2,706	1,686
Vance County	42,058	32	456	1,383	1,048	620
Wake County	570,353	235	6,451	19,567	14,836	7,451
Warren County	18,768	20	212	643	487	247
Washington County	13,527	6	146	442	335	203
Watauga County	40,904	32	500	1,516	1,149	403
Wayne County	111,853	95	1,228	3,725	2,824	1,592
Wilkes County	62,755	65	711	2,157	1,635	816
Wilson County	68,242	61	750	2,274	1,724	970
Yadkin County	34,892	16	399	1,211	918	439
Yancey County	16,590	17	191	580	440	204
NORTH DAKOTA CONSTITUENT: ALA OF NORTH DAKOTA	637,808	410	7,127	21,618	16,388	8,640
Adams County	2,707	1	31	94	71	34
Barnes County	11,960	10	138	420	318	145

TABLE 1 ESTIMATED PREVALENCE AND INCIDENCE OF LUNG DISEASE BY COUNTY,
STATE, AND LUNG ASSOCIATION, 1998 *(continued)*

| Association | Population | Lung Cancer[1] | CHRONIC LUNG DISEASES | | | |
			Emphysema	Chronic Bronchitis	Adult Asthma	Pediatric Asthma
ALA OF NORTH DAKOTA (cont.)						
Benson County	6,851	0	67	202	153	128
Billings County	1,068	0	11	34	26	17
Bottineau County	7,300	3	83	253	192	92
Bowman County	3,303	1	37	113	85	44
Burke County	2,269	3	27	81	61	26
Burleigh County	66,906	43	748	2,269	1,721	905
Cass County	116,888	60	1,343	4,075	3,090	1,451
Cavalier County	5,025	3	58	175	132	63
Dickey County	5,653	5	65	197	150	70
Divide County	2,368	4	28	85	65	26
Dunn County	3,551	1	38	116	88	54
Eddy County	2,850	6	33	99	75	36
Emmons County	4,330	5	50	153	116	52
Foster County	3,808	4	43	130	98	51
Golden Valley County	1,849	0	20	61	46	27
Grand Forks County	66,781	35	756	2,293	1,739	870
Grant County	2,960	3	34	103	78	37
Griggs County	2,846	1	33	99	75	35
Hettinger County	2,906	4	34	102	77	35
Kidder County	2,882	0	33	99	75	38
LaMoure County	4,775	3	54	163	124	63
Logan County	2,349	3	27	83	63	28
McHenry County	6,071	4	69	208	158	79
McIntosh County	3,458	5	42	129	98	33
McKenzie County	5,683	5	59	178	135	95
McLean County	9,712	8	107	324	245	138
Mercer County	9,399	8	99	299	227	150
Morton County	24,607	17	268	812	616	358
Mountrail County	6,593	9	70	213	161	102
Nelson County	3,725	5	44	134	102	41
Oliver County	2,202	0	23	69	52	36
Pembina County	8,483	8	94	286	217	116
Pierce County	4,646	9	53	161	122	59
Ramsey County	12,109	10	137	417	316	157
Ransom County	5,781	3	66	199	151	75
Renville County	2,814	1	31	95	72	38
Richland County	18,096	9	203	617	468	241
Rolette County	14,148	13	130	393	298	292
Sargent County	4,445	4	50	152	115	59
Sheridan County	1,692	0	20	61	46	19
Sioux County	4,148	0	35	106	80	97
Slope County	880	1	10	29	22	12
Stark County	22,707	8	249	755	572	325
Steele County	2,228	1	25	77	58	29
Stutsman County	20,981	20	241	732	555	260
Towner County	3,013	3	34	103	78	39
Traill County	8,538	4	97	294	223	110
Walsh County	13,557	8	151	459	348	184
Ward County	58,540	26	648	1,965	1,490	815
Wells County	5,208	5	61	185	140	61
Williams County	20,159	18	220	667	505	293

| Association | Population | Lung Cancer[1] | CHRONIC LUNG DISEASES | | | |
			Emphysema	Chronic Bronchitis	Adult Asthma	Pediatric Asthma
NORTHERN ROCKIES (MONTANA/ WYOMING) CONSTITUENT: *ALA OF NORTHERN ROCKIES*	1,359,578	887	15,064	45,687	34,641	18,875
MONTANA	879,533	617	9,803	29,730	22,543	12,006
Beaverhead County	8,809	14	99	299	227	119
Big Horn County	12,597	9	119	362	274	247
Blaine County	7,090	4	71	217	164	124
Broadwater County	4,131	1	45	138	105	58
Carbon County	9,402	9	105	319	242	127
Carter County	1,512	0	17	52	40	19
Cascade County	78,558	73	879	2,666	2,021	1,060
Chouteau County	5,187	5	58	176	133	70
Custer County	12,046	10	135	409	310	163
Daniels County	1,996	3	23	70	53	24
Dawson County	8,812	9	99	301	228	117
Deer Lodge County	9,961	5	117	354	268	116
Fallon County	2,957	1	32	98	74	43
Fergus County	12,276	14	139	422	320	160
Flathead County	71,888	46	798	2,420	1,835	994
Gallatin County	62,561	23	728	2,207	1,673	746
Garfield County	1,412	0	15	46	35	21
Glacier County	12,542	6	119	360	273	246
Golden Valley County	1,033	1	11	34	26	15
Granite County	2,665	4	30	92	69	35
Hill County	17,362	13	185	560	425	268
Jefferson County	10,118	3	110	334	253	148
Judith Basin County	2,294	1	26	80	61	28
Lake County	25,557	18	272	825	626	394
Lewis and Clark County	53,587	34	601	1,823	1,382	718
Liberty County	2,313	0	26	78	59	32
Lincoln County	18,717	17	206	625	474	265
Mc Cone County	1,961	1	22	67	51	26
Madison County	6,889	3	79	239	182	86
Meagher County	1,794	3	20	61	47	24
Mineral County	3,781	3	42	126	96	53
Missoula County	88,907	47	1,018	3,089	2,343	1,116
Musselshell County	4,572	4	52	158	120	58
Park County	15,795	17	181	548	415	199
Petroleum County	509	0	6	17	13	7
Phillips County	4,797	6	51	156	118	72
Pondera County	6,350	5	68	206	156	97
Powder River County	1,804	1	21	62	47	23
Powell County	7,004	5	84	254	192	76
Prairie County	1,352	0	16	48	36	16
Ravalli County	35,114	27	393	1,192	904	473
Richland County	10,161	8	109	329	250	155
Roosevelt County	10,997	5	108	326	247	203
Rosebud County	10,010	8	97	295	224	187
Sanders County	10,185	17	113	341	259	143
Sheridan County	4,244	3	49	148	112	53
Silver Bow County	34,540	29	399	1,210	918	422
Stillwater County	8,076	4	89	270	205	113
Sweet Grass County	3,391	3	38	116	88	45
Teton County	6,349	9	69	210	159	92

TABLE 1 ESTIMATED PREVALENCE AND INCIDENCE OF LUNG DISEASE BY COUNTY,
STATE, AND LUNG ASSOCIATION, 1998 *(continued)*

| Association | Population | Lung Cancer[1] | CHRONIC LUNG DISEASES | | | |
			Emphysema	Chronic Bronchitis	Adult Asthma	Pediatric Asthma
ALA OF NORTHERN						
ROCKIES (cont.)						
Toole County	4,738	8	51	154	117	72
Treasure County	876	0	10	29	22	12
Valley County	8,233	4	92	280	212	110
Wheatland County	2,345	1	26	80	61	31
Wibaux County	1,139	0	13	39	29	15
Yellowstone County	126,237	73	1,422	4,313	3,270	1,670
WYOMING	480,045	270	5,261	15,957	12,098	6,869
Albany County	29,251	9	356	1,080	819	293
Big Horn County	11,331	12	123	373	283	166
Campbell County	32,387	16	326	988	749	567
Carbon County	15,543	8	172	521	395	217
Converse County	12,280	6	129	393	298	194
Crook County	5,781	4	62	188	142	88
Fremont County	36,128	36	388	1,176	891	546
Goshen County	12,805	10	144	437	331	170
Hot Springs County	4,646	5	53	162	123	57
Johnson County	6,796	9	78	237	179	85
Laramie County	78,583	35	885	2,684	2,035	1,041
Lincoln County	13,809	6	136	412	312	252
Natrona County	63,241	47	705	2,137	1,621	864
Niobrara County	2,700	1	32	96	73	31
Park County	25,751	14	289	878	666	343
Platte County	8,618	3	96	292	221	117
Sheridan County	25,154	16	287	871	660	320
Sublette County	5,746	0	65	196	149	76
Sweetwater County	39,722	13	410	1,243	943	658
Teton County	14,193	4	166	504	382	166
Uinta County	20,394	8	192	583	442	402
Washakie County	8,686	5	95	287	218	126
Weston County	6,500	3	72	219	166	90
OHIO						
CONSTITUENT:	11,237,752	9,360	125,868	381,801	289,496	151,149
ALA OF OHIO						
Adams County	28,564	18	306	929	704	433
Allen County	107,246	86	1,181	3,584	2,717	1,513
Ashland County	51,634	30	569	1,725	1,308	728
Ashtabula County	103,242	91	1,133	3,436	2,605	1,472
Athens County	61,616	48	734	2,227	1,688	673
Auglaize County	47,042	32	507	1,539	1,167	702
Belmont County	71,860	88	838	2,541	1,927	850
Brown County	40,808	31	439	1,331	1,010	613
Butler County	330,892	248	3,686	11,182	8,479	4,520
Carroll County	29,088	14	320	969	735	413
Champaign County	38,349	42	427	1,295	982	525
Clark County	145,266	164	1,634	4,956	3,758	1,930
Clermont County	175,786	139	1,878	5,696	4,319	2,686
Clinton County	40,135	31	440	1,335	1,012	573
Columbiana County	111,407	84	1,240	3,760	2,851	1,527
Coshocton County	36,127	23	399	1,210	918	506
Crawford County	47,184	44	526	1,594	1,209	645
Cuyahoga County	1,380,428	1,256	15,772	47,841	36,275	17,469
Darke County	54,071	42	594	1,803	1,367	767

Association	Population	Lung Cancer[1]	CHRONIC LUNG DISEASES			
			Emphysema	Chronic Bronchitis	Adult Asthma	Pediatric Asthma
Defiance County	39,838	16	431	1,308	992	589
Delaware County	98,208	52	1,077	3,268	2,478	1,401
Erie County	78,226	83	878	2,665	2,020	1,044
Fairfield County	123,949	74	1,369	4,152	3,148	1,736
Fayette County	28,505	36	317	962	730	390
Franklin County	1,021,578	719	11,560	35,066	26,588	13,323
Fulton County	41,801	21	446	1,354	1,027	640
Gallia County	33,217	23	368	1,116	846	462
Geauga County	88,591	57	976	2,960	2,244	1,250
Greene County	147,942	120	1,668	5,061	3,837	1,950
Guernsey County	40,921	46	451	1,368	1,037	576
Hamilton County	847,202	788	9,442	28,640	21,716	11,562
Hancock County	69,009	39	763	2,315	1,755	963
Hardin County	31,691	26	356	1,079	818	424
Harrison County	16,119	22	182	552	419	212
Henry County	29,880	20	322	976	740	447
Highland County	40,427	36	442	1,341	1,017	581
Hocking County	28,926	27	322	975	740	398
Holmes County	37,848	20	368	1,116	846	707
Huron County	60,217	34	645	1,957	1,484	914
Jackson County	32,574	31	356	1,079	818	471
Jefferson County	74,596	83	867	2,630	1,994	892
Knox County	53,399	34	604	1,833	1,390	697
Lake County	226,825	187	2,593	7,866	5,964	2,865
Lawrence County	64,446	65	713	2,162	1,639	899
Licking County	134,962	122	1,507	4,572	3,466	1,831
Logan County	46,358	39	505	1,531	1,161	675
Lorain County	281,716	238	3,095	9,389	7,119	4,002
Lucas County	448,635	387	4,961	15,047	11,409	6,262
Madison County	41,089	36	469	1,423	1,079	521
Mahoning County	255,292	276	2,911	8,830	6,695	3,252
Marion County	67,087	53	756	2,294	1,739	885
Medina County	143,855	90	1,568	4,756	3,606	2,088
Meigs County	23,956	32	264	802	608	337
Mercer County	41,095	30	431	1,307	991	657
Miami County	98,208	74	1,091	3,310	2,510	1,352
Monroe County	15,377	17	174	527	400	201
Montgomery County	570,141	484	6,481	19,659	14,906	7,332
Morgan County	14,528	14	157	476	361	216
Morrow County	31,448	20	338	1,025	777	473
Muskingum County	84,635	78	938	2,844	2,156	1,175
Noble County	14,736	5	168	508	386	189
Ottawa County	41,011	30	469	1,424	1,080	516
Paulding County	20,082	25	213	648	491	311
Perry County	34,221	27	366	1,111	843	520
Pickaway County	53,278	42	613	1,859	1,409	660
Pike County	27,732	16	298	904	685	418
Portage County	150,829	121	1,714	5,199	3,942	1,942
Preble County	43,115	29	474	1,438	1,090	611
Putnam County	35,244	12	365	1,108	840	579
Richland County	129,697	112	1,462	4,434	3,362	1,712
Ross County	75,411	88	856	2,596	1,968	975
Sandusky County	62,077	39	676	2,051	1,556	902
Scioto County	80,777	87	890	2,700	2,047	1,138
Seneca County	59,975	55	650	1,973	1,496	882
Shelby County	47,547	42	505	1,532	1,162	737
Stark County	373,024	315	4,230	12,831	9,729	4,833
Summit County	537,160	477	6,112	18,541	14,059	6,885
Trumbull County	226,355	204	2,577	7,817	5,928	2,896

TABLE 1 ESTIMATED PREVALENCE AND INCIDENCE OF LUNG DISEASE BY COUNTY,
STATE, AND LUNG ASSOCIATION, 1998 *(continued)*

| Association | Population | Lung Cancer[1] | CHRONIC LUNG DISEASES | | | |
			Emphysema	Chronic Bronchitis	Adult Asthma	Pediatric Asthma
ALA OF OHIO (cont.)						
Tuscarawas County	88,543	70	988	2,997	2,272	1,204
Union County	39,883	29	440	1,334	1,011	561
Van Wert County	30,080	22	329	999	757	432
Vinton County	12,165	9	132	400	303	179
Warren County	146,027	96	1,621	4,916	3,728	2,016
Washington County	63,314	44	714	2,167	1,643	833
Wayne County	110,156	73	1,197	3,630	2,753	1,613
Williams County	37,858	42	412	1,249	947	553
Wood County	119,574	79	1,361	4,129	3,131	1,531
Wyandot County	22,819	10	251	760	577	324
OKLAHOMA						
CONSTITUENT:	3,339,478	3,069	36,851	111,772	84,754	46,877
ALA OF OKLAHOMA						
Adair County	20,404	21	214	649	492	326
Alfalfa County	6,025	5	71	215	163	69
Atoka County	13,302	21	148	450	341	182
Beaver County	6,045	6	65	198	150	90
Beckham County	19,949	13	214	648	491	303
Blaine County	10,420	14	113	343	260	153
Bryan County	34,717	38	390	1,183	897	463
Caddo County	30,881	25	335	1,016	771	454
Canadian County	85,424	57	902	2,735	2,074	1,344
Carter County	44,358	47	486	1,473	1,117	636
Cherokee County	39,019	44	429	1,302	987	553
Choctaw County	15,103	16	164	497	377	222
Cimarron County	2,990	4	32	98	74	44
Cleveland County	200,977	104	2,225	6,750	5,118	2,794
Coal County	6,030	4	66	201	153	85
Comanche County	108,143	70	1,149	3,486	2,643	1,674
Cotton County	6,641	6	74	223	169	92
Craig County	14,465	13	167	506	384	177
Creek County	67,117	72	735	2,230	1,691	961
Custer County	25,572	13	281	852	646	364
Delaware County	34,305	53	392	1,190	902	433
Dewey County	4,923	9	54	165	125	69
Ellis County	4,245	6	47	142	108	59
Garfield County	56,939	53	631	1,915	1,452	788
Garvin County	26,808	35	300	909	689	363
Grady County	45,765	39	492	1,493	1,132	688
Grant County	5,339	10	60	181	137	73
Greer County	6,357	6	76	230	174	69
Harmon County	3,476	4	37	112	85	54
Harper County	3,593	5	40	122	93	48
Haskell County	11,359	17	127	385	292	154
Hughes County	14,102	20	163	493	374	173
Jackson County	28,536	23	297	901	683	464
Jefferson County	6,578	10	74	225	170	87
Johnston County	10,302	14	113	343	260	147
Kay County	46,572	58	516	1,566	1,188	645
Kingfisher County	13,480	5	145	438	332	204
Kiowa County	10,671	8	116	352	267	155
Latimer County	10,276	12	113	342	259	147
Le Flore County	46,662	55	508	1,541	1,168	679
Lincoln County	31,318	14	339	1,027	779	465

Association	Population	Lung Cancer[1]	CHRONIC LUNG DISEASES			
			Emphysema	Chronic Bronchitis	Adult Asthma	Pediatric Asthma
Logan County	30,087	30	328	994	753	438
Love County	8,550	10	94	286	217	120
McClain County	26,206	31	286	869	659	377
McCurtain County	34,779	38	369	1,119	849	541
McIntosh County	19,006	18	220	668	507	229
Major County	7,804	1	86	260	197	111
Marshall County	12,251	14	142	430	326	149
Mayes County	37,635	38	418	1,267	961	520
Murray County	12,329	12	138	419	317	166
Muskogee County	70,091	81	768	2,328	1,765	1,005
Noble County	11,362	10	124	377	286	163
Nowata County	9,980	13	113	342	260	130
Okfuskee County	11,392	6	127	385	292	156
Oklahoma County	632,865	559	7,018	21,289	16,142	8,760
Okmulgee County	38,666	35	424	1,287	976	551
Osage County	42,896	40	467	1,418	1,075	623
Ottawa County	30,891	48	353	1,070	812	391
Pawnee County	16,392	17	180	546	414	233
Payne County	65,274	44	771	2,338	1,773	737
Pittsburg County	43,022	57	491	1,490	1,130	545
Pontotoc County	34,631	52	390	1,183	897	458
Pottawatomie County	62,291	68	685	2,077	1,575	884
Pushmataha County	11,474	17	129	390	296	154
Roger Mills County	3,581	4	39	118	90	52
Rogers County	68,013	53	746	2,262	1,715	972
Seminole County	24,756	48	274	830	630	345
Sequoyah County	37,546	40	407	1,234	936	554
Stephens County	43,527	52	483	1,466	1,112	600
Texas County	18,540	16	196	596	452	289
Tillman County	9,524	10	102	308	234	146
Tulsa County	543,417	452	6,036	18,308	13,882	7,489
Wagoner County	55,223	43	584	1,772	1,343	865
Washington County	47,523	34	535	1,622	1,230	630
Washita County	11,842	9	129	391	296	172
Woods County	8,300	4	98	296	225	95
Woodward County	18,624	16	201	610	463	277
OREGON CONSTITUENT: *ALA OF OREGON*	3,282,055	2,629	36,889	111,899	84,846	43,688
Baker County	16,411	25	184	560	424	218
Benton County	77,823	42	910	2,762	2,094	909
Clackamas County	334,773	208	3,732	11,320	8,583	4,565
Clatsop County	35,364	34	397	1,204	913	473
Columbia County	44,513	40	481	1,460	1,107	660
Coos County	62,156	103	711	2,157	1,636	783
Crook County	17,295	14	191	578	438	244
Curry County	21,071	40	257	778	590	211
Deschutes County	105,731	56	1,186	3,596	2,727	1,417
Douglas County	101,839	127	1,142	3,465	2,627	1,364
Gilliam County	2,020	1	22	68	52	28
Grant County	8,037	6	90	272	206	109
Harney County	7,201	4	80	242	183	100
Hood River County	19,595	16	212	644	489	289
Jackson County	173,243	160	1,964	5,958	4,517	2,247
Jefferson County	16,747	14	177	538	408	262
Josephine County	74,166	91	849	2,576	1,953	932
Klamath County	63,160	53	702	2,128	1,614	870
Lake County	7,157	10	79	239	181	101

TABLE 1   ESTIMATED PREVALENCE AND INCIDENCE OF LUNG DISEASE BY COUNTY,
STATE, AND LUNG ASSOCIATION, 1998 *(continued)*

Association	Population	Lung Cancer[1]	CHRONIC LUNG DISEASES			
			Emphysema	Chronic Bronchitis	Adult Asthma	Pediatric Asthma
ALA OF OREGON (cont.)						
Lane County	313,344	273	3,587	10,881	8,251	3,940
Lincoln County	45,282	49	526	1,596	1,210	542
Linn County	104,461	86	1,159	3,515	2,665	1,445
Malheur County	28,549	20	297	899	682	466
Marion County	268,910	207	2,947	8,940	6,779	3,846
Morrow County	9,953	10	105	318	241	158
Multnomah County	630,573	506	7,276	22,072	16,736	7,725
Polk County	61,403	40	686	2,082	1,579	831
Sherman County	1,795	3	20	60	46	25
Tillamook County	24,283	21	281	854	647	293
Umatilla County	65,591	58	709	2,150	1,630	974
Union County	24,874	21	274	830	629	352
Wallowa County	7,334	10	82	249	189	99
Wasco County	23,101	23	255	773	586	324
Washington County	400,715	200	4,419	13,405	10,164	5,634
Wheeler County	1,570	1	19	56	43	17
Yamhill County	82,015	57	881	2,674	2,027	1,235
PENNSYLVANIA CONSTITUENT: ALA OF PENNSYLVANIA	12,002,329	10,688	137,136	415,982	315,416	151,857
Adams County	86,660	62	972	2,948	2,235	1,162
Allegheny County	1,267,963	1,451	14,950	45,349	34,385	14,405
Armstrong County	73,313	48	834	2,530	1,918	941
Beaver County	184,287	216	2,121	6,434	4,878	2,277
Bedford County	49,405	42	556	1,686	1,279	655
Berks County	355,761	312	4,062	12,322	9,343	4,510
Blair County	130,547	126	1,479	4,486	3,401	1,697
Bradford County	62,386	49	683	2,071	1,570	896
Bucks County	587,863	434	6,581	19,962	15,136	7,919
Butler County	170,799	131	1,922	5,830	4,421	2,266
Cambria County	155,587	131	1,794	5,443	4,127	1,909
Cameron County	5,612	5	63	192	145	74
Carbon County	58,690	64	678	2,056	1,559	717
Centre County	131,997	58	1,610	4,883	3,703	1,310
Chester County	421,873	266	4,749	14,406	10,923	5,589
Clarion County	41,723	26	479	1,454	1,103	519
Clearfield County	80,722	61	911	2,764	2,095	1,061
Clinton County	36,937	34	424	1,287	976	459
Columbia County	63,906	57	749	2,273	1,723	741
Crawford County	89,266	84	992	3,010	2,283	1,227
Cumberland County	209,611	134	2,464	7,474	5,667	2,407
Dauphin County	245,456	203	2,793	8,473	6,425	3,146
Delaware County	542,592	507	6,232	18,905	14,335	6,749
Elk County	34,614	30	387	1,173	890	469
Erie County	278,114	230	3,082	9,348	7,088	3,858
Fayette County	144,362	125	1,636	4,963	3,763	1,874
Forest County	4,947	9	56	170	129	64
Franklin County	128,255	87	1,456	4,416	3,349	1,656
Fulton County	14,528	10	160	486	368	205
Greene County	42,228	39	474	1,439	1,091	563
Huntingdon County	44,755	22	515	1,562	1,185	553
Indiana County	88,389	65	1,012	3,071	2,329	1,109
Jefferson County	46,184	34	516	1,564	1,186	627

Association	Population	Lung Cancer[1]	CHRONIC LUNG DISEASES			
			Emphysema	Chronic Bronchitis	Adult Asthma	Pediatric Asthma
Juniata County	22,119	14	246	745	565	305
Lackawanna County	208,390	240	2,435	7,385	5,600	2,447
Lancaster County	456,679	309	5,023	15,238	11,554	6,467
Lawrence County	94,904	101	1,088	3,299	2,502	1,189
Lebanon County	117,631	103	1,336	4,052	3,073	1,517
Lehigh County	298,792	217	3,460	10,495	7,958	3,618
Luzerne County	314,609	272	3,704	11,235	8,519	3,594
Lycoming County	117,408	86	1,321	4,007	3,038	1,558
McKean County	46,319	53	522	1,583	1,200	612
Mercer County	121,760	105	1,399	4,245	3,219	1,512
Mifflin County	46,965	51	530	1,606	1,218	619
Monroe County	125,407	107	1,402	4,252	3,224	1,697
Montgomery County	719,569	528	8,374	25,401	19,260	8,565
Montour County	17,585	18	199	602	457	231
Northampton County	258,568	183	2,964	8,990	6,816	3,239
Northumberland County	93,950	64	1,087	3,298	2,501	1,140
Perry County	44,273	25	485	1,472	1,116	633
Philadelphia County	1,434,968	1,664	16,035	48,639	36,880	19,433
Pike County	40,149	20	448	1,360	1,031	545
Potter County	17,134	16	186	565	428	250
Schuylkill County	150,066	164	1,759	5,335	4,045	1,743
Snyder County	37,965	23	425	1,290	978	510
Somerset County	80,192	53	911	2,763	2,095	1,033
Sullivan County	6,074	5	70	212	161	75
Susquehanna County	42,082	35	462	1,401	1,062	600
Tioga County	41,522	34	465	1,410	1,069	559
Union County	40,270	25	476	1,444	1,095	453
Venango County	57,795	55	644	1,952	1,480	791
Warren County	43,793	35	493	1,494	1,133	582
Washington County	205,339	233	2,382	7,227	5,480	2,469
Wayne County	45,431	51	515	1,562	1,184	590
Westmoreland County	372,389	348	4,345	13,180	9,993	4,393
Wyoming County	29,212	25	319	969	735	421
York County	373,688	274	4,234	12,844	9,739	4,853
RHODE ISLAND CONSTITUENT: ALA OF RHODE ISLAND	987,704	951	11,258	34,151	25,896	12,591
Bristol County	49,194	43	572	1,736	1,317	586
Kent County	161,418	172	1,853	5,621	4,262	2,011
Newport County	82,586	87	942	2,856	2,166	1,052
Providence County	573,701	546	6,522	19,785	15,002	7,374
Washington County	120,805	103	1,369	4,153	3,149	1,568
SOUTH CAROLINA CONSTITUENT: ALA OF SOUTH CAROLINA	3,839,578	2,968	43,255	131,198	99,482	50,763
Abbeville County	24,641	9	280	849	644	317
Aiken County	134,008	104	1,493	4,528	3,433	1,831
Allendale County	11,406	10	125	380	288	162
Anderson County	160,711	110	1,839	5,577	4,229	2,025
Bamberg County	16,446	13	181	548	415	234
Barnwell County	21,821	23	233	707	536	333
Beaufort County	110,089	88	1,263	3,832	2,906	1,374
Berkeley County	137,591	79	1,434	4,351	3,299	2,229
Calhoun County	14,074	13	157	477	362	191

TABLE 1 ESTIMATED PREVALENCE AND INCIDENCE OF LUNG DISEASE BY COUNTY, STATE, AND LUNG ASSOCIATION, 1998 (continued)

Association	Population	Lung Cancer[1]	Emphysema	Chronic Bronchitis	Adult Asthma	Pediatric Asthma
				CHRONIC LUNG DISEASES		
ALA OF SOUTH CAROLINA (cont.)						
Charleston County	316,606	216	3,608	10,943	8,297	4,041
Cherokee County	49,223	36	553	1,676	1,271	657
Chester County	34,355	26	380	1,151	873	481
Chesterfield County	41,069	40	456	1,382	1,048	568
Clarendon County	30,767	23	340	1,031	782	430
Colleton County	37,350	30	406	1,231	934	546
Darlington County	66,334	64	731	2,217	1,681	935
Dillon County	29,705	23	312	948	718	472
Dorchester County	88,035	66	950	2,882	2,186	1,311
Edgefield County	20,006	14	221	671	509	279
Fairfield County	22,415	20	248	751	569	314
Florence County	124,682	120	1,371	4,158	3,153	1,768
Georgetown County	53,695	52	590	1,789	1,356	763
Greenville County	353,986	273	4,059	12,313	9,337	4,426
Greenwood County	63,594	52	727	2,204	1,672	804
Hampton County	19,147	9	203	615	466	299
Horry County	174,555	187	2,031	6,160	4,671	2,080
Jasper County	17,055	14	182	551	418	263
Kershaw County	48,613	42	544	1,649	1,250	657
Lancaster County	58,873	49	659	1,999	1,515	794
Laurens County	63,155	60	717	2,175	1,649	815
Lee County	20,302	14	224	680	516	284
Lexington County	205,044	159	2,297	6,969	5,284	2,755
Mc Cormick County	9,533	4	112	341	259	108
Marion County	34,546	18	368	1,116	846	532
Marlboro County	29,593	26	326	989	750	417
Newberry County	34,433	35	393	1,191	903	438
Oconee County	64,138	48	741	2,248	1,704	782
Orangeburg County	87,710	60	975	2,956	2,242	1,207
Pickens County	107,042	65	1,259	3,818	2,895	1,229
Richland County	304,891	208	3,528	10,701	8,114	3,701
Saluda County	17,036	10	192	584	443	223
Spartanburg County	247,206	202	2,838	8,608	6,527	3,081
Sumter County	112,325	75	1,231	3,733	2,830	1,608
Union County	30,523	23	351	1,065	808	377
Williamsburg County	36,980	36	388	1,178	893	588
York County	154,269	120	1,739	5,276	4,001	2,034
SOUTH DAKOTA CONSTITUENT:	730,789	502	7,958	24,136	18,298	10,640
ALA OF SOUTH DAKOTA						
Aurora County	3,018	5	33	99	75	45
Beadle County	17,134	16	193	585	443	228
Bennett County	3,385	0	32	96	73	67
Bon Homme County	7,257	4	84	254	193	89
Brookings County	25,956	8	305	924	701	300
Brown County	35,399	26	403	1,221	926	454
Brule County	5,530	1	57	172	130	93
Buffalo County	1,755	0	14	44	33	42
Butte County	8,923	5	96	292	221	133
Campbell County	1,877	1	22	68	51	21
Charles Mix County	9,305	8	95	289	219	157
Clark County	4,336	1	47	144	109	62
Clay County	13,192	5	159	481	365	139

Association	Population	Lung Cancer[1]	CHRONIC LUNG DISEASES			
			Emphysema	Chronic Bronchitis	Adult Asthma	Pediatric Asthma
Codington County	25,433	18	276	838	635	373
Corson County	4,181	4	40	120	91	82
Custer County	6,945	8	77	234	177	96
Davison County	17,732	16	196	596	452	246
Day County	6,398	9	71	214	163	90
Deuel County	4,502	0	50	153	116	60
Dewey County	5,870	4	51	155	118	130
Douglas County	3,517	9	38	115	87	52
Edmunds County	4,217	8	48	144	109	56
Fall River County	6,868	6	80	242	183	83
Faulk County	2,518	0	29	87	66	32
Grant County	8,051	1	87	263	200	120
Gregory County	4,954	6	54	165	125	71
Haakon County	2,359	0	24	72	54	42
Hamlin County	5,323	3	58	175	133	78
Hand County	4,161	5	46	140	106	58
Hanson County	2,955	3	31	95	72	46
Harding County	1,495	0	16	47	36	24
Hughes County	15,348	9	166	502	381	229
Hutchinson County	8,049	13	92	279	211	102
Hyde County	1,618	3	18	55	42	22
Jackson County	2,907	0	28	84	63	57
Jerauld County	2,209	1	25	76	58	28
Jones County	1,227	4	14	41	31	17
Kingsbury County	5,761	3	65	197	149	76
Lake County	10,679	6	120	363	275	144
Lawrence County	21,913	13	244	741	562	299
Lincoln County	20,448	8	214	648	492	329
Lyman County	3,775	3	37	113	86	68
McCook County	5,612	5	61	187	141	80
McPherson County	2,734	4	32	96	73	33
Marshall County	4,556	4	51	155	118	61
Meade County	21,614	13	224	681	516	353
Mellette County	2,040	3	19	59	44	40
Miner County	2,808	1	31	95	72	38
Minnehaha County	140,397	91	1,565	4,748	3,600	1,914
Moody County	6,496	5	68	206	156	104
Pennington County	87,323	57	949	2,878	2,182	1,279
Perkins County	3,492	1	40	120	91	45
Potter County	2,866	0	32	98	74	38
Roberts County	9,863	9	103	312	236	160
Sanborn County	2,719	1	30	91	69	39
Shannon County	12,198	12	97	295	224	303
Spink County	7,548	5	84	256	194	102
Stanley County	2,924	3	31	93	70	47
Sully County	1,477	0	16	50	38	21
Todd County	9,295	3	74	226	171	230
Tripp County	6,723	8	72	217	165	104
Turner County	8,620	5	96	292	222	117
Union County	12,260	6	132	400	304	184
Walworth County	5,595	6	62	188	142	78
Yankton County	20,989	17	236	715	542	280
Ziebach County	2,160	0	18	55	42	50
TENNESSEE CONSTITUENT: ALA OF TENNESSEE	5,432,679	4,957	61,466	186,452	141,378	70,880
Anderson County	70,893	84	818	2,480	1,881	870
Bedford County	34,528	29	387	1,175	891	463

TABLE 1 ESTIMATED PREVALENCE AND INCIDENCE OF LUNG DISEASE BY COUNTY,
STATE, AND LUNG ASSOCIATION, 1998 *(continued)*

| Association | Population | Lung Cancer[1] | CHRONIC LUNG DISEASES | | | |
			Emphysema	Chronic Bronchitis	Adult Asthma	Pediatric Asthma
ALA OF TENNESSEE						
(cont.)						
Benton County	16,291	18	190	576	437	193
Bledsoe County	10,762	12	123	374	283	135
Blount County	101,211	95	1,175	3,564	2,702	1,215
Bradley County	83,370	53	955	2,896	2,196	1,048
Campbell County	38,163	69	430	1,303	988	506
Cannon County	12,146	18	137	417	316	159
Carroll County	29,184	26	336	1,018	772	361
Carter County	53,321	46	629	1,907	1,446	606
Cheatham County	35,257	26	383	1,163	882	515
Chester County	14,677	17	168	510	386	185
Claiborne County	29,504	42	332	1,008	764	391
Clay County	7,273	8	84	255	194	88
Cocke County	31,953	42	368	1,116	846	394
Coffee County	45,815	48	516	1,564	1,186	607
Crockett County	14,017	18	159	482	365	182
Cumberland County	44,144	47	516	1,565	1,187	518
Davidson County	533,258	478	6,187	18,767	14,230	6,414
Decatur County	10,760	16	125	381	289	127
DeKalb County	16,007	21	183	555	421	202
Dickson County	42,283	31	462	1,403	1,064	608
Dyer County	36,577	31	409	1,240	940	495
Fayette County	30,406	25	321	973	738	479
Fentress County	16,153	21	181	549	417	217
Franklin County	37,606	30	431	1,308	992	470
Gibson County	48,016	69	551	1,671	1,267	600
Giles County	28,905	31	326	990	751	380
Grainger County	19,801	20	227	687	521	249
Greene County	60,257	57	705	2,140	1,622	703
Grundy County	14,048	14	153	466	353	203
Hamblen County	53,959	65	623	1,890	1,433	659
Hamilton County	294,494	272	3,381	10,254	7,775	3,670
Hancock County	6,808	16	77	233	177	90
Hardeman County	24,285	36	262	795	603	361
Hardin County	24,905	26	283	859	652	320
Hawkins County	49,524	44	573	1,738	1,318	602
Haywood County	19,534	20	208	630	478	302
Henderson County	24,418	30	277	840	637	316
Henry County	29,971	35	349	1,058	802	357
Hickman County	20,662	13	237	719	545	258
Houston County	7,841	13	90	272	207	98
Humphreys County	17,029	13	194	587	445	219
Jackson County	9,616	14	112	340	257	114
Jefferson County	43,609	39	514	1,560	1,183	495
Johnson County	16,709	14	198	601	456	186
Knox County	374,693	355	4,376	13,273	10,064	4,406
Lake County	8,205	6	101	306	232	78
Lauderdale County	24,172	25	263	799	606	351
Lawrence County	39,318	56	439	1,331	1,009	534
Lewis County	10,881	13	120	363	275	155
Lincoln County	29,678	35	337	1,023	776	382
Loudon County	39,023	38	454	1,378	1,045	463
McMinn County	46,210	44	528	1,602	1,214	585
McNairy County	23,987	29	275	833	631	302
Macon County	18,066	17	203	616	467	240

Association	Population	Lung Cancer[1]	CHRONIC LUNG DISEASES			
			Emphysema	Chronic Bronchitis	Adult Asthma	Pediatric Asthma
Madison County	85,825	58	953	2,892	2,193	1,182
Mario County	26,677	23	298	905	686	360
Marshall County	26,261	25	294	891	676	354
Maury County	69,590	58	772	2,343	1,777	961
Meigs County	9,969	9	113	343	260	129
Monroe County	34,846	36	393	1,192	904	460
Montgomery County	127,156	110	1,384	4,198	3,183	1,853
Moore County	5,155	3	58	177	134	67
Morgan County	18,675	25	210	636	482	249
Obion County	32,165	36	365	1,109	841	414
Overton County	19,519	29	224	679	515	244
Perry County	7,529	13	86	260	197	97
Pickett County	4,648	5	53	161	122	59
Polk County	14,931	20	172	521	395	184
Putnam County	59,050	55	691	2,097	1,590	688
Rhea County	27,825	43	315	954	723	364
Roane County	49,945	62	582	1,765	1,339	592
Robertson County	53,192	43	581	1,763	1,337	767
Rutherford County	166,086	101	1,814	5,502	4,172	2,399
Scott County	20,075	14	214	651	493	307
Sequatchie County	10,473	5	118	357	271	140
Sevier County	64,371	60	743	2,255	1,710	787
Shelby County	867,804	611	9,480	28,756	21,804	12,521
Smith County	16,354	17	185	560	425	215
Stewart County	11,521	10	135	409	310	134
Sullivan County	150,348	162	1,772	5,376	4,076	1,709
Sumner County	123,942	86	1,363	4,135	3,135	1,756
Tipton County	47,300	42	496	1,503	1,140	757
Trousdale County	6,861	9	78	236	179	89
Unicoi County	17,209	29	204	619	470	191
Union County	16,192	20	179	544	412	225
Van Buren County	5,026	4	56	171	130	67
Warren County	36,137	18	409	1,240	940	472
Washington County	102,192	112	1,204	3,653	2,770	1,163
Wayne County	16,439	18	190	577	438	199
Weakley County	32,907	38	386	1,170	887	382
White County	22,708	22	261	792	600	282
Williamson County	117,685	65	1,272	3,859	2,926	1,745
Wilson County	83,908	51	922	2,798	2,122	1,190
TEXAS CONSTITUENT: ALA OF TEXAS	19,712,389	12,294	210,848	639,570	484,947	300,326
Anderson County	52,121	51	602	1,825	1,383	638
Andrews County	14,047	9	138	418	317	258
Angelina County	77,290	64	828	2,511	1,904	1,174
Aransas County	22,819	39	256	775	588	307
Archer County	8,282	12	90	272	206	122
Armstrong County	2,156	1	23	70	53	33
Atascosa County	36,389	21	365	1,107	839	641
Austin County	23,401	12	255	773	586	341
Bailey County	6,846	3	70	212	161	116
Bandera County	15,816	8	182	553	419	195
Bastrop County	50,438	46	533	1,618	1,227	790
Baylor County	4,157	5	48	146	111	50
Bee County	27,739	13	298	903	684	420
Bell County	223,167	142	2,370	7,189	5,451	3,460
Bexar County	1,354,837	684	14,324	43,448	32,944	21,237
Blanco County	8,338	3	97	293	222	101

TABLE 1 ESTIMATED PREVALENCE AND INCIDENCE OF LUNG DISEASE BY COUNTY,
STATE, AND LUNG ASSOCIATION, 1998 *(continued)*

Association	Population	Lung Cancer[1]	CHRONIC LUNG DISEASES			
			Emphysema	Chronic Bronchitis	Adult Asthma	Pediatric Asthma
ALA OF TEXAS (cont.)						
Borden County	766	1	8	25	19	11
Bosque County	16,548	20	187	567	430	217
Bowie County	83,287	72	915	2,777	2,106	1,182
Brazoria County	228,859	187	2,424	7,352	5,575	3,572
Brazos County	132,919	51	1,545	4,686	3,553	1,590
Brewster County	8,830	3	101	306	232	112
Briscoe County	1,887	3	20	61	46	29
Brooks County	8,427	1	85	259	196	145
Brown County	36,834	27	403	1,224	928	528
Burleson County	15,560	13	169	512	389	228
Burnet County	32,272	36	357	1,083	821	450
Caldwell County	32,023	30	335	1,015	770	515
Calhoun County	20,590	16	219	663	503	319
Callahan County	12,796	13	139	423	321	186
Cameron County	324,046	127	3,139	9,521	7,219	6,095
Camp County	10,933	18	121	367	278	153
Carson County	6,707	5	70	213	161	108
Cass County	30,745	42	337	1,023	776	438
Castro County	8,314	4	80	241	183	160
Chambers County	23,791	18	251	763	578	373
Cherokee County	43,306	48	480	1,456	1,104	600
Childress County	7,586	6	88	267	202	92
Clay County	10,534	8	116	352	267	148
Cochran County	3,918	4	39	119	91	69
Coke County	3,375	6	38	116	88	43
Coleman County	9,514	9	107	326	247	125
Collin County	428,345	117	4,553	13,810	10,471	6,629
Collingsworth County	3,267	3	35	108	82	48
Colorado County	18,909	14	208	632	479	267
Comal County	73,519	77	820	2,486	1,885	1,002
Comanche County	13,530	16	153	465	352	176
Concho County	3,098	3	35	106	81	41
Cooke County	32,919	31	355	1,075	815	493
Coryell County	73,822	35	798	2,422	1,836	1,094
Cottle County	1,917	1	21	65	49	26
Crane County	4,445	3	43	131	99	84
Crockett County	4,503	3	47	142	108	73
Crosby County	7,225	4	74	224	170	122
Culberson County	3,006	4	30	91	69	53
Dallam County	6,553	10	68	205	155	109
Dallas County	2,045,309	1,188	22,378	67,880	51,469	29,388
Dawson County	14,630	12	155	471	357	227
Deaf Smith County	19,071	8	183	556	422	364
Delta County	4,946	3	55	168	127	67
Denton County	383,369	138	4,154	12,600	9,554	5,652
De Witt County	19,574	18	219	664	503	265
Dickens County	2,236	3	25	76	58	29
Dimmit County	10,410	9	101	306	232	196
Donley County	3,833	5	45	136	103	45
Duval County	13,624	13	140	426	323	227
Eastland County	17,628	32	201	610	463	224
Ector County	124,794	88	1,273	3,860	2,927	2,122
Edwards County	3,657	6	45	137	104	34
Ellis County	103,734	66	1,072	3,253	2,466	1,712
El Paso County	694,603	225	7,026	21,312	16,160	12,011

Association	Population	Lung Cancer[1]	CHRONIC LUNG DISEASES			
			Emphysema	Chronic Bronchitis	Adult Asthma	Pediatric Asthma
Erath County	31,367	21	354	1,074	814	412
Falls County	17,500	18	193	587	445	244
Fannin County	28,366	29	324	982	744	361
Fayette County	21,276	9	241	732	555	275
Fisher County	4,273	9	47	144	109	59
Floyd County	8,201	1	83	252	191	142
Foard County	1,676	0	19	57	43	23
Fort Bend County	336,822	124	3,410	10,344	7,843	5,813
Franklin County	9,736	9	109	330	250	132
Freestone County	17,646	17	197	599	454	238
Frio County	15,837	12	162	490	372	269
Gaines County	14,871	8	141	429	325	289
Galveston County	244,993	199	2,671	8,102	6,143	3,554
Garza County	4,602	4	47	143	108	78
Gillespie County	19,994	16	230	698	529	247
Glasscock County	1,382	0	13	41	31	26
Goliad County	6,989	4	76	230	174	103
Gonzales County	17,485	12	186	563	427	271
Gray County	23,593	25	265	803	609	316
Grayson County	102,019	109	1,137	3,450	2,616	1,391
Gregg County	112,948	87	1,233	3,739	2,835	1,634
Grimes County	23,336	16	255	774	587	335
Guadalupe County	80,453	56	858	2,601	1,973	1,236
Hale County	36,702	21	373	1,131	857	629
Hall County	3,630	4	41	124	94	48
Hamilton County	7,651	9	86	262	199	100
Hansford County	5,349	3	55	168	128	88
Hardeman County	4,565	5	50	152	115	66
Hardin County	49,147	32	521	1,582	1,199	764
Harris County	3,202,021	1,699	34,248	103,886	78,771	48,789
Harrison County	59,781	51	643	1,949	1,478	900
Hartley County	5,142	0	60	183	139	60
Haskell County	6,125	5	69	208	158	82
Hays County	89,304	43	996	3,022	2,292	1,215
Hemphill County	3,527	1	36	110	84	58
Henderson County	68,988	116	789	2,393	1,814	871
Hidalgo County	519,661	162	4,936	14,974	11,354	10,119
Hill County	30,559	40	340	1,032	783	418
Hockley County	23,705	20	240	728	552	409
Hood County	37,259	47	423	1,284	974	480
Hopkins County	30,350	39	334	1,012	768	430
Houston County	22,033	39	248	752	570	293
Howard County	32,076	25	351	1,063	806	462
Hudspeth County	3,192	3	33	99	75	54
Hunt County	70,239	58	775	2,350	1,782	988
Hutchinson County	24,041	22	257	780	591	366
Irion County	1,724	1	19	57	43	26
Jack County	7,440	6	81	246	187	108
Jackson County	13,671	8	147	447	339	204
Jasper County	33,438	40	361	1,095	830	497
Jeff Davis County	2,364	1	26	79	60	34
Jefferson County	241,219	256	2,674	8,110	6,149	3,344
Jim Hogg County	5,011	0	51	155	118	85
Jim Wells County	40,055	32	409	1,239	940	681
Johnson County	118,200	86	1,260	3,823	2,898	1,815
Jones County	18,625	16	212	643	488	238
Karnes County	15,188	9	169	512	389	209
Kaufman County	65,535	47	694	2,105	1,596	1,024
Kendall County	21,190	17	234	711	539	296

TABLE 1 ESTIMATED PREVALENCE AND INCIDENCE OF LUNG DISEASE BY COUNTY,
STATE, AND LUNG ASSOCIATION, 1998 *(continued)*

Association	Population	Lung Cancer[1]	CHRONIC LUNG DISEASES			
			Emphysema	Chronic Bronchitis	Adult Asthma	Pediatric Asthma
ALA OF TEXAS (cont.)						
Kenedy County	452	0	5	14	11	7
Kent County	879	1	10	30	23	12
Kerr County	42,667	53	492	1,491	1,131	525
Kimble County	4,141	8	46	140	106	56
King County	359	0	4	11	8	6
Kinney County	3,474	4	40	120	91	44
Kleberg County	30,103	21	320	971	736	465
Knox County	4,225	5	45	138	104	64
Lamar County	45,880	46	509	1,544	1,170	635
Lamb County	14,762	12	154	467	354	239
Lampasas County	17,738	22	191	579	439	266
La Salle County	6,036	4	63	192	146	96
Lavaca County	18,838	23	211	641	486	252
Lee County	14,885	12	156	473	359	238
Leon County	14,481	26	162	490	372	197
Liberty County	65,154	70	707	2,143	1,625	958
Limestone County	20,747	23	227	690	523	296
Lipscomb County	2,962	1	32	96	73	45
Live Oak County	10,149	20	110	335	254	148
Llano County	13,449	23	169	512	388	117
Loving County	116	0	1	4	3	2
Lubbock County	228,220	148	2,502	7,590	5,755	3,260
Lynn County	6,714	4	69	209	159	112
McCulloch County	8,715	9	94	284	216	131
McLennan County	203,214	164	2,240	6,793	5,151	2,863
McMullen County	795	1	9	27	21	10
Madison County	11,852	9	139	420	319	139
Marion County	10,894	16	123	374	284	142
Martin County	5,019	4	50	150	114	91
Mason County	3,673	0	42	126	96	48
Matagorda County	37,987	29	391	1,186	899	633
Maverick County	47,660	10	448	1,360	1,031	944
Medina County	36,910	29	395	1,198	909	561
Menard County	2,323	4	26	79	60	31
Midland County	119,120	94	1,229	3,727	2,826	1,975
Milam County	24,197	27	260	789	598	365
Mills County	4,748	6	54	163	124	61
Mitchell County	8,832	5	100	305	231	113
Montague County	18,573	20	209	633	480	248
Montgomery County	271,801	194	2,875	8,720	6,612	4,256
Moore County	19,582	13	194	590	447	351
Morris County	13,360	16	147	445	337	190
Motley County	1,330	3	15	46	35	17
Nacogdoches County	56,243	46	642	1,947	1,477	714
Navarro County	41,600	46	454	1,378	1,045	600
Newton County	14,258	21	153	463	351	217
Nolan County	16,433	12	177	536	406	247
Nueces County	315,723	178	3,293	9,988	7,573	5,108
Ochiltree County	8,791	9	91	276	209	145
Oldham County	2,158	3	19	58	44	47
Orange County	84,769	94	917	2,783	2,110	1,253
Palo Pinto County	25,889	32	285	866	657	364
Panola County	23,047	25	250	759	576	338
Parker County	82,266	57	894	2,711	2,056	1,204
Parmer County	10,299	5	102	311	236	184

Association	Population	Lung Cancer[1]	CHRONIC LUNG DISEASES Emphysema	Chronic Bronchitis	Adult Asthma	Pediatric Asthma
Pecos County	16,087	9	170	515	390	253
Polk County	50,182	44	582	1,766	1,339	604
Potter County	108,289	92	1,164	3,532	2,678	1,628
Presidio County	8,554	0	87	264	200	147
Rains County	8,589	14	97	293	222	114
Randall County	98,779	57	1,063	3,223	2,444	1,484
Reagan County	4,232	5	39	118	89	87
Real County	2,701	4	31	94	72	33
Red River County	13,740	22	156	474	359	176
Reeves County	14,308	14	145	439	333	248
Refugio County	7,899	12	87	263	199	113
Roberts County	936	1	10	30	23	15
Robertson County	15,613	12	167	507	384	238
Rockwall County	37,202	23	401	1,215	921	557
Runnels County	11,518	16	124	377	286	172
Rusk County	45,743	43	497	1,509	1,144	668
Sabine County	10,513	10	125	380	288	115
San Augustine County	8,101	10	93	281	213	103
San Jacinto County	21,828	29	243	737	559	299
San Patricio County	70,737	44	727	2,206	1,672	1,182
San Saba County	5,817	4	61	184	139	94
Schleicher County	2,970	6	30	91	69	51
Scurry County	18,001	22	195	592	449	265
Shackelford County	3,288	3	36	108	82	49
Shelby County	22,882	32	253	766	581	321
Sherman County	2,866	0	31	94	71	43
Smith County	168,070	129	1,857	5,633	4,271	2,350
Somervell County	6,385	4	65	198	150	108
Starr County	55,443	13	509	1,545	1,172	1,140
Stephens County	9,732	13	108	326	247	136
Sterling County	1,384	0	14	41	31	25
Stonewall County	1,796	4	20	61	46	25
Sutton County	4,468	3	47	141	107	73
Swisher County	8,280	0	89	271	206	123
Tarrant County	1,354,040	771	14,722	44,658	33,861	19,783
Taylor County	122,036	90	1,329	4,030	3,056	1,777
Terrell County	1,174	3	13	38	29	18
Terry County	12,892	1	132	400	304	217
Throckmorton County	1,704	3	19	59	44	22
Titus County	25,423	35	270	819	621	394
Tom Green County	102,685	75	1,117	3,390	2,570	1,497
Travis County	709,182	334	7,975	24,190	18,342	9,427
Trinity County	12,611	22	146	444	337	152
Tyler County	20,373	23	237	720	546	241
Upshur County	35,821	32	391	1,186	899	518
Upton County	3,767	0	37	112	85	70
Uvalde County	25,448	22	258	784	594	437
Val Verde County	43,637	20	432	1,310	993	788
Van Zandt County	43,961	57	492	1,493	1,132	592
Victoria County	81,672	73	855	2,594	1,967	1,309
Walker County	54,802	48	661	2,004	1,519	571
Waller County	27,248	12	303	918	696	376
Ward County	11,795	9	119	360	273	206
Washington County	29,119	18	326	989	750	392
Webb County	186,798	48	1,775	5,384	4,083	3,635
Wharton County	40,120	36	422	1,280	970	637
Wheeler County	5,286	1	58	175	133	76
Wichita County	128,497	129	1,434	4,351	3,299	1,745
Wilbarger County	14,076	17	153	464	352	205

TABLE 1 ESTIMATED PREVALENCE AND INCIDENCE OF LUNG DISEASE BY COUNTY,
STATE, AND LUNG ASSOCIATION, 1998 *(continued)*

Association	Population	Lung Cancer[1]	CHRONIC LUNG DISEASES			
			Emphysema	Chronic Bronchitis	Adult Asthma	Pediatric Asthma
ALA OF TEXAS (cont.)						
Willacy County	19,599	3	189	573	434	372
Williamson County	223,665	110	2,294	6,958	5,275	3,757
Wilson County	31,304	9	322	976	740	523
Winkler County	7,971	6	79	240	182	143
Wise County	44,326	20	476	1,445	1,096	667
Wood County	34,317	61	393	1,193	905	430
Yoakum County	7,969	5	78	238	180	146
Young County	17,555	27	194	587	445	247
Zapata County	11,446	5	110	335	254	217
Zavala County	11,887	4	116	351	266	221
UTAH						
CONSTITUENT:	2,100,562	451	20,954	63,558	48,191	37,367
ALA OF UTAH						
Beaver County	5,901	5	58	177	134	107
Box Elder County	41,930	8	395	1,198	908	828
Cache County	87,227	6	871	2,643	2,004	1,548
Carbon County	21,021	8	215	651	494	356
Daggett County	722	0	7	22	17	12
Davis County	233,600	44	2,224	6,746	5,115	4,532
Duchesne County	14,514	3	132	400	303	304
Emery County	11,013	6	101	306	232	228
Garfield County	4,294	1	44	133	101	73
Grand County	8,070	9	86	260	197	125
Iron County	28,777	12	293	889	674	491
Juab County	7,602	4	72	217	165	150
Kane County	6,219	3	63	190	144	108
Millard County	12,280	0	111	336	255	260
Morgan County	7,032	3	66	200	152	140
Piute County	1,407	0	15	45	34	22
Rich County	1,858	0	17	51	38	40
Salt Lake County	845,913	194	8,613	26,125	19,809	14,429
San Juan County	13,640	0	124	377	286	284
Sanpete County	21,590	6	210	638	484	401
Sevier County	18,435	6	176	534	405	355
Summit County	26,798	1	277	842	638	441
Tooele County	33,474	9	334	1,012	767	597
Uintah County	25,637	10	240	729	553	511
Utah County	339,904	35	3,337	10,123	7,675	6,235
Wasatch County	13,273	3	127	384	291	257
Washington County	82,276	26	824	2,501	1,896	1,451
Wayne County	2,358	0	23	69	53	44
Weber County	183,797	49	1,899	5,760	4,367	3,038
VERMONT						
CONSTITUENT:	590,579	451	6,741	20,446	15,505	7,500
ALA OF VERMONT						
Addison County	35,150	13	398	1,208	916	457
Bennington County	35,936	36	413	1,253	950	446
Caledonia County	28,562	20	318	964	731	392
Chittenden County	142,487	112	1,664	5,047	3,827	1,676
Essex County	6,585	5	74	226	171	86
Franklin County	43,973	32	475	1,440	1,092	655
Grand Isle County	6,229	4	70	213	162	82
Lamoille County	21,638	14	245	743	563	282

Association	Population	Lung Cancer[1]	CHRONIC LUNG DISEASES			
			Emphysema	Chronic Bronchitis	Adult Asthma	Pediatric Asthma
Orange County	27,866	26	310	939	712	384
Orleans County	25,366	21	279	846	642	359
Rutland County	62,543	51	726	2,201	1,669	753
Washington County	56,178	48	642	1,946	1,476	712
Windham County	42,699	30	488	1,481	1,123	539
Windsor County	55,367	39	639	1,939	1,471	677
VIRGINIA CONSTITUENT: *ALA OF VIRGINIA*	6,789,225	4,975	77,081	233,821	177,294	87,625
Accomack County	32,252	49	370	1,123	851	402
Albemarle County	79,417	49	930	2,820	2,138	926
Alleghany County	12,197	9	140	424	321	153
Amelia County	10,400	1	116	353	267	141
Amherst County	29,978	26	347	1,053	798	363
Appomattox County	13,146	12	149	451	342	172
Arlington County	174,607	91	2,187	6,635	5,031	1,529
Augusta County	60,296	48	685	2,077	1,575	778
Bath County	4,911	1	58	177	134	54
Bedford County	56,728	49	650	1,972	1,495	711
Bland County	6,805	6	80	242	184	78
Botetourt County	28,657	23	334	1,013	768	340
Brunswick County	17,388	13	203	616	467	204
Buchanan County	28,986	27	323	978	742	397
Buckingham County	14,629	12	172	521	395	168
Campbell County	50,102	53	573	1,738	1,318	632
Caroline County	21,989	18	245	743	564	300
Carroll County	27,776	32	327	991	751	318
Charles City County	7,153	1	83	250	190	88
Charlotte County	12,323	20	141	427	323	157
Chesterfield County	250,161	160	2,660	8,070	6,119	3,866
Clarke County	12,718	13	149	452	343	148
Craig County	4,877	1	56	171	130	59
Culpeper County	33,107	22	369	1,119	848	453
Cumberland County	7,846	8	87	265	201	108
Dickenson County	16,868	16	186	564	427	238
Dinwiddie County	25,477	21	294	893	677	310
Essex County	9,081	9	105	317	240	112
Fairfax County	927,895	364	10,549	31,998	24,262	11,929
Fauquier County	53,939	38	597	1,810	1,372	752
Floyd County	13,063	8	152	460	349	157
Fluvanna County	18,908	17	214	650	493	246
Franklin County	44,604	27	518	1,572	1,192	534
Frederick County	55,667	29	616	1,868	1,416	776
Giles County	16,244	16	191	579	439	187
Gloucester County	34,942	39	383	1,160	880	501
Goochland County	17,406	13	208	632	479	186
Grayson County	16,399	20	192	583	442	190
Greene County	14,044	5	154	467	354	201
Greensville County	10,908	13	131	398	302	115
Halifax County	36,736	44	420	1,273	965	465
Hanover County	82,302	62	936	2,840	2,154	1,056
Henrico County	241,766	220	2,796	8,482	6,432	2,939
Henry County	55,842	43	650	1,971	1,494	665
Highland County	2,486	4	29	89	68	28
Isle of Wight County	29,181	25	326	990	750	395
James City County	44,488	20	510	1,548	1,174	556
King and Queen County	6,500	8	74	223	169	84
King George County	17,187	18	186	565	429	253

TABLE 1 ESTIMATED PREVALENCE AND INCIDENCE OF LUNG DISEASE BY COUNTY, STATE, AND LUNG ASSOCIATION, 1998 *(continued)*

Association	Population	Lung Cancer[1]	Emphysema	Chronic Bronchitis	Adult Asthma	Pediatric Asthma
ALA OF VIRGINIA (cont.)						
King William County	12,819	8	141	429	325	180
Lancaster County	11,339	16	137	415	315	118
Lee County	23,862	34	265	805	611	327
Loudoun County	144,514	48	1,583	4,803	3,642	2,068
Louisa County	24,540	21	275	835	633	328
Lunenburg County	11,989	21	139	421	319	145
Madison County	12,636	12	143	433	328	166
Mathews County	9,105	16	109	331	251	98
Mecklenburg County	31,046	29	360	1,091	827	376
Middlesex County	9,633	10	116	352	267	101
Montgomery County	76,884	46	941	2,854	2,164	751
Nelson County	13,901	20	160	484	367	173
New Kent County	12,870	10	147	446	338	162
Northampton County	12,721	20	143	435	330	168
Northumberland County	11,473	17	139	421	319	118
Nottoway County	15,168	14	178	540	410	175
Orange County	25,374	17	291	883	669	317
Page County	23,056	22	266	806	611	284
Patrick County	18,446	23	217	660	500	210
Pittsylvania County	56,536	46	646	1,958	1,485	716
Powhatan County	21,492	13	247	751	569	265
Prince Edward County	19,234	17	229	693	526	212
Prince George County	28,333	17	312	946	717	400
Prince William County	262,414	101	2,744	8,324	6,312	4,219
Pulaski County	34,405	39	404	1,226	930	396
Rappahannock County	7,329	4	86	261	198	84
Richmond County	8,680	5	105	318	242	89
Roanoke County	81,264	72	950	2,881	2,185	953
Rockbridge County	19,275	5	225	683	518	227
Rockingham County	63,234	35	719	2,180	1,653	813
Russell County	28,890	29	326	987	749	382
Scott County	22,644	25	266	807	612	260
Shenandoah County	34,721	32	408	1,236	938	401
Smyth County	32,789	30	381	1,156	876	392
Southampton County	17,524	14	203	616	467	212
Spotsylvania County	83,846	55	878	2,664	2,020	1,343
Stafford County	89,668	43	940	2,852	2,162	1,433
Surry County	6,496	13	72	218	165	90
Sussex County	10,054	18	115	350	265	126
Tazewell County	46,659	60	526	1,596	1,210	616
Warren County	30,083	23	340	1,033	783	392
Washington County	49,574	66	581	1,764	1,337	574
Westmoreland County	16,319	23	188	571	433	200
Wise County	39,123	47	433	1,315	997	543
Wythe County	26,270	26	304	921	698	320
York County	57,554	34	617	1,871	1,419	872
Alexandria City[2]	114,978	66	1,452	4,403	3,338	967
Bedford City[2]	6,590	3	78	237	180	73
Bristol City[2]	16,988	25	203	616	467	184
Buena Vista City[2]	6,624	10	78	238	181	74
Charlottesville City[2]	36,988	32	455	1,379	1,046	354
Chesapeake City[2]	199,407	140	2,143	6,501	4,929	3,002
Clifton Forge City[2]	4,249	9	50	153	116	47
Colonial Heights City[2]	16,431	25	194	589	447	185
Covington City[2]	6,924	9	83	251	190	75

Association	Population	Lung Cancer[1]	CHRONIC LUNG DISEASES			
			Emphysema	Chronic Bronchitis	Adult Asthma	Pediatric Asthma
Danville City[2]	51,710	70	605	1,835	1,391	605
Emporia City[2]	5,747	9	65	198	150	74
Fairfax City[2]	20,774	21	252	764	580	211
Falls Church City[2]	9,763	5	119	361	274	97
Franklin City[2]	8,474	9	94	284	215	118
Fredericksburg City[2]	19,028	18	233	706	535	186
Galax City[2]	6,651	5	79	240	182	74
Hampton City[2]	136,706	108	1,547	4,694	3,559	1,781
Harrisonburg City[2]	33,931	9	426	1,293	981	292
Hopewell City[2]	22,962	30	258	782	593	306
Lexington City[2]	7,343	8	97	295	224	46
Lynchburg City[2]	64,261	58	755	2,290	1,737	739
Manassas City[2]	32,656	10	351	1,065	808	491
Manassas Park City[2]	7,736	5	80	242	184	128
Martinsville City[2]	15,282	13	181	550	417	170
Newport News City[2]	178,001	135	1,936	5,873	4,453	2,598
Norfolk City[2]	227,108	208	2,592	7,863	5,962	2,883
Norton City[2]	4,057	3	45	138	104	55
Petersburg City[2]	34,853	40	401	1,216	922	431
Poquoson City[2]	11,431	4	125	378	287	166
Portsmouth City[2]	99,049	116	1,091	3,309	2,509	1,397
Radford City[2]	15,559	5	202	613	464	111
Richmond City[2]	191,001	209	2,285	6,930	5,255	2,055
Roanoke City[2]	93,797	98	1,102	3,343	2,535	1,079
Salem City[2]	24,225	27	292	887	673	251
Staunton City[2]	24,619	31	296	899	682	258
Suffolk City[2]	62,675	36	685	2,079	1,577	901
Virginia Beach City[2]	430,656	194	4,648	14,100	10,691	6,412
Waynesboro City[2]	19,064	20	222	673	510	227
Williamsburg City[2]	12,363	8	169	512	388	59
Winchester City[2]	22,396	25	266	807	612	248
WASHINGTON CONSTITUENT: ALA OF WASHINGTON	5,687,832	3,695	63,216	191,748	145,393	78,244
Adams County	15,339	9	148	448	340	292
Asotin County	21,286	14	231	701	531	312
Benton County	136,132	96	1,433	4,348	3,297	2,155
Chelan County	60,169	43	648	1,966	1,490	901
Clallam County	64,273	68	739	2,242	1,700	797
Clark County	327,418	228	3,521	10,679	8,098	4,923
Columbia County	4,158	5	47	142	108	55
Cowlitz County	91,409	84	1,004	3,044	2,308	1,301
Douglas County	33,600	22	368	1,115	846	483
Ferry County	7,163	6	75	226	172	116
Franklin County	46,511	21	450	1,364	1,034	878
Garfield County	2,317	3	26	78	59	32
Grant County	70,667	40	724	2,198	1,666	1,188
Grays Harbor County	67,463	96	743	2,254	1,709	951
Island County	71,747	43	794	2,410	1,827	997
Jefferson County	26,275	36	309	937	711	301
King County	1,654,329	954	19,246	58,378	44,265	19,715
Kitsap County	232,933	133	2,525	7,659	5,808	3,430
Kittitas County	31,403	22	369	1,120	850	360
Klickitat County	19,361	10	206	624	473	300
Lewis County	68,094	57	734	2,228	1,689	1,016
Lincoln County	9,766	8	109	330	250	134
Mason County	49,826	61	563	1,707	1,294	654
Okanogan County	38,286	38	412	1,249	947	575

TABLE 1 ESTIMATED PREVALENCE AND INCIDENCE OF LUNG DISEASE BY COUNTY,
STATE, AND LUNG ASSOCIATION, 1998 (continued)

| Association | Population | Lung Cancer[1] | CHRONIC LUNG DISEASES | | | |
			Emphysema	Chronic Bronchitis	Adult Asthma	Pediatric Asthma
ALA OF WASHINGTON (cont.)						
Pacific County	20,855	34	239	726	551	260
Pend Oreille County	11,523	10	123	372	282	177
Pierce County	675,962	391	7,392	22,424	17,003	9,724
San Juan County	12,545	12	150	456	346	133
Skagit County	99,389	77	1,100	3,336	2,529	1,385
Skamania County	9,779	6	104	315	239	151
Snohomish County	585,487	303	6,395	19,398	14,708	8,451
Spokane County	408,221	309	4,517	13,702	10,389	5,686
Stevens County	39,591	30	411	1,247	946	646
Thurston County	202,264	133	2,226	6,752	5,120	2,860
Wahkiakum County	3,862	3	44	132	100	51
Walla Walla County	53,671	39	605	1,835	1,391	708
Whatcom County	157,244	92	1,769	5,365	4,068	2,089
Whitman County	38,706	17	476	1,442	1,094	372
Yakima County	218,808	142	2,241	6,799	5,155	3,685
WEST VIRGINIA CONSTITUENT:	1,811,688	2,040	21,030	63,797	48,372	21,746
ALA OF WEST VIRGINIA						
Barbour County	16,106	9	184	560	424	202
Berkeley County	71,021	56	808	2,451	1,859	911
Boone County	26,164	32	295	896	679	344
Braxton County	13,220	23	151	457	347	169
Brooke County	26,015	27	311	944	716	280
Cabell County	94,112	117	1,132	3,434	2,603	990
Calhoun County	7,945	5	89	270	205	107
Clay County	10,519	8	114	347	263	154
Doddridge County	7,503	5	84	255	193	101
Fayette County	47,094	49	541	1,642	1,245	584
Gilmer County	7,180	10	85	256	194	82
Grant County	11,114	4	129	390	296	135
Greenbrier County	35,349	40	416	1,262	957	404
Hampshire County	19,148	17	218	661	501	246
Hancock County	34,010	36	406	1,230	933	370
Hardy County	11,857	16	139	422	320	137
Harrison County	70,808	84	822	2,492	1,890	851
Jackson County	27,980	25	322	977	741	345
Jefferson County	41,445	35	477	1,446	1,096	513
Kanawha County	201,477	292	2,386	7,238	5,488	2,251
Lewis County	17,609	26	205	620	470	211
Lincoln County	22,185	42	247	750	569	303
Logan County	41,023	62	459	1,392	1,056	554
Mc Dowell County	29,997	34	330	1,001	759	424
Marion County	56,466	74	670	2,033	1,541	626
Marshall County	35,235	43	409	1,242	942	421
Mason County	25,933	35	298	903	685	323
Mercer County	64,342	72	755	2,290	1,737	744
Mineral County	27,044	27	313	950	720	328
Mingo County	31,911	40	344	1,045	792	475
Monongalia County	77,452	42	950	2,882	2,185	750
Monroe County	13,191	16	153	464	352	159
Morgan County	13,706	16	164	497	376	148
Nicholas County	27,557	35	309	938	711	369
Ohio County	48,232	47	578	1,754	1,330	514

Association	Population	Lung Cancer[1]	CHRONIC LUNG DISEASES			
			Emphysema	Chronic Bronchitis	Adult Asthma	Pediatric Asthma
Pendleton County	8,066	3	95	287	218	93
Pleasants County	7,498	10	86	260	197	94
Pocahontas County	9,093	5	107	326	247	103
Preston County	29,805	29	337	1,021	774	391
Putnam County	51,195	40	580	1,761	1,335	664
Raleigh County	79,232	77	902	2,737	2,075	1,013
Randolph County	28,672	31	335	1,017	771	335
Ritchie County	10,381	17	120	363	276	127
Roane County	15,323	13	173	525	398	201
Summers County	13,919	20	164	498	378	157
Taylor County	15,359	23	177	537	407	189
Tucker County	7,592	6	89	271	205	87
Tyler County	9,789	12	113	342	260	120
Upshur County	23,546	27	271	822	623	291
Wayne County	41,978	52	483	1,467	1,112	518
Webster County	10,238	10	115	347	263	138
Wetzel County	18,307	21	211	640	485	225
Wirt County	5,710	6	64	195	148	76
Wood County	86,694	105	1,011	3,067	2,325	1,024
Wyoming County	27,341	32	304	923	700	375
WISCONSIN CONSTITUENT: *ALA OF WISCONSIN*	5,222,124	3,498	58,099	176,232	133,623	71,626
Adams County	18,427	16	220	666	505	201
Ashland County	16,443	9	181	548	415	234
Barron County	43,839	29	479	1,452	1,101	634
Bayfield County	15,187	12	168	510	387	211
Brown County	214,942	120	2,370	7,188	5,450	3,025
Buffalo County	14,240	8	157	477	362	200
Burnett County	14,639	13	167	505	383	188
Calumet County	38,468	12	403	1,223	927	615
Chippewa County	54,566	31	593	1,799	1,364	798
Clark County	33,139	18	349	1,060	804	523
Columbia County	51,148	53	570	1,728	1,310	699
Crawford County	16,598	10	179	542	411	249
Dane County	424,665	178	4,946	15,004	11,377	5,039
Dodge County	83,007	73	917	2,783	2,110	1,160
Door County	27,049	21	305	925	701	357
Douglas County	43,128	43	482	1,461	1,107	586
Dunn County	39,036	9	440	1,335	1,012	515
Eau Claire County	89,235	34	1,010	3,063	2,323	1,163
Florence County	5,179	0	57	174	132	72
Fond du Lac County	94,559	60	1,045	3,169	2,403	1,323
Forest County	9,677	13	106	321	244	139
Grant County	49,292	40	547	1,658	1,257	683
Green County	33,465	18	368	1,117	847	473
Green Lake County	19,508	14	218	662	502	263
Iowa County	22,333	12	242	733	556	330
Iron County	6,346	12	75	228	173	71
Jackson County	17,735	12	195	591	448	252
Jefferson County	73,601	49	824	2,500	1,895	991
Juneau County	23,800	36	263	796	604	334
Kenosha County	144,388	94	1,589	4,819	3,654	2,043
Kewaunee County	19,875	8	216	656	497	290
La Crosse County	102,425	58	1,160	3,518	2,667	1,333
Lafayette County	16,177	21	174	529	401	241
Langlade County	20,486	12	227	689	522	284
Lincoln County	29,750	22	329	999	757	414

TABLE 1 ESTIMATED PREVALENCE AND INCIDENCE OF LUNG DISEASE BY COUNTY, STATE, AND LUNG ASSOCIATION, 1998 *(continued)*

Association	Population	Lung Cancer[1]	CHRONIC LUNG DISEASES			
			Emphysema	Chronic Bronchitis	Adult Asthma	Pediatric Asthma
ALA OF WISCONSIN *(cont.)*						
Manitowoc County	82,454	57	917	2,782	2,109	1,132
Marathon County	123,082	58	1,337	4,056	3,075	1,802
Marinette County	43,009	39	477	1,447	1,097	595
Marquette County	15,125	22	173	524	398	191
Menominee County	4,977	9	44	134	101	108
Milwaukee County	911,536	710	10,153	30,797	23,352	12,461
Monroe County	39,513	22	422	1,280	970	605
Oconto County	33,878	26	371	1,127	854	484
Oneida County	35,750	38	415	1,259	955	429
Outagamie County	156,395	101	1,693	5,134	3,893	2,313
Ozaukee County	81,132	40	909	2,758	2,092	1,089
Pepin County	7,145	5	77	233	176	108
Pierce County	35,527	12	391	1,186	899	503
Polk County	38,786	43	419	1,272	965	575
Portage County	64,818	34	727	2,206	1,673	867
Price County	15,715	12	174	529	401	217
Racine County	185,537	134	2,029	6,155	4,667	2,669
Richland County	17,859	14	196	595	452	253
Rock County	150,720	131	1,663	5,046	3,826	2,115
Rusk County	15,194	12	167	506	383	217
St. Croix County	58,915	30	626	1,898	1,439	914
Sauk County	53,373	27	588	1,782	1,351	754
Sawyer County	16,083	20	178	540	409	224
Shawano County	38,818	22	429	1,301	986	543
Sheboygan County	109,986	90	1,216	3,687	2,796	1,537
Taylor County	19,247	6	204	618	469	301
Trempealeau County	26,493	14	295	896	679	361
Vernon County	27,364	13	300	911	691	390
Vilas County	21,257	20	250	759	575	243
Walworth County	85,481	65	978	2,966	2,249	1,077
Washburn County	15,427	16	173	525	398	207
Washington County	113,899	53	1,243	3,771	2,859	1,647
Waukesha County	353,035	211	3,934	11,934	9,049	4,818
Waupaca County	50,515	43	558	1,691	1,283	708
Waushara County	21,648	23	247	748	567	277
Winnebago County	149,995	116	1,721	5,221	3,959	1,871
Wood County	76,084	40	834	2,530	1,918	1,088

Notes:
(1) Lung cancer estimates are for 1997. 1998 data has not been released as of this printing.
(2) City population estimates overlap with county population estimates. Please do not add the two population estimates to calculate disease prevalence or incidence, as the existing overlap would overestimate disease in your community.
(3) Does not include the population of Holliston Town, Natick Town, Newton City, and Sherborn Town. These are in the territory serviced by the ALA of Greater Norfolk County.

Sources:
(1) U.S. Census Bureau, Population Estimates Branch: County Resident Population by Age Group, July 1, 1998.
(2) U.S. Census Bureau, Population Estimates Branch: Estimates of Population of Minor Civil Divisions: Annual Time Series, July 1, 1998.

Reprinted by permission of the American Lung Association.

APPENDIX III
TRENDS IN LUNG CANCER MORBIDITY AND MORTALITY

INTRODUCTION[1]

Lung cancer is the leading cause of cancer mortality in both men and women in the United States and will cause an estimated 157,400 deaths in 2001, accounting for 28 percent of all cancer deaths. The incidence and mortality attributed to this disorder has been rising steadily since the 1930s. Lung cancer has been the leading cause of cancer deaths among men since the early 1950s and, in 1987, surpassed breast cancer to become the leading cause of cancer deaths in women.

MORTALITY TRENDS[2]

Table 1 depicts the age-adjusted death rates for the most common cancer sites by sex between 1979 and 1998. This table indicates that mortality rates for most cancers are decreasing in both sexes. The main exception to this trend is deaths due to malignant neoplasms of respiratory and intrathoracic organs in females. During the period 1979–98, the respiratory cancer death rate has decreased in males by 11.8 percent, but has increased 63.3 percent in females. By contrast, mortality for cancer at all sites has decreased by 9.6 percent in males and 1.5 percent in females.

Table 2 delineates the number of deaths and age-adjusted mortality rates for lung cancer, specifically, between 1979 and 1998. The number of deaths due to lung cancer has increased 57 percent, from 98,541 in 1979 to 154,561 in 1998. In 1998, 91,447 males and 63,114 females died from lung cancer. Overall the age-adjusted mortality rate increased from 33.6 per 100,000 to 37.0 per 100,000, an increase of 10.1 percent. The rate in males has fluctuated; however, the rate reported in 1998 was 11.1 percent lower than that reported in 1979. Conversely, over the same time period the mortality rate in females has grown by over 65 percent. Despite the increase observed in women, the mortality rate in males is still almost double the rate in females.

Table 3 delineates mortality data by race and sex for 1979–98. Mortality in whites has increased by almost 12 percent during this time, from 33.0 per 100,000 to 36.8 per 100,000. However, the mortality rate in white males decreased (-10.9 percent) over this time span. The overall increase in whites

is, therefore, due entirely to the 68 percent increase observed in white females. Overall, mortality among blacks has increased by 7.2 percent, from 41.6 per 100,000 to 44.6 per 100,000. Mortality among black females has increased by almost 66 percent, from 16.6 per 100,000 to 27.5 per 100,000. The mortality rate in black males decreased 7.7 percent during this time. However, the mortality rate in black males (68.5 per 100,000) is almost 42 percent higher than that of white males (48.4 per 100,000). In contrast, mortality reported among females of both races has been similar since 1973. In 1998, the mortality rate was reported at 27.5 per 100,000 for both white and black females.

Figure 1 graphically depicts the trend in age-adjusted death rates discussed above. The disparity in death rates between black and white males is clearly displayed here, as is the congruence in the rates of black and white females.

Table 4 shows the age-specific mortality rates for lung cancer by sex and race for selected years from 1980–98. Age-specific mortality attributed to lung cancer increases with age and is greatest in the oldest age groups. If we examine the age-specific data for the most recent year, we see the rates are greater in black males than in white males across all age groups, as is expected based on the overall mortality differential. The difference in rates between black and white males is much more pronounced in the younger age groups. When we examine the trend in females, the mortality rates are only higher in black females in the younger age groups. Above age 65, the trend shifts and mortality is higher in white females.

Figure 2 depicts the death rate for respiratory system neoplasms by age for 1998. Mortality rates increase with age and reach their peak at 378.4 per 100,000 persons aged 75 to 84.

Table 5 delineates the age-adjusted death rates for cancer of the trachea and lung by sex and state for 1998. Overall, Kentucky experienced the greatest death rate (52.3 per 100,000) and Utah had the lowest (16.6 per 100,000). Mississippi experienced the greatest death rate for males (74.7 per 100,000) and Nevada had the greatest death rate for females (37.3 per 100,000). The lowest state-specific mortality rates for males (22.2 per 100,000) and females

(11.9 per 100,000) were seen in Utah. Figure 3 portrays 1998 lung cancer death rates by state.

Table 6 depicts 1998 data on state-specific age-adjusted mortality rates by race. For whites, the greatest state-specific death rate is reported in Kentucky (52.1 per 100,000). When we examine the rate in blacks, the small number of deaths in some states makes the corresponding data unreliable. Among the states with more than 20 deaths, high mortality rates among blacks are reported in Iowa (68.4 per 100,000) and Nebraska (66.7 per 100,000). The overall mortality rate in blacks (44.6 per 100,000) is 17.5 percent greater than the rate observed in whites (36.8 per 100,000). Figure 4 examines 1998 age-adjusted lung cancer death rates in blacks by state.

INCIDENCE TRENDS

Data on cancer incidence is collected by the Surveillance, Epidemiology, and End Results (SEER) program of the National Cancer Institute. The SEER Program is a continuing project of the National Cancer Institute that collects cancer data on a routine basis from designated population-based cancer registries in various areas of the country. Trends in cancer incidence and patient survival in the United States are derived from the SEER database.

Cancer of the Trachea, Bronchus, and Lung

The American Cancer Society estimates that there will be 169,500 new cases of the lung cancer in 2001. These new cases will account for 13 percent of all cancer diagnoses. Table 7 delineates the age-adjusted cancer incidence rates for the lung and bronchus, as well as cancer of all sites between 1973 and 1998. Lung cancer incidence increased by 29 percent over this time period; the incidence rate for cancer at all sites increased by 23.5 percent. The lung cancer incidence rate in 1998 was 54.8 per 100,000.

When the incidence rate is examined by race and sex (Figure 5 and Table 8), varying trends emerge. Overall, the incidence rates for lung cancer in men and women were 69.8 per 100,000 and 43.4 per 100,000, respectively. The rate in white males decreased by 5.5 percent while the rate in black males decreased by 4.0 percent between 1973 and 1998. However, the 1998 incidence rate in black men is more than 47 percent higher than that of white men. The incidence rate among females has increased at a much greater rate than the rate in males over this time period. Lung cancer in both white and black women has more than doubled between 1973 and 1998, +152 percent and +129 percent, respectively. Unlike the rates in males, lung cancer rates in white women (44.8 per 100,000) and black women (47.9 per 100,000) were similar.

The SEER Program has examined trends in lung cancer incidence during the period 1973–98. Evaluation of the estimated annual percentage change (EAPC) in incidence indicates that the EAPC was different from zero p<.05 for white males, and white and black females. Between 1973 and 1998, the EAPC was -0.4 in white males, 3.2 percent in white females, and 2.9 percent in black females. During the same time period, black males saw an estimated annual percentage change of -0.1 percent.

Cancer of the Oral Cavity and Pharynx

Table 8 also reports the incidence rates for respiratory cancer by site, race, and sex for 1973–98. Overall, cancer of the oral cavity and pharynx for both races decreased during this time period. However, the rate in black males has increased (+9.6 percent) since 1973. Between 1997 and 1998, the rate of oral cavity and pharynx cancer in blacks has increased while rates overall and in whites have declined.

Cancer of the Larynx

The overall incidence rate for cancer of the larynx has decreased 26.7 percent between 1973 and 1998. However, if we examine the data by race and sex specifically, white and black females have experienced an increase in incidence of 14 percent and 33 percent, respectively. White and black males have experienced a decrease in incidence of 37 percent and 18 percent, respectively. The 1998 incidence rate in black females (2.4 per 100,000) is 71 percent higher than white females (1.4 per 100,000). Black males had an incidence rate that was 85 percent higher than that of white males, 9.8 per 100,000 vs. 5.3 per 100,000, respectively.

HOSPITALIZATION TRENDS

Table 9 delineates age-specific hospital discharge data derived from the National Hospital Discharge survey for 1979–99. Of the more than 1.27 million discharges attributed to cancer in 1999, 13.0 percent were attributed to lung cancer. The total number of discharges reported for lung cancer was 164,000. This represents a discharge rate of 6.0 per 10,000 and is almost a 38 percent decrease from the discharge rate of 9.7 per 10,000 reported in 1988. The hospital discharge rate attributed to lung cancer is the second highest among all malignant neoplasms, with the exception of colorectal cancer. The greatest number of discharges is experienced in the population over age 65. In 1999 all age groups experienced declines in the number of discharges and the discharge rate except for the over 65 age group.

When examined by sex, the number of discharges and discharge rate between 1979 and 1999 has decreased in males and females, -41 percent and -34 percent, respectively. The trend in hospital discharges by sex is portrayed in Figure 6. Table 10 displays the race-specific number of discharges and discharge rate between 1988 and 1999. The 1999 discharge rate for lung cancer was highest in all other races (6.3 per 10,000), followed by whites (5.1 per 10,000) and then blacks (3.5 per 10,000). These rates, however, should be interpreted with caution due to the large percentage of discharges (17.2 percent) for which race was not reported.

TRENDS IN SURVIVAL RATES

Table 11 depicts trends in survival rate for lung and other types of cancer by race from 1960 through 1997. Survival rates for lung cancer tend to be much lower than those of most other cancers. In whites, survival rates for all cancers listed have experienced statistically significant increases since 1974–76. However, the survival rate for lung cancer has increased by only 18.4 percent, which is a relatively low increase when compared to the other cancers listed. With the exception of the survival rate for lung cancer (11.7 percent), the sur-

vival rates in blacks for all listed cancers showed statistically significant increases since 1974–76.

Compared to whites, blacks experienced lower five-year survival rates for each type of cancer listed. The five-year survival rate for lung cancer in blacks during the period spanning 1992–97 was 11.7 percent. The survival rate for lung cancer in whites was only slightly better at 14.4 percent. Black men and women have poorer survival rates for lung cancer than whites, even when controlling for age at diagnosis.

The prognosis (outlook for survival) for a patient with lung cancer depends, to a large extent, on the cancer's stage. Staging is used to determine whether the cancer has spread and, if so, to what parts of the body. Stages include localized (within lungs), regional (spread to lymph nodes), and distant (spread to other organs). Figure 7 displays the five-year survival rates for all stages by type of lung cancer. The average five-year survival rate between 1992 and 1997 for localized lung cancer was 48 percent compared to 14.5 percent overall and 2.5 percent for a distant tumor. Unfortunately, only 15 percent of people are diagnosed at an early, localized stage.

LUNG CANCER TYPES[3]

There are two major types of lung cancer: small cell lung cancer (SCLC) and non-small cell lung cancer (NSCLC). Sometimes a lung cancer may have characteristics of both types, which is known as mixed small cell/large cell carcinoma.

SCLC is less common, accounting for 20 percent of all lung cancer. This type of lung cancer grows more quickly and is more likely to spread to other organs in the body. Small cell lung cancer often starts in the bronchi and toward the center of the lungs. Smoking almost always causes it.

NSCLC accounts for the remaining 80 percent of all lung cancer cases. It generally grows and spreads more slowly. There are three main types of NSCLC. They are named for the type of cells in which the cancer develops: squamous cell carcinoma, adenocarcinoma, and large cell carcinoma.

Figure 8 delineates the stage distribution for the most common lung cancer types. Between 1992 and 1997, 62 percent of all SCLC cases were diagnosed during the distant stage and only 6 percent were diagnosed in the local stage. This compares to the 45 percent of NSCLC diagnosed in the distant stage and the 16 percent of cases diagnosed in the localized stage.

SMOKING-ATTRIBUTABLE LUNG CANCER DEATHS

The most important cause of lung cancer in the United States is cigarette smoking. It is estimated that 87 percent of lung cancer cases are caused by smoking. Table 12 delineates, by sex and age, the estimated number and proportion of smoking-attributable lung cancer deaths in the United States in 1990 and 1995. In males, the overall expected number of smoking-attributable deaths has increased between 1990 and 1995, although the percentage of deaths caused by smoking remained the same. In females, both the number of deaths and the proportion of deaths caused by smoking increased. Overall, for both sexes combined, the percentage of lung cancer deaths attributed to smoking increased slightly (1 percent). However, the overall estimated number of deaths attributed to smoking increased by 19 percent.

LIFETIME RISK OF BEING DIAGNOSED WITH CANCER

Using data from the Surveillance, Epidemiology, and End Results registry, the National Cancer Institute has calculated the lifetime risk of being diag-

nosed with lung cancer, as well as the lifetime risk of dying from lung cancer. This risk is calculated for the entire population and includes smokers and nonsmokers. These data are displayed in Table 13 by race and sex for 1996–98. As shown in the table, the lifetime risk of a lung cancer diagnosis is highest in black males (8.47 percent) and white males (7.83 percent). The lifetime risk of dying from lung cancer is highest in whites.

REFERENCES

1. American Cancer Society. Cancer Facts and Figures, 2001.
2. National Center for Health Statistics. Report of Final Mortality Statistics, 1979–1998.
3. CDC Wonder: Unpublished Mortality Data, 1998.
4. National Cancer Institute SEER Program: Cancer Statistics Review, 1973–1998.
5. National Center for Health Statistics. Detailed Diagnoses & Procedures, National Hospital Discharge Survey, 1999.

FOOTNOTES:

(1) Unless otherwise noted, terms such as higher or less are not intended to indicate statistical significance.
(2) Information on mortality for lung cancer is available from two different sources: the National Center for Health Statistics (NCHS) and the Surveillance, Epidemiology, and End Results (SEER) program of the National Cancer Institute. Since these mortality numbers are age-adjusted to different populations (SEER adjusts to the 1970 U.S. Population; NCHS adjusts to the 1940 U.S. population), the mortality rates from different sources should not be compared to each other.
(3) Information on lung cancer types and stages comes from the Surveillance, Epidemiology, and End Results (SEER) program of the National Cancer Institute and the American Cancer Society.

TABLE 1 AGE-ADJUSTED DEATH RATES[1] FOR SELECTED CANCER SITES BY SEX, 1979–1998

SITES	SEX	1979	1981	1983	1985	1987	1989	1991	1993	1995	1997	1998	Percent Change 1979–1987	Percent Change 1987–1998	Percent Change 1979–1998
All Sites[2]	Male	163.4	163.8	165.3	166.1	165.5	165.5	165.0	161.9	156.8	150.4	147.7	1.3	-10.8	-9.6
	Female	107.1	108.7	110.1	111.7	111.4	112.3	112.6	111.4	110.4	107.3	105.5	4.0	-5.3	-1.5
Digestive[3]	Male	41.8	41.3	40.8	40.6	39.7	39.3	38.7	37.9	37.4	36.5	36.2	-5.0	-8.8	-13.4
	Female	26.4	25.7	25.2	24.8	24.1	23.2	23.0	22.7	22.3	21.4	21.4	-8.7	-11.2	-18.9
Respiratory[4]	Male	58.6	59.6	60.1	60.7	61.1	60.5	60.1	58.1	55.3	52.8	51.7	4.3	-15.4	-11.8
	Female	16.9	18.8	21.0	22.5	23.8	25.6	26.5	27.2	27.5	27.5	27.6	40.8	16.0	63.3
Breast[5]	Male	0.2	0.2	0.2	0.2	0.2	0.2	0.1	0.2	0.2	0.2	0.2	0.0	0.0	0.0
	Female	22.3	22.7	22.7	23.3	23.0	23.1	22.7	21.5	21.0	19.4	18.8	3.1	-18.3	-15.7
Genital[6]	Male	14.8	14.9	15.2	15.3	15.6	16.4	17.1	16.8	15.8	14.3	13.6	5.4	-12.8	-8.1
	Female	13.8	13.4	13.0	12.6	12.3	12.1	12.2	11.7	11.6	11.3	11.1	-10.9	-9.8	-19.6

Source: Division of Vital Statistics, National Center for Health Statistics, 1998.
Notes:
(1) Rates are per 100,000 persons and age-adjusted to the 1940 U.S. Census population.
(2) Includes ICD Codes 140–208.
(3) Includes ICD Codes 150–159.
(4) Includes ICD Codes 160–165.
(5) Includes ICD Codes 174–175.
(6) Includes ICD Codes 179–187.

TABLE 2   NUMBER OF DEATHS AND AGE-ADJUSTED MORTALITY RATES[1] FOR CANCER OF THE TRACHEA, BRONCHUS, AND LUNG (ICD-9-CM CODE 162) BY SEX, 1979–1998

YEAR	TOTAL NUMBER	TOTAL RATE	MALE NUMBER	MALE RATE	FEMALE NUMBER	FEMALE RATE
1979	98,541	33.6	72,803	55.7	25,648	16.3
1980	103,844	34.8	75,535	56.9	28,309	17.6
1981	106,561	35.1	76,764	56.9	29,797	18.2
1982	111,393	35.9	79,228	57.6	32,165	19.2
1983	115,023	36.4	80,338	57.3	34,685	20.3
1984	118,730	37.0	82,491	58.0	36,239	20.8
1985	122,566	37.6	83,854	58.1	38,702	21.8
1986	125,522	37.8	85,057	57.9	40,465	22.3
1987	130,009	38.5	87,261	58.5	42,748	23.1
1988	133,284	38.9	88,059	58.2	45,225	24.0
1989	137,150	39.3	89,052	57.9	48,098	24.9
1990	141,285	39.9	91,091	58.5	50,194	25.6
1991	143,758	39.6	91,690	57.5	52,068	25.8
1992	145,943	39.3	91,405	56.0	54,538	26.4
1993	148,855	39.3	92,564	55.7	56,291	26.6
1994	149,482	38.7	91,893	54.2	57,589	26.6
1995	151,200	38.3	91,856	52.9	59,344	26.9
1996	152,015	37.8	91,620	51.8	60,395	26.8
1997	153,310	37.4	91,352	50.5	61,958	27.0
1998	154,561	37.0	91,447	49.5	63,114	27.0

Source: National Center for Health Statistics, Mortality Data, 1979–1998.
CDC Wonder, Unpublished Mortality Data, 1998.
Note:
(1) Rates are per 100,000 persons and age-adjusted to the 1940 U.S. Census population.

TABLE 3   AGE-ADJUSTED MORTALITY RATES[1] FOR CANCER OF THE TRACHEA, BRONCHUS, AND LUNG (ICD-9-CM CODE 162) BY RACE AND SEX, 1979–1998

YEAR	ALL RACES TOTAL	ALL RACES MALE	ALL RACES FEMALE	WHITE TOTAL	WHITE MALE	WHITE FEMALE	ALL OTHER RACES[2] TOTAL TOTAL	ALL OTHER RACES[2] TOTAL MALE	ALL OTHER RACES[2] TOTAL FEMALE	ALL OTHER RACES[2] BLACK TOTAL	ALL OTHER RACES[2] BLACK MALE	ALL OTHER RACES[2] BLACK FEMALE
1979	33.6	55.7	16.3	33.0	54.3	16.4	38.4	67.4	15.7	41.6	74.2	16.6
1980	34.8	56.9	17.6	34.2	55.5	17.6	39.8	69.2	17.1	43.9	77.2	18.5
1981	35.1	56.9	18.2	34.4	55.3	18.2	40.2	70.0	17.2	44.7	79.0	18.9
1982	35.9	57.6	19.2	35.3	56.0	19.4	40.6	70.6	17.6	45.6	80.4	19.5
1983	36.4	57.3	20.3	35.8	55.7	20.5	41.3	70.6	19.1	46.5	80.4	21.2
1984	37.0	58.0	20.8	36.4	56.2	21.0	41.9	72.5	18.9	47.2	83.1	20.7
1985	37.6	58.1	21.8	37.0	56.4	22.1	41.9	71.6	19.5	47.6	82.6	21.8
1986	37.8	57.9	22.3	37.2	56.2	22.5	42.1	71.4	20.2	48.0	82.8	22.6
1987	38.5	58.5	23.1	37.9	56.8	23.3	42.8	71.9	21.3	49.0	84.0	23.7
1988	38.9	58.2	24.0	38.3	56.5	24.3	42.5	71.0	21.6	48.9	83.1	24.3
1989	39.3	57.9	24.9	38.6	56.0	25.3	43.4	72.3	22.1	50.2	85.3	25.0
1990	39.9	58.5	25.6	39.3	56.6	25.9	43.9	72.3	23.2	51.3	86.2	26.4
1991	39.6	57.5	25.8	39.1	55.8	26.1	42.7	70.0	22.8	49.9	83.2	26.1
1992	39.3	56.0	26.4	38.8	54.4	26.7	42.4	68.1	23.6	49.8	81.4	27.3
1993	39.3	55.7	26.6	38.9	54.0	27.0	41.7	67.7	22.9	48.9	80.8	26.2
1994	38.7	54.2	26.6	38.4	52.7	27.1	40.7	64.9	23.1	47.9	77.6	26.7
1995	38.3	53.0	26.9	38.0	51.6	27.4	40.1	63.0	23.5	47.3	75.8	26.9
1996	37.8	51.8	26.8	37.6	50.5	27.5	40.7	64.8	23.3	46.2	73.2	26.5

TABLE 3   AGE-ADJUSTED MORTALITY RATES[1] FOR CANCER OF THE TRACHEA, BRONCHUS, AND LUNG (ICD-9-CM CODE 162) BY RACE AND SEX, 1979-1998 (continued)

| YEAR | ALL RACES | | | WHITE | | | ALL OTHER RACES[2] | | | | | |
| | | | | | | | TOTAL | | | BLACK | | |
	TOTAL	MALE	FEMALE	TOTAL	MALE	FEMALE	TOTAL	MALE	FEMALE	TOTAL	MALE	FEMALE
1997	37.4	50.5	27.0	37.1	49.3	27.5	39.4	61.4	23.8	45.3	70.6	27.4
1998	37.0	49.5	27.0	36.8	48.4	27.5	39.2	56.8	23.6	44.6	68.5	27.5

Source: CDC Wonder, 1979–1998.
Notes:
(1) Rates are per 100,000 persons and age-adjusted to the 1940 U.S. Census population.
(2) All other races includes blacks and all races other than white.

TABLE 4   CANCER OF THE LUNG AND BRONCHUS: AVERAGE ANNUAL AGE-SPECIFIC MORTALITY RATES[1] BY RACE, SEX, AND AGE, SELECTED YEARS, 1980-1998

YEAR	SEX & RACE	<1	1-4	5-9	10-14	15-19	20-24	25-29	30-34	35-39	40-44	45-49	50-54	55-59	60-64	65-69	70-74	75-79	80-84	85+
1980	WHITE MALE	0.1	0.0	**	0.0	0.0	0.1	0.3	1.1	5.5	17.3	45.4	95.1	162.7	255.6	358.7	458.6	502.4	477.7	374.1
	BLACK MALE	0.4	0.1	0.1	**	0.1	0.3	0.9	2.6	12.2	39.3	93.9	174.6	274.8	377.2	460.3	489.2	485.8	446.5	311.3
	WHITE FEMALE	0.1	0.0	0.0	**	0.0	0.0	0.2	0.8	3.3	10.4	22.7	42.5	60.7	84.5	103.2	106.4	100.7	86.8	92.4
	BLACK FEMALE	0.4	**	**	**	**	0.1	0.4	0.8	3.6	11.5	34.6	52.3	74.4	86.2	84.9	92.2	77.5	83.1	85.8
1985	WHITE MALE	*	*	*	*	*	*	0.3	1.0	4.3	15.0	40.1	87.0	167.6	262.8	364.7	468.7	541.5	538.0	440.0
	BLACK MALE	*	*	*	*	*	*	*	*	2.5	9.5	34.4	75.5	175.8	294.7	416.0	495.9	602.0	560.6	548.3	382.3
	WHITE FEMALE	*	*	*	*	*	*	0.2	0.9	2.9	8.7	23.9	47.5	75.5	109.3	138.6	153.6	140.9	125.4	99.3
	BLACK FEMALE	*	*	*	*	*	*	*	*	3.0	12.8	25.1	54.8	87.9	120.6	107.1	129.3	100.7	101.9	114.3
1990	WHITE MALE	*	*	*	*	*	*	0.3	1.1	3.8	11.6	34.6	80.5	159.3	268.1	373.9	485.5	565.0	584.8	516.3
	BLACK MALE	*	*	*	*	*	*	*	*	3.5	9.0	30.6	79.7	157.6	293.9	429.8	544.0	644.4	659.2	620.2	449.5
	WHITE FEMALE	*	*	*	*	*	*	0.2	0.8	2.8	7.5	22.9	48.5	82.4	127.8	165.5	200.2	206.4	177.6	138.3
	BLACK FEMALE	*	*	*	*	*	*	*	*	4.8	10.9	27.8	57.2	96.7	140.2	158.9	171.4	152.9	140.6	134.9
1991	WHITE MALE	*	*	*	*	*	*	0.3	0.9	3.6	10.8	33.5	75.9	154.6	263.4	377.3	475.3	550.5	603.5	532.5
	BLACK MALE	*	*	*	*	*	*	*	*	1.7	8.9	25.5	79.9	153.9	272.2	388.9	545.0	626.1	643.6	721.8	510.1
	WHITE FEMALE	*	*	*	*	*	*	0.2	0.9	2.8	7.5	21.8	45.8	84.9	126.3	171.6	201.4	217.2	190.9	148.9
	BLACK FEMALE	*	*	*	*	*	*	*	*	4.2	11.2	26.7	57.1	85.0	132.7	159.7	178.4	178.9	156.6	152.1
1992	WHITE MALE	*	*	*	*	*	*	*	0.9	3.5	10.9	31.4	75.2	146.8	253.3	378.9	490.7	547.9	591.5	522.5
	BLACK MALE	*	*	*	*	*	*	*	*	2.5	9.0	25.7	68.0	150.9	270.2	385.5	523.2	631.6	631.4	694.1	529.7
	WHITE FEMALE	*	*	*	*	*	*	0.3	0.8	2.9	7.4	20.6	45.2	82.7	130.9	176.3	215.7	224.1	206.2	156.0
	BLACK FEMALE	*	*	*	*	*	*	*	*	4.7	12.0	26.7	55.6	94.0	135.6	172.1	194.6	179.4	150.4	154.7
1993	WHITE MALE	*	*	*	*	*	*	*	1.0	3.9	10.2	28.7	70.5	147.8	255.7	376.2	463.6	540.9	591.4	531.8
	BLACK MALE	*	*	*	*	*	*	*	*	2.8	7.7	25.3	71.8	141.9	245.0	348.0	510.7	670.1	662.6	708.4	565.9
	WHITE FEMALE	*	*	*	*	*	*	*	0.8	2.5	7.0	20.2	44.0	82.3	132.7	180.8	221.0	234.6	215.3	168.9
	BLACK FEMALE	*	*	*	*	*	*	*	*	1.5	3.4	10.2	29.3	49.7	86.9	124.6	165.0	194.3	180.5	177.2	163.5
1994	WHITE MALE	*	*	*	*	*	*	*	1.0	3.6	10.1	26.6	68.6	136.8	251.2	369.1	461.8	530.7	589.5	528.5
	BLACK MALE	*	*	*	*	*	*	*	*	1.7	7.3	23.8	60.4	141.5	239.1	367.8	488.2	645.0	647.4	726.8	584.0
	WHITE FEMALE	*	*	*	*	*	*	*	0.9	2.7	10.1	26.6	68.6	136.8	251.2	369.1	461.8	530.7	589.5	528.5
	BLACK FEMALE	*	*	*	*	*	*	*	*	4.1	9.4	24.1	47.9	89.2	127.2	172.4	211.0	196.3	189.0	152.0
1995	WHITE MALE	*	*	*	*	*	*	*	1.2	3.3	9.5	26.2	66.1	132.7	233.6	359.6	470.9	529.9	580.6	542.4
	BLACK MALE	*	*	*	*	*	*	*	*	6.6	24.0	54.8	132.3	230.6	371.3	476.9	647.5	647.5	684.9	573.2
	WHITE FEMALE	*	*	*	*	*	*	*	0.9	3.1	6.7	18.7	43.1	80.4	130.9	182.2	229.1	251.2	239.2	184.0
	BLACK FEMALE	*	*	*	*	*	*	*	*	3.3	10.5	25.2	47.7	83.5	132.6	177.6	217.6	191.1	185.0	163.7

TABLE 4   CANCER OF THE LUNG AND BRONCHUS: AVERAGE ANNUAL AGE-SPECIFIC MORTALITY RATES[1] BY RACE, SEX, AND AGE, SELECTED YEARS, 1980-1998 *(continued)*

YEAR	SEX & RACE	<1	1-4	5-9	10-14	15-19	20-24	25-34	34-44	45-54	55-64	65-74	75-84	85+
1996[2]	WHITE MALE	**	**	*	*	**	*	0.7	6.5	42.7	174.4	404.9	543.7	524.5
	BLACK MALE	**	**	**	**	**	0.1	0.9	14.7	85.3	287.0	520.8	660.8	544.7
	WHITE FEMALE	*	**	*	*	*	*	0.6	4.9	28.4	102.9	209.9	251.5	188.2
	BLACK FEMALE	**	**	**	**	0.1	**	0.6	7.4	33.0	99.3	196.1	209.3	162.1
1997	WHITE MALE	*	**	**	**	*	*	0.6	6.3	39.6	167.4	400.4	540.1	549.1
	BLACK MALE	**	**	**	*	*	**	0.8	13.7	79.4	270.1	507.9	660.1	553.8
	WHITE FEMALE	**	*	**	**	*	*	0.5	5.2	26.8	100.9	213.2	259.7	200.5
	BLACK FEMALE	**	**	**	**	*	*	*	7.8	33.6	101.8	200.5	220.1	184.2
1998	WHITE MALE	*	**	**	**	*	*	0.6	6.4	37.5	162.5	399.2	531.7	516.6
	BLACK MALE	**	**	**	**	*	*	*	12.4	78.8	263.2	487.5	647.5	533.1
	WHITE FEMALE	**	**	*	*	*	*	0.6	5.1	25.8	99.7	216.6	263.1	200.3
	BLACK FEMALE	**	**	**	**	*	*	*	7.7	33.4	102.6	202.5	222.4	176.6

Source: CDC Wonder, 1979–1998.
Notes:
(1) Rates are per 100,000 population.
(2) As of 1996, data are only available for the age groups indicated in charts.
*Figure does not meet standards for reliability or precision (number of deaths is less than 20).
**Quantity is zero.
0.0 Quantity is more than zero but less than 0.05.

TABLE 5   AGE-ADJUSTED MORTALITY RATES[1] FOR CANCER OF THE TRACHEA, BRONCHUS, AND LUNG (ICD-9-CM CODE 162) BY STATE AND SEX, 1996–1998

STATE	1996			1997			1998			PERCENT CHANGE[2] 1996-1998	PERCENT CHANGE[2] 1997-1998
	TOTAL	MALE	FEMALE	TOTAL	MALE	FEMALE	TOTAL	MALE	FEMALE		
Alabama	42.3	63.4	26.3	43.1	67.0	24.5	42.7	64.1	26.5	0.9	-0.9
Alaska	37.6	45.5	30.3	37.9	49.3	26.7	36.9	41.9	32.2	-1.9	-2.6
Arizona	33.5	44.6	24.3	32.3	41.4	24.9	31.8	40.1	24.8	-5.1	-1.5
Arkansas	47.1	70.4	28.7	48.2	71.5	29.7	46.8	67.3	30.7	-0.6	-2.9
California	31.4	39.2	25.1	31.0	38.6	25.0	29.9	37.1	24.0	-4.8	-3.5
Colorado	26.1	35.3	19.1	24.7	31.9	19.2	25.6	31.7	20.9	-1.9	3.6
Connecticut	34.3	44.2	26.8	33.6	41.3	28.0	33.3	42.6	26.1	-2.9	-0.9
Delaware	47.4	60.6	37.2	43.0	57.3	31.7	42.8	56.0	32.6	-9.7	-0.5
District of Columbia	36.9	56.1	23.0	40.9	58.7	28.3	40.1	54.0	29.7	8.7	-2.0
Florida	39.4	53.6	27.9	39.4	52.2	28.9	37.9	49.4	28.2	-3.8	-3.8
Georgia	40.9	62.1	25.0	41.6	61.2	27.2	41.3	60.2	27.0	1.0	-0.7
Hawaii	25.2	33.9	17.6	25.9	35.3	17.8	27.3	36.9	19.2	8.3	5.4
Idaho	28.5	36.9	21.1	29.8	40.2	20.8	30.4	39.3	22.8	6.7	2.0
Illinois	39.2	53.5	28.1	37.5	51.0	26.9	37.3	49.8	27.6	-4.8	-0.5
Indiana	42.9	60.2	29.5	41.8	57.1	29.8	43.6	60.3	30.4	1.6	4.3
Iowa	35.1	49.4	23.9	34.6	48.2	23.9	33.6	45.5	24.1	-4.3	-2.9
Kansas	36.4	49.1	26.4	37.3	53.4	24.5	34.5	46.7	25.0	-5.2	-7.5
Kentucky	54.1	76.8	36.5	53.3	75.3	36.0	52.3	72.2	36.8	-3.3	-1.9
Louisiana	45.2	67.5	28.1	45.4	65.6	30.3	45.3	65.5	29.7	0.2	-0.2
Maine	43.1	55.8	33.3	41.0	51.9	32.7	41.1	52.1	32.5	-4.6	0.2
Maryland	41.6	56.1	30.2	39.5	53.3	28.8	39.9	52.0	30.5	-4.1	1.0
Massachusetts	37.0	47.8	29.2	35.9	45.4	28.9	36.6	46.5	29.3	-1.1	1.9
Michigan	39.5	53.6	28.6	38.2	50.6	28.4	37.5	49.1	28.4	-5.1	-1.8

TABLE 5   AGE-ADJUSTED MORTALITY RATES[1] FOR CANCER OF THE TRACHEA, BRONCHUS, AND LUNG (ICD-9-CM CODE 162) BY STATE AND SEX, 1996-1998 *(continued)*

STATE	1996 TOTAL	1996 MALE	1996 FEMALE	1997 TOTAL	1997 MALE	1997 FEMALE	1998 TOTAL	1998 MALE	1998 FEMALE	PERCENT CHANGE[2] 1996–1998	PERCENT CHANGE[2] 1997–1998
Minnesota	31.0	40.0	24.1	30.8	40.3	23.1	30.6	38.8	24.1	-1.3	-0.6
Mississippi	44.8	70.7	25.4	45.9	70.8	26.9	47.2	74.7	26.5	5.4	2.8
Missouri	43.2	61.1	29.0	43.1	58.0	31.5	43.9	60.0	31.2	1.6	1.9
Montana	32.7	41.3	25.9	31.8	38.6	25.7	34.8	45.0	26.6	6.4	9.4
Nebraska	33.2	46.3	22.4	32.7	46.9	21.1	32.7	45.7	22.4	-1.5	0.0
Nevada	44.6	53.4	36.5	42.6	57.1	34.8	43.2	49.6	37.3	-3.1	1.4
New Hampshire	38.8	47.4	32.4	38.8	48.6	31.3	40.2	50.2	32.1	3.6	3.6
New Jersey	36.3	47.5	27.9	35.5	45.0	28.3	35.4	46.5	26.8	-2.5	-0.3
New Mexico	24.1	30.2	19.2	28.0	35.0	21.8	24.7	32.0	18.6	2.5	-11.8
New York	34.1	45.9	25.0	32.6	43.3	24.5	32.5	42.8	24.7	-4.7	-0.3
North Carolina	43.1	65.9	25.5	41.8	62.4	26.3	41.2	60.7	26.5	-4.4	-1.4
North Dakota	30.3	39.9	22.5	29.8	39.9	21.2	30.9	42.3	21.5	2.0	3.7
Ohio	41.5	56.6	30.1	40.5	55.3	29.2	41.2	55.7	30.0	-0.7	1.7
Oklahoma	42.9	61.3	28.2	44.3	61.5	30.7	43.3	60.3	29.9	0.9	-2.3
Oregon	37.8	47.9	29.6	38.1	48.3	30.0	37.6	46.4	30.3	-0.5	-1.3
Pennsylvania	37.6	53.6	25.3	37.7	52.3	26.5	37.0	50.3	27.0	-1.6	-1.9
Rhode Island	41.9	55.7	31.8	43.6	55.8	35.0	39.3	56.1	26.5	-6.2	-9.9
South Carolina	41.7	62.3	25.9	42.3	63.3	25.9	40.2	58.3	26.3	-3.6	-5.0
South Dakota	35.1	50.6	22.1	30.8	47.5	16.8	30.0	37.1	24.5	-14.5	-2.6
Tennessee	47.5	72.1	28.3	47.4	70.5	29.5	46.9	69.0	29.7	-1.3	-1.1
Texas	38.5	53.4	26.5	37.6	52.5	25.8	36.8	50.8	25.6	-4.4	-2.1
Utah	17.0	22.4	12.2	14.4	20.4	9.5	16.6	22.2	11.9	-2.4	15.3
Vermont	36.3	48.3	26.6	40.0	54.7	28.1	38.0	49.2	29.1	4.7	-5.0
Virginia	40.1	55.6	28.5	40.1	56.3	27.6	38.7	54.2	26.7	-3.5	-3.5
Washington	35.9	44.6	28.9	34.7	41.9	29.1	36.1	44.1	29.5	0.6	4.0
West Virginia	44.7	61.6	31.9	48.1	65.4	35.0	47.6	66.8	32.7	6.5	-1.0
Wisconsin	32.2	42.8	23.6	32.4	41.9	24.8	33.3	43.4	25.3	3.4	2.8
Wyoming	28.7	37.6	21.0	29.8	37.4	23.7	30.5	36.8	25.3	6.3	2.3
U.S. Total	**37.8**	**51.8**	**26.8**	**37.4**	**50.5**	**27.0**	**37.0**	**49.5**	**27.0**	**-2.1**	**-1.1**

Source: CDC Wonder, 1996, 1997, 1998.
Notes:
(1) Rates are per 100,000 persons and are adjusted to the 1940 U.S. population.
(2) Due to rounding, U.S. total rates presented in this table may differ from those in Table 2.

TABLE 6   AGE-ADJUSTED MORTALITY RATES[1] FOR CANCER OF THE TRACHEA, BRONCHUS AND LUNG (ICD-9-CODE 162) BY STATE AND RACE, 1998

STATE	BLACK	WHITE	OTHER[2]
Alabama	39.7	43.5	23.8*
Alaska	44.4*	36.4	38.4
Arizona	35.6	32.7	9.4
Arkansas	50.2	46.6	22.1*
California	40.6	30.8	17.0
Colorado	26.4	25.8	16.6*
Connecticut	39.1	33.3	7.3*
District of Columbia	41.1	43.4	11.4*

TABLE 6 AGE-ADJUSTED MORTALITY RATES (1) FOR CANCER OF THE TRACHEA,
BRONCHUS, AND LUNG (ICD-9-CODE 162) BY STATE AND RACE, 1998 *(continued)*

STATE	BLACK	WHITE	OTHER[2]
Delaware	49.1	23.1	15.4*
Florida	36.9	38.2	14.3
Georgia	40.5	41.8	19.5
Hawaii	15.3*	27.0	27.7
Idaho	0.0*	30.5	21.3*
Illinois	54.6	35.4	12.8
Indiana	54.1	43.1	16.1*
Iowa	68.4	33.3	24.1*
Kansas	39.7	34.1	56.4
Kentucky	58.3	52.1	6.2*
Louisiana	54.7	42.4	18.6*
Maine	0.0*	41.3	38.3*
Maryland	45.7	39.4	11.0
Massachusetts	35.2	37.1	15.9
Michigan	45.2	36.7	29.0
Minnesota	49.5	30.0	45.6
Mississippi	49.9	46.4	24.3*
Missouri	58.3	42.7	30.0
Montana	64.2*	34.4	49.6
Nebraska	66.7	31.8	36.8*
Nevada	43.9	44.3	21.4
New Hampshire	0.0*	40.5	20.4*
New Jersey	44.0	35.3	9.7
New Mexico	31.0*	25.6	7.5*
New York	32.2	33.3	15.0
North Carolina	43.1	41.1	24.7
North Dakota	0.0*	30.6	52.7*
Ohio	49.9	40.5	15.2
Oklahoma	47.3	44.3	25.9
Oregon	29.9*	38.0	25.7
Pennsylvania	53.4	36.0	13.1
Rhode Island	52.8	39.3	4.0*
South Carolina	40.9	40.1	25.9*
South Dakota	0.0*	29.3	53.5*
Tennessee	51.1	46.6	18.7*
Texas	49.2	36.0	12.0
Utah	47.3*	16.6	12.5*
Vermont	59.9*	38.2	0.0*
Virginia	46.8	37.8	14.1
Washington	49.0	36.6	21.9
West Virginia	38.2	48.0	6.9*
Wisconsin	54.8	32.7	29.7
Wyoming	0.0*	31.1	0.0*
United States Total [3]	**44.6**	**36.8**	**18.5**

Source: CDC Wonder, 1998
Notes:
*These rates should be interpreted with caution as they represent 20 or fewer deaths.
(1) Rates are per 100,000 persons and age-adjusted to the 1940 U.S. population.
(2) Includes races other than black and white.
(3) Due to rounding, U.S. total rates presented in this table may differ from those in Table 3.

TABLE 7   AGE-ADJUSTED INCIDENCE RATES[1] FOR LUNG AND
BRONCHUS CANCER AND ALL CANCER SITES, 1973-1998

YEAR OF DIAGNOSIS	LUNG & BRONCHUS	ALL SITES
1973	42.4	320.0
1974	43.9	332.9
1975	45.3	333.7
1976	47.8	338.0
1977	48.9	337.6
1978	50.2	337.7
1979	50.9	341.3
1980	52.3	345.8
1981	53.9	352.0
1982	54.9	351.7
1983	55.0	357.4
1984	56.8	364.5
1985	56.2	372.4
1986	56.9	374.4
1987	58.5	387.5
1988	58.7	384.9
1989	58.0	387.8
1990	58.6	399.5
1991	59.7	417.5
1992	59.8	426.2
1993	58.0	412.5
1994	57.2	403.4
1995	56.8	399.1
1996	56.0	399.5
1997	55.8	403.8
1998	54.8	395.3

Source: National Cancer Institute: SEER Cancer Statistics Review, 1973–1998.
Note:
(1) Rates are per 100,000 persons and are age-adjusted to the 1970 U.S. population.

TABLE 8   RESPIRATORY CANCER: AGE-ADJUSTED INCIDENCE RATES[1]
BY SITE, RACE, AND SEX: ALL SEER AREAS COMBINED, 1973–1998

YEAR/SITE	ALL RACES			WHITES			BLACKS		
	TOTAL	MALES	FEMALES	TOTAL	MALES	FEMALES	TOTAL	MALES	FEMALES
ORAL CAVITY & PHARYNX									
1973	11.3	17.6	6.3	11.2	17.6	6.1	11.0	16.6	6.0
1974	11.1	17.4	6.1	11.2	17.6	6.1	10.8	16.1	6.3
1975	11.4	18.0	6.2	11.4	18.3	6.0	11.7	17.2	7.3
1976	11.5	17.8	6.5	11.4	17.8	6.4	13.2	20.4	7.4
1977	11.1	17.4	6.1	11.0	17.1	6.1	12.8	21.1	6.0
1978	11.6	17.7	6.7	11.4	17.6	6.7	13.2	21.5	6.7
1979	12.1	18.7	6.9	11.8	18.3	6.6	16.5	24.9	9.8
1980	11.6	17.4	6.8	11.2	17.0	6.6	15.3	23.1	8.6
1981	11.8	18.0	6.9	11.6	17.5	6.9	14.9	25.1	6.7
1982	11.5	17.4	6.8	11.3	17.0	6.7	15.4	24.7	7.9
1983	11.6	18.2	6.3	11.5	18.1	6.3	14.3	23.4	7.1
1984	11.8	17.9	6.9	11.3	17.2	6.7	17.0	27.1	8.9
1985	11.5	17.1	7.0	11.4	16.8	7.1	14.1	22.6	7.5
1986	11.0	16.8	6.2	10.8	16.4	6.2	14.2	24.8	5.2
1987	11.6	17.8	6.5	11.5	17.5	6.6	14.8	26.1	6.1
1988	10.8	16.2	6.3	10.4	15.7	6.1	14.9	23.5	8.0
1989	10.7	16.2	6.3	10.5	15.6	6.3	14.2	24.2	6.4
1990	11.1	17.0	6.3	10.9	16.3	6.3	14.3	24.8	6.2
1991	10.8	16.3	6.2	10.7	16.1	6.2	13.0	21.3	6.5
1992	10.5	16.1	6.0	10.3	15.7	5.9	13.4	22.7	6.2
1993	10.9	16.5	6.2	10.6	16.0	6.1	14.3	23.0	7.2
1994	10.3	15.7	5.8	10.0	14.9	5.8	14.6	25.1	6.4
1995	10.0	14.7	6.0	10.0	14.5	6.2	12.2	20.6	5.9
1996	10.2	15.1	6.0	9.8	14.6	5.8	14.0	22.7	7.0
1997	9.9	14.7	5.7	9.8	14.4	5.8	10.6	17.1	5.5
1998	9.3	13.6	5.6	9.2	13.3	5.6	11.1	18.2	5.7
LARYNX									
1973	4.5	8.4	1.3	4.4	8.4	1.2	6.3	11.9	1.8
1974	4.5	8.2	1.4	4.5	8.3	1.4	6.0	10.1	2.4
1975	4.5	8.3	1.3	4.4	8.3	1.3	6.4	11.9	1.8
1976	4.7	8.9	1.2	4.7	8.9	1.3	6.5	12.9	1.3
1977	4.5	8.5	1.2	4.4	8.5	1.2	6.4	11.9	2.0
1978	4.7	8.6	1.6	4.7	8.6	1.7	6.3	11.7	2.0
1979	4.8	8.9	1.5	4.8	9.0	1.5	6.7	11.8	2.7
1980	4.7	8.8	1.4	4.6	8.6	1.4	6.6	12.6	1.8
1981	4.8	8.6	1.7	4.7	8.4	1.8	7.2	14.5	1.6
1982	4.7	8.6	1.6	4.7	8.6	1.6	7.2	13.0	2.6
1983	4.8	8.8	1.6	4.9	9.0	1.6	6.1	10.9	2.4
1984	4.6	8.5	1.4	4.4	8.4	1.3	7.9	14.1	3.1
1985	4.9	8.7	1.8	4.8	8.7	1.8	7.5	13.4	3.0
1986	4.5	8.2	1.5	4.4	8.0	1.5	7.0	13.8	1.9
1987	4.7	8.3	1.8	4.6	8.2	1.7	7.3	13.3	2.8
1988	4.6	8.3	1.7	4.6	8.3	1.6	7.3	13.2	3.0
1989	4.5	7.8	1.8	4.5	7.8	1.9	7.0	12.6	2.9
1990	4.5	8.1	1.7	4.4	7.9	1.6	8.4	15.4	3.2
1991	4.2	7.4	1.6	4.2	7.4	1.7	5.9	11.3	1.9
1992	4.5	7.9	1.6	4.3	7.7	1.5	7.8	14.2	3.0

TABLE 8   RESPIRATORY CANCER: AGE-ADJUSTED INCIDENCE RATES[1]
BY SITE, RACE, AND SEX: ALL SEER AREAS COMBINED, 1973–1998 *(continued)*

YEAR/SITE	ALL RACES			WHITES			BLACKS		
	TOTAL	MALES	FEMALES	TOTAL	MALES	FEMALES	TOTAL	MALES	FEMALES
1993	3.9	7.0	1.3	3.8	6.8	1.4	6.2	12.6	1.4
1994	4.1	7.3	1.6	4.0	7.1	1.5	8.0	14.0	3.4
1995	3.8	6.8	1.4	3.9	6.7	1.4	5.8	10.9	2.0
1996	3.9	6.5	1.4	3.8	6.6	1.4	5.6	10.2	2.6
1997	3.7	6.4	1.4	3.6	6.2	1.4	6.3	11.6	2.3
1998	3.3	5.6	1.4	3.1	5.3	1.4	5.6	9.8	2.4

LUNG & BRONCHUS

YEAR/SITE	ALL RACES			WHITES			BLACKS		
	TOTAL	MALES	FEMALES	TOTAL	MALES	FEMALES	TOTAL	MALES	FEMALES
1973	42.4	73.2	18.2	41.6	72.4	17.85	8.8	104.8	20.9
1974	43.9	74.5	19.9	43.4	74.2	19.85	8.9	102.0	21.7
1975	45.3	76.2	21.5	45.1	75.9	21.85	6.5	101.0	20.6
1976	47.8	79.4	23.8	47.2	78.4	23.86	2.6	110.9	25.2
1977	48.9	80.7	24.7	48.3	80.0	24.66	4.2	108.7	28.9
1978	50.2	82.0	26.2	49.7	81.1	26.56	5.0	113.5	27.1
1979	50.9	81.4	27.8	50.4	80.7	27.96	5.4	111.6	29.4
1980	52.3	84.4	28.1	51.2	82.2	28.27	6.0	131.0	33.8
1981	53.9	84.5	30.9	53.4	83.4	31.37	3.3	126.1	33.1
1982	54.9	85.1	32.3	54.6	83.8	33.37	1.1	123.5	31.4
1983	55.0	84.1	33.3	54.5	82.2	34.47	5.9	130.9	34.7
1984	56.8	86.5	34.6	55.7	84.2	34.88	2.8	140.5	39.7
1985	56.2	83.9	35.3	55.5	82.0	35.97	9.0	131.3	40.2
1986	56.9	83.6	37.0	56.3	81.9	37.78	1.3	134.0	43.0
1987	58.5	85.3	38.6	58.6	84.3	39.87	4.5	124.1	38.4
1988	58.7	83.3	40.4	58.9	82.3	41.77	7.9	125.9	42.9
1989	58.0	82.2	40.0	58.0	81.1	41.17	8.2	123.1	45.7
1990	58.6	81.7	41.5	58.7	80.9	42.57	6.6	118.6	46.9
1991	59.5	81.8	43.2	59.4	80.4	44.28	1.9	126.0	49.8
1992	59.8	81.9	43.2	59.2	79.5	44.48	2.5	128.7	49.1
1993	58.0	78.8	42.4	58.0	77.2	43.87	5.2	115.7	46.0
1994	57.2	75.6	43.4	57.3	74.7	44.57	6.3	112.9	49.3
1995	56.8	74.7	43.1	57.0	73.0	44.97	2.9	116.6	43.2
1996	56.0	72.6	43.5	56.3	71.2	45.17	1.8	105.5	48.4
1997	55.8	70.8	44.3	56.2	69.3	46.36	8.4	106.6	43.4
1998	54.8	69.8	43.4	55.0	68.4	44.87	0.1	100.6	47.9

Source: National Cancer Institute: SEER Cancer Statistics Review, 1973–1998.
Note:
(1) Rates are per 100,000 persons and are age-adjusted to the 1970 U.S. standard population.

TABLE 9   LUNG CANCER: TOTAL NUMBER OF FIRST-LISTED HOSPITAL DISCHARGES AND
RATE PER 10,000 POPULATION BY AGE (ICD-9-CODE 162, 197.0, 197.3), 1979–1999[1]

YEAR	<15 NUMBER OF DISCHARGES	<15 RATE PER 10,000	15–44 NUMBER OF DISCHARGES	15–44 RATE PER 10,000	45–64 NUMBER OF DISCHARGES	45–64 RATE PER 10,000	65+ NUMBER OF DISCHARGES	65+ RATE PER 10,000	TOTAL[2] NUMBER OF DISCHARGES	TOTAL[2] RATE PER 10,000
1979	1,000*	0.2*	12,000	1.2	130,000	29.3	131,000	52.1	274,000	12.7
1980	—	—*	12,000	1.2	123,000	27.8	142,000	55.3	277,000	12.4
1981	—*	—*	11,000	1.0	134,000	30.2	145,000	55.2	293,000	12.9
1982	—*	—	15,000	1.4	147,000	33.2	155,000	58.0	319,000	13.9
1983	—*	—*	12,000	1.1	151,000	34.0	176,000	64.1	339,000	14.6
1984	—*	—*	13,000	1.2	155,000	34.1	172,000	61.2	340,000	14.5
1985	—*	—*	13,000	1.2	132,000	29.4	169,000	59.4	315,000	13.3
1986	—*	—*	15,000	1.3	120,000	26.7	155,000	53.3	290,000	12.1
1987	0.	0.1*	12,000	1.1	129,000	28.5	169,000	54.9	305,000	12.6
1988[3]	—*	—	8,000*	0.7*	102,000	22.2	125,000	41.2	236,000	9.7
1989	—*	—*	11,000	1.0	101,000	21.8	127,000	40.9	239,000	9.7
1990	—*	—*	12,000	1.0	101,000	21.4	119,000	37.7	231,000	9.3
1991	—*	—*	10,000	0.8	101,000	21.6	125,000	39.3	236,000	9.4
1992	—*	—	7,000*	0.6*	86,000	17.8	122,000	37.8	215,000	8.5
1993	—*	—	7,000*	0.6*	75,000	15.1	110,000	33.9	194,000	7.6
1994	—*	—*	9,000*	0.7*	73,000	14.3	126,000	37.9	199,000	7.6
1995	—*	—*	8,000*	0.7*	75,000	14.4	110,000	32.8	197,000	7.5
1996	—*	—*	10,000	0.8	72,000	13.4	122,000	36.0	210,000	8.0
1997	—*	—*	—*	—*	60,000	10.9	123,000	36.4	192,000	7.1
1998	—*	—	9,000	0.7*	55,000	9.6	99,000	29.0	165,000	6.0
1999	—*	—*	5,000	0.4*	54,000	9.2	104,000	30.5	164,000	6.0

Source: National Center for Health Statistics: National Hospital Discharge Survey, 1979–98, and National Hospital Discharge Survey, Advanced
Data 1999.
Notes:
*Estimates of 5,000–10,000 and corresponding rates to be used with caution.
— Figure does not meet standards of reliability or precision.
(1) Includes malignant neoplasms of the trachea, bronchus, and lung.
(2) Due to rounding and the exclusion of numbers that do not meet standards of reliability, numbers across may not sum to the total of
hospital discharges.
(3) Data from 1988–99 may not be comparable to earlier years due to the redesign of the survey in 1988.

TABLE 10   LUNG CANCER: TOTAL NUMBER OF FIRST-LISTED HOSPITAL DISCHARGES
AND RATE PER 10,000 PERSONS BY RACE (ICD-9-CODE 162, 197.0, 197.3), 1988–1999

YEAR	NUMBER OF DISCHARGES				RATE PER 10,000 POPULATION			
	TOTAL[1]	WHITE	BLACK	ALL OTHER	TOTAL (1)	WHITE	BLACK	ALL OTHER
1988	236,000	193,000	N/A	N/A	9.7	9.3	N/A	N/A
1989	239,000	194,000	N/A	N/A	9.7	9.3	N/A	N/A
1990	231,000	183,000	19,000	*	9.3	8.7	6.3	*
1991	236,000	181,000	21,000	7,000*	9.4	8.6	6.9	7.1*
1992	215,000	161,000	16,000	5,000*	8.5	7.6	5.2	4.7*
1993	194,000	149,000	16,000	*	7.6	7.0	5.1	*
1994[2]	208,000	151,000	21,000	7,000*	8.0	7.0	6.4	6.0*
1995	199,000	140,000	21,000	*	7.6	6.5	6.4	*
1996	210,000	156,000	17,000	5,000*	8.0	7.1	5.3	4.4*
1997	193,000	142,000	20,000	*	7.1	6.4	5.6	*
1998	65,000	114,000	14,000	7,000	6.0	5.1	3.8	5.1
1999	64,000	115,000	13,000	8,000	6.0	5.1	3.5	6.3

Source: National Center for Health Statistics National Hospital Discharge Survey 1988–1999.
Notes:
(1) Total includes white, black, other race and unspecified race discharges.
(2) In 1994 discharges for ICD-9-CM Code 176.4 were added to this category.
*Figure does not meet standard of reliability or precision.
N/A Not available.

TABLE 11   TRENDS IN SURVIVAL RATES BY SELECTED CANCER SITES, BY RACE, CASES DIAGNOSED IN
1960–1963, 1970–1973, 1974–1976, 1977–1979, 1980–1982, 1983–1985, 1986–1988, 1989–1991, 1992–1997

SITE	TOTAL RELATIVE 5-YEAR SURVIVAL								
	1960–63[1]	1970–73[1]	1974–76[2]	1977–79[2]	1980–82[2]	1983–85[2]	1986–88[2]	1989–91[2]	1992–97[2]
Lung and Bronchus	*	*	12.4	13.4	13.4	13.6	13.3	13.9	14.5[3]
Colon	*	*	50.4	52.9	55.4	57.7	60.9	62.5	61.2[3]
Rectum	*	*	48.5	49.9	52.1	55.0	58.5	60.0	60.8[3]
Breast	*	*	74.7	74.7	76.3	78.1	82.8	84.8	85.5[3]
Esophagus	*	*	4.8	5.1	6.7	8.3	9.8	10.8	13.7[3]
Prostate	*	*	67.1	71.1	73.4	74.8	81.1	90.4	96.2[3]

SITE	WHITE RELATIVE 5-YEAR SURVIVAL								
	1960–63[1]	1970–73[1]	1974–76[2]	1977–79[2]	1980–82[2]	1983–85[2]	1986–88[2]	1989–91[2]	1992–97[2]
Lung and Bronchus	8.0	10.0	12.5	13.7	13.5	14.0	13.8	14.3	14.8[3]
Colon	43.0	49.0	50.6	52.9	55.6	58.4	61.5	63.1	62.1[3]
Rectum	38.0	45.0	48.9	50.8	52.9	55.9	59.1	60.5	61.5[3]
Breast	63.0	68.0	75.3	75.4	77.1	79.2	83.8	86.1	86.8[3]
Esophagus	4.0	4.0	5.1	5.6	7.4	9.3	10.8	11.6	15.1[3]
Prostate	50.0	63.0	68.1	72.2	74.5	76.2	82.6	91.7	97.0[3]

TABLE 11   TRENDS IN SURVIVAL RATES BY SELECTED CANCER SITES, BY RACE, CASES DIAGNOSED IN 1960–1963, 1970–1973, 1974–1976, 1977–1979, 1980–1982, 1983–1985, 1986–1988, 1989–1991, 1992–1997
(continued)

| | BLACK RELATIVE 5-YEAR SURVIVAL | | | | | | | | |
SITE	1960–63[1]	1970–73[1]	1974–76[2]	1977–79[2]	1980–82[2]	1983–85[2]	1986–88[2]	1989–91[2]	1992–97[2]
Lung and Bronchus	5.0	7.0	11.5	11.1	12.2	11.5	11.8	10.7	11.7
Colon	34.0	37.0	45.9	48.1	49.2	49.2	52.5	53.7	51.3[3]
Rectum	27.0	30.0	42.1	38.8	38.2	43.8	51.0	54.1	51.9[3]
Breast	46.0	51.0	63.1	63.2	65.9	63.5	69.2	71.2	72.0[3]
Esophagus	1.0	4.0	4.0	2.8	5.4	6.3	7.3	8.8	9.0[3]
Prostate	35.0	55.0	58.3	62.5	64.7	64.1	69.0	80.4	91.8[3]

Source: National Cancer Institute: SEER Cancer Statistics Review, 1973–1998.
Notes:
(1) Rates are based on data from a series of hospital registries and one population based registry.
(2) Rates are from the SEER program and are based on follow-up of all patients through 1998.
(3) The difference in rates between 1974-76 and 1992-97 is statistically significant (p<0.05).

TABLE 12   ESTIMATES OF SMOKING-ATTRIBUTABLE LUNG CANCER DEATHS, UNITED STATES, 1990, 1995

AGE/SEX	1990		1995	
	NUMBER OF DEATHS	PERCENTAGE	NUMBER OF DEATHS	PERCENTAGE
MALES				
0-34	0	0	0	0
35-69	45,367	94	46,244	94
70+	39,085	92	46,880	92
ALL AGES	84,452	93	93,124	93
FEMALES				
0-34	0	0	0	0
35-69	22,451	86	26,719	87
70+	20,096	84	31,232	88
ALL AGES	42,457	85	57,951	88
BOTH SEXES				
0-34	0	0	0	0
35-69	67,818	91	72,963	91
70+	59,181	89	78,112	91
ALL AGES	126,999	90	151,075	91

Source: Mortality from smoking in developed countries, 1950–2000.
    Indirect estimates from National Vital Statistics, 1994.

TABLE 13   LIFETIME RISK (PERCENT) OF BEING DIAGNOSED WITH LUNG CANCER AND
LIFETIME RISK (PERCENT OF DYING FROM LUNG CANCER) BY RACE AND SEX, 1996–1998

TYPE OF RISK	ALL RACES		WHITES		BLACKS	
	MALES	FEMALES	MALES	FEMALES	MALES	FEMALES
LIFETIME RISK OF DIAGNOSIS	7.85	5.75	7.83	6.04	8.47	5.06
LIFETIME RISK OF DYING	7.61	4.84	7.67	5.02	7.68	3.98

Source: SEER Cancer Statistics Review, 1973–1998.

APPENDIX IV
TRENDS IN ASTHMA MORBIDITY AND MORTALITY

Table of Contents

INTRODUCTION[1,2]

Asthma is a serious chronic condition affecting many Americans. Public attention has recently focused on this condition because its prevalence and the associated mortality rate have increased over the last decade. The following delineates information available from national surveys and reports on trends in asthma morbidity and mortality. As an overview of the widespread and growing nature of the asthma problem in the United States, we have examined data on hospitalization, prevalence, mortality, and economic costs.

ASTHMA MORTALITY TRENDS, 1970–1998

Due to decennial revisions of the International Classification of Diseases (ICD) coding system, there is a lack of comparability in cause of death statistics. The number and rate of asthma deaths reported prior to 1979 are not directly comparable to those reported after 1979. Although time trends covering different revisions of the code should be examined separately, it is important to note that increases in mortality attributed to asthma have been sustained through changes in the code and have been consistent since 1979.

Table 1 documents the trend in age-adjusted asthma mortality between 1970 and 1998. Overall, the age-adjusted death rate increased from 0.9 per 100,000 in 1979 to 1.4 per 100,000 in 1998, a 55.6 percent increase. In contrast, the age-adjusted death rate attributed to all causes decreased 18 percent and seven out of the ten leading causes of death experienced decreases in age-adjusted mortality.

Trends in Sex and Race-Specific Mortality Rates

Between 1979 and 1998, the age-adjusted mortality rate for asthma increased 33 percent in males, from 0.9 to 1.2, and increased 67 percent in females, from 0.9 to 1.5 per 100,000 population. Females tend to have higher asthma mortality rates. In 1998, the female death rate was 25 percent greater than the rate seen in males. Figure 1 illustrates the age-adjusted death rate by sex from 1970 to 1998.

In 1998, the age-adjusted death rate for asthma in the black population (3.7 per 100,000) was more than three times the rate in the white population (1.1 per 100,000). Between 1979 and 1998, the age-adjusted asthma mortality rate has increased 12.5 percent in white males and 50 percent in white females. During the same period, the age-adjusted mortality rate increased by 78.9 percent in black males and 90 percent in black females. Age-adjusted mortality rates in nonwhites (all races other than white) increased 61 percent in males and 72 percent in females over this time span.

Table 2 summarizes the trend in the crude death rate by sex and race from 1970 to 1998. Table 3 depicts the number of asthma deaths from 1979 to 1998 by sex and race. The number of deaths due to asthma has increased from 2,598 to 5,438 over this time period, an increase of 109 percent. This trend of increase in the number of asthma deaths is depicted by sex in Figure 2.

Trends in Age-Specific Mortality

Table 4 delineates mortality rates for asthma by 10-year age groups from 1979 through 1998. Between 1979 and 1998, increases in age-specific mortality were seen in all age groups. The death rate increases with age and is highest in those over age 85. Between 1979 and 1998, the death rate in those over 85 increased by 131.4 percent. Table 5 shows the number of deaths by 10-year age groups from 1979 to 1998.

ASTHMA PREVALENCE TRENDS, 1982–1996 AND 1997–1998

The National Health Interview Survey (NHIS) is a multipurpose health survey conducted by the National Center for Health Statistics (NCHS), Centers for Disease Control and Prevention (CDC). It is the principal source of information on the health of the civilian, noninstitutionalized, household population of the United States.

Despite the periodic revision of the NHIS Core questionnaire, Supplements began to play an increasingly important role in the survey as a means of enhancing topic coverage in the Core section. The unintended result was an increasingly unwieldy survey instrument and longer interviewing sessions: recent questionnaires (Core and Supplements combined) ran almost 300 pages, while the interviews averaged two hours. This imposed an unacceptable burden on NCHS staff, U.S.

Bureau of Census interviewers, the data collection budget, and on the NHIS respondents. Furthermore, the excessive length of NHIS interviews contributed to declines in both response rate and data quality. For all these reasons, NCHS implemented a redesigned NHIS questionnaire in 1997.

The new questionnaire design has made it impossible to compare current asthma estimates with those prior to 1997. The revised questionnaire evaluates both period and point prevalence of asthma. Asking respondents or their proxies if they have been diagnosed with asthma by a health professional within their lifetime assessed the period prevalence of asthma. The point prevalence of asthma was measured by asking all those diagnosed if they had an asthmatic attack or episode in the past 12 months. Between 1982 and 1996, respondents were asked to self-report asthma prevalence by letting interviewers know if any family member had asthma during the past 12 months. In contrast with the prior questionnaire, the redesigned survey measures physician-diagnosed asthma and produces a more specific estimate than self-report. In addition, estimating asthma attack prevalence is more helpful for planning public health interventions by measuring the population at risk for serious outcomes from asthma. These new estimates most likely continue to reflect an underestimate of true asthma prevalence, since studies have shown that there are many individuals suffering from undiagnosed asthma.

Period Prevalence

Based on the 1997 NHIS sample, it was estimated that 25.7 million people had been diagnosed with asthma by a health professional within their lifetime. That estimated number increased to 26.3 million people in 1998. The highest prevalence rate was seen in children 5–17 years of age for both years: 130.1 per 1,000 in 1997 and 135.0 per 1,000 in 1998. Females had higher rates than males, 99.0 vs. 94.0 per 1,000 persons in 1997 and 100.3 vs. 95.8 per 1,000 in 1998, but this difference was not significant in either year. The prevalence rate in blacks was 15 percent higher in 1997 and 30 percent higher in 1998 compared to the rate seen in whites. The difference between races was significant for both 1997 and 1998. This data is displayed in Table 6.

Point Prevalence

For simplicity, Tables 7, 8, and 9 will display point prevalence estimates for both trend phases—1982 to 1996 and 1997 to 1998, but again the data should not be compared to each other. In addition, this trend report will mainly focus on the revised survey data. Data from 1982 to 1996 will be highlighted but more detailed information on this trend series can be found in past versions of the morbidity and mortality reports.

Age-Specific Prevalence

Age-specific asthma prevalence trends are shown in Table 7. Between 1982 and 1996 the asthma prevalence rate increased 58.6 percent. There were significant differences seen in the rate increases for those under 45 but not for those in older age groups. The greatest increase was seen in those 18–44 (123.4%) and the smallest increase was seen in those over 65 (39.6%). The trend in age specific prevalence for 1982–1996 is delineated in Figure 3.

The new revised NHIS trends show that between 1997 and 1998 the asthma attack prevalence rate for all ages decreased 5.3 percent. However, the prevalence rate in those under five increased 12.9 percent and by 5 percent in those over 65+. In 1997 and 1998 5–17 year olds had the highest prevalence rates (59.5 and 55.6 per 1,000 population) while those over 65 had the lowest (27.3 and 28.7 per 1,000 population). For both years the rate in those under 18 was significantly greater than those over 18. Overall, an estimated 10.6 million people (3.8 million children under 18) had an asthma attack or episode in 1998. This trend in age-specific prevalence is delineated in Figure 4.

Sex-Specific Prevalence

Sex-specific prevalence trends are delineated in Table 8. Between 1982 and 1996, the prevalence rate increased by almost 22 percent in males and 97 percent in females. The 1996 rate was 44.4 per 1,000 in males and 65.3 per 1,000 persons in females. These rates were significantly different from each other. The trend in sex-specific prevalence is depicted in Figure 5.

Between 1997 and 1998, the prevalence rate decreased 2.0 percent in males and 7.7 percent in females. In 1997, 4.6 males (35.3 per 1,000) and

6.5 million females (47.8 per 1,000) had an asthma attack or episode. In 1998, an estimated 4.6 million males had an asthma attack or episode (34.5 per 1,000) compared to 6.1 million females (43.9 per 1,000). The difference between sexes was significant for both years. This trend in sex-specific prevalence is depicted in Figure 7.

Race-Specific Prevalence

Race-specific prevalence trends are displayed in Table 9. In 1996 the prevalence rate in whites was 53.5 per 1,000 persons while the prevalence rate in blacks was 69.6 per 1,000 persons. Both of these rates represent significant differences from the rates reported in 1982, when they were 34.6 and 39.2 for whites and blacks, respectively. This trend in race-specific prevalence is also shown in Figure 6.

Between 1997 and 1998 the prevalence rate among whites decreased 6.8 percent from 41.0 to 38.2 per 1,000, while the prevalence rate among blacks increased 2.5 percent from 48.9 to 50.1 per 1,000. During both years, the prevalence rate for whites was highest in the 5–17 age group and lowest in those over 65. In 1997 the prevalence rate for blacks was highest in the 5–17 age group and lowest in the 18 to 44 group. In 1998 the rate was highest in those under five and lowest in those over 65. This trend in race-specific prevalence is also shown in Figure 7.

Percentage Distribution of Conditions, 1998

The percentage distribution of asthma cases in 1998 is displayed in Figure 8. Four pie charts show the distribution of asthma by sex, age group, race, and geographic region.

ASTHMA TRENDS IN HOSPITAL DISCHARGES, 1970–1998

Tables 10, 11, and 12 delineate the number of first-listed hospital discharges and discharge rate by sex, age, and race for asthma from 1970–1998, respectively. The first listed diagnosis is the diagnosis identified as the principal diagnosis or listed first on the medical record.

Although data are presented for 1970 through 1998, due to the 1979 change in disease classification, the data on hospital discharges between 1970 and 1978 are not directly comparable to years 1979 and after. In addition, due to a second change in the design of the survey, data from 1988–1998 is not directly comparable to that of earlier years. We have restricted our analysis to estimates made since 1988.

Hospital Discharges: 1988–1998

The hospital discharge rate for asthma increased dramatically from 1970 to 1988, it then plateaued into the mid-1990s and has been on the decline since 1996. In 1998, 423,000 discharges (15.5 per 10,000 people) were due to asthma.

Sex-Specific Trends

Table 10 delineates the trend in the hospital discharge rate by sex from 1970–1998. Between 1988 and 1995 the number of hospital discharges stayed relatively the same. However, since 1995 the number of hospital discharges decreased 17 percent overall, 20 percent in males and 15 percent in females. In 1998, a total of 255,000 discharges were reported in females and 168,000 were reported in males. The discharge rate in females (18.3 per 10,000) was significantly different from that reported in males (12.6 per 10,000).

Age-Specific Trends

As shown in Table 11, hospital discharge rates for asthma decreased in all age groups between 1995 and 1998. Those under 15 and those 15–44 years of age exhibited a 25 percent decline in rate followed by a 23 percent drop in those over age 65 and a 3 percent decline among those 45–64 years old. Unlike other chronic lung diseases, asthma discharges are very common among the pediatric population. Over 39 percent of asthma discharges in 1998 were in those under 15, whereas only 22 percent of the population were less than 15 years old. However, the discharge rate in the population <15 was only statistically greater than the rate in those 15–44. Figure 9 depicts this age-specific trend.

Race-Specific Trends

The trend in hospital discharges by race is delineated in Table 12. The 1998 discharge rate for asthma was highest in blacks (32.2 per 10,000) and lowest in whites (10.0 per 10,000). The rate in all other races was 21.0 per 10,000. These rates, however, should be interpreted with caution due to the large percentage of discharges (13.7% in 1998) for which race was not reported. Figure 10 also displays this race-specific trend.

ECONOMIC COST OF ASTHMA

Estimates of direct medical expenditures and indirect costs (in 2000 dollars) attributed to asthma are shown in Table 13. Asthma entails an annual economic cost to our nation in direct health care costs of $8.1 billion; indirect costs (lost productivity) add another $4.6 billion for a total of $12.7 billion. Inpatient hospital services represented the largest single direct medical expenditure, over $3.5 billion. The value of reduced productivity due to loss of school days represented the largest single indirect cost at $1.5 billion.

SUMMARY

Asthma is a serious chronic condition affecting many Americans. Asthma accounts for an estimated 3 million lost work days for adults and 10.1 million lost school days in children annually.

Over the past 20 years mortality, morbidity, and hospital discharge rates attributed to asthma have substantially increased. Between 1979 and 1998, the age-adjusted mortality rate increased 56 percent, while the prevalence rate increased by almost 22 percent in males and 97 percent in females between 1982 and 1996.

However, new evidence suggests that these asthma mortality and morbidity rates may be beginning to plateau. The age-adjusted mortality rate for asthma has remained the same over the past two years and the asthma attack prevalence rate decreased 5.3 percent between 1997 and 1998. Since the National Health Interview Survey revised their questionnaire in 1997, more years of data are needed to accurately assess this prevalence trend.

Hospital discharges have been declining over the past few years. The rate peaked at 19.5 per 10,000 in 1995 and has declined since then.

Although asthma estimates seem to be declining, it is still a major public health concern. Asthma ranks within the top ten prevalent conditions causing limitation of activity and costs our nation $12.7 billion in health care costs annually.

GLOSSARY

Prevalence: The number of existing cases of a particular condition, disease, or other occurrence (e.g., persons smoking) at a given time.

Period Prevalence: The proportion of cases that exist within a population at any point during a specified period of time.

Point Prevalence: The proportion of cases that exist within a population at a single point in time.

Crude Rate: Cases in a particular population quantity (e.g., per hundred).

Age-Adjusted Rate: A figure that is statistically corrected to remove the distorting effect of age when comparing populations of different age structures.

P value: The probability of observing a result as extreme as that observed solely to chance. If p=0.05, then there is no more than a 5% chance of seeing that result again, but if p=0.05, then chance cannot be excluded as a likely explanation and the findings are said to be not significant at that level.

REFERENCES:

1. National Center for Health Statistics. *Current Estimates from the National Health Interview Survey,* U.S., selected years, 1970–1996.
2. National Center for Health Statistics. *National Hospital Discharge Survey: 1980–1998* and data provided upon special request to the NCHS.
3. National Center for Health Statistics. *Raw Data from the National Health Interview Survey,* U.S., 1997–1998. (Analysis by the American Lung Association Best Practices Division, using SPSS and SUDAAN software)
4. National Center for Health Statistics. *Report of Final Mortality Statistics: 1970–1998.*
5. National Heart, Lung and Blood Institute Chartbook, U.S. Department of Health and Human Services, National Institute of Health, 2000.
6. Weiss, Kevin B., M.D.; Peter J. Gergen, M.D. M.P.H.; and Thomas A. Hodgson, Ph.D. "An Economic Evaluation of Asthma in the U.S." *The New England Journal of Medicine,* 1992, 326: 862-6.

FOOTNOTES:

[1]Unless otherwise noted, terms such as *higher* or *less* are not intended to indicate statistical significance.
[2]In this document, an association is considered statistical significance if the p value is less than or equal to 0.05

TABLE 1 ASTHMA: AGE-ADJUSTED MORTALITY RATE BY RACE AND SEX
PER 100,000 POPULATION, 1970–1998[1]

| | TOTAL | | | WHITE | | | ALL OTHER[2] | | | | | |
| | | | | | | | TOTAL | | | BLACK | | |
YEAR	BOTH SEXES	MALE	FEMALE	BOTH SEXES	MALE	FEMALE	BOTH SEXES	MALE	FEMALE	BOTH SEXES	MALE	FEMALE
1970[3]	1.0	0.9	1.1	0.8	0.8	0.9	2.6	2.4	2.7	2.8	2.6	2.9
1971	1.0	0.8	1.0	0.8	0.7	0.8	2.2	2.1	2.4	2.3	2.2	2.4
1972	1.0	0.9	1.0	0.8	0.7	0.9	2.1	2.1	2.1	2.2	2.3	2.2
1973	0.8	0.7	0.8	0.6	0.6	0.7	1.9	1.9	1.9	2.0	2.0	2.0
1974	0.7	0.7	0.8	0.6	0.6	0.7	1.6	1.7	1.6	1.8	1.7	1.8
1975	0.8	0.7	0.8	0.6	0.6	0.7	1.8	1.6	1.8	1.9	1.9	1.9
1976	0.8	0.7	0.8	0.6	0.6	0.7	1.6	1.3	1.6	1.7	1.7	1.8
1977	0.6	0.6	0.6	0.5	0.5	0.5	1.3	1.4	1.3	1.5	1.4	1.4
1978	0.7	0.6	0.8	0.6	0.5	0.7	1.4	1.3	1.3	1.5	1.5	1.4
1979[4]	0.9	0.9	0.9	0.8	0.8	0.8	1.8	1.8	1.8	1.9	1.9	2.0
1980	1.0	1.0	1.0	0.8	0.8	0.8	2.0	2.1	1.9	2.2	2.2	2.2
1981	1.0	1.0	1.1	0.9	0.8	0.9	2.1	2.2	1.9	2.3	2.4	2.1
1982	1.0	1.0	1.1	0.9	0.8	0.9	2.2	2.3	2.2	2.5	2.5	2.5
1983	1.2	1.1	1.3	0.9	0.9	1.0	2.5	2.5	2.5	2.8	2.8	2.8
1984	1.1	1.1	1.2	1.0	0.9	1.0	2.3	2.4	2.3	2.6	2.5	2.6
1985	1.2	1.1	1.3	1.0	0.9	1.2	2.5	2.6	2.3	2.8	3.0	2.7
1986	1.2	1.1	1.3	1.0	0.9	1.1	2.6	2.5	2.7	2.9	2.9	3.0
1987	1.3	1.2	1.4	1.1	1.0	1.2	2.9	2.9	2.8	3.2	3.3	3.2
1988	1.4	1.2	1.5	1.1	1.0	1.2	3.0	3.1	3.0	3.5	3.5	3.4
1989	1.4	1.2	1.6	1.2	1.0	1.3	2.8	2.8	2.9	3.3	3.2	3.3
1990	1.4	1.3	1.5	1.2	1.0	1.3	2.9	3.0	2.8	3.4	3.5	3.3
1991	1.5	1.3	1.6	1.2	1.0	1.4	3.0	3.0	3.0	3.5	3.5	3.5
1992	1.4	1.2	1.5	1.1	0.9	1.3	2.8	2.8	2.9	3.3	3.1	3.5
1993	1.4	1.3	1.6	1.2	1.0	1.3	2.9	2.8	3.0	3.5	3.3	3.7
1994	1.5	1.4	1.7	1.2	1.0	1.4	3.1	3.1	3.1	3.7	3.6	3.7
1995	1.5	1.3	1.7	1.3	1.0	1.5	3.2	3.1	3.3	3.8	3.6	3.9
1996	1.5	1.3	1.7	1.2	1.0	1.4	3.3	3.1	3.5	3.9	3.6	4.1
1997	1.4	1.2	1.6	1.1	1.0	1.3	3.0	2.9	3.1	3.5	3.2	3.6
1998	1.4	1.2	1.5	1.1	0.9	1.2	3.0	2.9	3.1	3.7	3.4	3.8

Source: National Center for Health Statistics, Final Mortality Statistics Report, 1970–1998.
Notes:
(1) Rates are age-adjusted to the 1940 U.S. standard population.
(2) All races other than white.
(3) International Classification of Diseases, 8th Revision (ICD-8) Code 493.
(4) International Classification of Diseases, 9th Revision (ICD-9) Code 493.

TABLE 2   ASTHMA: CRUDE MORTALITY RATE BY RACE AND SEX
PER 100,000 POPULATION, 1970–1998

| | TOTAL | | | WHITE | | | ALL OTHER[1] | | | | | |
| | | | | | | | TOTAL | | | BLACK | | |
YEAR	BOTH SEXES	MALE	FEMALE	BOTH SEXES	MALE	FEMALE	BOTH SEXES	MALE	FEMALE	BOTH SEXES	MALE	FEMALE
1970[2]	1.1	1.0	1.3	1.0	0.8	1.1	2.3	2.1	2.4	2.5	2.3	2.6
1971	1.0	0.9	1.2	0.9	0.8	1.0	2.0	1.8	2.1	2.0	1.9	2.2
1972	1.1	1.0	1.2	1.0	0.9	1.1	1.9	1.9	1.9	2.0	2.0	2.0
1973	0.9	0.8	1.0	0.8	0.7	0.9	1.7	1.6	1.7	1.8	1.8	1.8
1974	0.9	0.8	1.0	0.8	0.7	0.9	1.5	1.4	1.5	1.6	1.5	1.6
1975	0.9	0.8	1.0	0.8	0.7	0.9	1.6	1.5	1.6	1.7	1.6	1.7
1976	0.9	0.8	1.0	0.8	0.7	1.0	1.5	1.4	1.5	1.6	1.5	1.7
1977	0.8	0.7	0.8	0.7	0.6	0.8	1.2	1.2	1.3	1.3	1.3	1.4
1978	0.8	0.7	1.0	0.8	0.6	0.9	1.3	1.3	1.3	1.4	1.4	1.4
1979[3]	1.2	1.1	1.3	1.1	1.0	1.2	1.7	1.6	1.7	1.8	1.7	1.9
1980	1.3	1.2	1.4	1.2	1.1	1.3	1.9	1.9	1.9	2.1	2.1	2.1
1981	1.3	1.2	1.5	1.2	1.0	1.4	1.9	2.0	1.9	2.1	2.2	2.1
1982	1.4	1.2	1.5	1.2	1.0	1.4	2.1	2.1	2.1	2.3	2.3	2.4
1983	1.5	1.3	1.8	1.4	1.1	1.6	2.4	2.3	2.4	2.6	2.5	2.7
1984	1.5	1.3	1.7	1.4	1.1	1.6	2.2	2.2	2.3	2.5	2.3	2.6
1985	1.6	1.3	1.9	1.5	1.2	1.8	2.4	2.4	2.4	2.7	2.7	2.7
1986	1.6	1.3	1.9	1.5	1.2	1.8	2.5	2.3	2.7	2.8	2.6	3.0
1987	1.8	1.5	2.1	1.6	1.2	2.0	2.7	2.7	2.8	3.1	3.0	3.1
1988	1.9	1.5	2.2	1.7	1.3	2.1	2.9	2.9	3.0	3.4	3.2	3.5
1989	2.0	1.5	2.4	1.8	1.3	2.3	2.8	2.6	3.0	3.2	3.0	3.4
1990	1.9	1.6	2.3	1.8	1.3	2.2	2.8	2.8	2.9	3.2	3.2	3.3
1991	2.0	1.6	2.5	1.9	1.3	2.3	2.9	2.7	3.0	3.3	3.2	3.5
1992	1.9	1.5	2.4	1.8	1.3	2.2	2.8	2.5	3.0	3.3	2.9	3.6
1993	2.0	1.5	2.5	1.8	1.3	2.3	2.9	2.7	3.2	3.5	3.0	3.8
1994	2.1	1.7	2.5	1.9	1.4	2.4	3.1	2.9	3.2	3.6	3.4	3.8
1995	2.1	1.6	2.6	1.9	1.4	2.5	3.2	2.9	3.4	3.8	3.4	4.1
1996	2.1	1.6	2.7	1.9	1.3	2.4	3.4	3.0	3.8	4.0	3.4	4.5
1997	2.0	1.5	2.5	1.8	1.3	2.3	3.1	2.7	3.4	3.5	3.1	3.9
1998	2.0	1.5	2.5	1.8	1.2	2.3	3.2	2.8	3.5	3.7	3.3	4.2

Source: National Center for Health Statistics, Final Mortality Statistics Report, 1970–1998.
Notes:
(1) Rates are age-adjusted to the 1940 U.S. standard population.
(2) All races other than white.
(3) International Classification of Diseases, 8th Revision (ICD-8) Code 493.
(4) International Classification of Diseases, 9th Revision (ICD-9) Code 493.

TABLE 3   ASTHMA: NUMBER OF DEATHS BY RACE AND SEX, 1979–1998

| | TOTAL | | | WHITE | | | ALL OTHER[1] TOTAL | | | BLACK | | |
YEAR	BOTH SEXES	MALE	FEMALE	BOTH SEXES	MALE	FEMALE	BOTH SEXES	MALE	FEMALE	BOTH SEXES	MALE	FEMALE
1979	2,598	1,133	1,465	2,095	898	1,197	503	235	268	470	214	256
1980	2,891	1,292	1,599	2,291	1,008	1,283	600	284	316	557	260	297
1981	3,054	1,287	1,767	2,426	977	1,449	628	310	318	576	281	295
1982	3,154	1,314	1,840	2,450	983	1,467	704	331	373	647	301	346
1983	3,561	1,455	2,106	2,751	1,084	1,667	810	371	439	732	336	396
1984	3,564	1,467	2,097	2,779	1,106	1,673	785	361	424	701	312	389
1985	3,880	1,551	2,329	3,026	1,140	1,886	854	411	443	778	371	407
1986	3,955	1,584	2,371	3,036	1,178	1,858	919	406	513	828	360	468
1987	4,360	1,730	2,630	3,327	1,244	2,083	1,033	486	547	920	428	492
1988	4,597	1,822	2,775	3,473	1,299	2,174	1,124	523	601	1,012	460	552
1989	4,869	1,848	3,021	3,761	1,352	2,409	1,108	496	612	984	434	550
1990	4,819	1,885	2,934	3,696	1,358	2,338	1,123	527	596	986	460	526
1991	5,106	1,927	3,179	3,915	1,388	2,527	1,191	539	652	1,043	472	571
1992	4,964	1,869	3,095	3,789	1,362	2,427	1,175	507	668	1,036	433	603
1993	5,167	1,928	3,239	3,910	1,384	2,526	1,257	544	713	1,112	465	647
1994	5,487	2,101	3,386	4,134	1,492	2,642	1,353	609	744	1,186	525	661
1995	5,637	2,079	3,558	4,208	1,454	2,754	1,429	625	804	1,247	538	709
1996	5,667	2,075	3,592	4,110	1,426	2,684	1,557	649	908	1,325	540	785
1997	5,434	1,986	3,448	4,002	1,383	2,619	1,432	603	829	1,200	498	702
1998	5,438	2,000	3,438	3,947	1,366	2,581	1,491	634	857	1,290	536	754

Source: National Center for Health Statistics, Monthly Vital Statistics Report, 1979–1998.
Note:
(1) All races other than white.

TABLE 4 ASTHMA: MORTALITY RATE BY 10-YEAR AGE GROUPS PER 100,000 POPULATION, 1979–1998

YEAR	TOTAL	<1	1-4	5-14	15-24	25-34	35-44	45-54	55-64	65-74	75-84	85+
1979	1.2	—	—	0.1	0.2	0.3	0.6	1.2	2.3	4.5	6.6	8.6
1980	1.3	—	0.2	0.2	0.2	0.4	0.6	1.4	2.4	4.9	7.7	9.9
1981	1.3	—	—	0.2	0.3	0.4	0.7	1.4	2.8	5.1	7.2	9.7
1982	1.4	—	0.2	0.2	0.4	0.4	0.6	1.5	2.6	4.9	7.2	9.6
1983	1.5	—	0.2	0.2	0.4	0.5	0.8	1.7	3.1	5.1	8.2	11.5
1984	1.5	—	—	0.2	0.3	0.4	0.7	1.6	3.0	5.4	8.1	11.7
1985	1.6	—	0.1	0.3	0.4	0.4	0.7	1.7	3.4	5.6	8.8	12.4
1986	1.6	—	—	0.3	0.4	0.5	0.8	1.6	3.1	5.7	9.2	12.8
1987	1.8	—	—	0.3	0.5	0.5	1.0	1.9	3.3	6.2	9.3	14.5
1988	1.9	—	—	0.3	0.4	0.5	1.0	1.8	3.6	6.2	10.3	14.9
1989	2.0	—	0.2	0.3	0.4	0.6	1.0	1.9	3.5	6.8	11.1	15.9
1990	1.9	—	0.2	0.3	0.4	0.5	0.9	2.0	3.5	6.2	10.7	16.9
1991	2.0	—	0.2	0.3	0.5	0.7	1.0	2.0	3.5	6.3	11.3	17.5
1992	1.9	—	0.2	0.2	0.5	0.5	0.9	1.8	3.3	6.3	10.4	18.7
1993	2.0	—	0.2	0.3	0.5	0.6	1.0	1.8	3.5	6.4	10.4	18.3
1994	2.1	—	0.2	0.3	0.6	0.7	1.0	2.0	3.7	6.5	10.6	18.3
1995	2.1	—	0.1	0.3	0.6	0.7	1.2	2.1	3.7	6.1	10.7	18.3
1996	2.1	—	0.2	0.4	0.6	0.7	1.1	2.0	3.8	5.9	10.3	19.6
1997	2.0	—	0.2	0.3	0.5	0.8	1.1	1.9	3.5	5.4	10.1	19.4
1998	2.0	—	0.2	0.3	0.6	0.7	1.1	1.9	3.0	5.3	10.0	19.9

Source: National Center for Health Statistics, Monthly Vital Statistics Report, 1979–1998.
Note:
— Figure does not meet standard of reliability or precision (estimate based on fewer than 20 deaths)

TABLE 5 ASTHMA: NUMBER OF DEATHS IN 10-YEAR AGE GROUPS, 1979–1998

YEAR	TOTAL	<1	1-4	5-14	15-24	25-34	35-44	45-54	55-64	65-74	75-84	85+	NOT STATED
1979	2,598	5	19	39	99	111	157	282	502	695	499	190	—
1980	2,891	8	21	61	105	130	145	309	529	765	596	222	—
1981	3,054	3	12	72	112	155	178	308	607	803	575	229	—
1982	3,154	8	26	70	162	169	176	341	582	793	593	234	—
1983	3,561	5	28	78	144	186	231	384	686	836	693	290	—
1984	3,564	10	17	79	132	159	227	355	674	905	702	303	1
1985	3,880	6	21	98	156	182	231	378	755	936	785	332	—
1986	3,955	13	17	92	166	197	251	356	688	982	843	350	—
1987	4,360	4	19	101	181	199	341	443	709	1,081	873	408	1

TABLE 5   ASTHMA: NUMBER OF DEATHS IN 10-YEAR AGE GROUPS, 1979–1998 *(continued)*

YEAR	TOTAL	<1	1-4	5-14	15-24	25-34	35-44	45-54	55-64	65-74	75-84	85+	NOT STATED
1988	4,597	7	19	93	162	231	343	440	785	1,097	991	429	—
1989	4,869	6	26	95	148	256	346	472	743	1,208	1,094	473	2
1990	4,819	12	24	102	160	237	332	502	738	1,125	1,074	512	1
1991	5,106	5	30	106	183	280	386	510	737	1,155	1,161	553	—
1992	4,964	9	38	88	168	232	373	495	692	1,164	1,097	608	—
1993	5,167	6	32	118	186	240	405	508	738	1,196	1,114	623	1
1994	5,487	5	24	118	215	304	421	597	780	1,223	1,155	644	1
1995	5,637	13	21	130	224	298	498	663	785	1,147	1,195	663	0
1996	5,667	8	34	149	214	288	496	649	816	1,095	1,177	739	2
1997	5,434	5	30	119	174	298	489	636	757	992	1,183	751	1
1998	5,438	7	33	131	214	277	487	647	673	972	1,190	807	—

Source: National Center for Health Statistics, Final Vital Statistics Report, 1979–1998.

TABLE 6   ASTHMA: NUMBER OF PEOPLE EVER TOLD BY A DOCTOR OR OTHER HEALTH PROFESSIONAL THAT THEY HAD ASTHMA AND RATES PER 1,000 PEOPLE BY AGE, SEX, AND RACE, 1997–1998[1] (PERIOD PREVALENCE)

	1997			1998		
	NUMBER	RATE	CI OF RATE	NUMBER	RATE	CI OF RATE
AGE						
TOTAL	25,747,105	96.6	(93.3–99.8)	26,394,037	98.1	(94.7–101.6)
<5	1,398,233	70.9	(61.0–80.8)	1,627,352	82.6	(71.2–94.1)
5–17	6,719,692	130.1	(122.2–138.1)	7,022,501	135.0	(127.0–143.0)
<18	8,117,925	113.8	(107.3–120.3)	8,649,853	120.6	(113.8–127.5)
18–44	10,377,177	95.7	(90.7–100.8)	9,935,452	91.6	(86.4–96.9)
45–64	4,810,974	87.7	(81.0–94.3)	5,304,135	93.6	(86.4–100.7)
65+	2,441,029	76.3	(68.9–83.6)	2,504,597	77.7	(70.7–84.8)
SEX						
MALE	12,238,763	94.0	(89.3–98.7)	12,589,221	95.8	(90.8–100.8)
FEMALE	13,508,342	99.0	(94.6–103.5)	13,804,816	100.3	(95.5–105.2)
RACE						
WHITE	20,799,967	95.5	(91.9–99.0)	20,827,971	95.3	(91.5–99.1)
<5	944,392	62.1	(50.9–73.2)	1,064,697	70.5	(58.4–82.6)
5–17	5,120,714	128.3	(119.5–137.1)	5,287,332	131.6	(122.8–140.5)
18–44	8,514,352	97.4	(91.7–103.0)	7,869,545	90.9	(85.0–96.9)
45–64	4,067,545	87.3	(80.0–94.6)	4,437,937	92.1	(84.2–99.9)
65+	2,152,964	75.1	(67.3–83.0)	2,168,460	76.0	(68.6–83.4)

TABLE 6   ASTHMA: NUMBER OF PEOPLE EVER TOLD BY A DOCTOR OR OTHER HEALTH PROFESSIONAL THAT THEY HAD ASTHMA AND RATES PER 1,000 PEOPLE BY AGE, SEX AND RACE, 1997–1998[1] (PERIOD PREVALENCE)

	1997			1998		
	NUMBER	RATE	CI OF RATE	NUMBER	RATE	CI OF RATE
BLACK	3,659,349	109.8	(101.3–118.3)	4,165,356	124.2	(115.4–132.9)
<5	331,716	108.0	(82.3–133.7)	397,810	134.4	(100.3–168.5)
5–17	1,205,433	148.7	(130.4–167.1)	1,311,478	160.7	(136.6–184.7)
18–44	1,350,218	97.0	(84.4–109.7)	1,529,102	109.5	(96.2–122.7)
45–64	536,779	95.7	(78.7–112.8)	685,390	118.4	(96.5–140.2)
65+	235,203	89.4	(65.0–113.7)	241,576	90.7	(68.5–112.9)

Source: National Center for Health Statistics, National Health Interview Survey, 1997–1998.
  Calculation of rates and confidence intervals performed by the Epidemiology and Statistics Unit.
Note:
(1) In 1997, the National Health Interview Survey's questionnaire was completely redesigned. Therefore, estimates prior to 1997 cannot be compared with later estimates.

TABLE 7   ASTHMA: NUMBER OF CONDITIONS AND AGE-SPECIFIC PREVALENCE RATE PER 1,000 PERSONS, 1982–1996, 1997–1998[1,2] (ATTACK PREVALENCE)

	ALL AGES		UNDER 5		5-17		<18		18-44		45-64		65+	
YEAR	NO.	RATE	NO.	RATE	NO.	RATE	NO.	RATE	NO.	RATE	RATE	NO.	RATE	NO.
1982	7,899,000	34.8	*	*	*	*	2,513,000	40.1	2,749,000	29.0	36.3	1,603,000	40.8	1,035,000
1983	8,787,000	38.3	*	*	*	*	2,828,000	45.2	3,487,000	36.1	34.6	1,529,000	36.4	943,000
1984	8,388,000	36.2	*	*	*	*	2,668,000	42.5	3,152,000	32.1	33.5	1,485,000	41.3	1,093,000
1985	8,612,000	36.8	*	*	*	*	2,997,000	47.8	3,323,000	33.4	28.2	1,255,000	38.3	1,036,000
1986	9,690,000	41.0	*	*	*	*	3,223,000	51.1	3,672,000	36.4	36.3	1,622,000	42.6	1,173,000
1987	9,565,000	40.1	*	*	*	*	3,323,000	52.5	3,522,000	34.5	36.3	1,633,000	38.6	1,087,000
1988	9,934,000	41.2	*	*	*	*	3,171,000	49.9	3,989,000	38.7	34.8	1,587,000	41.4	1,188,000
1989	11,621,000	47.7	*	*	*	*	3,901,000	61.0	4,302,000	41.3	41.5	1,914,000	51.5	1,504,000
1990	10,311,000	41.9	*	*	*	*	3,725,000	57.6	3,703,000	35.2	38.6	1,800,000	36.3	1,082,000
1991	11,735,000	47.2	*	*	*	*	4,094,000	62.5	4,594,000	43.4	40.7	1,921,000	37.2	1,126,000
1992	12,375,000	49.2	*	*	*	*	4,218,000	63.4	4,748,000	44.9	45.0	2,183,000	39.8	1,226,000
1993	13,074,000	51.4	*	*	*	*	4,830,000	71.6	4,495,000	42.5	45.0	2,242,000	48.2	1,506,000
1994	14,562,000	56.1	*	*	*	*	4,837,000	69.1	5,598,000	51.7	50.8	2,561,000	50.5	1,566,000
1995	14,878,000	56.8	*	*	*	*	5,294,000	74.9	5,577,000	51.6	53.3	2,754,000	39.8	1,253,000
1996	14,596,000	55.2	*	*	*	*	4,429,000	62.0	6,141,000	56.9	48.6	2,581,000	45.5	1,445,000
1997	11,113,225	41.7	812,410	41.2	3,072,538	59.5	3,884,948	54.4	4,367,913	40.3	36.2	1,985,366	27.3	874,998
1998	10,613,056	39.5	914,961	46.5	2,894,220	55.6	3,809,181	53.1	3,817,945	36.2	36.4	2,061,312	28.7	924,618

Source: National Center for Health Statistics, National Health Interview Survey, 1982–1996, 1997–1998.
  Calculations performed by the Epidemiology and Statistics Unit.
Notes:
*Data for these age groups were not calculated.
(1) Due to rounding, numbers across may not sum up to totals.
(2) In 1997, the National Health Interview Survey's questionnaire was completely redesigned. Therefore, estimates prior to 1997 cannot be compared with later estimates.

TABLE 8   ASTHMA: TRENDS IN SEX-SPECIFIC PREVALENCE PER 1,000 PERSONS,
1982–1996, 1997–1998[1] (ATTACK PREVALENCE)

YEAR	MALE		FEMALE	
	NUMBER	RATE	NUMBER	RATE
1982	3,994,000	36.5	3,906,000	33.2
1983	3,818,000	34.5	4,968,000	41.9
1984	3,924,000	35.1	4,464,000	37.3
1985	3,864,000	34.2	4,748,000	39.3
1986	4,670,000	40.8	5,019,000	41.1
1987	4,609,000	39.9	4,956,000	40.3
1988	4,650,000	39.9	5,285,000	42.5
1989	5,593,000	47.4	6,028,000	48.0
1990	4,741,000	39.7	5,570,000	44.0
1991	5,724,000	47.4	6,011,000	47.0
1992	5,516,000	45.1	6,859,000	53.1
1993	5,946,000	48.1	7,127,000	54.6
1994	6,542,000	51.7	8,019,000	60.2
1995	6,687,000	52.4	8,190,000	61.0
1996	5,751,000	44.4	8,845,000	65.3
1997	4,591,616	35.3	6,521,609	47.8
1998	4,550,372	34.6	6,062,684	44.1

Source: National Center for Health Statistics, National Health Interview Survey, 1982–1996, 1997–1998. Calculations performed by the Epidemiology and Statistics Unit.
Note:
(1) In 1997, the National Health Interview Survey's questionnaire was completely redesigned. Therefore, estimates prior to 1997 cannot be compared with later estimates.

**TABLE 9   ASTHMA: NUMBER OF CONDITIONS AND PREVALENCE RATE
PER 1,000 PERSONS BY RACE AND AGE, 1982–1996, 1997–1998[1]** *(continued)*

WHITE

YEAR	ALL AGES #	RATE	UNDER 5 #	RATE	5-17 #	RATE	18-44 #	RATE	UNDER 45 #	RATE	45-64 #	RATE	65+ #	RATE
1982	6,711,000	34.6	*	*	*	*	*	*	4,393,000	33.3	1,423,000	36.5	895,000	39.0
1983	7,412,000	37.7	*	*	*	*	*	*	5,197,000	38.8	1,367,000	35.0	848,000	36.2
1984	7,296,000	36.9	*	*	*	*	*	*	4,982,000	37.0	1,295,000	33.1	1,019,000	42.6
1985	7,425,000	37.2	*	*	*	*	*	*	5,372,000	39.6	1,121,000	28.7	932,000	38.1
1986	8,190,000	40.9	*	*	*	*	*	*	5,758,000	42.2	1,451,000	37.2	981,000	39.6
1987	8,126,000	40.3	*	*	*	*	*	*	5,676,000	41.3	1,463,000	37.4	987,000	38.8
1988	8,101,000	39.9	*	*	*	*	*	*	5,728,000	41.6	1,327,000	33.5	1,046,000	40.5
1989	9,675,000	47.1	*	*	*	*	*	*	6,619,000	47.6	1,743,000	43.6	1,313,000	49.9
1990	8,544,000	41.3	*	*	*	*	*	*	6,033,000	43.1	1,585,000	39.3	926,000	34.6
1991	9,660,000	46.4	*	*	*	*	*	*	6,958,000	49.6	1,689,000	41.6	1,013,000	37.2
1992	10,309,000	49.2	*	*	*	*	*	*	7,341,000	52.4	1,900,000	45.5	1,068,000	38.8
1993	10,616,000	50.2	*	*	*	*	*	*	7,338,000	52.2	1,904,000	44.5	1,374,000	49.2
1994	12,052,000	56.2	*	*	*	*	*	*	8,353,000	58.2	2,258,000	52.3	1,441,000	51.9
1995	12,198,000	56.2	*	*	*	*	*	*	8,834,000	61.0	2,323,000	52.5	1,041,000	37.0
1996	11,764,000	53.5	*	*	*	*	*	*	8,301,000	56.9	2,168,000	47.4	1,295,000	45.3
1997	8,924,460	41.0	562,767	37.0	2,316,765	58.0	3,657,439	41.8	6,536,971	45.8	1,653,314	35.5	734,175	25.6
1998	8,351,811	38.2	600,960	39.8	2,191,663	54.6	3,001,924	34.7	5,794,547	40.9	1,755,150	36.4	802,114	28.1

BLACK

YEAR	ALL AGES #	RATE	UNDER 5 #	RATE	5-17 #	RATE	18-44 #	RATE	UNDER 45 #	RATE	45-64 #	RATE	65+ #	RATE
1982	1,055,000	39.2	*	*	*	*	*	*	796,000	38.6	156,000	37.2*	103,000	48.7*
1983	1,230,000	45.1	*	*	*	*	*	*	985,000	47.1	150,000	35.5*	95,000	44.5*
1984	965,000	34.8	*	*	*	*	*	*	750,000	35.2	153,000	35.9*	62,000	28.4*
1985	1,119,000	39.8	*	*	*	*	*	*	913,000	42.5	122,000	27.5	84,000	37.2*
1986	1,212,000	42.5	*	*	*	*	*	*	902,000	41.5	164,000	36.5	146,000	63.5*
1987	1,281,000	44.3	*	*	*	*	*	*	1,033,000	46.9	148,000	32.5	100,000	42.5*
1988	1,631,000	55.5	*	*	*	*	*	*	1,301,000	58.2	225,000	48.5	105,000	43.7*
1989	1,586,000	53.1	*	*	*	*	*	*	1,304,000	57.4	112,000	23.8*	170,000	69.3
1990	1,414,000	46.6	*	*	*	*	*	*	1,107,000	48.0	180,000	37.6	127,000	50.7*
1991	1,740,000	56.3	*	*	*	*	*	*	1,462,000	62.3	195,000	40.1	83,000	32.4*
1992	1,787,000	56.8	*	*	*	*	*	*	1,393,000	58.4	249,000	49.9	145,000	55.3*
1993	1,967,000	61.4	*	*	*	*	*	*	1,554,000	64.2	315,000	61.3	98,000	36.7*
1994	1,861,000	56.3	*	*	*	*	*	*	1,495,000	58.9	255,000	49.7	111,000	44.0*
1995	2,217,000	67.7	*	*	*	*	*	*	1,726,000	69.0	313,000	60.0	178,000	70.1*
1996	2,310,000	69.6	*	*	*	*	*	*	1,926,000	76.6	275,000	50.7*	109,000	41.7*
1997	1,629,383	48.9	176,626	57.5	596,741	73.6	483,297	34.7	1,256,664	50.1	251,084	44.8	121,635	46.2
1998	1,679,906	50.1	208,240	70.4	528,300	64.7	614,097	44.0	1,350,637	53.8	265,660	45.9	63,609	23.9

Source: National Center for Health Statistics, National Health Interview Survey, 1982–1996, 1997–1998.
NOTES:
* Estimate for which the numerator has a relative standard error of more than 30%.
(1) In 1997, the National Health Interview Survey's questionnaire was completely redesigned. Therefore, estimates prior to 1997 cannot be compared with later estimates.

TABLE 10   ASTHMA: NUMBER OF FIRST-LISTED HOSPITAL DISCHARGES AND RATE PER 10,000 POPULATION BY SEX, 1970–1998[1]

YEAR	TOTAL		MALE		FEMALE	
	NUMBER OF DISCHARGES	RATE PER 10,000	NUMBER OF DISCHARGES	RATE PER 10,000	NUMBER OF DISCHARGES	RATE PER 10,000
1970[2]	133,000	6.7	53,866	5.4	79,126	7.6
1971	134,000	6.7	54,037	5.4	79,223	7.5
1972	162,000	7.9	67,365	6.6	93,995	8.8
1973	161,000	7.8	73,111	7.1	87,024	8.0
1974	159,000	7.6	67,041	6.5	91,495	8.4
1975	183,000	8.7	71,799	6.8	111,371	10.1
1976	190,000	9.0	78,718	7.4	111,730	10.0
1977	199,000	9.4	86,391	8.1	112,125	10.0
1978	201,000	9.4	82,939	7.7	117,928	10.3
1979[3]	339,000	15.7	143,000	13.1	196,000	17.0
1980	408,000	18.0	180,000	16.3	228,000	19.6
1981	418,000	18.4	180,000	16.2	237,000	20.1
1982	434,000	18.9	190,000	17.1	245,000	20.6
1983	459,000	19.8	190,000	17.0	269,000	22.4
1984	465,000	19.8	197,000	17.1	268,000	22.0
1985	462,000	19.5	195,000	17.0	266,000	21.8
1986	477,000	19.9	206,000	17.8	271,000	21.9
1987	454,000	18.8	193,000	16.5	261,000	20.9
1988[4]	479,000	19.6	210,000	17.7	270,000	21.4
1989	475,000	19.3	204,000	17.1	271,000	21.3
1990	476,000	19.1	191,000	15.8	285,000	22.2
1991	490,000	19.6	221,000	18.2	269,000	20.9
1992	463,000	18.3	201,000	16.3	263,000	20.1
1993	468,000	18.3	191,000	15.3	278,000	21.1
1994	451,000	17.4	189,000	15.0	262,000	19.7
1995	511,000	19.5	210,000	16.5	301,000	22.4
1996	474,000	17.9	195,000	15.1	279,000	20.6
1997	484,000	17.9	204,000	15.4	279,000	20.2
1998	423,000	15.5	168,000	12.6	255,000	18.3

Source: National Center for Health Statistics, National Hospital Discharge Survey, 1970–1998.
Notes:
(1) Due to rounding, numbers across may not add up to the total number of hospital discharges.
(2) International Classification of Diseases, 8th Revision (ICD-8) Code 493.
(3) International Classification of Diseases, 9th Revision (ICD-9) Code 493.
(4) Data from 1988–98 may not be comparable to earlier years due to the redesign of the survey.

TABLE 11   ASTHMA: NUMBER OF FIRST-LISTED HOSPITAL DISCHARGES AND RATE
PER 10,000 POPULATION BY AGE, 1970–1998[1]

YEAR	<15 NUMBER OF DISCHARGES	<15 RATE PER 10,000	15-44 NUMBER OF DISCHARGES	15-44 RATE PER 10,000	45-64 NUMBER OF DISCHARGES	45-64 RATE PER 10,000	65+ NUMBER OF DISCHARGES	65+ RATE PER 10,000	TOTAL NUMBER OF DISCHARGES	TOTAL RATE PER 10,000
1970[2]	33,000	5.8	36,000	4.4	38,000	9.0	26,000	13.6	133,000	6.7
1971	32,000	5.5	38,000	4.5	41,000	9.7	24,000	12.1	134,000	6.7
1972	48,000	8.6	41,000	4.8	40,000	9.5	32,000	16.1	162,000	7.9
1973	55,000	9.9	36,000	4.1	42,000	9.7	29,000	14.1	161,000	7.8
1974	56,000	10.2	38,000	4.2	36,000	8.3	29,000	14.1	159,000	7.6
1975	58,000	10.9	49,000	5.3	49,000	11.4	27,000	12.9	183,000	8.7
1976	60,000	11.5	49,000	5.3	48,000	11.4	33,000	14.9	190,000	9.0
1977	69,000	13.3	51,000	5.4	46,000	10.6	33,000	14.8	199,000	9.4
1978	61,000	12.1	60,000	6.2	50,000	11.6	29,000	12.9	201,000	9.4
1979[3]	99,000	19.8	94,000	9.5	83,000	19.1	63,000	27.0	339,000	15.7
1980	124,000	24.2	99,000	9.5	101,000	22.7	84,000	32.7	408,000	18.0
1981	128,000	25.0	12,000	10.6	104,000	23.4	74,000	28.2	418,000	18.4
1982	151,000	29.3	104,000	9.7	98,000	22.1	81,000	30.4	434,000	18.9
1983	136,000	26.4	110,000	10.1	119,000	26.7	94,000	34.2	459,000	19.8
1984	150,000	29.0	109,000	9.9	102,000	22.8	105,000	37.4	466,000	19.8
1985	144,000	27.8	241,000	11.1	97,000	21.5	97,000	34.1	462,000	19.5
1986	158,000	30.3	122,000	10.8	99,000	22.0	98,000	33.7	477,000	19.9
1987	149,000	28.4	112,000	9.8	92,000	20.4	101,000	33.8	454,000	18.8
1988[4]	164,000	31.0	110,000	9.6	93,000	20.3	112,000	36.8	479,000	19.6
1989	168,000	31.2	127,000	11.0	88,000	19.0	93,000	29.9	475,000	19.3
1990	169,000	30.8	119,000	10.3	86,000	18.2	102,000	32.4	476,000	19.1
1991	187,000	33.9	128,000	10.9	85,000	18.2	90,000	28.5	490,000	19.6
1992	193,000	34.4	117,000	10.0	78,000	16.1	76,000	23.6	463,000	18.3
1993	159,000	28.0	128,000	10.9	94,000	19.0	87,000	26.6	468,000	18.3
1994	169,000	29.5	125,000	10.6	80,000	15.7	76,000	22.9	451,000	17.4
1995	212,000	36.7	135,000	11.4	87,000	16.7	77,000	23.0	511,000	19.5
1996	195,000	33.8	132,000	11.1	88,000	16.4	59,000	17.4	474,000	17.9
1997	214,000	35.8	117,000	9.6	98,000	15.9	65,000	19.2	484,000	17.9
1998	166,000	27.7	104,000	8.6	92,000	16.2	60,000	17.7	423,000	15.5

Source: National Center for Health Statistics, National Hospital Discharge Survey, 1970–1998.
Notes:
(1) Due to rounding, numbers across may not add up to the total number of hospital discharges.
(2) International Classification of Diseases, 8th Revision (ICD-8) Code 493.
(3) International Classification of Diseases, 9th Revision (ICD-9) Code 493.
(4) Data from 1988–98 may not be comparable to earlier years due to the redesign of the survey.

TABLE 12   ASTHMA: NUMBER OF FIRST-LISTED HOSPITAL DISCHARGES AND RATE
PER 10,000 POPULATION BY RACE, 1988–1998

YEAR	NUMBER OF DISCHARGES					RATE PER 10,000 POPULATION[1]			
	TOTAL[2]	WHITE	BLACK	ALL OTHER	RACE NOT REPORTED[3]	TOTAL	WHITE	BLACK	ALL OTHER
1988	479,000	295,000	116,000	31,000	37,000	19.6	14.4	39.4	36.1
1989	475,000	286,000	117,000	22,000	50,000	19.3	13.9	39.2	24.2
1990	476,000	263,000	116,000	19,000	78,000	19.1	12.7	38.3	19.8
1991	490,000	269,000	120,000	23,000	78,000	19.6	12.8	38.9	22.9
1992	463,000	215,000	134,000	25,000	89,000	18.3	10.2	42.8	23.8
1993	468,000	246,000	103,000	22,000	97,000	18.3	11.5	32.3	20.1
1994	451,000	227,000	125,000	29,000	70,000	17.4	10.5	38.6	26.0
1995	511,000	256,000	140,000	25,000	90,000	19.5	11.6	42.7	21.4
1996	474,000	237,000	133,000	33,000	70,000	17.9	10.8	40.1	27.6
1997	484,000	262,000	125,000	39,000	58,000	17.9	11.8	35.5	30.7
1998	423,000	222,000	115,000	28,000	58,000	15.5	10.0	32.2	21.0

Source: National Center for Health Statistics: National Hospital Discharge Survey, 1988–1998.
Notes:
1. Rates shown here may differ from previously published rates due to adjustments made to population used.
2. Total includes white, black and other race discharges as well as discharges of an unspecified race.
3. Between 1988 and 1998, the number of discharges not reporting race increased dramatically. It appears that hospital discharges in whites might be disproportionately underestimated, particularly in later years. For this reason, comparisons between races should be made with caution.

TABLE 13   ECONOMIC COST OF ASTHMA:
DIRECT MEDICAL AND INDIRECT EXPENDITURES, UNITED STATES, 2000

CATEGORY	DOLLAR COST (in billions)
Direct Medical Expenditures:	
Hospital Care	
Inpatient	3,474.90
Emergency Room	656.10
Outpatient	421.20
Physicians' Services	
Inpatient	324.00
Outpatient	769.50
Medications	2,446.20
All Direct Expenditures	8,091.90
Indirect Costs:	
School Days Lost	1,495.00
Loss of Work	
Outside Employment	
Men	225.40
Women	349.60
Housekeeping	837.20
Mortality	
Men	805.00
Women	887.80
All Indirect Costs	4,600.00
All Costs:	12,691.90

Sources: New England Journal of Medicine, Vol. 326, No. 13, March 26, 1992.
    Morbidity and Mortality, Chartbook on Cardiovascular, Lung and Blood Diseases, NHLBI, 2000.
Note: Estimates of direct medical expenditures and indirect costs were derived using mortality and health survey data available from the National Center for Health Statistics, health expenditure data from the Health Care Financing Administration, and income data from the U.S. Bureau of Census. The cost estimates were projected to 2000 dollars. These numbers are estimates and should be cited as such.

APPENDIX V

GUIDELINES FOR THE DIAGNOSIS AND MANAGEMENT OF ASTHMA

Excerpted from the Expert Panel Report 2, National Institutes of Health and National Heart, Lung, and Blood Institute, April 1997 (some illustrations have been omitted)

INTRODUCTION

Asthma is a chronic inflammatory disease of the airways. In the United States, asthma affects 14 million to 15 million persons. It is the most common chronic disease of childhood, affecting an estimated 4.8 million children (Adams and Marano 1995; Centers for Disease Control and Prevention 1995). People with asthma collectively have more than 100 million days of restricted activity and 470,000 hospitalizations annually. More than 5,000 people die of asthma annually. Asthma hospitalization rates have been highest among blacks and children, while death rates for asthma were consistently highest among blacks aged 15 to 24 years (Centers for Disease Control and Prevention 1996). These rates have increased or remained stable over the past decade. This report describes the appropriate use of the available therapies in the management of asthma.

To help health care professionals bridge the gap between current knowledge and practice, the National Heart, Lung, and Blood Institute's (NHLBI) National Asthma Education and Prevention Program (NAEPP) has convened two Expert Panels to prepare guidelines for the diagnosis and management of asthma. The NAEPP Coordinating Committee, under the leadership of Claude Lenfant, M.D., director of the NHLBI, convened the first Expert Panel in 1989. The charge to this panel was to develop a report that would provide a gen-

eral approach to diagnosing and managing asthma based on current science. The *Expert Panel Report: Guidelines for the Diagnosis and Management of Asthma* (NAEPP 1991) was published in 1991, and the recommendations for the treatment of asthma were organized around four components of effective asthma management:

- Use of objective measures of lung function to assess the severity of asthma and to monitor the course of therapy

- Environmental control measures to avoid or eliminate factors that precipitate asthma symptoms or exacerbations

- Comprehensive pharmacologic therapy for long-term management designed to reverse and prevent the airway inflammation characteristic of asthma as well as pharmacologic therapy to manage asthma exacerbations

- Patient education that fosters a partnership among the patient, his or her family, and clinicians

The principles addressed within these four components of asthma management served as the starting point for the development of two additional reports prepared by asthma experts from many countries in cooperation with the NHLBI: the *International Consensus Report on Diagnosis and Management of Asthma* (NHLBI 1992) and the *Global Initiative for Asthma* (NHLBI/WHO 1995). The *Expert Panel Report 2 Guidelines for the Diagnosis and Management of Asthma* (EPR-2) is the latest report from the NAEPP and updates the 1991 Expert Panel Report. The second Expert Panel critically reviewed and built upon the reports listed above.

This report presents basic recommendations for the diagnosis and management of asthma that will help clinicians and patients make appropriate decisions about asthma care. Of course, the clinician and patient need to develop individual treatment plans that are tailored to the specific needs and circumstances of the patient. The NAEPP, and all who participated in the development of this latest report, hope that the patient with asthma will be the beneficiary of the recommendations in this document. This report is not an official regulatory document of any government agency.

METHODS USED TO DEVELOP THIS REPORT

The NAEPP Coordinating Committee established a Science Base Committee of U.S. asthma experts who began work in early 1994 to monitor the scientific literature and advise the Coordinating Committee when an update of the 1991 *Expert Panel Report: Guidelines for the Diagnosis and Management of Asthma* was needed. The Science Base Committee, along with international members of the *Global Initiative for Asthma*, examined all the relevant literature on asthma in human subjects published in English between 1991 and mid-1995, obtained through a series of MEDLINE database searches. More than 5,000 abstracts were reviewed. In 1995, the Science Base Committee recommended to the NAEPP Coordinating Committee that sufficient new information had been published since 1991 to convene a panel of experts to update the first Expert Panel Report.

The second Expert Panel is a multidisciplinary group of clinicians and scientists with expertise in asthma management. The panel includes health care professionals in the areas of general medicine, family practice, pediatrics, emergency medicine, allergy, pulmonary medicine, nursing, pharmacy, and health education. Among the panel members are individuals who served on either the Science Base Committee or the 1991 Expert Panel. Other members were chosen based on names submitted by NAEPP Coordinating Committee member organizations. Several Expert Panel members are themselves members of the Coordinating Committee.

Representatives from several Federal agencies also have participated.

The charge to the panel was to prepare recommendations for use by clinicians working in diverse health care settings that address the practical decision-making issues in the diagnosis and management of asthma. The panel also was requested to develop specific aids to facilitate implementation of the recommendations.

Panel members were asked to base their recommendations on their review of the scientific literature and to cite studies that support the recommendations. When a clear recommendation could not be extracted from the studies (e.g., studies were not available, were conflicting, or were equivocal), the panel was asked to label the recommendation as "based on the opinion of the Expert Panel," "recommended by the Expert Panel," or similar terminology. When a whole section was "based on the opinion of the Expert Panel," this was indicated at the beginning of the section (e.g., see component 1-Initial Assessment and Diagnosis).

This report was prepared in a systematic and iterative process. In addition to the Science Base Committee review of the scientific literature, the panel conducted in-depth reviews of the literature in selected areas it considered controversial. In interpreting the literature, the panel considered the nature and quality of the study designs and analyses. Given the complexities of several issues, the panel chose not to use the strict evidence ranking system used in the guidelines development procedures of the U.S. Preventive Services Task Force. However, this procedure was applied in the area of peak flow monitoring. The panel submitted their interpretation of the literature and related recommendations for multiple reviews by their fellow Expert Panel members and outside reviewers.

The development of EPR-2 was directed by an Executive Committee; each member of the Executive Committee headed a subcommittee assigned to prepare a specific chapter. Each member of the panel was assigned to one of the subcommittees. The subcommittees were responsible for reviewing the pertinent literature and drafting the recommendations with the supporting evidence for the full panel to review. Once the subcommittee reports were prepared, the full panel critically reviewed the evidence and rationale for each recommendation, discussed revisions, and reached final agreement on each recommendation. A vote was taken to confine the consensus of the panel. The final report was approved by the NAEPP Coordinating Committee via mail. . . .

The development of this report was *entirely* funded by the National Heart, Lung, and Blood Institute, National Institutes of Health. Panel members and reviewers participated as volunteers and were compensated only for travel expenses related to the two Expert Panel meetings and the Executive Committee meetings.

The goal of the EPR-2: *Guidelines for the Diagnosis and Management of Asthma* is to serve as a comprehensive guide to diagnosing and managing asthma. Implementation of EPR-2 recommendations is likely to increase some costs of asthma care by increasing the number of primary care visits for asthma and the use of asthma medications, environmental control products and services, and equipment (e.g., spacer/holding chamber devices). However, asthma diagnosis and management are expected to improve, which should reduce the numbers of lost school and work days, hospitalizations and emergency department visits, and deaths due to asthma. A net reduction in total health care costs should result. The NAEPP encourages research to evaluate the impact of implementing the recommendations in this report.

OVERVIEW OF THE REPORT

Each section of EPR-2 begins with a list of "Key Points" and "Differences from the 1991 *Expert Panel Report: Guidelines for the Diagnosis and Management of Asthma.'* A brief overview of each section is provided below.

Pathogenesis and Definition

In the 1991 Expert Panel Report, the role of inflammation in the pathogenesis of asthma was emphasized although the scientific evidence for the involvement of inflammation in asthma was just emerging. Now in 1997, although the role of inflammation is still evolving as a concept, a much firmer scientific basis exists to indicate that asthma results from complex interactions among inflammatory cells, mediators, and the cells and tissues resident in the airways.

Thus, asthma is now defined as a chronic inflammatory disorder of the airways in which many cells and cellular elements play a role, in particular, mast cells, eosinophils, T lymphocytes, neutrophils, and epithelial cells. In susceptible individuals, this inflammation causes recurrent episodes of wheezing, breathlessness, chest tightness, and cough, particularly at night and in the early morning. These episodes are usually associated with widespread but variable airflow obstruction that is often reversible either spontaneously or with treatment. The inflammation also causes an associated increase in the existing bronchial hyperresponsiveness to a variety of stimuli.

Component 1: Measures of Assessment and Monitoring

Initial Assessment and Diagnosis of Asthma
Making the correct diagnosis of asthma is extremely important. Clinical judgment is required because signs and symptoms vary widely from patient to patient as well as within each patient over time. To establish the diagnosis of asthma, the clinician must determine that:

- Episodic symptoms of airflow obstruction are present.
- Airflow obstruction is at least partially reversible.
- Alternative diagnoses are excluded.

This section differs from the 1991 Expert Panel Report in several ways. Asthma severity classifications have been changed from mild, moderate, and severe to mild intermittent, mild persistent, moderate persistent, and severe persistent to more accurately reflect the clinical manifestations of asthma. The panel emphasizes that patients at any level of severity can have mild, moderate, or severe exacerbations. In addition, information on wheezing in infancy and vocal cord dysfunction has been expanded in the differential diagnosis section in Component 1. Situations that may warrant referral to an asthma specialist have been refined with input from specialty and primary care physicians.

Periodic Assessment and Monitoring

To establish whether the goals of asthma therapy have been achieved, ongoing monitoring and periodic assessment are needed. The goals of asthma therapy are to:

- Prevent chronic and troublesome symptoms

- Maintain (near) "normal" pulmonary function

- Maintain normal activity levels (including exercise and other physical activity)

- Prevent recurrent exacerbations of asthma and minimize the need for emergency department visits or hospitalizations

- Provide optimal pharmacotherapy with minimal or no adverse effects

- Meet patients' and families' expectations of and satisfaction with asthma care

Several types of monitoring are recommended: signs and symptoms, pulmonary function, quality of life/functional status history of asthma exacerbations, pharmacotherapy, patient-provider communication, and patient satisfaction.

The panel recommends that patients, especially those with moderate to severe persistent asthma or a history of severe exacerbations, be given a written action plan based on signs and symptoms and/or peak expiratory flow. As in the 1991 report, daily peak flow monitoring is recommended for patients with moderate to severe persistent asthma. In addition, the panel states that any patient who develops severe exacerbations may benefit from peak flow monitoring. A complete review of the literature on peak flow monitoring was conducted, evidence tables were prepared, and the results of this analysis are summarized in the report.

Component 2: Control of Factors Contributing to Asthma Severity

Exposure of sensitive patients to inhalant allergens has been shown to increase airway inflammation, airway hyperresponsiveness, asthma symptoms, need for medication, and death due to asthma. Substantially reducing exposures significantly reduces these outcomes. Environmental tobacco smoke is a major precipitant of asthma symptoms in children, increases symptoms and the need for medications, and reduces lung function in adults. Increased air pollution levels of respirable particulates, ozone, SO_2, and NO_2 have been reported to precipitate asthma symptoms and increase emergency department visits and hospitalizations for asthma. Other factors that can contribute to asthma severity include rhinitis and sinusitis, gastroesophageal reflux, some medications, and viral respiratory infections. EPR-2 discusses environmental control and other measures to reduce the effects of these factors.

Component 3: Pharmacologic Therapy

EPR-2 offers an extensive discussion of the pharmacologic management of patients at all levels of asthma severity. It is noted that asthma pharmacotherapy should be instituted in conjunction with environmental control measures that reduce exposure to factors known to increase the patient's asthma symptoms.

As in the 1991 report, a stepwise approach to pharmacologic therapy is recommended, with the type and amount of medication dictated by asthma severity. EPR-2 continues to emphasize that persistent asthma requires daily long-term therapy in addition to appropriate medications to manage asthma exacerbations. To clarify this concept, the EPR-2 now categorizes medications into two general classes: *long-term control medications* to achieve and maintain control of persistent asthma and *quick-relief medications* to treat symptoms and exacerbations.

Observations into the basic mechanisms of asthma have had a tremendous influence on therapy. Because inflammation is considered an early and persistent component of asthma, therapy for persistent asthma must be directed toward long-term suppression of the inflammation. Thus EPR-2 continues to emphasize that the most effective medications for long-term control are those shown to have anti-inflammatory effects. For example, early intervention with inhaled corticosteroids can improve asthma control and normalize lung function, and preliminary studies suggest that it may prevent irreversible airway injury.

An important addition to EPR-2 is a discussion of the management of asthma in infants and young children that incorporates recent studies on wheezing in early childhood. Another addition is discussions of long-term–control medications that have become available since 1991—long-acting inhaled beta$_2$-agonists, nedocromil, zafirlukast, and zileuton.

Recommendations for managing asthma exacerbations are similar to those in the 1991 Expert Panel Report. However, the treatment recommendations are now on a much firmer scientific basis because of the number of studies addressing the treatment of asthma exacerbations in children and adults in the past six years.

Component 4: Education for a Partnership in Asthma Care

As in the 1991 Expert Panel Report, education for an active partnership with patients remains the cornerstone of asthma management and should be carried out by health care providers delivering asthma care. Education should start at the time of asthma diagnosis and be integrated into every step of clinical asthma care. Asthma self-management education should be tailored to the needs of each patient, maintaining a sensitivity to cultural beliefs and practices. New emphasis is placed on evaluating outcomes in terms of patient perceptions of improvement, especially quality of life and the ability to engage in usual activities. Health care providers need to systematically teach and frequently review with patients how to manage and control their asthma. Patients also should be provided with and taught to use a written daily self-management plan and an action plan for exacerbations. It is especially important to give a written action plan to patients with moderate to severe persistent asthma or a history of severe exacerbations. Appropriate patients should also receive a daily asthma diary. Adherence should be encouraged by promoting open communication; individualizing, reviewing, and adjusting plans as needed; emphasizing goals and outcomes; and encouraging family involvement.

In summary, the 1997 *Expert Panel Report 2: Guidelines for the Diagnosis and Management of Asthma* reflects the experience of the past six years as well as the increasing scientific base of published articles on asthma. The Expert Panel hopes this new report will assist the clinician in forming a valuable partnership with patients to achieve excellent asthma treatment and outcomes.

REFERENCES

Adams PF, Marano MA. Current estimates from the National Health Interview Survey, 1994. *Vital Health Stat* 1995; 10:94.

Centers for Disease Control and Prevention. Asthma mortality and hospitalization among children and young adults—United States, 1990–1995. *MMWR* 1996;45:350–353.

Centers for Disease Control and Prevention. Asthma-United States, 1989–1992. *MMWR* 1995;43:952–955.

National Asthma Education and Prevention Program. *Expert Panel Report: Guidelines for the Diagnosis and Management of Asthma.* National Institutes of Health publication 91-3642. Bethesda, Md., 1991.

National Heart, Lung, and Blood Institute. *International Consensus Report on Diagnosis and Management of Asthma.* National Institutes of Health publication 92-3091. Bethesda, Md., 1992.

National Heart, Lung, and Blood Institute and World Health Organization. *Global Initiative for Asthma.* National Institutes of Health Publication 95-3659. Bethesda, Md., 1995.

U.S. Preventive Services Task Force. *Guide to Clinical Preventive Health Services.* Baltimore, Md.: Williams and Wilkins, 1989.

PATHOGENESIS AND DEFINITION

Key Points

- Asthma, whatever the severity, is a chronic inflammatory disorder of the airways. This has implications for the diagnosis, management, and potential prevention of the disease.

- The immunohistopathologic features of asthma include:

  - Denudation of airway epithelium

  - Collagen deposition beneath basement membrane

  - Edema

  - Mast cell activation

  - Inflammatory cell infiltration

  - Neutrophils (especially in sudden-onset, fatal asthma exacerbations)

- Eosinophils
- Lymphocytes (TH2-like cells)
- Airway inflammation contributes to airway hyperresponsiveness, airflow limitation, respiratory symptoms, and disease chronicity.
- Airway inflammation also contributes to several forms of airflow limitation, including acute bronchoconstriction, airway edema, mucus plug formation, and airway wall remodeling. These features lead to bronchial obstruction.
- Atopy, the genetic predisposition for the development of an IgE-mediated response to 10 common aeroallergens, is the strongest identifiable predisposing factor for developing asthma.

Differences from 1991 *Expert Panel Report: Guidelines for the Diagnosis and Management of Asthma*

- The critical role of inflammation in asthma has been further substantiated by research. It is recognized that asthma results from complex interactions among inflammatory cells, mediators, and other cells and tissues resident in the airway.
- Evidence indicates that subbasement membrane fibrosis may occur in some patients and that these changes contribute to persistent abnormalities in lung function. The importance of airway remodeling and the development of persistent airflow limitation need further exploration and may have significant implications for the treatment of asthma.

The clinician, physiologist, immunologist, and pathologist all may have different perspectives on asthma based on their individual viewpoints and experience. The merging of these different perspectives into an acceptable definition of asthma has occurred and is important for more specific and effective treatment of this disease and for investigation into its pathogenesis. Furthermore, even though this disorder affects virtually the entire spectrum of life, asthma has certain age-specific characteristics and differential diagnosis issues that need to be considered in both its treatment and its etiology.

Based on current knowledge, a working definition of asthma is: *a chronic inflammatory disorder of the airways in which many cells and cellular elements play a role, in particular mast cells, eosinophils, T lymphocytes, macrophages, neutrophils, and epithelial cells. In susceptible individuals, this inflammation causes recurrent episodes of wheezing, breathlessness, chest tightness, and coughing, particularly at night or in the early morning. These episodes are usually associated with widespread but variable airflow obstruction that is often reversible either spontaneously or with treatment. The inflammation also causes an associated increase in the existing bronchial hyperresponsiveness to a variety of stimuli* (NHLBI 1995). Moreover, recent evidence indicates that subbasement membrane fibrosis may occur in some patients with asthma and that these changes contribute to persistent abnormalities in lung function (Roche 1991).

This working definition and its expanded recognition of key features of asthma have been derived from studying how airway changes in asthma relate to various factors associated with the development of allergic inflammation (e.g., allergens, respiratory viruses, and some occupational exposures. . . . From this approach has come a more comprehensive understanding of asthma pathogenesis, the development of persistent airway inflammation, and the profound implications these issues have for the diagnosis, treatment, and potential prevention of asthma.

AIRWAY PATHOLOGY AND ASTHMA

Until recently, information on airway pathology in asthma has come largely from postmortem examination (Dunnill 1960), which shows that both large and small airways often contain plugs composed of mucus, serum proteins, inflammatory cells, and cellular debris. Viewed microscopically, airways are infiltrated with eosinophils and mononuclear cells, and there is vasodilation and evidence of microvascular leakage and epithelial disruption. The airway smooth muscle is often hypertrophied, which is characterized by new vessel formation, increased numbers of epithelial goblet cells, and deposition of interstitial collagens beneath the epithelium. These features of airway wall remodeling further underscore the importance of chronic, recurrent inflammation in asthma and its effects on the airway. Moreover, these morphologic changes may not be completely reversible. Consequently, research is currently focused on determining whether these changes can be prevented or modified by early diagnosis, avoidance of factors that contribute to asthma severity, and pharmacologic therapy directed at suppressing airway inflammation.

Establishing the relationship between the pathologic changes and the clinical features of asthma has been difficult. Fiber-optic bronchoscopy with lavage and biopsy provide new insight into mechanisms of airway disease and features that link altered lung function to a specific type of mucosal inflammation (Laitinen et al. 1985; Beastey et al. 1989; Jeffery et al. 1989). From such studies, evidence has emerged that mast cells, eosinophils, epithelial cells, macrophages, and activated T cells are key features of the inflammatory process of asthma (Djukanovic et al. 1990). . . . These cells can influence airway function through secretion of preformed and newly synthesized mediators that act either directly on the airway or indirectly through neural mechanisms (Emanuel and Howarth 1995). Furthermore, with the use of cellular and molecular biological techniques, subpopulations of T lymphocytes (TH2) have been identified as important cells that may regulate allergic inflammation in the airway through the release of selective cytokines and also establish disease chronicity (Robinson et al. 1992). In addition, constituent cells of the airway, including fibroblasts, endothelial cells, and epithelial cells, also contribute to this process by releasing cytokines and chemokines.

The above factors may be important in both initiating and maintaining the level of airway inflammation (Robinson et al. 1993). It is hypothesized that airway inflammation can be acute, subacute, and chronic. The acute inflammatory response is represented by the early recruitment of cells to the airway. In the subacute phase, recruited and resident cells are activated to cause a more persistent pattern of inflammation. Chronic inflammation is characterized by a persistent level of cell damage and an ongoing repair process, changes that may

cause permanent abnormalities in the airway.

Finally, it is recognized that specific adhesion proteins, found in the vascular tissue, lung matrix, and bronchial epithelium, may be critical in directing and anchoring cells in the airway, thus causing the inflammatory changes noted (Albelda 1991). From these studies of the histological features associated with asthma has come evidence of an association between airway inflammation and markers of airway disease severity and an indication that this process is multicellular, redundant, and self-amplifying.

Cell-derived mediators can influence airway smooth muscle tone, modulate vascular permeability, activate neurons, stimulate mucus secretion, and produce characteristic structural changes in the airway (Horwitz and Busse 1995). These mediators can target ciliated airway epithelium to cause injury or disruption. As a consequence, epithelial cells and myofibroblasts present beneath the epithelium proliferate and begin to deposit interstitial collagens in the lamina reticularis of the basement membrane. This may explain apparent basement membrane thickening and the irreversible airway changes that may occur in some asthma patients (Roche 1991). Other changes, including hypertrophy and hyperplasia of airway smooth muscle, increases in goblet cell number, enlargement of submucous glands, and remodeling of the airway connective tissue, are components of asthma that need to be recognized in both its pathogenesis and treatment. This inflammatory process is redundant in its ability to alter airway physiology and architecture.

Child-Onset Asthma

Asthma often begins in childhood, and when it does, it is frequently found in association with atopy, which is the genetic susceptibility to produce IgE directed toward common environmental allergens, including house-dust mites, animal proteins, and fungi (Larsen 1992). With the production of IgE antibodies, mast cells and possibly other airway cells (e.g., lymphocytes) are sensitized and become activated when they encounter specific antigens. Although atopy has been found in 30 to 50 percent of the general population, it is frequently found in the absence of asthma. Nevertheless, atopy is one of the strongest predisposing factors in the development of asthma (Sporik et al. 1990). Furthermore, among infants and young children who have wheezing with viral infections, allergy or family history of allergy is the factor that is most strongly associated with continuing asthma through childhood (Martinez et al. 1995).

Adult-Onset Asthma

Although asthma begins most frequently in childhood and adolescence, it can develop at any time in life. Adult-onset asthma can occur in a variety of situations. In adult-onset asthma, allergens may continue to play an important role. However, in some adults who develop asthma, IgE antibodies to allergens or a family history of asthma are not detected. These individuals often have coexisting sinusitis, nasal polyps, and sensitivity to aspirin or related nonsteroidal anti-inflammatory drugs. The mechanisms of nonallergic, or intrinsic, asthma are less well established, although the inflammatory process is similar (but not identical) to that seen in atopic asthma (Walker et al. 1992).

Occupational exposure to workplace materials (animal products; biological enzymes; plastic resin; wood dusts, particularly cedar; and metals) (see Component 2) can cause airway inflammation, bronchial hyperresponsiveness, and clinical signs of asthma (Chan-Yeung and Malo 1994; Fabbri et al. 1994). Identification of the causative agent and its removal from the workplace can reduce symptoms; however, some individuals will have persistent asthma even though exposure to the causative agent is eliminated. The mechanisms of this form of asthma are not clearly established.

RELATIONSHIP OF AIRWAY INFLAMMATION AND LUNG FUNCTION

Airway Hyperresponsiveness

An important feature of asthma is an exaggerated bronchoconstrictor response to a wide variety of stimuli. The propensity for airways to narrow too easily and too much is a major, but not necessarily unique, feature of asthma. Airway hyperresponsiveness leads to clinical symptoms of wheezing and dyspnea after exposure to allergens, environmental irritants, viral infections, cold air, or exercise. Research indicates that airway hyperresponsiveness is important in the pathogenesis of asthma and that the level of airway responsiveness usually correlates with the clinical severity of asthma.

Airway hyperresponsiveness can be measured by inhalation challenge testing with methacholine or histamine, as well as after exposure to such nonpharmacologic stimuli as hyperventilation with cold dry air, inhalation of hypotonic or hypertonic aerosols, or after exercise (O'Connor et al. 1989). In addition, variability between morning and evening peak expiratory flow (PEF) appears to reflect airway hyperresponsiveness and may serve as a measure of airway hyperresponsiveness, asthma instability, or asthma severity.

The factors contributing to airway inflammation in asthma are multiple and involve a variety of different inflammatory cells (as illustrated in Figure 2) (Busse et al. 1993). It is also apparent that asthma is not caused by either a single cell or a single inflammatory mediator but rather results from complex interactions among inflammatory cells, mediators, and other cells and tissues resident in airways. An initial trigger in asthma may be the release of inflammatory mediators from bronchial mast cells, macrophages, T lymphocytes, and epithelial cells. These substances direct the migration and activation of other inflammatory cells, such as eosinophils and neutrophils, to the airway where they cause injury, such as alterations in epithelial integrity, abnormalities in autonomic neural control of airway tone, mucus hypersecretion, change in mucociliary function, and increased airway smooth muscle responsiveness.

The importance of the airway inflammatory response to airway hyperresponsiveness is substantiated by several observations. First, airway markers of inflammation correlate with bronchial hyperresponsiveness. Second, treatment of asthma and modification of airway inflammatory markers not only reduce symptoms but also diminish airway responsiveness. However, the relationship between airway inflammation and airway responsiveness is complex. Some investigations have shown that although anti-inflammatory therapy reduced airway hyperresponsiveness, it did not eradicate it. A small study found that control of airway inflammation did not control bronchial hyperresponsiveness (Lundgren et al. 1988). Thus, factors in addition to inflammation may contribute to airway hyperresponsiveness.

Airflow Obstruction

Airflow limitation in asthma is recurrent and caused by a variety of changes in the airway. These include:

- Acute bronchoconstriction. Allergen-induced acute bronchoconstriction results from an IgE-dependent release of mediators from the mast cell that include histamine, tryptase, leukotrienes, and prostaglandins (Marshall and Bienenstock 1994), which directly contract airway smooth muscle. Aspirin and other nonsteroidal anti-inflammatory drugs (see Component 2) can also cause acute airflow obstruction in some patients, and evidence indicates that this non–IgE-dependent response also involves mediator release from airway cells (Fischer et al. 1994). In addition, other stimuli, including exercise, cold air, and irritants, can cause acute airflow obstruction. The mechanisms regulating the airway response to these factors are less well-defined, but the intensity of the response appears related to underlying airway inflammation (Busse et al. 1993). There is emerging evidence that stress can play a role in precipitating asthma exacerbations. The mechanisms involved have yet to be established and may include enhanced generation of proinflammatory cytokines (Friedman et al. 1994).

- Airway edema. Airway wall edema, even without smooth muscle contraction or bronchoconstriction, limits airflow in asthma. Increased microvascular permeability and leakage caused by released mediators also contribute to mucosal thickening and swelling of the airway. As a consequence, swelling of the airway wall causes the airway to become more rigid and interferes with airflow.

- Chronic mucous plug formation. In severe intractable asthma, airflow limitation is often persistent. In part, this change may arise as a consequence of mucous secretion and the formation of inspissated mucous plugs.

- Airway remodeling. In some patients with asthma, airflow limitation may be only partially reversible. The etiology of this component is not as well studied as other features of asthma but may relate to structural changes in the airway matrix that may accompany long-standing and severe airway inflammation. There is evidence that a histological feature of asthma in some patients is an alteration in the amount and composition of the extracellular matrix in the airway wall (Djukanovic et al. 1990; Laitinen and Laitinen 1994). As a consequence of these changes, airway obstruction may be persistent and not responsive to treatment. Regulation of this repair and remodeling process is not well established, but both the process of repair and its regulation are likely to be key events in explaining the persistent nature of the disease and limitations to a therapeutic response. Although yet to be fully explored, the importance of airway remodeling and the development of persistent airflow limitation suggest a rationale for early intervention with anti-inflammatory therapy.

RELEVANCE OF CHRONIC AIRWAY INFLAMMATION TO ASTHMA THERAPY

Although inflammation can be used to describe a variety of conditions in various diseases, the inflammatory response in asthma has special features that include eosinophil infiltration, mast cell degranulation, interstitial airway wall injury, and lymphocyte activation. Furthermore, there is evidence that a TH2 lymphocyte cytokine profile (i.e., IL-4 and IL-5) is instrumental in initiating and sustaining the inflammatory process (James and Kay 1995; Ricci et al. 1993) . . . These observations also have become important in directing treatment in asthma.

It is hypothesized that inflammation is an early and persistent component of asthma. As a consequence, therapy to suppress the inflammation must be long term. Furthermore, preliminary evidence suggests that early intervention with anti-inflammatory therapy may modify the disease process (Agertoft and Pedersen 1994; Laitinen et al. 1992; Djukanovic et al. 1992).

Observations into the basic mechanisms of asthma have had tremendous impact and influence on therapy. Studies have shown that improvements in asthma control achieved with high doses of inhaled corticosteroids are associated with improvement in markers of airway inflammation (Laitinen et al. 1992; Djukanovic et al. 1992). These observations indicate that a strong link may exist between features of airway inflammation, bronchial hyperresponsiveness, asthma symptoms, and severity. Furthermore, insight into the mechanisms of asthma with airway inflammation and bronchial wall repair has become a driving factor in designing logical, and hopefully, effective, treatment paradigms.

Another area that needs clarification is the classification of compounds as anti-inflammatory in nature. Because many factors contribute to the inflammatory response in asthma, many drugs may fit this category. At present, corticosteroids are the anti-inflammatory compounds that have been demonstrated to modify histopathological features of asthma (Barnes 1995). It may be necessary to evaluate each new compound for the specificity of its "anti-inflammatory" action and determine from appropriate observations whether the compound is indeed anti-inflammatory and what consequences this has on the clinical features of the disease.

REFERENCES

Agertoft L, Pedersen S. Effects of long-term treatment with an inhaled corticosteroid on growth and pulmonary function in asthmatic children. *Respir Med* 1994;88:373–381.

Albelda SM. Endothelial and epithelial cell adhesion molecules. *Am J Respir Cell Mol Biol* 1991;4:195–203.

Barnes PJ. Inhaled glucocorticosteroid for asthma. *N Engl J Med* 1995;332:868–875.

Beasley R, Roche WR, Roberts TA, Holgate ST. Cellular events in the bronchi in mild asthma and bronchial provocation. *Am Rev Respir Dis* 1989;139:806–817.

Busse WW, Calhoun WI, Sedgwick JD. Mechanisms of airway inflammation in asthma. *Am Rev Respir Dis* 1993;147:S20–S24.

Chan-Yeung M, Malo JL. Aetiological agents in occupational asthma. *Eur Respir J* 1994;7:346–371.

Djukanovic R, Roche WR, Wilson JW, et al. Mucosal inflammation in asthma. *Am Rev Respir Dis* 1990;142:434–457.

Djukanovic R, Wilson TW, Britten Icil, et al. Affect of an inhaled corticosteroid on airway inflammation and

symptoms of asthma. *Am Rev Respir Dis* 1992; 145:669–674.

Dunnill MS. The pathology of asthma, with special reference to changes in the bronchial mucosa. *J Clin Pathol* 1960;13:27–33.

Emanuel MB, Howarth PH. Asthma and anaphylaxis: a relevant model for chronic disease? An historical analysis of directions in asthma research. *Clin Exp Allergy* 1995;25:15–26.

Fabbri IM, Maestrelli F, Saetta M, Mapp CM. Mechanisms of occupational asthma. *Clin Exp Allergy* 1994;24:628–635.

Fischer AR, Rosenherg MA, Lilly CM, et al. Direct evidence for a role of the mast cell in the nasal response to aspirin in aspirin-sensitive asthma. *J Allergy Clin Immunol* 1994;94:1046–1056.

Friedman EM, Cue CL, Ershler WB. Bidirectional effects of interleukin-1 on immune responses in rhesus monkeys. *Brain Behav Immunol* 1994;8: 87–99.

Horwitz RJ, Busse WW. Inflammation and asthma. *Clin Chest Med* 1995;16:583–602.

James DG, Kay AB. Are you TH-1 or TH-2? [editorial] *Clin Exp Allergy* 1995;25:389–90.

Jeffery PK, Wardlaw AJ, Nelson FC, Collins JV, Kay AB. Bronchial biopsies in asthma. An ultrastructural, qualitative study and correlation with hyperreactivity. *Am Rev Respir Dis* 1989;140:1745–1753.

Laitinen A, Laitinen LA. Airway morphology: endothelial/basement membrane. *Am J Respir Crit Care Med* 1994;150:514–517.

Laitinen IA, Heino M, Leitinen A, Kava T, Haahtela T. Damage of the airway epithelium and bronchial reactivity in patients with asthma. *Am Rev Respir Dis* 1985;131:599–606.

Laitinen LA, Laitinen A, Haahtela T. A comparative study of the effects of an inhaled corticosteroid, budesonide, and a beta$_2$-agonist, terbutaline, on airway inflammation in newly diagnosed asthma: a randomized, double-blind, parallel-group controlled trial. *J Allergy Clin Immunol* 1992;90:32–42.

Larsen GL. Asthma in children. *N Engl J Med* 1992; 326:1540–1545.

Lundgren R, Stiderherg M, Horstedt P, et al. Morphological studies of bronchial biopsies from asthmatics before and after 10 years of treatment with inhaled steroids. *Eur Respir J* 1988;1:853–859.

Marshall JS, Bienenstock J. The role of mast cells in inflammatory reactions of the airways, skin and intestine. *Curr Opin Immunol* 1994;6:853–859.

Martinez PD, Wright AL, Taussig IM, Holberg CJ, Halonen M, Morgan WI, Group Health Medical Associates.

Asthma and wheezing in the first six years of life. *N Engl J Med* 1995;332:133–138.

National Heart, Lung, and Blood Institute. *Global Initiative for Asthma*. National Institutes of Health publication 95–3659. 1995.

O'Connor GT, Sparrow D, Weiss ST. The role of allergy and nonspecific airway hyperresponsiveness in the pathogenesis of chronic obstructive pulmonary disease. *Am Rev Respir Dis* 1959;140:225–252.

Ricci M, Rossi O, Bertoni M, Matucci A. The importance of TH2-like cells in the pathogenesis of airway allergic inflammation. *Clin Exp Allergy* 1993; 23:360–369.

Robinson DS, Durham SR, Kay AB. Cytokines in asthma. *Thorax* 1993;48:845–853.

Robinson DS, Hamid Q, Ying S, et al. Predominant TH2-like broncheoalveolar T-lymphocyte population in atopic asthma. *N Engl J Med* 1992;326: 298–304.

Roche WR. Fibroblasts and asthma. *Clin Exp Allergy* 1991;21:545–548.

Sporik R, Holgate ST, Platts-Mills TA, Cogswell JJ. Exposure to house-dust mite allergen (Der pI) and the development of asthma in childhood. A prospective study. *N Engl J Med* 1990;323:502–507.

Walker C, Bode E, Boer L, Hausel TT, Blaser K, Virchow JC Jr. Allergic and nonallergic asthmatics have distinct patterns of T-cell activation and cytokine production in peripheral blood and bronchoalveolar lavage. *Am Rev Respir Dis* 1992;146:109–115.

COMPONENT 1
MEASURES OF ASSESSMENT AND MONITORING: INITIAL ASSESSMENT AND DIAGNOSIS OF ASTHMA

Key Points

- To establish a diagnosis of asthma, the clinician should determine that:
  Episodic symptoms of airflow obstruction are present.
  Airflow obstruction is at least partially reversible.
  Alternative diagnoses are excluded.
- Recommended mechanisms to establish the diagnosis are:
  Detailed medical history
  Physical exam focusing on the upper respiratory tract, chest, and skin
  Spirometry to demonstrate reversibility

- Additional studies may be considered to:
  Evaluate alternative diagnoses
  Identify precipitating factors
  Assess severity
  Investigate potential complications
- Recommendations are presented for referral for consultation or care to a specialist in asthma care.

Differences from 1991 *Expert Panel Report: Guidelines for the Diagnosis and Management of Asthma*

- Severity classifications were changed from mild, moderate, and severe to mild intermittent, mild persistent, moderate persistent, and severe persistent.
- Examples of questions to use for diagnosis and initial assessment of asthma were added.
- Information on wheezing in infancy and vocal cord dysfunction was expanded in the differential diagnosis section.
- Criteria for referral were refined with input from specialty and primary care physicians.
- More specific recommendations for measuring peak expiratory flow (PEF) diurnal variation are made.

The guidelines to help establish a diagnosis of asthma presented in this component are based on the opinion of the Expert Panel.

The clinician trying to establish a diagnosis of asthma should determine that:

- Episodic symptoms of airflow obstruction are present.
- Airflow obstruction is at least partially reversible.
- Alternative diagnoses are excluded.

A careful medical history, physical examination, pulmonary function tests, and additional tests will provide the information needed to ensure a correct diagnosis of asthma . . . Each of these methods of assessment is described in this section.

Clinical judgment is needed in conducting the assessment for asthma. Patients with asthma are heterogeneous and present signs and symptoms that vary widely from patient to patient as well as within each patient over time.

Medical History

A detailed medical history of the new patient known or thought to have asthma should address the items listed in Figure 1-1. The medical history can help:

- *Identify the symptoms likely to be due to asthma.* See Figure 1-2 for sample questions.

- *Support the likelihood of asthma* (e.g., patterns of symptoms, family history of asthma or allergies).

- *Assess the severity of asthma* (e.g., symptom frequency and severity, exercise tolerance, hospitalizations, current medications). See Figure 1-3 for a description of the levels of asthma severity.

- *Identify possible precipitating factors* (e.g., viral respiratory infections; exposure at home, work, day care, or school to inhalant allergens or irritants such as tobacco smoke). See Component 2, Control of Factors Contributing to Asthma Severity, for more details.

Physical Examination

The upper respiratory tract, chest, and skin are the focus of the physical examination for asthma. Physical findings that increase the probability of asthma include:

- *Hyperexpansion of the thorax,* especially in children; use of accessory muscles; appearance of hunched shoulders; and chest deformity.

- *Sounds of wheezing during normal breathing or a prolonged phase of forced exhalation* (typical of airflow obstruction). Wheezing during forced exhalation is not a reliable indicator of airflow limitation. In mild intermittent asthma, or between exacerbations, wheezing may be absent.

- *Increased nasal secretion, mucosal swelling, and nasal polyps.*

- *Atopic dermatitis/eczema* or any other manifestation of an allergic skin condition.

Pulmonary Function Testing (Spirometry)

Spirometry measurements (FEV_1, FVC, FEV_1/FVC) before and after the patient inhales a short-acting bronchodilator should be undertaken for patients

---

BOX 1. KEY INDICATORS FOR CONSIDERING A DIAGNOSIS OF ASTHMA

Consider asthma and performing spirometry if any of these indicators are present.* These indicators are not diagnostic by themselves, but the presence of multiple key indicators increases the probability of a diagnosis of asthma. Spirometry is needed to establish a diagnosis of asthma.

- Wheezing—high-pitched whistling sounds when breathing out—especially in children. (Lack of wheezing and a normal chest examination do not exclude asthma.)

- History of any of the following:
  Cough, worse particularly at night
  Recurrent wheeze
  Recurrent difficulty in breathing
  Recurrent chest tightness

- Reversible airflow limitation and diurnal variation as measured by using a peak flow meter, for example:
  Peak expiratory flow (PEF) varies 20 percent or more from PEF measurement on arising in the morning (before taking

an inhaled short-acting beta$_2$-agonist) to PEF measurement in the early afternoon (after taking an inhaled short-acting beta$_2$-agonist).

- Symptoms occur or worsen in the presence of:
  Exercise
  Viral infection
  Animals with fur or feathers
  House-dust mites (in mattresses, pillows, upholstered furniture, carpets)
  Mold
  Smoke (tobacco, wood)
  Pollen
  Changes in weather
  Strong emotional expression (laughing or crying hard)
  Airborne chemicals or dusts
  Menses

- Symptoms occur or worsen at night, awakening the patient.

---

*Eczema, hay fever, or a family history of asthma or atopic diseases are often associated with asthma, but they are not key indicators.

in whom the diagnosis of asthma is being considered (Bye et al. 1992; Li and O'Connell 1996). This helps determine whether there is airflow obstruction and whether it is reversible over the short term (see Box 2 for further information). Spirometry is generally valuable in children over age four; however, some children cannot conduct the maneuver adequately until after age seven.

Spirometry typically measures the maximal volume of air forcibly exhaled from the point of maximal inhalation (forced vital capacity, FVC) and the volume of air exhaled during the first second of the FVC (forced expiratory volume in 1 second, FEV_1). Airflow obstruction is indicated by reduced FEV_1 and FEV_1/FVC values relative to reference or predicted values. Significant reversibility is indicated by an increase of >12 percent and 200 ml in FEV, after inhaling a short-acting bronchodilator (American Thoracic Society 1991) (see Figure 14 [omitted] for example of a spirometric curve for this test). A two- to three-week trial of oral corticosteroid therapy may be required to demonstrate reversibility. The spirometry measurements that establish reversibility may not indicate the patient's best lung function.

Abnormalities of lung function are categorized as restrictive and obstructive defects. A reduced ratio of FEV_1/FVC (i.e., <65 percent) indicates obstruction to the flow of air from the lungs, whereas a reduced FVC with a normal FEV_1/FVC ratio suggests a restrictive pattern. The severity of abnormality of spirometric measurements is evaluated by comparison of the patient's results with reference values based on age, height, sex, and race (American Thoracic Society 1991).

Although asthma is typically associated with an obstructive impairment that is reversible, neither this finding nor any other single test or measure is adequate to diagnose asthma. Many diseases are associated with this pattern of abnormality. The patient's pattern of symptoms (along with other information from the patient's medical history) and exclusion of other possible diagnoses also are needed to establish a diagnosis of asthma. In severe cases, the FVC may also be reduced, due to trapping of air in the lungs.

Office-based physicians who care for asthma patients should have access to spirometry, which is useful in both diagnosis and periodic monitoring. Spirometry should be performed using equipment and techniques that meet standards developed by the American Thoracic Society (1995). Correct technique, calibration methods, and maintenance of equipment are necessary to achieve consistently accurate test results. Maximal patient effort in performing the test is required to avoid important errors in diagnosis and management.

Training courses in the performance of spirometry that are approved by the National Institute for Occupational Safety and Health are available (800)35NIOSH. When office spirometry shows severe abnormalities, or if questions arise regarding test accuracy or interpretation, the Expert Panel recommends further assessment in a specialized pulmonary function laboratory.

FIGURE 1-1. SUGGESTED ITEMS FOR MEDICAL HISTORY*

A detailed medical history of the new patient who is known or thought to have asthma should address the following items:

1. Symptoms
   - Cough
   - Wheezing
   - Shortness of breath
   - Chest tightness
   - Sputum production

2. Pattern of symptoms
   - Perennial, seasonal, or both
   - Continual, episodic, or both
   - Onset, duration, frequency (number of days or nights, per week or month)
   - Diurnal variations, especially nocturnal and on awakening in early morning

3. Precipitating and/or aggravating factors
   - Viral respiratory infections
   - Environmental allergens, indoor (e.g., mold, house-dust mite, cockroach, animal dander, or secretory products) and outdoor (e.g., pollen)
   - Exercise
   - Occupational chemicals or allergens
   - Environmental change (e.g., moving to new home; going on vacation; and/or alterations in workplace, work processes, or materials used)
   - Irritants (e.g., tobacco smoke, strong odors, air pollutants, occupational chemicals, dusts and particulates, vapors, gases, and aerosols)
   - Emotional expressions (e.g., fear, anger, frustration, hard crying or laughing)

- Drugs (e.g., aspirin; beta-blockers, including eyedrops; nonsteroidal anti-inflammatory drugs; others)
- Food, food additives, and preservatives (e.g., sulfites)
- Changes in weather, exposure to cold air
- Endocrine factors (e.g., menses, pregnancy, thyroid disease)

4. Development of disease and treatment
   - Age of onset and diagnosis
   - History of early-life injury to airways (e.g., bronchopulmonary dysplasia, pneumonia, parental smoking)
   - Progress of disease (better or worse)
   - Present management and response, including plans for managing exacerbations
   - Need for oral corticosteroids and frequency of use
   - Comorbid conditions

5. Family history
   - History of asthma, allergy, sinusitis, rhinitis, or nasal polyps in close relatives

6. Social history
   - Characteristics of home including age, location, cooling and heating system, wood-burning stove, humidifier, carpeting over concrete, presence of molds or mildew, characteristics of rooms where patient spends time (e.g., bedroom and living room with attention to bedding, floor covering, stuffed furniture), smoking (patient and others in home or day care)
   - Day care, workplace, and school characteristics that may interfere with adherence
   - Social factors that interfere with adherence, such as substance abuse
   - Social support/social networks
   - Level of education completed
   - Employment (if employed, characteristics of work environment)

7. Profile of typical exacerbation
   - Usual prodromal signs and symptoms
   - Usual patterns and management (what works?)

8. Impact of asthma on patient and family
   - Episodes of unscheduled care (emergency department, urgent care, hospitalization)
   - Life-threatening exacerbations (e.g., intubation, intensive care unit admission)
   - Number of days missed from school/work
   - Limitation of activity, especially sports and strenuous work
   - History of nocturnal awakening
   - Effect on growth, development, behavior, school or work performance, and lifestyle
   - Impact on family routines, activities, or dynamics
   - Economic impact

9. Assessment of patient's and family's perceptions of disease
   - Patient, parental, and spouse's or partner's knowledge of asthma and belief in the chronicity of asthma and in the efficacy of treatment

- Patient perception and beliefs regarding use and long-term effects of medications
- Ability of patient and parents, spouse, or partner to cope with disease
- Level of family support and patient's and parents', spouse's, or partner's capacity to recognize severity of an exacerbation
- Economic resources
- Sociocultural beliefs

---

*This list does not represent a standardized assessment or diagnostic instrument. The validity and reliability of this list have not been assessed.

Additional Studies

Even though additional studies are not routine, they may be considered. No one test or set of tests is appropriate for every patient. However, the following procedures may be useful when considering alternative diagnoses, identifying precipitating factors, assessing severity, and investigating potential complications:

- *Additional pulmonary function studies* (e.g., lung volumes and inspiratory and expiratory flow volume loops) may be indicated, especially if there are questions about coexisting chronic obstructive pulmonary disease, a restrictive defect, or possible central airway obstruction. A *diffusing capacity test* is helpful in differentiating between asthma and emphysema in patients at risk for both illnesses, such as smokers and older patients.

- *Assessment of diurnal variation in peak expiratory flow over one to two weeks* is recommended when patients have asthma symptoms but normal spirometry (Enright et al. 1994). PEF is generally lowest on first awakening and highest several hours before the midpoint of the waking day (e.g., between noon and 2 P.M.) (Quackenboss et al. 1991). Optimally, PEF should be measured close to those two times, before taking an inhaled short-acting beta$_2$-agonist in the morning and after taking one in the afternoon. A 20 percent difference between morning and afternoon measurements suggests asthma. Measuring PEF on waking and in the evening may be more practical and feasible, but values will tend to underestimate the actual diurnal variation.

- *Bronchoprovocation* with methacholine, histamine, or exercise challenge may be useful when asthma is suspected and spirometry is normal or near normal. For safety reasons, bronchoprovocation testing should be carried out by a trained individual in an appropriate facility and is not generally recommended if the FEV_1 is <65 percent predicted. A negative bronchoprovocation may be helpful to rule out asthma.

- *Chest X ray* may be needed to exclude other diagnosis.

- *Allergy testing* (see Component 2).

- *Evaluation of the nose for nasal polyps and sinuses for sinus disease.*

- *Evaluation for gastroesophageal reflux* (Harding and Richter 1992) (see Component 2).

The usefulness of measurements of biomarkers of inflammation (e.g., total and differential cell count and mediator assays) in sputum, blood, or urine as aids to the diagnosis of asthma is currently being evaluated in clinical research trials.

Differential Diagnosis of Asthma

Recurrent episodes of cough and wheezing are almost always due to asthma in both children and adults. Underdiagnosis of asthma is a frequent problem, especially in children who wheeze when they have respiratory infections. These children are often labeled as having bronchitis, bronchiolitis, or pneumonia even though the signs and symptoms are most compatible with a diagnosis of asthma.

However, the clinician needs to be aware of other causes of airway obstruction leading to wheezing (see Figure 1-5).

There are two general patterns of wheezing in infancy: nonallergic and allergic. Nonallergic infants wheeze when they have an acute upper respiratory viral infection, but as their airways grow larger in the preschool years, the wheezing disappears. Allergic infants also wheeze with viral infections, but they are more likely to have asthma that will continue throughout childhood. This group may have eczema, allergic rhinitis, or food allergy as other manifestations of allergy. Both groups may benefit from asthma treatment.

FIGURE 1-3. CLASSIFICATION OF ASTHMA SEVERITY TABLE

Clinical Features Before Treatment*

	Symptoms**	Nighttime Symptoms	Lung Function
STEP 4 Severe Persistent	■ Continual symptoms ■ Limited physical activity ■ Frequent exacerbations	Frequent	■ FEV_1 or PEF ≤60% predicted ■ PEF variability >30%
STEP 3 Moderate Persistent	■ Daily symptoms ■ Daily use of inhaled short-acting beta₂-agonist ■ Exacerbations affect activity ■ Exacerbations ≥2 times a week; may last days	>1 time a week	■ FEV_1 or PEF >60% - <80% predicted ■ PEF variability >30%
STEP 2 Mild Persistent	■ Symptoms >2 times a week but <1 time a day ■ Exacerbations may affect activity	>2 times a month	■ FEV_1 or PEF ≥80% predicted ■ PEF variability 20-30%
STEP 1 Mild Intermittent	■ Symptoms ≤2 times a week ■ Asymptomatic and normal PEF between exacerbations ■ Exacerbations brief (from a few hours to a few days); intensity may vary	≤2 times a month	■ FEV_1 or PEF ≥80% predicted ■ PEF variability <20%

*The presence of one of the features of severity is sufficient to place a patient in that category. An individual should be assigned to the most severe grade in which any feature occurs. The characteristics noted in this figure are general and may overlap because asthma is highly variable. Furthermore, an individual's classification may change over time.

**Patients at any level of severity can have mild, moderate, or severe exacerbations. Some patients with intermittent asthma experience severe and life-threatening exacerbations separated by long periods of normal lung function and no symptoms.

Vocal cord dysfunction often mimics asthma. Patients with vocal cord dysfunction can present with recurrent severe shortness of breath and wheezing. Vocal cord dysfunction may even cause alveolar hypoventilation, with increases in Pco_2 that prompt urgent intubation and mechanical ventilation. Vocal cord dysfunction that mimics asthma is more common in young adults with psychological disorders. It should be suspected when physical examination reveals a monophonic wheeze heard loudest over the glottis. Further evaluation by flow-volume curve revealing inspiratory flow limitation strongly supports the diagnosis of vocal cord dysfunction. Definitive diagnosis—and exclusion of organic causes of vocal cord narrowing—requires direct visualization of the vocal cords. Treatment with speech therapy that teaches techniques for relaxed throat breathing is often effective (Newman et al. 1995; Bucca et al. 1995; Christopher et al. 1983).

FIGURE 1-2. SAMPLE QUESTIONS* FOR THE DIAGNOSIS AND INITIAL ASSESSMENT OF ASTHMA

A "yes" answer to any question suggests that an asthma diagnosis is likely. In the past 12 months . . .

- Have you had a sudden severe episode or recurrent episodes of coughing, wheezing (high-pitched whistling sounds when breathing out), or shortness of breath?

- Have you had colds that "go to the chest" or take more than 10 days to get over?

- Have you had coughing, wheezing, or shortness of breath during a particular season or time of the year?

- Have you had coughing, wheezing, or shortness of breath in certain places or when exposed to certain things (e.g., animals, tobacco smoke, perfumes)?

- Have you used any medications that help you breathe better? How often?

- Are your symptoms relieved when the medications are used?

In the past 4 weeks, have you had coughing, wheezing, or shortness of breath . . .

- At night that has awakened you?
- In the early morning?
- After running, moderate exercise, or other physical activity?

---

*These questions are examples and do not represent a standardized assessment or diagnostic instrument. The validity and reliability of these questions have not been assessed.

BOX 2.   IMPORTANCE OF SPIROMETRY IN ASTHMA DIAGNOSIS

Objective assessments of pulmonary function are necessary for the diagnosis of asthma because medical history and physical examination are not reliable means of excluding other diagnoses or of characterizing the status of lung impairment. Although physicians generally seem able to identify a lung abnormality as obstructive (Russell et al. 1986), they have a poor ability to assess the degree of airflow obstruction (Shim and Williams 1980) or to predict whether the obstruction is reversible (Russell et al. 1986).

For diagnostic purposes, spirometry is generally recommended over measurements by a peak flow meter in the clinician's office because there is wide variability even in the best published peak expiratory flow reference values. Reference values need to be specific to each brand of peak flow meter, and such normative brand-specific values currently are not available for most brands. Peak flow meters are designed as monitoring, not as diagnostic, tools in the office (see Component 1—Periodic Assessment and Monitoring: Essential for Asthma Monitoring). However, peak flow monitoring can establish peak flow variability and thus aid in the determination of asthma severity when patients have asthma symptoms and normal spirometry (see Additional Studies section).

General Guidelines for Referral to an Asthma Specialist

Criteria for the referral of an asthma patient have been developed (Spector and Nicklas 1995; Shuttari 1995). Based on the opinion of the Expert Panel, referral for consultation or care to a specialist in asthma care (usually, a fellowship-trained allergist or pulmonologist; occasionally, other physicians with expertise in asthma management developed through additional training and experience) is recommended when:

- Patient has had a life-threatening asthma exacerbation.

- Patient is not meeting the goals of asthma therapy (see Component 1—Periodic Assessment and Monitoring) after three to six months of treatment. An earlier referral or consultation is appropriate if the physician concludes that the patient is unresponsive to therapy.

- Signs and symptoms are atypical or there are problems in differential diagnosis.

- Other conditions complicate asthma or its diagnosis (e.g., sinusitis, nasal polyps, aspergillosis, severe rhinitis, vocal cord dysfunction, gastroesophageal reflux, chronic obstructive pulmonary disease).

- Additional diagnostic testing is indicated (e.g., allergy skin testing, rhinoscopy, complete pulmonary function studies, provocative challenge, bronchoscopy).

- Patient requires additional education and guidance on complications of therapy, problems with adherence, or allergen avoidance.

- Patient is being considered for immunotherapy.

- Patient has severe persistent asthma, requiring step 4 care (referral may be considered for patients requiring step care; see Component 3—Managing Asthma Long Term).

- Patient requires continuous oral corticosteroid therapy or high-dose inhaled corticosteroids or has required more than two bursts of oral corticosteroids in one year.

- Patient is under age three and requires step 3 or 4 care (see Component 3—Managing Asthma Long Term). When patient is under age three and requires step 2 care initiation of daily long-term therapy, referral should be considered.

- Patient requires confirmation of a history that suggests that an occupational or environmental inhalant or ingested substance is provoking or contributing to asthma. Depending on the complexities of diagnosis, treatment, or the intervention required in the work environment, it may be appropriate in some cases for the specialist to manage the patient over a period of time or co-manage with the primary care provider.

In addition, patients with significant psychiatric, psychosocial, or family problems that interfere with their asthma therapy may need referral to an appropriate mental health professional for counseling or treatment. These characteristics have been shown to interfere with a patient's ability to adhere to treatment (Strunk 1987; Strunk et al. 1985).

FIGURE 1-5. DIFFERENTIAL DIAGNOSTIC POSSIBILITIES FOR ASTHMA

Infants and Children

Upper airway diseases
- Allergic rhinitis and sinusitis

Obstruction involving large airways
- Foreign body in trachea or bronchus
- Vocal cord dysfunction
- Vascular rings or laryngeal webs
- Laryngotracheomalacia, tracheal stenosis, or bronchostenosis
- Enlarged lymph nodes or tumor

Obstructions involving small airways
- Viral bronchiolitis or obliterative bronchiolitis
- Cystic fibrosis
- Bronchopulmonary dysplasia
- Heart disease

Other causes
- Recurrent cough not due to asthma
- Aspiration from swallowing mechanism dysfunction or gastroesophageal reflux

Adults

- Chronic obstructive pulmonary disease (chronic bronchitis or emphysema)
- Congestive heart failure
- Pulmonary embolism
- Laryngeal dysfunction
- Mechanical obstruction of the airways (benign and malignant tumors)
- Pulmonary infiltration with eosinophilia
- Cough secondary to drugs (angiotensin-converting enzyme [ACE] inhibitors)
- Vocal cord dysfunction

REFERENCES

American Thoracic Society. Lung function testing: selection of reference values and interpretive strategies. *Am Rev Respir Dis* 1991;144:1202–1218.

American Thoracic Society. Standardization of spirometry: 1994 update. *Am J Respir Crit Care Med* 1995; 152: 1107–1136.

Bucca C, Rolla G, Brussino L, De Rose V, Bugiani M. Are asthma-like symptoms due to bronchial or extrathoracic airway dysfunction? *Lancet* 1995;346:791–795.

Bye MR, Kerstein D, Barsh B. The importance of spirometry in the assessment of childhood asthma. *Am J Dis Child* 1992;146:977–978.

Christopher KL, Wood RP 2nd, Eckert RC, Blager FB, Raney RA, Souhrada JF. Vocal cord dysfunction presenting as asthma. *N Engl J Med* 1983; 308: 1566–1570.

Enright PL, Lebowitz MD, Cockroft DW. Physiologic measures: pulmonary function tests. Asthma outcome. *Am J Respir Crit Care Med* 1994;149:59–68.

Harding SM, Richter JE. Gastroesophageal reflux disease and asthma. *Semin Gastrointest Dis* 1992;3:139–150.

Knudson RJ, Lebowitz MD, Holberg CJ, Burrows B. Changes in the normal maximal expiratory flow-volume curve with growth and aging. *Am Rev Respir Dis* 1983;127:725–734.

Li JT, O'Connell EJ. Clinical evaluation of asthma. *Ann Allergy Asthma Immunol* 1996;76:1–13.

Newman KB, Mason UG 3rd, Schmaling KB. Clinical features of vocal cord dysfunction. *Am J Respir Crit Care Med* 1995;152:1382–1386.

Quackenboss JJ, Lebowitz MD, Krzyzanowski M. The normal range of diurnal changes in peak expiratory flow rates. Relationship to symptoms and respiratory disease. *Am Rev Respir Dis* 1991;143:323–330.

Russell NJ, Crichton NJ, Emerson PA, Morgan AD. Quantitative assessment of the value of spirometry. *Thorax* 1986;41:360–363.

Shim CS, Williams MH Jr. Evaluation of the severity of asthma: patients versus physicians. *Am J Med* 1980;68:11–13.

Shuttari MF. Asthma: diagnosis and management. *Am Fam Physician* 1995;52:2225–2235.

Spector SL, Nicklas RA, eds. Practice parameters for the diagnosis and treatment of asthma. *J Allergy Clin Immunol* 1995;96:729–731.

Strunk RC. Asthma deaths in childhood: identification of patients at risk and intervention. *J Allergy Clin Immunol* 1997;80:472–477.

Strunk RC, Mrazek DA, Wolfson Fuhrmann GS, LaBrecque JR. Physiologic and psychological characteristics associated with deaths due to asthma in childhood. A case-controlled study. *JAMA* 1985; 254:1193–1198.

PERIODIC ASSESSMENT AND MONITORING: ESSENTIAL FOR ASTHMA MANAGEMENT

Key Points

- The goals of therapy are to:
    Prevent chronic and troublesome symptoms (e.g., coughing or breathlessness in the night, in the early morning, or after exertion)
    Maintain (near) "normal" pulmonary function
    Maintain normal activity levels (including exercise and other physical activity)
    Prevent recurrent exacerbations of asthma and minimize the need for emergency department visits or hospitalizations
    Provide optimal pharmacotherapy with the least amount of adverse effects
    Meet patients' and families' expectations of and satisfaction with asthma care

- Periodic assessments and ongoing monitoring of asthma are recommended to determine if the goals of therapy are being met. Measurements of the following are recommended:
    Signs and symptoms of asthma
    Pulmonary function
    Quality of life/functional status
    History of asthma exacerbations
    Pharmacotherapy
    Patient-provider communication and patient satisfaction

- Clinician assessment and patient self-assessment are the primary methods for monitoring asthma. Population-based assessment is beginning to be used by managed care organizations.

- Spirometry tests are recommended (1) at the time of initial assessment, (2) after treatment is initiated and symptoms and PEF have stabilized, and (3) at least every 1 to 2 years.

- Patients should be given a written action plan based on signs and symptoms and/or PEF: This is especially important for patients with moderate-to-severe persistent asthma or a history of severe exacerbations.

- Patients should be trained to recognize symptom patterns indicating inadequate asthma control and the need for additional therapy.

- Recommendations on how and when to do peak flow monitoring are presented.

Differences from 1991 *Expert Panel Report: Guidelines for the Diagnosis and Management of Asthma*

- The new report includes an additional goal of therapy (meet patients' and families' expectations of and satisfaction with asthma care) that was not listed in the 1991 report.

- Periodic assessment of six domains of patient health that correspond with the goals of asthma therapy are now recommended, including signs and symptoms, pulmonary function, quality of life, history of exacerbations, pharmacotherapy, and patient-provider communication and patient satisfaction.

- The following changes affecting peak flow monitoring have been made:

  The recommendation for peak flow monitoring was changed from twice daily to morning. If the morning reading is less than 80 percent of personal best PEF, more frequent peak flow monitoring may be desired.

  Discussion of inconsistencies in measurement among peak flow meters was added.

  Use of the individual patient's personal best PEF is emphasized strongly.

- The recommendation for patients at all severity levels to monitor symptoms to recognize early signs of deterioration is emphasized.

- Sample questions to use in periodic assessments were added.

Goals of Therapy

The purpose of periodic assessment and ongoing monitoring is to determine whether the goals of asthma therapy are being achieved. The goals of therapy are as follows:

- Prevent chronic and troublesome symptoms (e.g., coughing or breathlessness in the night, in the early morning, or after exertion)
- Maintain (near) "normal" pulmonary function
- Maintain normal activity levels (including exercise and other physical activity)
- Prevent recurrent exacerbations of asthma and minimize the need for emergency department visits or hospitalizations
- Provide optimal pharmacotherapy with minimal or no adverse effects
- Meet patients' and families' expectations of and satisfaction with asthma care

Assessment Measures

The Expert Panel recommends ongoing monitoring in the six areas listed below to determine whether the goals of therapy are being met. The assessment measures for monitoring these six areas are described in this section and are recommended based on the opinion of the Expert Panel.

- Monitoring signs and symptoms of asthma
- Monitoring pulmonary function
- Spirometry
- Peak flow monitoring
- Monitoring quality of life/functional status
- Monitoring history of asthma exacerbations
- Monitoring patient-provider communication and patient satisfaction

Monitoring Signs and Symptoms of Asthma

Every patient with asthma should be taught to recognize symptom patterns that indicate inadequate asthma control (see Patient Self-Assessment section and Component 4). Symptom monitoring should be used as a means to determine the need for intervention, including additional medication, in the context of an action plan (see Figure 4-5 [omitted]).

Symptoms and clinical signs of asthma should be assessed at each health care visit through physical examination and appropriate questions. This is crucial to optimal asthma care. A description of the important elements of an asthma-related physical examination can be found in Component 1—Initial Assessment and Diagnosis, which also discusses the variability in the types of symptoms associated with asthma.

Detailed patient recall of symptoms decreases over time; therefore, the Expert Panel recommends that any detailed symptoms history be based on a short (two to four weeks) recall period. For example, the clinician may choose to assess over a two-week, three-week, or four-week recall period (see Figure 1-6 [omitted]). Symptom assessment for periods longer than four weeks should reflect more global symptom assessment, such as inquiring whether the patient's asthma has been better or worse since the last visit and inquiring whether the patient has encountered any particular difficulties during specific seasons or events. Figure 1-6 provides an example of a set of questions that can be used to characterize both global (long-term recall) and recent (short-term recall) asthma symptoms.

In addition, any assessment of the patient's symptom history should include at least three key symptom expressions:

- Daytime asthma symptoms (including wheezing, cough, chest tightness, or shortness of breath)
- Nocturnal awakening as a result of asthma symptoms
- Monitoring pharmacotherapy
- Asthma symptoms early in the morning that are not improved 15 minutes after inhaling a short-acting beta$_2$-agonist

Monitoring Pulmonary Function

In addition to assessing symptoms, it is also important to periodically assess pulmonary function. The main methods are spirometry and peak flow monitoring.

Regular monitoring of pulmonary function is particularly important for asthma patients who do not perceive their symptoms until airflow obstruction is severe. Currently, there is no readily available method of detecting the "poor perceivers." The literature reports that patients who had a near fatal asthma exacerbation, as well as older patients, are more likely to have poor perception of airflow obstruction (Kikuchi et al. 1994; Connolly et al. 1992).

Spirometry

The Expert Panel recommends that spirometry tests be done (1) at the time of initial assessment; (2) after treatment is initiated and symptoms and peak expiratory flow (PEF) have stabilized, to document attainment of (near) "normal" airway function; and (3) at least every one to two years to assess the maintenance of airway function.

Spirometry may be indicated more often than every one to two years, depending on the clinical severity and response to management. Spirometry with measurement of the FEV$_1$ is also useful:

- As a periodic (e.g., yearly) check on the accuracy of the peak flow meter (Miles et al. 1995)

- When more precision is desired in measuring lung function (e.g., when evaluating response to bronchodilator or nonspecific airway responsiveness or when assessing response to a "step down" in pharmacotherapy)
- When PEF results are unreliable (e.g., in some very young or elderly patients or when neuromuscular or orthopedic problems are present) and the physician needs the quality checks that are available only with spirometry (Hankinson and Wagner 1993).

For routine monitoring at most outpatient visits, measurement of PEF with a peak flow meter is generally a sufficient assessment of pulmonary function, particularly in mild intermittent, mild persistent, and moderate persistent asthma.

Peak Flow Monitoring

Peak expiratory flow provides a simple, quantitative, and reproducible measure of the existence and severity of airflow obstruction. PEF can be measured with inexpensive and portable peak flow meters. *It must be stressed that peak flow meters are designed as tools for ongoing monitoring, not diagnosis.* Because the measurement of PEF is dependent on effort and technique, patients need instructions, demonstrations, and frequent reviews of technique (see Figure 1-7 [omitted], the patient handout How to Use Your Peak Flow Meter).

Peak flow monitoring can be used for short-term monitoring, managing exacerbations, and daily long-term monitoring. When used in these ways, the patient's measured personal best is the most appropriate reference value. Four studies (Woolcock et al. 1988; Ignacio-Garcia and Gonzalez-Santos 1995; Lahdensuo et al. 1996; Beasley et al. 1989) have found that comprehensive asthma self-management programs, in which peak flow monitoring was a component, achieved significant improvements in health outcomes. Thus far, the few studies that have isolated a comparison of peak flow and symptom monitoring have not been sufficient to assess the relative contributions of each to asthma management (see Box 1, Peak Flow Monitoring Literature Review). The literature does suggest which patients may benefit most from peak flow monitoring. The Expert Panel concludes, on the basis of this literature and the panel's opinion, that:

- Patients with moderate-to-severe persistent asthma should learn how to monitor their PEF and have a peak flow meter at home.
- Peak flow monitoring during exacerbations of asthma is recommended for patients with moderate-to-severe persistent asthma to:
  Determine severity of the exacerbation
  Guide therapeutic decisions (see Component 3 [omitted]—Managing Exacerbations and Figure 4-5) in the home, clinician's office, or emergency department
- Long-term daily peak flow monitoring is helpful in managing patients with moderate-to-severe persistent asthma to:
  Detect early changes in disease status that require treatment
  Evaluate responses to changes in therapy
  Provide assessment of severity for patients with poor perception of airflow obstruction
  Afford a quantitative measure of impairment
- If long-term daily peak flow monitoring is not used, a short-term (two to three weeks) period of peak flow monitoring is recommended to:
  Evaluate responses to changes in chronic maintenance therapy
  Identify temporal relationship between changes in PEF and exposure to environmental or occupational irritants or allergens. It may be necessary to record PEF four or more times a day (Chan-Yeung 1995).
- The Expert Panel does not recommend long-term daily peak flow monitoring for patients with mild intermittent or mild persistent asthma unless the patient/family and/or clinician find it useful in guiding therapeutic decisions. Any patient who develops severe exacerbations may benefit from peak flow monitoring.

Limitations of long-term peak flow monitoring include:

- Difficulty in maintaining adherence to monitoring (Reeder et al. 1990; Chmelik and Doughty 1994; Mao et al. 1993), often due to inconve-

nience, lack of required level of motivation, or lack of a specific treatment plan based on PEF
- Potential for incorrect readings related to poor technique, misinterpretation, or device failure

Whether peak flow monitoring, symptom monitoring, or a combination of approaches is used, the Expert Panel believes that self-monitoring is important to the effective self-management of asthma The nature and intensity of self-monitoring should be individualized, based on such factors as asthma severity, patient's ability to perceive airflow obstruction, availability of peak flow meters, and patient preferences.

It is the opinion of the Expert Panel that, regardless of the type of monitoring used, patients should be given a written action plan and be instructed to use it . . . The panel believes it is especially important to give a written action plan to patients with moderate-to-severe persistent asthma and any patient with a history of severe exacerbations. The action plan will describe the actions patients should take based on their signs and symptoms and/or PEF. The clinician should periodically review the plan, revise it as necessary, and confirm that the patient knows what to do if his or her asthma gets worse.

Recommendations on How to Monitor Peak Flow
The Expert Panel recommends that patients who are using a peak flow meter be instructed on how to establish their personal best peak expiratory flow (figure 1-7 [omitted]) and use it as the basis of their action plan (figure 4-5 [omitted]). Meters used to measure PEF should meet American Thoracic Society recommendations for monitoring devices (American Thoracic Society 1995).

The patients personal best PEF can be estimated after a two to three week period in which the patient records PEF two to four times per day. The personal best value is usually achieved in the early afternoon measurement after maximal therapy has stabilized the patient (Quackenboss et al. 1991). A course of oral corticosteroids may be needed to establish the personal best PEF. The patient's personal best value should be reassessed periodically to account for progression of disease in children and adults and for growth in children. Occasionally, a PEF value is recorded that is markedly higher than other values. This may be due to "spitting" (especially if the peak flow meter mouthpiece is small) or coughing into the peak flow meter, as well as other reasons that are not well understood.

Therefore, caution should be used in establishing a personal best value when an outlying value is observed. Children with moderato-to-severe persistent asthma should repeat the short-term monitoring period every six months to establish changes in personal best PEF that occur with growth.

Patients requiring daily peak flow monitoring should measure their PEF on waking from sleep in the morning before taking a bronchodilator, if the patient uses a bronchodilator (Reddel et al. 1995; Morris et al. 1994). When the morning PEF is below 80 percent of the patient's personal best, PEF should be measured more than once a day (again, before taking a bronchodilator). This recommendation is based, not on scientific data, but on the logic of reducing delays in treatment. The additional measurements of PEF during the day will enable patients to detect if their asthma is continuing to worsen or is improving after taking medication. If their asthma is worsening, they will have the opportunity to quickly respond to this. In addition, periodically having patients take their PEF first thing in the morning and in the early afternoon for one to two weeks will assess airflow variability, which is an indicator of the current level of the patient's asthma severity (see figure 1-3 and Additional Studies section, page 19 [omitted]).

It is the Expert Panel's opinion that, in general, PEF below 80 percent of the patient's personal best before bronchodilator inhalation indicates a need for additional medication. PEF below 50 percent indicates a severe asthma exacerbation (see Component 3 for recommended treatment). These cutpoints of 80 and 50 percent of the personal best are somewhat arbitrary. The emphasis is not on a specific PEF value but, rather, on a patient's change from personal best or from one reading to the next. Cutpoints should be tailored to individual patients' needs and PEF patterns.

Cutpoints may be easier to use and remember when they are adapted to a traffic light system . . . (Lewis et al. 1984; Mendoza et al. 1988; Plaut 1995). In this system, for example, the green zone (80 to 100 percent of personal best) signals good control, the yellow zone (50 to less than 80 percent of personal best) signals caution, and the red zone (below 50 percent of personal best) signals a medical alert (see figure 1-7 [omitted]). Because the yellow zone includes a wide spectrum of asthma severity, clinicians may consider recommending different interventions for a high yellow zone (e.g., 65 to less than 80 percent of personal best) and a low yellow zone (e.g., 50 to less than 65 percent of personal best).

—Excerpted from the Expert Panel Report

APPENDIX VI
EDUCATION FOR A PARTNERSHIP
IN ASTHMA CARE

(Adapted from the *Expert Panel Report 2: Guidelines for the Diagnosis and Management of Asthma* published in April 1997 by the National Institutes of Health, National Heart, Lung, and Blood Institute, NIH Publication No. 97-4051)

Patient education is an essential component of successful asthma management. Current management approaches require patients and families to effectively carry out complex pharmacologic regimens, institute environmental control strategies, detect and self-treat most asthma exacerbations, and communicate appropriately with health care providers. Patient education is the mechanism through which patients learn to successfully accomplish those tasks. It is also a powerful tool for helping patients gain the motivation, skill, and confidence to control their asthma.

Research shows that asthma education can be cost-effective and can reduce morbidity for both adults and children, especially among high-risk patients. The following are strategies for enhancing the delivery of patient education and improving the likelihood that patients will follow clinical recommendations, as well as key messages to communicate to the patient.

Establish a partnership. Patient education should begin at the time of diagnosis and be integrated into every step of medical care, in the context of medical appointments and other clinician-patient communication. When clinicians take the time to provide education, it sends a powerful message to patients and families about the importance of knowledgeable self-management of asthma. From the time of diagnosis, the clinician and other members of the health care team should begin to build a partnership with the patient and family. Building the partnership requires that clin-

icians promote open communication and ensure that patients have a basic and accurate foundation of knowledge about asthma, understand the treatment approach, and have the self-management skills necessary to monitor the disease objectively, and take medication effectively.

When nurses, pharmacists, respiratory therapists, and other health care professionals are available to support and expand patient education, a team approach should be used. The principal clinician should introduce the key educational messages and negotiate agreements with patients. Team members should document in the patient's record the key educational points, patient concerns, and actions the patient agrees to take.

Clinicians should teach basic facts about asthma so that the patient and family understand the rationale for needed actions. Give a brief verbal description of what asthma is and the intended role of each medication. Do not overwhelm the patient with too much information all at once, but repeat the important messages at each visit. Ask the patient to bring all medications to each appointment for review.

Teach the patient necessary medication skills, such as correct use of the inhaler and spacer/holding chamber and knowing when and how to take quick-relief medications.

Teach self-monitoring skills: symptom monitoring, peak flow monitoring as appropriate, and recognizing early signs of deterioration.

Teach relevant environmental control/avoidance strategies. Teach how environmental precipitants or exposures can make the patient's asthma worse (e.g., allergens and irritants) at home, school, and work, and how to recognize both immediate and delayed reactions.

Jointly develop treatment goals. Fundamental to building a partnership is for clinicians and patients to jointly develop and agree on both short- and long-term treatment goals. Such agreements can encourage active participation, enhance the partnership, and improve asthma management. It is the opinion of the Expert Panel that clinicians should:

Determine the patient's personal treatment goals. Ask how the asthma interferes with the patient's life (e.g., inability to sleep through the night, play a sport) and incorporate the responses into personal treatment goals. Asthma-specific quality-of-life instruments may be useful.

Share the general goals of asthma treatment with the patient and family. Tell patients, "Our goals are to have you: *Be free from severe symptoms day and night, including sleeping through the night; Have the best possible lung function; Be able to participate fully in any activities of your choice; Not miss work or school because of asthma symptoms; Need fewer or no urgent care visits and hospitalizations for asthma; Use medications to control asthma with as few side effects as possible; and Be satisfied with your asthma care.*"

Agree on the goals of treatment. The clinicians, the patient, and when appropriate, the patient's family should agree on the goals of asthma management, which include both the patient's personal goals and the general goals suggested by the clinicians.

Provide the patient with tools for self-management. It is the opinion of the Expert Panel that, at the first visit, clinicians should develop a written, individualized, daily self-management plan in consultation with the patient. Include the recommended doses and frequencies of daily medications and the daily self-management activities needed to achieve the agreed-on goals. Review and refine the plan at subsequent follow-up visits. List the treatment goals in the plan and explain how following the plan will help the patient reach those goals. Emphasizing the patient's personal goals is

essential to enhancing adherence. For example, ask, "Have you had any problems taking your bronchodilator immediately before playing basketball? Has it helped you stay in the game?"

Discuss the long-term benefits of following the written, daily self-management plan. For some patients, focusing on long-term treatment goals and discussing "the big picture" of asthma control and how medications can be adjusted over time may improve adherence.

Also at the first visit, jointly develop a written action plan to help the patient manage asthma exacerbations. This is especially important for patients with moderate-to-severe persistent asthma and patients with a history of severe exacerbations. Review and refine the plan at follow-up visits. The action plan directs the patient to adjust medicines at home in response to particular signs, symptoms, and peak flow measurements. It should also list the PEF levels and symptoms indicating the need for acute care and emergency telephone numbers for the physician, emergency department, rapid transportation, and family/friend for aid and support. Clinicians should choose an action plan that suits their practice, patients, and style.

It is the opinion of the Expert Panel that clinicians should provide an asthma diary to appropriate patients for self-monitoring symptoms, peak flow measurements, frequency of daily quick-relief inhaler medication use, and activity restriction.

Encourage adherence. Use effective techniques to promote open communication. Early in each visit, elicit the patient's concerns, perceptions, and unresolved questions about his or her asthma. A question such as "What worries you most about your asthma?" which cannot be answered yes or no, encourages patients and families to voice issues, personal beliefs, or concerns they may be apprehensive about discussing or may not think are of interest to the clinician. These potential barriers to adherence can be dealt with only if they are identified. By asking about and discussing such concerns, clinicians build trust and a sense of partnership with the patient. Most nonadherence originates in personal beliefs or concerns about asthma that have not been discussed with the clinician. Until such fears and worries are identified and addressed, patients will not be able to adhere to the clinician's recommendations.

Assess the patient's and family's perceptions of the severity level of the disease. Two questions may prove useful: "How severe do you think your asthma is?" and "How much danger do you believe you are in from your asthma?" When patients are identified who are overwhelmed by fear of death, put their fears in perspective by providing them with the results of objective assessments and expert opinion. A clearly written, detailed action plan that directs the patient how to respond to worsening asthma may be extremely helpful in reducing anxiety. Patients' perceptions about their disease severity and its threat to their well-being influence self-management behavior and use of the health care system.

Assess the patient's and family's level of social support. Ask, "Who among your family or friends can you turn to for help if your asthma worsens?" Counsel patients to identify an asthma "partner" among their family or friends who is willing to be educated and provide support. Include at least one of these individuals in follow-up appointments so that he or she can hear what is expected of the patient in following the self-management and action plans.

Encourage or enlist family involvement. Ask patients to identify ways their family members can help them follow the plans. Ask the patient to share the plans with family members, elicit their input, and agree on actions they can help with. It may be helpful for children and parents to discuss this with a clinician present.

Consider referral to a psychologist, social worker, psychiatrist, or other licensed professional when stress seems to unduly interfere with daily asthma management. As with other chronic diseases, emotional and social stress may be a confounding factor for many patients struggling with asthma control. Although stress does not cause asthma, it can play a role in precipitating asthma exacerbations and can complicate an individual's attempts at self-management. Referral to a local support group may be useful.

Use methods to increase the chances that the patient will adhere to the written, daily self-management plan. For instance, adherence to the self-

management plan is enhanced when the plan is simplified as much as possible, when the number of medications and frequency of daily doses are minimized, when the medication doses and frequency fit into the patient's and family's daily routine, and when the plan considers the patient's ability to afford the medications. Because nonadherence is difficult for clinicians to detect, it is prudent to explore potential barriers to adherence with every patient by asking what concerns they have about medicines (e.g., safety) or other aspects of treatment.

Tailor education to the needs of the individual patient. Assess cultural or ethnic beliefs or practices that may influence and modify educational approaches, as needed. Cultural variables may affect patient understanding of and adherence to medical regimens. Open-ended questions such as "In your community, what does having asthma mean?" can elicit informative responses. The culturally sensitive clinician should attempt to find ways to incorporate harmless or potentially beneficial remedies with the pharmacologic plan. For example, a prevalent belief among the Latino population is that illnesses are either "hot" or "cold." Asthma is viewed as a "cold" illness amenable to "hot" treatment. Suggesting that asthma medications be taken with hot tea or hot water incorporates this belief into the therapeutic regimen and helps build the therapeutic partnership. When harmful home remedies are being used, clinicians should discourage their use of suggesting a culturally acceptable alternative as a replacement or recommending a safer route of administration. These and other strategies may be useful in working with ethnic minorities.

Every effort should be made to discuss asthma care, especially the self-management plan, in the patient's native language so that educational messages are fully understood. Research suggests that lack of language concordance between the clinician and the patient affects adherence and appropriate use of health care services. Language barriers also may complicate the assessment of cultural differences. If interpreters are used, they should be equally competent in both English and the patient's language and knowledgeable about medical terms.

Maintain the partnership. As part of ongoing care, the clinician should continue to build the partnership by being a sympathetic coach and by helping the patient follow the self-management plan and take other needed actions. Educational efforts should be continuous, because it may take up to six months for the impact of education to be evident. Furthermore, it is necessary to periodically review information and skills covered previously because patient self-management behavior is likely to decline over time.

In particular, it is essential that clinicians demonstrate, review, evaluate, and correct inhaler/spacer/holding chamber technique at each visit because these skills deteriorate rapidly. Written instructions are helpful, but insufficient. Research suggests that patients tend to make specific mistakes in using inhalers that need to be corrected. Patients especially need to be reminded to inhale slowly and to activate the inhaler only once for each breath.

Clinicians should continue to promote open communication with the patient and family by addressing the following elements in each follow-up visit:

- Continue asking patients early in each visit what concerns they have about their asthma and what they especially want addressed during the visit.

- Review the short-term goals agreed upon in the initial visit. Assess how well they are being achieved (e.g., was the patient's wish to engage in physical activity achieved?). Revise the goals as needed. Achievement of short-term goals should be discussed as indicators that the patient is moving toward long-term goals. Give positive verbal reinforcement for achievement of a goal and recognize the patient's success in moving closer to full control of the disease.

- Review the daily self-management plan and the steps the patient was to take. Adjust the plan as needed (e.g., the recommendations of how to use medicines if the dose or type is not working). Identify other problems the patient has in following the agreed-upon steps (e.g., disguising the bad taste of medicine); treat these as areas needing more work, not as adherence failures. Write a self-management plan to help school personnel manage a child's asthma.

- Periodically review the asthma action plan and revise as necessary. Confirm that the patient knows what to do if his or her asthma gets worse.

- Continue teaching and reinforcing educational messages. Provide information skills over several visits so as not to overwhelm the patient with too much information at one time. Repeat important points often.

- Give patients simple, brief written materials that reinforce the actions recommended and skills taught. Many organizations distribute patient education materials, including some Spanish-language materials.

Supplement patient education delivered by clinicians. All patients may benefit from a formal asthma education program that has been evaluated and reported in the literature to be effective. These programs should be taught by qualified asthma educators who are knowledgeable about asthma and experienced in patient education. Communication among the asthma educator, the clinicians providing direct care, and the patient/family is critical. When formal programs are available in local communities, *they can supplement, but not replace,* patient education provided in the office. Individual and group programs have been developed and tested for patients of all ages, including parents of very young children (birth to four years). These patient education programs should be delivered as designed. Some validity and effectiveness may be compromised when segments of various programs are pieced together or when programs are condensed. In the interest of saving time, educators should not delete educational strategies, such as using small groups or scheduling multiple sessions spaced with "homework" assignments, because these strategies have demonstrated effectiveness in motivating individuals to make significant behavior changes.

A variety of other educational formats, such as videotapes and interactive computer software may also *enhance, but not replace,* education delivered by clinicians.

Provide patient education in other clinical settings. Patient education also should be delivered in the context of emergency department visits and hospitalization. Asthma exacerbations may represent teachable moments when patients are more receptive to educational message. Research on adults with asthma who are referred to emergency department providers to an asthma education program shows that education can decrease utilization of emergency services. Educational programs delivered to hospitalized children and adult asthma patients show increased knowledge and use of self-management behaviors, reduced length of hospital stay, and overall reduction in asthma readmissions.

Asthma Daily Self-Management Plan (EXAMPLE 1)

ASTHMA SELF-MANAGEMENT PLAN FOR _____
(Name)

YOUR TREATMENT GOALS
■ Be free from severe symptoms day and night, including sleeping through the night
■ Have the best possible lung function
■ Be able to participate fully in any activities of your choice
■ Not miss work or school because of asthma symptoms
■ Not need emergency visits or hospitalizations for asthma
■ Use asthma medications to control asthma with as few side effects as possible

Add personal goals here: _____

_____

_____

YOUR DAILY MEDICATIONS

Daily Medication   How Much To Take   When To Take It

_____

_____

_____

_____

RECORD DAILY SELF-MONITORING ACTIONS in the asthma diary your doctor gives you.

Peak flow: At least every morning when you wake up, before taking your medication, measure your peak flow and record it in your diary. Bring these records to your next appointment with your doctor.

Symptoms: Note if you had asthma symptoms (shortness of breath, wheezing, chest tightness, or cough) and rate how severe they were during the day or night: mild, moderate, severe.

Use of your quick-relief inhaler (bronchodilator): Keep a record of the number of puffs you needed to use each day or night to control your symptoms.

Actual use of daily medications

Activity restriction

This plan is provided as an example to clinicians.

Asthma Daily Self-Management Plan (EXAMPLE 2)

Long-Term Self-Management Plan for Persistent Asthma

Introduction: This long-term plan provides four benefits to the clinician and patient, who complete it together during an early visit and review it periodically. The chart (1) reflects the step-up/step-down concept of pharmacotherapy; (2) enables patient and clinician to negotiate which medicines will be used and how often; (3) combines symptoms and/or peak flow monitoring as the basis for patient's adding or deleting medicines at home and self-adjusting doses; and (4) gives the patient a view of what the clinician recommends over the long term—under what future circumstances the clinician intends that the regimen be increased or decreased.

Directions: The clinician writes the patient's medicines in the first column. Based on the symptoms and peak flow specified in the top row, the clinician then writes the doses and frequency of administration for each medication. (Some clinicians may prefer to print standard recommendations on the form to save time.)

Medication	At the FIRST sign of a cold or exposure to known trigger	If cough or wheeze is present or peak flow is between 50 and 80% of personal best	If cough or wheeze worsen or peak flow is below 50% of personal best	As soon as cough and wheeze have stopped or peak flow is above 80% of personal best	When there is no cough or wheeze for 2 weeks, even with activity or peak flow is above 80% of personal best for 2 weeks	When there is no cough or wheeze for ___ months or peak flow is above 80% of personal best for ___ months	Before exercise or physical activity	For rapidly worsening asthma (severe exacerbation)
Times per day								

(Adapted from NHLBI 1995c).

This plan is provided as an example to clinicians.

Please note that the following long-term plan is included only as an example of how to fill out the plan. The treatment regimen itself does not correspond to recommendations made in the *Expert Panel Report II: Guidelines for the Diagnosis and Management of Asthma.*

Long-Term Self-Management Plan for Persistent Asthma (EXAMPLE ONLY)

Medication	At the FIRST sign of a cold or exposure to known trigger	If cough or wheeze is present / or / peak flow is between 50 and 80% of personal best	If cough or wheeze worsen / or / peak flow is below 50% of personal best	As soon as cough and wheeze have stopped / or / peak flow is above 80% of personal best	When there is no cough or wheeze for 2 weeks, even with activity / or / peak flow is above 80% of personal best for 2 weeks	When there is no cough or wheeze for ___ months / or / peak flow is above 80% of personal best for ___ months	Before exercise or physical activity	For rapidly worsening asthma (severe exacerbation)
Short-acting beta$_2$-agonist	2 puffs	2 puffs	2 puffs	2 puffs	0	0	2 puffs	2 puffs
Nonsteroidal anti-inflammatory	2 puffs	2 puffs	2 puffs	2 puffs	2 puffs	2 puffs	0	0
Inhaled corticosteroid	2 puffs	4 puffs	4 puffs	2 puffs	2 puffs	0	0	0
Antibiotic								
TIMES PER DAY	3	4 (every 4 hours)	4 (every 4 hours)	3	3	3	5-10 minutes before exercise	every 20 minutes for 3 doses*
Oral corticosteroid	0	0	2 mg/kg/day x 2 days then 1 mg/kg/day x 3 days	0	0	0	0	0

*If there is not a good response, seek emergency care immediately. If there is a good response, return to the third column.

Asthma Action Plan (EXAMPLE 1)

Name _____   Date _____

ASTHMA ACTION PLAN

It is important in managing asthma to keep track of your symptoms, medications, and peak expiratory flow (PEF). You can use the colors of a traffic light to help learn your asthma medications:

A. Green means Go - use preventive (anti-inflammatory) medicine
B. Yellow means Caution - use quick-relief (short-acting bronchodilator) medicine in addition to the preventive medicine.
C. Red means STOP! - get help from a doctor.

---

a. Your GREEN ZONE is _____ 80 to 100% of your personal best. GO!
Breathing is good with no cough, wheeze, or chest tightness during work, school, exercise, or play.
ACTION:
■ Continue with medications listed in your daily treatment plan.

---

b. Your YELLOW ZONE is _____ 50 to less than 80% of your personal best. CAUTION!
Asthma symptoms are present (cough, wheeze, chest tightness).
Your peak flow number drops below _____ or you notice:
　■ Increased need for inhaled quick-relief medicine
　■ Increased asthma symptoms upon awakening
　■ Awakening at night with asthma symptoms
　■ _____
ACTIONS:
■ Take _____ puffs of your quick-relief (bronchodilator) medicine _____ .
　Repeat _____ times.
■ Take _____ puffs of _____ (anti-inflammatory) _____ times/day.
■ Begin/increase treatment with oral steroids:
　Take _____ mg of _____ every a.m. _____ p.m. _____ .
■ Call your doctor (phone)_____ or emergency room (phone)_____ .

---

c. Your RED ZONE is _____ 50% or less of your best. DANGER!!
Your peak flow number drops below _____, or you continue to get worse after increasing treatment according to the directions above.
ACTIONS:
■ Take _____ puffs of your quick-relief (bronchodilator) medicine _____ .
　Repeat _____ times.
■ Begin/increase treatment with oral steroids: Take _____ mg now.
■ Call your doctor now (phone)_____ .
　If you cannot contact your doctor, go directly to the emergency room (phone)_____ .
　Other important phone numbers for transportation _____ .

AT ANY TIME, CALL YOUR DOCTOR IF:
　■ Asthma symptoms worsen while you are taking oral steroids, or
　■ Inhaled bronchodilator treatments are not lasting 4 hours, or
　■ Your peak flow number remains or falls below _____ in spite of following the plan.

Physician Signature_____   Patient's/Family Member's Signature_____

This plan is provided as an example to clinicians.

Asthma Action Plan (EXAMPLE 2)

Name:

Doctor's Name:

Doctor's Phone:

Baseline/Personal Best Peak Flow:

Medicines:

← Fold Here

Asthma
Action
Plan

ZONE	ACTIONS
GREEN	
YELLOW	
RED	

Adapted with permission from Cecilia Vicuña-Keady, R.N.
This plan is provided as an example to clinicians.

Asthma Action Plan (EXAMPLE 3)

**ADULT SELF-MANAGEMENT INSTRUCTIONS
FOR ASTHMA ACTION PLAN**
DATE -_____.

When to Monitor Peak Flow Numbers
- ☐ In the morning soon after waking up.
- ☐ Before supper.
- ☐ Before bed.
- ☐ Before and 5-15 minutes after inhaled treatments.
- ☐ With increased respiratory symptoms.
- ☐ _____.

Important Peak Flow Numbers
Baseline _____.
_____ % baseline _____.
_____ % baseline _____.

If your peak flow number drops below_____ or you notice:
- • Increased use of inhaled treatments to manage asthma
- • Increased asthma symptoms upon awakening
- • Awakening at night with asthma symptoms
- • _____.

Follow these treatment steps:
- ☐ Increase inhaled steroids.
  Take_____ puffs of _____ _____times a day.
- ☐ Begin/increase treatment with oral steroids.
  Take_____ mg of _____.
  In the ☐ morning and /or ☐ before supper.
- ☐ _____.

If your peak flow number drops below_____ or you continue to get worse after increasing treatment according to the directions above, follow these treatment steps:
- ☐ Begin/increase treatment with oral steroids.
  Take_____mg of _____.
  In the ☐ morning and /or ☐ before supper.
- ☐ Contact your health care provider.

Contact your health care provider if:
- ☐ Asthma symptoms worsen while you are taking oral steroids or,
- ☐ Inhaled bronchodilator treatments are not lasting 4 hours or,
- ☐ Your peak flow number falls below_____.
- ☐ If you cannot contact your health care provider go directly to the Emergency Room.

Directions for Resuming Normal Treatment:
- ☐ Continue increased treatment until symptoms and peak flow number have returned to normal, then continue increased inhaled steroids or _____ mg of oral steroids for the same number of days it took to return to normal. If your peak flow number has not returned to normal in 5 days contact your health care provider.
- ☐ Call your health care provider for specific instructions.

If you have questions please call:
- ☐   ☐ Other_____ After hours
- ☐ Your home physician.

Physician Signature _____ Date _____

Patient/Family Signature_____ Staff Signature _____

T-101 1/95

Asthma Action Plan (EXAMPLE 4)

ASTHMA ACTION PLAN (Peak Flow monitoring)

ZONE	LEVEL	STATUS	ACTION
Green Zone: All Clear My best peak Flow: _____ **Peak Flow:** _____ to _____ (100 - 80% of My Best Peak Flow) • No symptoms of an asthma episode • Able to do usual activities • Usual medications control asthma	**1**	DOING WELL	**TAKE:** Medicine Dose Max # times/day _____ _____ _____ _____ _____ _____ _____ _____ _____
Yellow Zone: Caution Peak Flow: _____ to _____ (80 - 50% of My Best Peak Flow) • Increased asthma symptoms (including wakening at night due to asthma) • Usual activities somewhat limited • Increased need for asthma medications	**2**	INCREASE IN SYMPTOMS	**ADD:** Medicine Dose Max # times/day _____ _____ _____ Return to Level 1 when symptoms improve
Red Zone: Medical Alert Peak Flow: Less than _____ (50% of My Best Peak Flow) • Increased symptoms longer than 24 hrs • Very short of breath • Usual activities severely limited • Asthma medications haven't reduced symptoms	**3**	NO IMPROVEMENT AFTER ____ HRS or EVEN MORE SYMPTOMS	**ADD:** Medicine Dose _____ _____ _____ _____ **AND CALL YOUR PROVIDER**

DANGER SIGNS:
- DIFFICULTY WALKING AND TALKING DUE TO SHORTNESS OF BREATH
- LIPS OR FINGERNAILS ARE BLUE

☞ GO TO THE HOSPITAL NOW
☞ OR CALL 911 NOW

Used with permission from Kaiser Permanente Center for Health Research, Portland, OR.
This plan is provided as an example to clinicians.

Asthma Action Plan (EXAMPLE 5)

ASTHMA ACTION PLAN (Symptom monitoring)

LEVEL	STATUS	ACTION
All Clear • No symptoms of an asthma episode • Able to do usual activities • Usual medications control asthma **1**	DOING WELL	**TAKE:** Medicine Dose Max # times/day _____ _____ _____ _____ _____ _____ _____ _____ _____
Caution • Increased asthma symptoms (including wakening at night due to asthma) • Usual activities somewhat limited • Increased need for asthma medications **2**	INCREASE IN SYMPTOMS	**ADD:** Medicine Dose Max # times/day _____ _____ _____ Return to Level 1 when symptoms improve
Medical Alert • Increased symptoms longer than 24 hrs • Very short of breath • Usual activities severely limited • Asthma medications haven't reduced symptoms **3**	NO IMPROVEMENT AFTER ____ HRS or EVEN MORE SYMPTOMS	**ADD:** Medicine Dose _____ _____ _____ _____ **AND CALL YOUR PROVIDER**

DANGER SIGNS:
- DIFFICULTY WALKING AND TALKING DUE TO SHORTNESS OF BREATH
- LIPS OR FINGERNAILS ARE BLUE

☞ GO TO THE HOSPITAL NOW
☞ OR CALL 911 NOW

Adapted with permission from Kaiser Permanente Center for Health Research, Portland, OR.
This plan is provided as an example to clinicians.

Asthma Action Plan (EXAMPLE 6)

For adults, teens, and children age 5 and over
PEAK FLOW-BASED HOME TREATMENT PLAN

Name: _____   Date: _____   Best Peak Flow: _____

GREEN ZONE: Peak flow between _____ and _____.

Normal activity. (Insert brand name in blanks.)

❑ Adrenaline-like medicine: albuterol (_____), pirbuterol (_____), or terbuterol (_____): 1 or 2 puffs 15 minutes before exercise.

❑ Nedocromil (_____) or cromolyn (_____): 2 puffs before contact with cat or other allergen.

Medicine to be taken every day:

❑ Nedocromil (_____) or cromolyn (_____): ____ puffs ____ times a day (a total of ____ puffs daily).

❑ Inhaled steroid (_____): ____ puffs ____ times a day (a total of ____ puffs daily).

❑ Adrenaline-like medicine (see above): ____ puffs before each *nedocromil, cromolyn,* or *inhaled steroid* dose for the first month.

❑ Other:

HIGH YELLOW ZONE: Peak flow between _____ and _____.

Eliminate triggers and change medicines. No strenuous exercise.

Medicine to be taken:

❑ Adrenaline-like medicine: ____ puffs by holding chamber. Give three to six times in 24 hours. Continue until peak flow is in the *Green Zone* for 2 days.

❑ Double *inhaled steroid* to ____ puffs daily until peak flow is in the *Green Zone* for as long as it was in the *Yellow Zone.*

❑ Other:

LOW YELLOW ZONE: Peak flow between _____ and _____.

Follow this plan if peak flow does not reach *High Yellow Zone* within 10 minutes after taking inhaled adrenaline-like medicine, or drops back into *Low Yellow Zone* within 4 hours:

❑ Continue adrenaline-like medicine treatment as above.

❑ Add *oral steroid** ____ mg immediately. Continue each morning (8:00 a.m.) until peak flow is in the *Green Zone* for at least 24 hours.

❑ Please call the office before starting oral steroid.

* If your condition does not improve within 2 days after starting oral steroid, or if peak flow does not reach the *Green Zone* within 7 days of treatment, see your doctor.

RED ZONE: Peak flow less than _____.

Follow this plan if peak flow does not reach *Low Yellow Zone* within 10 minutes after taking inhaled adrenaline-like medicine, or drops back into *Red Zone* within 4 hours.

✔ Adrenaline-like medicine: ____ puffs by holding chamber.

✔ Give oral steroid ____ mg.

✔ Visit your doctor or go to the emergency room.

Green Zone

Yellow Zone

Red Zone

Adapted with permission from Plaut and Brennan 1996.
This plan is provided as an example to clinicians.

Asthma and Allergy
Foundation of America
1125 15th St., N.W., Suite 502
Washington, DC 20005

STUDENT ASTHMA
ACTION CARD

Endorsed by

National Asthma
Education Program

ID Photo

Name: _____ Grade: _____ Age: _____

Teacher: _____ Room: _____

Parent/Guardian Name: _____ Ph: (H) _____

Address:_____ Ph: (W) _____

Parent/Guardian Name: _____ Ph: (H) _____

Address:_____ Ph: (W) _____

Emergency Phone Contact #1 _____

Name   Relationship   Phone

Emergency Phone Contact #2 _____

Name   Relationship   Phone

Physician Student Sees for Asthma: _____ Ph: _____

Other Physician: _____ Ph: _____

DAILY ASTHMA MANAGEMENT PLAN

- **Identify the things which start an asthma episode (Check each that applies to the student.)**

  ☐ Exercise   ☐ Strong odors or fumes   ☐ Other _____

  ☐ Respiratory infections   ☐ Chalk dust   _____

  ☐ Change in temperature   ☐ Carpets in the room

  ☐ Animals   ☐ Pollens

  ☐ Food _____ ☐ Molds

  Comments _____

- **Control of School Environment**

  (List any environmental control measures, pre-medications, and/or dietary restrictions that the student needs to prevent an asthma episode.)

  _____

  _____

  _____

- **Peak Flow Monitoring**

  Personal Best Peak Flow number: _____

  Monitoring Times: _____ _____ _____

- **Daily Medication Plan**

	Name	Amount	When to Use
1.	_____	_____	_____
2.	_____	_____	_____
3.	_____	_____	_____
4.	_____	_____	_____

EMERGENCY PLAN

Emergency action is necessary when the student has symptoms such as _____, _____, _____, _____ or has a peak flow reading of _____.

- **Steps to take during an asthma episode:**

  1. Give medications as listed below.

  2. Have student return to classroom if _____ _____

  3. Contact parent if _____

  4. Seek emergency medical care if the student has any of the following:

     ✔ No improvement 15-20 minutes after initial treatment with medication and a relative cannot be reached.

     ✔ Peak flow of _____

     ✔ Hard time breathing with:

       · Chest and neck pulled in with breathing

       · Child is hunched over

       · Child is struggling to breathe

     ✔ Trouble walking or talking

     ✔ Stops playing and can't start activity again

     ✔ Lips or fingernails are gray or blue

     } *IF THIS HAPPENS, GET EMERGENCY HELP NOW!*

- **Emergency Asthma Medications**

	Name	Amount	When to Use
1.	_____	_____	_____
2.	_____	_____	_____
3.	_____	_____	_____
4.	_____	_____	_____

COMMENTS / SPECIAL INSTRUCTIONS

_____
_____
_____

FOR INHALED MEDICATIONS

☐ I have instructed _____ in the proper way to use his/her medications. It is my professional opinion that _____ should be allowed to carry and use that medication by him/herself.

☐ It is my professional opinion that _____ should not carry his/her inhaled medication by him/herself.

_____   _____
Physician Signature   Date

_____   _____
Parent Signature   Date

This plan is provided as an example.

APPENDIX VII

STEPWISE APPROACHES FOR MANAGING ACUTE OR CHRONIC ASTHMA SYMPTOMS IN INFANTS AND CHILDREN UNDER AGE FIVE AND ADULTS AND CHILDREN OVER AGE FIVE

Stepwise Approach for Managing Asthma in Adults and Children Older Than 5 Years of Age

Goals of Asthma Treatment
- Prevent chronic and troublesome symptoms (e.g., coughing or breathlessness in the night, in the early morning, or after exertion)
- Maintain (near) "normal" pulmonary function
- Maintain normal activity levels (including exercise and other physical activity)
- Prevent recurrent exacerbations of asthma and minimize the need for emergency department visits or hospitalizations
- Provide optimal pharmacotherapy with minimal or no adverse effects
- Meet patients' and families' expectations of and satisfaction with asthma care

Classify Severity of Asthma

Clinical Features Before Treatment*

	Symptoms**	Nighttime Symptoms	Lung Function
STEP 4 **Severe Persistent**	■ Continual symptoms ■ Limited physical activity ■ Frequent exacerbations	Frequent	■ FEV_1 or PEF ≤60% predicted ■ PEF variability >30%
STEP 3 **Moderate Persistent**	■ Daily symptoms ■ Daily use of inhaled short-acting beta$_2$-agonist ■ Exacerbations affect activity ■ Exacerbations ≥2 times a week; may last days	>1 time a week	■ FEV_1 or PEF >60% - <80% predicted ■ PEF variability >30%
STEP 2 **Mild Persistent**	■ Symptoms >2 times a week but <1 time a day ■ Exacerbations may affect activity	>2 times a month	■ FEV_1 or PEF ≥80% predicted ■ PEF variability 20-30%
STEP 1 **Mild Intermittent**	■ Symptoms ≤2 times a week ■ Asymptomatic and normal PEF between exacerbations ■ Exacerbations brief (from a few hours to a few days); intensity may vary	≤2 times a month	■ FEV_1 or PEF ≥80% predicted ■ PEF variability <20%

* The presence of one of the features of severity is sufficient to place a patient in that category. An individual should be assigned to the most severe grade in which any feature occurs. The characteristics noted in this figure are general and may overlap because asthma is highly variable. Furthermore, an individual's classification may change over time.

** Patients at any level of severity can have mild, moderate, or severe exacerbations. Some patients with intermittent asthma experience severe and life-threatening exacerbations separated by long periods of normal lung function and no symptoms.

Stepwise Approach for Managing Asthma in Adults and Children Older Than 5 Years of Age

	Treatment		Preferred treatments are in bold print.
	Long-Term Control	**Quick Relief**	**Education**
STEP 4 **Severe** **Persistent**	Daily medications: ■ **Anti-inflammatory: inhaled cortico-steroid (high dose)** AND ■ Long-acting bronchodilator: either **long-acting inhaled beta₂-agonist,** sustained-release theophylline, or long-acting beta₂-agonist tablets AND ■ Corticosteroid tablets or syrup long term (2 mg/kg/day, generally do not exceed 60 mg per day).	■ Short-acting bronchodilator: **inhaled beta₂-agonists** as needed for symptoms. ■ Intensity of treatment will depend on severity of exacerbation; see component 3-Managing Exacerbations. ■ Use of short-acting inhaled beta₂-agonists on a daily basis, or increasing use, indicates the need for additional long-term-control therapy.	Steps 2 and 3 actions plus: ■ Refer to individual education/counseling
STEP 3 **Moderate** **Persistent**	Daily medication: ■ Either 　　**Anti-inflammatory: inhaled cortico-steroid (medium dose)** 　OR 　　**Inhaled corticosteroid (low-medium dose)** and add a long-acting bronchodilator, especially for nighttime symptoms: either **long-acting inhaled beta₂-agonist,** sustained-release theophylline, or long-acting beta₂-agonist tablets. ■ If needed 　　Anti-inflammatory: **inhaled cortico-steroids (medium-high dose)** 　　AND 　　**Long-acting bronchodilator,** especially for nighttime symptoms; either **long-acting inhaled beta₂-agonist,** sustained-release theophylline, or long-acting beta₂-agonist tablets.	■ Short-acting bronchodilator: **inhaled beta₂-agonists** as needed for symptoms. ■ Intensity of treatment will depend on severity of exacerbation; see component 3-Managing Exacerbations. ■ Use of short-acting inhaled beta₂-agonists on a daily basis, or increasing use, indicates the need for additional long-term-control therapy.	Step 1 actions plus: ■ Teach self-monitoring ■ Refer to group education if available ■ Review and update self-management plan
STEP 2 **Mild** **Persistent**	One daily medication: ■ **Anti-inflammatory:** either **inhaled corticosteroid** (low doses) or **cromolyn or nedocromil** (children usually begin with a trial of cromolyn or nedocromil). ■ Sustained-release theophylline to serum concentration of 5-15 mcg/mL is an alternative, but not preferred, therapy. Zafirlukast or zileuton may also be considered for patients ≥12 years of age, although their position in therapy is not fully established.	■ Short-acting bronchodilator: **inhaled beta₂-agonists** as needed for symptoms. ■ Intensity of treatment will depend on severity of exacerbation; see component 3-Managing Exacerbations. ■ Use of short-acting inhaled beta₂-agonists on a daily basis, or increasing use, indicates the need for additional long-term-control therapy.	
STEP 1 **Mild** **Intermittent**	■ No daily medication needed.	■ Short-acting bronchodilator: **inhaled beta₂-agonists** as needed for symptoms. ■ Intensity of treatment will depend on severity of exacerbation; see component 3-Managing Exacerbations. ■ Use of short-acting inhaled beta₂-agonists more than 2 times a week may indicate the need to initiate long-term-control therapy.	■ Teach basic facts about asthma ■ Teach inhaler/spacer/holding chamber technique ■ Discuss roles of medications ■ Develop self-management plan ■ Develop action plan for when and how to take rescue actions, especially for patients with a history of severe exacerbations ■ Discuss appropriate environmental control measures to avoid exposure to known allergens and irritants (See component 4.)

↓ **Step down**
Review treatment every 1 to 6 months; a gradual stepwise reduction in treatment may be possible.

↑ **Step up**
If control is not maintained, consider step up. First, review patient medication technique, adherence, and environmental control (avoidance of allergens or other factors that contribute to asthma severity).

NOTE:
■ **The stepwise approach presents general guidelines to assist clinical decisionmaking; it is not intended to be a specific prescription. Asthma is highly variable; clinicians should tailor specific medication plans to the needs and circumstances of individual patients.**
■ Gain control as quickly as possible; then decrease treatment to the least medication necessary to maintain control. Gaining control may be accomplished by either starting treatment at the step most appropriate to the initial severity of the condition or starting at a higher level of therapy (e.g., a course of systemic corticosteroids or higher dose of inhaled corticosteroids).
■ A rescue course of systemic corticosteroids may be needed at any time and at any step.
■ Some patients with intermittent asthma experience severe and life-threatening exacerbations separated by long periods of normal lung function and no symptoms. This may be especially common with exacerbations provoked by respiratory infections. A short course of systemic corticosteroids is recommended.
■ At each step, patients should control their environment to avoid or control factors that make their asthma worse (e.g., allergens, irritants); this requires specific diagnosis and education.
■ Referral to an asthma specialist for consultation or comanagement is *recommended* if there are difficulties achieving or maintaining control of asthma or if the patient requires step 4 care. Referral may be *considered* if the patient requires step 3 care (see also component 1-Initial Assessment and Diagnosis).

Stepwise Approach for Managing Infants and Young Children (5 Years of Age and Younger) With Acute or Chronic Asthma Symptoms

	Long-Term Control	Quick Relief
STEP 4 **Severe** **Persistent**	■ Daily anti-inflammatory medicine- 　　High-dose inhaled corticosteroid with spacer/holding chamber 　　　and face mask 　　If needed, add systemic corticosteroids 2 mg/kg/day and reduce 　　　to lowest daily or alternate-day dose that stabilizes symptoms	■ Bronchodilator as needed for symptoms (see step 1) up to 3 times a day
STEP 3 **Moderate** **Persistent**	■ Daily anti-inflammatory medication. Either: 　　Medium-dose inhaled corticosteroid with spacer/holding 　　　chamber and face mask 　　OR, once control is established: 　　Medium-dose inhaled corticosteroid and nedocromil 　　OR 　　Medium-dose inhaled corticosteroid and long-acting bron- 　　　chodilator (theophylline)	■ Bronchodilator as needed for symptoms (see step 1) up to 3 times a day
STEP 2 **Mild** **Persistent**	■ Daily anti-inflammatory medication. Either: 　　Cromolyn (nebulizer is preferred; or MDI) or nedocromil (MDI 　　　only) tid-qid 　　Infants and young children usually begin with a trial of cro- 　　　molyn or nedocromil 　　OR 　　Low-dose inhaled corticosteroid with spacer/holding cham- 　　　ber and face mask	■ Bronchodilator as needed for symptoms (see step 1)
STEP 1 **Mild** **Intermittent**	■ No daily medication needed.	■ Bronchodilator as needed for symptoms <2 times a week. Intensity of treatment will depend upon severity of exacerbation (see component 3-Managing Exacerbations). Either: 　　Inhaled short-acting beta$_2$-agonist by nebulizer or face mask 　　　and spacer/holding chamber 　　OR 　　Oral beta$_2$-agonist for symptoms ■ With viral respiratory infection: 　　Bronchodilator q 4-6 hours up to 24 hours (longer with 　　　physician consult) but, in general, repeat no more than 　　　once every 6 weeks 　　Consider systemic corticosteroid if 　　　Current exacerbation is severe 　　　OR 　　　Patient has history of previous severe exacerbations

NOTES:
■ **The stepwise approach presents guidelines to assist clinical decisionmak-**
ing. Asthma is highly variable; clinicians should tailor specific medica-
tion plans to the needs and circumstances of individual patients.
■ Gain control as quickly as possible; then decrease treatment to the least medication necessary to maintain control. Gaining control may be accomplished by
either starting treatment at the step most appropriate to the initial severity of
their condition or by starting at a higher level of therapy (e.g., a course of systemic corticosteroids or higher dose of inhaled corticosteroids).
■ A rescue course of systemic corticosteroid (prednisolone) may be needed at any
time and step.
■ In general, use of short-acting beta$_2$-agonist on a daily basis indicates the need
for additional long-term-control therapy.
■ It is important to remember that there are very few studies on asthma therapy
for infants.
■ Consultation with an asthma specialist is *recommended* for patients with moderate or severe persistent asthma in this age group. Consultation should be *con-*
sidered for all patients with mild persistent asthma.

Step down
Review treatment every 1 to 6 months. If contol is sustained for at least 3
months, a gradual stepwise reduction in treatment may be possible.

Step up
If control is not achieved, consider step up. But first, review patient medication technique, adherence, and environmental control (avoidance of allergens
or other precipitant factors).

APPENDIX VIII

USUAL DOSAGES FOR QUICK-RELIEF MEDICATIONS AND LONG-TERM CONTROL MEDICATIONS

Quick-Relief Medications

Name/Products	Indications/Mechanisms	Potential Adverse Effects	Therapeutic Issues
Short-Acting Inhaled Beta$_2$-Agonists Albuterol Bitolterol Pirbuterol Terbutaline	*Indications* ■ Relief of acute symptoms; quick-relief medication. ■ Preventive treatment prior to exercise for exercise-induced bronchospasm. *Mechanisms* ■ **Bronchodilation.** Smooth muscle relaxation following adenylate cyclase activation and increase in cyclic AMP producing functional antagonism of bronchoconstriction.	Tachycardia, skeletal muscle tremor, hypokalemia, increased lactic acid, headache, hyperglycemia. Inhaled route, in general, causes few systemic adverse effects. Patients with preexisting cardiovascular disease, especially the elderly, may have adverse cardiovascular reactions with inhaled therapy.	■ Drugs of choice for acute bronchospasm. Inhaled route has faster onset, fewer adverse effects, and is more effective than systemic routes. The less beta$_2$-selective agents (isoproterenol, metaproterenol, isoetharine, and epinephrine) are not recommended due to their potential for excessive cardiac stimulation, especially in high doses. Albuterol liquid is not recommended. ■ For patients with mild intermittent asthma, regularly scheduled daily use neither harms nor benefits asthma control (Drazen et al. 1996). Regularly scheduled daily use is not generally recommended. ■ Increasing use or lack of expected effect indicates inadequate asthma control. >1 canister a month (e.g., albuterol-200 puffs per canister) may indicate overreliance on this drug; ≥2 canisters in 1 month poses additional adverse risks. ■ For patients frequently using beta$_2$-agonist, anti-inflammatory medication should be initiated or intensified.
Anticholinergics Ipratropium bromide	*Indications* ■ Relief of acute bronchospasm (see Therapeutic Issues column). *Mechanisms* ■ **Bronchodilation.** Competitive inhibition of muscarinic cholinergic receptors. ■ Reduces intrinsic vagal tone to the airways. May block reflex bronchoconstriction secondary to irritants or to reflux esophagitis. ■ May decrease mucus gland secretion.	Drying of mouth and respiratory secretions, increased wheezing in some individuals, blurred vision if sprayed in eyes.	■ Reverses only cholinergically mediated bronchospasm; does not modify reaction to antigen. Does not block exercise-induced bronchospasm. ■ May provide additive effects to beta$_2$-agonist but has slower onset of action. ■ Is an alternative for patients with intolerance to beta$_2$-agonists. ■ Treatment of choice for bronchospasm due to beta-blocker medication.
Corticosteroids ***Systemic:*** Methylprednisolone Prednisolone Prednisone	*Indications* ■ For moderate-to-severe exacerbations to prevent progression of exacerbation, reverse inflammation, speed recovery, and reduce rate of relapse. *Mechanisms* ■ **Anti-inflammatory.** See figure 3-1.	■ Short-term use: reversible abnormalities in glucose metabolism, increased appetite, fluid retention, weight gain, mood alteration, hypertension, peptic ulcer, and rarely aseptic necrosis of femur. ■ Consideration should be given to coexisting conditions that could be worsened by systemic corticosteroids, such as herpes virus infections, *Varicella*, tuberculosis, hypertension, peptic ulcer, and *Strongyloides*.	■ Short-term therapy should continue until patient achieves 80% PEF personal best or symptoms resolve. This usually requires 3 to 10 days but may require longer. ■ There is no evidence that tapering the dose following improvement prevents relapse.

Usual Dosages for Quick-Relief Medications

Medication	Dosage Form	Adult Dose	Child Dose	Comments
Short-Acting Inhaled Beta₂-Agonists				
Albuterol Albuterol HFA Bitolterol Pirbuterol Terbutaline	**MDIs** 90 mcg/puff, 200 puffs 90 mcg/puff, 200 puffs 370 mcg/puff, 300 puffs 200 mcg/puff, 400 puffs 200 mcg/puff, 300 puffs	■ 2 puffs q 5 minutes prior to exercise ■ 2 puffs tid-qid prn	■ 1-2 puffs 5 minutes prior to exercise ■ 2 puffs tid-qid prn	■ An increasing use or lack of expected effect indicates diminished control of asthma. ■ Not generally recommended for long-term treatment. Regular use on a daily basis indicates the need for additional long-term-control therapy. ■ Differences in potency exist so that all products are essentially equipotent on a per puff basis. ■ May double usual dose for mild exacerbations. ■ Nonselective agents (i.e., epinephrine, isoproterenol, metaproterenol) are not recommended due to their potential for excessive cardiac stimulation, especially in high doses.
Albuterol Rotahaler	**DPI** 200 mcg/capsule	1-2 capsules q 4-6 hours as needed and prior to exercise	1 capsule q 4-6 hours as needed and prior to exercise	
Albuterol	**Nebulizer solution** 5 mg/mL (0.5%)	1.25-5 mg (.25-1 cc) in 2-3 cc of saline q 4-8 hours	0.05 mg/kg (min 1.25 mg, max 2.5 mg) in 2-3 cc of saline q 4-6 hours	May mix with cromolyn or ipratropium nebulizer solutions. May double dose for mild exacerbations.
Bitolterol	2 mg/mL (0.2%)	0.5-3.5mg (.25-1 cc) in 2-3 cc of saline q 4-8 hours	Not established	May not mix with other nebulizer solutions.
Anticholinergics Ipratropium	**MDI** 18 mcg/puff, 200 puffs **Nebulizer solution** .25 mg/mL (0.025%)	2-3 puffs q 6 hours 0.25-0.5 mg q 6 hours	1-2 puffs q 6 hours 0.25 mg q 6 hours	Evidence is lacking for anticholinergics producing added benefit to beta₂-agonists in long-term asthma therapy.
Systemic Corticosteroids		(Applies to all three systemic corticosteroids)		
Methylprednisolone Prednisolone Prednisone	2, 4, 8, 16, 32 mg tablets 5 mg tabs, 5 mg/5 cc, 15 mg/5 cc 1, 2.5, 5, 10, 20, 25 mg tabs; 5 mg/cc, 5 mg/5 cc	■ Short course "burst": 40-60 mg/day as single or 2 divided doses for 3-10 days	■ Short course "burst": 1-2 mg/kg/day, maximum 60 mg/day, for 3-10 days	■ Short courses or "bursts" are effective for establishing control when initiating therapy or during a period of gradual deterioration. ■ The burst should be continued until patient achieves 80% PEF personal best or symptoms resolve. This usually requires 3-10 days but may require longer. There is no evidence that tapering the dose following improvement prevents relapse.

Long-Term-Control Medications

Name/Products	Indications/Mechanisms	Potential Adverse Effects	Therapeutic Issues
Corticosteroids (Glucocorticoids) **Inhaled:** Beclomethasone dipropionate Budesonide Flunisolide Fluticasone propionate Triamcinolone acetonide	*Indications* ■ Long-term prevention of symptoms; suppression, control, and reversal of inflammation. ■ Reduce need for oral corticosteroid. *Mechanisms* ■ **Anti-inflammatory.** Block late reaction to allergen and reduce airway hyperresponsiveness. Inhibit cytokine production, adhesion protein activation, and inflammatory cell migration and activation. ■ Reverse beta$_2$-receptor down-regulation. Inhibit microvascular leakage.	■ Cough, dysphonia, oral thrush (candidiasis). ■ In high doses (see figure 3-5b), systemic effects may occur, although studies are not conclusive, and clinical significance of these effects has not been established (e.g., adrenal suppression, osteoporosis, growth suppression, and skin thinning and easy bruising) (Barnes and Pedersen 1993; Kamada et al. 1996).	■ Spacer/holding chamber devices and mouth washing after inhalation decrease local side effects and systemic absorption. ■ Preparations are not absolutely interchangeable on a mcg or per puff basis (see figure 3-5c for estimated clinical comparability). New delivery devices may provide greater delivery to airways, which may affect dose. ■ The risks of uncontrolled asthma should be weighed against the limited risks of inhaled corticosteroids. The potential but small risk of adverse events is well balanced by their efficacy. (See text.) ■ Dexamethasone is not included because it is highly absorbed and has long-term suppressive side effects.
Systemic: Methylprednisolone Prednisolone Prednisone	*Indications* ■ For short-term (3-10 days) "burst": to gain prompt control of inadequately controlled persistent asthma. ■ For long-term prevention of symptoms in severe persistent asthma: suppression, control, and reversal of inflammation. *Mechanisms* ■ Same as inhaled.	■ Short-term use: reversible abnormalities in glucose metabolism, increased appetite, fluid retention, weight gain, mood alteration, hypertension, peptic ulcer, and rarely aseptic necrosis of femur. ■ Long-term use: adrenal axis suppression, growth suppression, dermal thinning, hypertension, diabetes, Cushing's syndrome, cataracts, muscle weakness, and–in rare instances–impaired immune function. ■ Consideration should be given to coexisting conditions that could be worsened by systemic corticosteroids, such as herpes virus infections, *Varicella*, tuberculosis, hypertension, peptic ulcer, and *Strongyloides*.	Use at lowest effective dose. For long-term use, alternate-day a.m. dosing produces least toxicity. If daily doses are required, one study shows improved efficacy with no increase in adrenal suppression when administered at 3 p.m. rather than in the morning (Beam et al. 1992).
Cromolyn Sodium and Nedocromil Cromolyn Nedocromil	*Indications* ■ Long-term prevention of symptoms; may modify inflammation. ■ Preventive treatment prior to exposure to exercise or known allergen. *Mechanisms* ■ **Anti-inflammatory.** Block early and late reaction to allergen. Interfere with chloride channel function. Stabilize mast cell membranes and inhibit activation and release of mediators from eosinophils and epithelial cells. ■ Inhibit acute response to exercise, cold dry air, and SO$_2$.	15 to 20 percent of patients complain of an unpleasant taste from nedocromil.	■ Therapeutic response to cromolyn and nedocromil often occurs within 2 weeks, but a 4- to 6-week trial may be needed to determine maximum benefit. ■ Dose of cromolyn MDI (1 mg/puff) may be inadequate to affect airway hyperresponsiveness. Nebulizer delivery (20 mg/ampule) may be preferred for some patients. ■ Safety is the primary advantage of these agents.
Long-Acting Beta$_2$-Agonists **Inhaled:** Salmeterol	*Indications* ■ Long-term prevention of symptoms, especially nocturnal symptoms, *added to anti-inflammatory therapy*. ■ Prevention of exercise-induced bronchospasm. ■ *Not to be used to treat acute symptoms or exacerbations.* *Mechanisms* ■ **Bronchodilation.** Smooth muscle relaxation following adenylate cyclase activation and increase in cyclic AMP producing functional antagonism of bronchoconstriction. ■ In vitro, inhibit mast cell mediator release, decrease vascular permeability, and increase mucociliary clearance. ■ Compared to short-acting inhaled beta$_2$-agonist, salmeterol (but not formoterol) has slower onset of action (15 to 30 minutes) but longer duration (>12 hours).	■ Tachycardia, skeletal muscle tremor, hypokalemia, prolongation of QT$_C$ interval in overdose. ■ A diminished bronchoprotective effect may occur within 1 week of chronic therapy. Clinical significance has not been established. ■ See text for additional discussion.	■ *Not to be used to treat acute symptoms or exacerbations.* ■ Clinical significance of potentially developing tolerance is uncertain because studies show symptom control and bronchodilation are maintained. ■ Should not be used in place of anti-inflammatory therapy. ■ May provide more effective symptom control when added to standard doses of inhaled corticosteroid compared to increasing the corticosteroid dosage.

Long-Term-Control Medications *(continued)*

Name/Products	Indications/Mechanisms	Potential Adverse Effects	Therapeutic Issues
Long-Acting Beta₂-Agonists ***Oral:*** Albuterol, sustained-release			■ *Inhaled long-acting beta₂-agonists are preferred because they are longer acting and have fewer side effects than oral sustained-release agents.*
Methylxanthines Theophylline, sustained-release tablets and capsules	*Indications* ■ Long-term control and prevention of symptoms, especially nocturnal symptoms. *Mechanisms* ■ Bronchodilation. Smooth muscle relaxation from phosphodiesterase inhibition and possibly adenosine antagonism. ■ May affect eosinophilic infiltration into bronchial mucosa as well as decrease T-lymphocyte numbers in epithelium. ■ Increases diaphragm contractility and mucociliary clearance.	■ Dose-related acute toxicities include tachycardia, nausea and vomiting, tachyarrhythmias (SVT), central nervous system stimulation, headache, seizures, hematemesis, hyperglycemia, and hypokalemia. ■ Adverse effects at usual therapeutic doses include insomnia, gastric upset, aggravation of ulcer or reflux, increase in hyperactivity in some children, difficulty in urination in elderly males with prostatism.	■ Maintain steady-state serum concentrations between 5 and 15 mcg/mL. Routine serum concentration monitoring is essential due to significant toxicities, narrow therapeutic range, and individual differences in metabolic clearance. Absorption and metabolism may be affected by numerous factors (see figure 3-5a), which can produce significant changes in steady-state serum theophylline concentrations. ■ Not generally recommended for exacerbations. There is minimal evidence for added benefit to optimal doses of inhaled beta₂-agonists. Serum concentration monitoring is mandatory.
Leukotriene Modifiers Zafirlukast tablets	*Indications* ■ Long-term control and prevention of symptoms in mild persistent asthma for patients ≥12 years of age. *Mechanisms* ■ **Leukotriene receptor antagonist;** selective competitive inhibitor of LTD4 and LTE4 receptors.	■ No specific adverse effects to date. As with any new drug, there is possibility of rare hypersensitivity or idiosyncratic reactions that cannot usually be detected in initial premarketing trials. One reported case of reversible hepatitis and hyperbilirubinemia; high concentrations may develop in patients with liver impairment.	■ Administration with meals decreases bioavailability; take at least 1 hour before or 2 hours after meals. ■ Inhibits the metabolism of warfarin and increases prothrombin time; it is a competitive inhibitor of the CYP2C9 hepatic microsomal isozymes. (It has not affected elimination of terfenadine, theophylline, or ethinyl estradiol drugs metabolized by the CYP3A4 isozymes.)
Zileuton tablets	*Indications* ■ Long-term control and prevention of symptoms in mild persistent asthma for patients ≥12 years of age. *Mechanisms* ■ **5-lipoxygenase inhibitor.**	■ Elevation of liver enzymes has been reported. Limited case reports of reversible hepatitis and hyperbilirubinemia.	■ Zileuton is microsomal CYP3A4 enzyme inhibitor that can inhibit the metabolism of terfenadine, warfarin, and theophylline. Doses of these drugs should be monitored accordingly. ■ Monitor hepatic enzymes (ALT).

APPENDIX IX
MANAGEMENT OF ASTHMA EXACERBATIONS— EMERGENCY DEPARTMENT AND HOSPITAL-BASED CARE

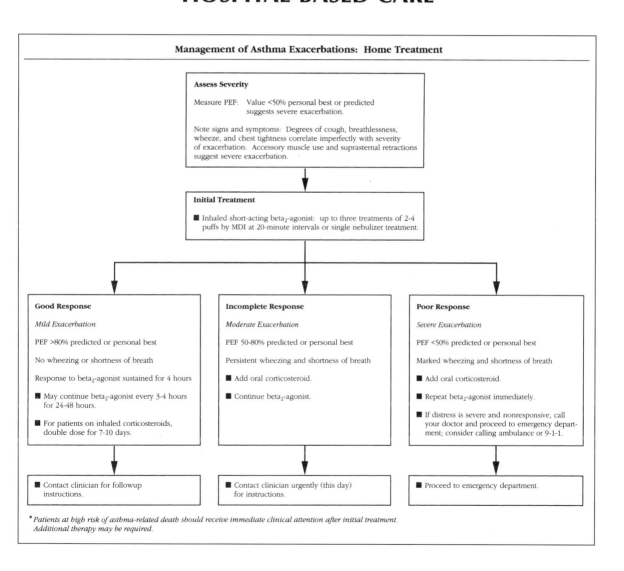

Management of Asthma Exacerbations: Home Treatment

Assess Severity

Measure PEF: Value <50% personal best or predicted
    suggests severe exacerbation.

Note signs and symptoms: Degrees of cough, breathlessness,
wheeze, and chest tightness correlate imperfectly with severity
of exacerbation. Accessory muscle use and suprasternal retractions
suggest severe exacerbation.

Initial Treatment

■ Inhaled short-acting beta$_2$-agonist: up to three treatments of 2-4
 puffs by MDI at 20-minute intervals or single nebulizer treatment.

Good Response

Mild Exacerbation

PEF >80% predicted or personal best

No wheezing or shortness of breath

Response to beta$_2$-agonist sustained for 4 hours

■ May continue beta$_2$-agonist every 3-4 hours
 for 24-48 hours.

■ For patients on inhaled corticosteroids,
 double dose for 7-10 days.

■ Contact clinician for followup
 instructions.

Incomplete Response

Moderate Exacerbation

PEF 50-80% predicted or personal best

Persistent wheezing and shortness of breath

■ Add oral corticosteroid.

■ Continue beta$_2$-agonist.

■ Contact clinician urgently (this day)
 for instructions.

Poor Response

Severe Exacerbation

PEF <50% predicted or personal best

Marked wheezing and shortness of breath

■ Add oral corticosteroid.

■ Repeat beta$_2$-agonist immediately.

■ If distress is severe and nonresponsive, call
 your doctor and proceed to emergency department; consider calling ambulance or 9-1-1.

■ Proceed to emergency department.

*Patients at high risk of asthma-related death should receive immediate clinical attention after initial treatment.
Additional therapy may be required.

Classifying Severity of Asthma Exacerbations

	Mild	Moderate	Severe	Respiratory Arrest Imminent
Symptoms				
Breathlessness	While walking	While talking (infant–softer, shorter cry; difficulty feeding)	While at rest (infant–stops feeding)	
	Can lie down	Prefers sitting	Sits upright	
Talks in	Sentences	Phrases	Words	
Alertness	May be agitated	Usually agitated	Usually agitated	Drowsy or confused
Signs				
Respiratory rate	Increased	Increased	Often >30/min	
		Guide to rates of breathing in awake children: Age　　　　　　Normal rate <2 months　　　<60/minute 2-12 months　　<50/minute 1-5 years　　　<40/minute 6-8 years　　　<30/minute		
Use of accessory muscles; suprasternal retractions	Usually not	Commonly	Usually	Paradoxical thoracoabdominal movement
Wheeze	Moderate, often only end expiratory	Loud; throughout exhalation	Usually loud; throughout inhalation and exhalation	Absence of wheeze
Pulse/minute	<100	100-120	>120	Bradycardia
		Guide to normal pulse rates in children: Age　　　　　　Normal rate 2-12 months　　<160/minute 1-2 years　　　<120/minute 2-8 years　　　<110/minute		
Pulsus paradoxus	Absent <10 mm Hg	May be present 10-25 mm Hg	Often present >25 mm Hg (adult) 20-40 mm Hg (child)	Absence suggests respiratory muscle fatigue
Functional Assessment				
PEF % predicted or % personal best	80%	Approx. 50-80%	<50% predicted or personal best or response lasts <2 hrs	
PaO_2 (on air) and/or	Normal (test not usually necessary)	>60 mm Hg (test not usually necessary)	<60 mm Hg: possible cyanosis	
PCO_2	<42 mm Hg (test not usually necessary)	<42 mm Hg (test not usually necessary)	≥42 mm Hg: possible respiratory failure (see text)	
SaO_2% (on air) at sea level	>95% (test not usually necessary)	91-95%	<91%	

Hypercapnia (hypoventilation) develops more readily in young children than in adults and adolescents.

NOTE:
■ The presence of several parameters, but not necessarily all, indicates the general classification of the exacerbation.
■ Many of these parameters have not been systematically studied, so they serve only as general guides.

Dosages of Drugs for Asthma Exacerbations in Emergency Medical Care or Hospital

Medications	Dosages		Comments
	Adult Dose	**Child Dose**	
Inhaled Short-Acting Beta₂-Agonists			
Albuterol			
Nebulizer solution (5 mg/mL)	2.5-5 mg every 20 minutes for 3 doses, then 2.5-10 mg every 1-4 hours as needed, or 10-15 mg/hour continuously	0.15 mg/kg (minimum dose 2.5 mg) every 20 minutes for 3 doses, then 0.15-0.3 mg/kg up to 10 mg every 1-4 hours as needed, or 0.5 mg/kg/hour by continuous nebulization	Only selective beta₂-agonists are recommended. For optimal delivery, dilute aerosols to minimum of 4 mL at gas flow of 6-8 L/min.
MDI (90 mcg/puff)	4-8 puffs every 20 minutes up to 4 hours, then every 1-4 hours as needed	4-8 puffs every 20 minutes for 3 doses, then every 1-4 hours as needed	As effective as nebulized therapy if patient is able to coordinate inhalation maneuver. Use spacer/holding chamber.
Bitolterol			
Nebulizer solution (2 mg/mL)	See albuterol dose	See albuterol dose; thought to be half as potent as albuterol on a mg basis	Has not been studied in severe asthma exacerbations. Do not mix with other drugs.
MDI (370 mcg/puff)	See albuterol dose	See albuterol dose	Has not been studied in severe asthma exacerbations.
Pirbuterol			
MDI (200 mcg/puff)	See albuterol dose	See albuterol dose; thought to be one-half as potent as albuterol on a mg basis.	Has not been studied in severe asthma exacerbations.
Systemic (Injected) Beta₂-Agonists			
Epinephrine 1:1000 (1 mg/mL)	0.3-0.5 mg every 20 minutes for 3 doses sq	0.01 mg/kg up to 0.3-0.5 mg every 20 minutes for 3 doses sq	No proven advantage of systemic therapy over aerosol.
Terbutaline (1 mg/mL)	0.25 mg every 20 minutes for 3 doses sq	0.01 mg/kg every 20 minutes for 3 doses then every 2-6 hours as needed sq	No proven advantage of systemic therapy over aerosol.
Anticholinergics			
Ipratropium bromide Nebulizer solution (.25 mg/mL)	0.5 mg every 30 minutes for 3 doses then every 2-4 hours as needed	.25 mg every 20 minutes for 3 doses, then every 2 to 4 hours	May mix in same nebulizer with albuterol. Should not be used as first-line therapy; should be added to beta₂-agonist therapy.
MDI (18 mcg/puff)	4-8 puffs as needed	4-8 puffs as needed	Dose delivered from MDI is low and has not been studied in asthma exacerbations.
Corticosteroids			
Prednisone Methylprednisolone Prednisolone	120-180 mg/day in 3 or 4 divided doses for 48 hours, then 60-80 mg/day until PEF reaches 70% of predicted or personal best	1 mg/kg every 6 hours for 48 hours then 1-2 mg/kg/day (maximum = 60 mg/day) in 2 divided doses until PEF 70% of predicted or personal best	For outpatient "burst" use 40-60 mg in single or 2 divided doses for adults (children, 1-2 mg/kg/day, maximum 60 mg/day) for 3-10 days

NOTE:

■ No advantage has been found for higher dose corticosteroids in severe asthma exacerbations, nor is there any advantage for intravenous administration over oral therapy provided gastrointestinal transit time or absorption is not impaired. The usual regimen is to continue the frequent multiple daily dosing until the patient achieves an FEV₁ or PEF of 50 percent of predicted or personal best and then lower the dose to twice daily. This usually occurs within 48 hours. Therapy following a hospitalization or emergency department visit may last from 3 to 10 days. If patients are then started on inhaled corticosteroids, studies indicate there is no need to taper the systemic corticosteroid dose. If the followup systemic corticosteroid therapy is to be given once daily, one study indicates that it may be more clinically effective to give the dose in the afternoon at 3:00 p.m., with no increase in adrenal suppression (Beam et al. 1992).

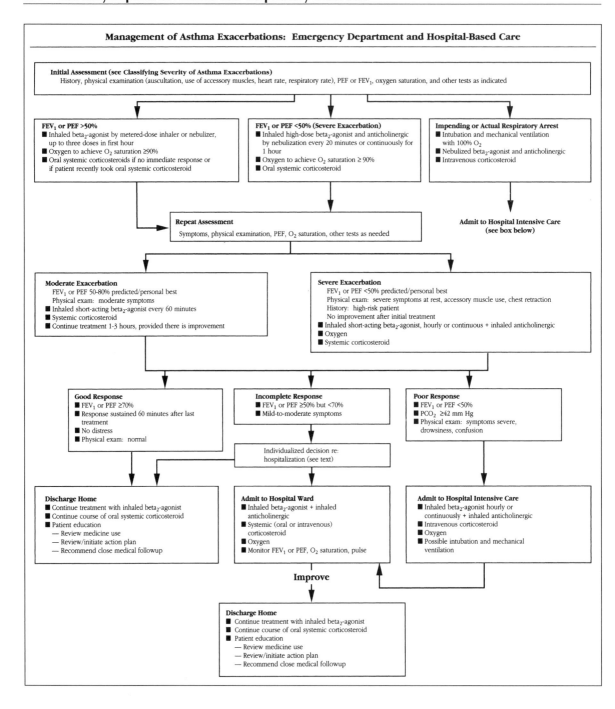

Management of Asthma Exacerbations: Emergency Department and Hospital-Based Care

Initial Assessment (see Classifying Severity of Asthma Exacerbations)
History, physical examination (auscultation, use of accessory muscles, heart rate, respiratory rate), PEF or FEV$_1$, oxygen saturation, and other tests as indicated

FEV$_1$ or PEF >50%
- Inhaled beta$_2$-agonist by metered-dose inhaler or nebulizer, up to three doses in first hour
- Oxygen to achieve O$_2$ saturation ≥90%
- Oral systemic corticosteroids if no immediate response or if patient recently took oral systemic corticosteroid

FEV$_1$ or PEF <50% (Severe Exacerbation)
- Inhaled high-dose beta$_2$-agonist and anticholinergic by nebulization every 20 minutes or continuously for 1 hour
- Oxygen to achieve O$_2$ saturation ≥ 90%
- Oral systemic corticosteroid

Impending or Actual Respiratory Arrest
- Intubation and mechanical ventilation with 100% O$_2$
- Nebulized beta$_2$-agonist and anticholinergic
- Intravenous corticosteroid

Repeat Assessment
Symptoms, physical examination, PEF, O$_2$ saturation, other tests as needed

Admit to Hospital Intensive Care
(see box below)

Moderate Exacerbation
FEV$_1$ or PEF 50-80% predicted/personal best
Physical exam: moderate symptoms
- Inhaled short-acting beta$_2$-agonist every 60 minutes
- Systemic corticosteroid
- Continue treatment 1-3 hours, provided there is improvement

Severe Exacerbation
FEV$_1$ or PEF <50% predicted/personal best
Physical exam: severe symptoms at rest, accessory muscle use, chest retraction
History: high-risk patient
No improvement after initial treatment
- Inhaled short-acting beta$_2$-agonist, hourly or continuous + inhaled anticholinergic
- Oxygen
- Systemic corticosteroid

Good Response
- FEV$_1$ or PEF ≥70%
- Response sustained 60 minutes after last treatment
- No distress
- Physical exam: normal

Incomplete Response
- FEV$_1$ or PEF ≥50% but <70%
- Mild-to-moderate symptoms

Poor Response
- FEV$_1$ or PEF <50%
- PCO$_2$ ≥42 mm Hg
- Physical exam: symptoms severe, drowsiness, confusion

Individualized decision re: hospitalization (see text)

Discharge Home
- Continue treatment with inhaled beta$_2$-agonist
- Continue course of oral systemic corticosteroid
- Patient education
  — Review medicine use
  — Review/initiate action plan
  — Recommend close medical followup

Admit to Hospital Ward
- Inhaled beta$_2$-agonist + inhaled anticholinergic
- Systemic (oral or intravenous) corticosteroid
- Oxygen
- Monitor FEV$_1$ or PEF, O$_2$ saturation, pulse

Admit to Hospital Intensive Care
- Inhaled beta$_2$-agonist hourly or continuously + inhaled anticholinergic
- Intravenous corticosteroid
- Oxygen
- Possible intubation and mechanical ventilation

Improve

Discharge Home
- Continue treatment with inhaled beta$_2$-agonist
- Continue course of oral systemic corticosteroid
- Patient education
  — Review medicine use
  — Review/initiate action plan
  — Recommend close medical followup

APPENDIX X

TRAVELING WITH ALLERGIES OR ASTHMA

Traveling may trigger allergy or asthma attacks because of exposure to allergens usually avoided at home, increased stress level, and other factors, including change of climate and quality of air. Persons with allergies and/or asthma should be prepared for a possible attack while away from home.

- Take extra medication with you; don't forget your inhaler or any other equipment you normally use at home.

- If you are severely allergic to bee (or other insect, such as fire ant) stings, a food, or other substance and you have experienced anaphylactic shock because of one of these triggers, wear a medical alert bracelet engraved with important information about your allergy and the treatment. This will help a doctor in an emergency room offer you more immediate treatment. You may even need to carry a syringe and adrenaline for emergency use.

- Travel with a companion who is aware of your condition and knows what to do in case you have an attack.

- Carry a copy of your asthma chart listing episodes and treatments. Carry a letter from your doctor explaining your condition and how he or she has treated it so far.

- When children are traveling on their own, they should have a doctor's letter, including clear instructions for medications or other treatment.

- Avoid smoking sections on airplanes or trains, in restaurants, and other places if smoke irritates your respiratory system.

- Avoid traveling to places notorious for air pollution, certain species of weeds, grasses, or trees, or other characteristics that could exacerbate your condition, such as going to the home of a relative who has cats.

- Know the difference between hyperventilation and an asthma attack. Learn relaxation and deep-breathing techniques before you travel. They can help ward off an asthma attack or possibly relieve one.

- Get in shape before you travel. Regular, appropriate exercise facilitates optimal body functioning. Losing excess weight makes it easier for you to breathe and your body to function well. If you find yourself in a strenuous situation while traveling, make sure you take your medication before exertion, if your doctor advises it.

- Understand that as long as you can manage your condition, you can travel successfully. Ask your allergist for advice specific to your symptoms.

APPENDIX XI
ALTERNATIVE TREATMENTS AND REMEDIES FOR RESPIRATORY DISORDERS

Asthma

1. Ginger, stramonium, elecampane, grindelia, hyssop, wild cherry bark, motherwort, almond, ephedra, and turmeric are among Ayurvedic, Chinese, and Western herbal remedies for asthma.
2. Homeopathic remedies for asthma include ipecac, arsenicum, bryonia, natrium sulfuricum (nat. sulf.), and lachesis.
3. Vitamin B_6.
4. Aromatherapy includes steam inhalation of chamomile, eucalyptus, or lavender essential oils, vaporized pine oil, and bergamot, clary sage, neroli, chamomile, and roses.

Bronchitis

1. Heated mustard oil compress applied to the head, and ginger, hollyhock, bitter orange, and stramonium are among Ayurvedic treatments.
2. Fritillary bulb, plantain seed, balloon flower root, honeysuckle flowers, mulberry leaves, gardenia fruit, anise, wild cherry bark, coltsfoot, garlic oil chest rub, ginseng tea, peppermint tea, honey and lemon, and onions are among Chinese, traditional, and Western herbal remedies.
3. Aromatherapy includes eucalyptus, ginger and thyme oils, juniper, myrrh, and rosemary.
4. Vitamins B, C, and A, and zinc.
5. Homeopathic remedies include pulsatilla, ipecac, bryonia, phosphorus, and aconite.

Common Cold

1. Sunflower, coriander seeds, ginger, plantain seed, peppermint, mulberry, honeysuckle, skullcap, barley water, honey and lemon, cinnamon, garlic, ginseng powder, echinacea, and a mustard poultice or foot bath are among Ayurvedic, Chinese, traditional, and Western herbal remedies.
2. Homeopathic remedies include aconite, belladonna, mercurius, gelsemium, allium, pulsatilla, natrum muriaticum (nat. mur.), dulcamara, kali bichronicum, and bryonia.
3. Vitamin C, zinc, royal jelly.
4. Aromatherapy includes tea tree, lemon, lavender, and eucalyptus oils.

Cough

1. Coriander seeds, root ginger, sunflower, henbane, stramonium, fresh garlic or garlic tincture, ginseng, honey and lemon, mustard powder or onion poultice, peppermint tea, licorice root, aniseed, marshmallow, wild cherry bark, goldenseal, plantain, and thyme are among Ayurvedic, Chinese, traditional, and Western herbal remedies.
2. Aromatherapy includes eucalyptus oil, pine oil, oil of myrrh, frankincense, and sandalwood.
3. Homeopathic remedies include pulsatilla, rumex, bryonia, phosphorus, drosera, chamomilla, and antimonium tartaricum (ant. tart.).

Emphysema

1. Garlic, stramonium, peppermint tea, and slippery elm bark are among Ayurvedic and herbal remedies.
2. Homeopathic treatment includes cough, asthma, and bronchitis remedies.
3. Aromatherapy includes cedarwood, peppermint, and eucalyptus oils.

Hiccups

1. Berilla stems, rhubarb, ginger, lemon juice, water with honey, nux vomica, arsenicum, ignatia, cicuta, and magnesia phosphorica (mag. phos.) are among Chinese and traditional herbal remedies and homeopathic treatment.

Hyperventilation

1. Ayurvedic treatment involves balancing the tridoshas.
2. Chinese, traditional, and Western herbalism include ginseng, Chinese angelica, white peony root, thorowax root, oats, skullcap, valerian, lady's slipper, and limeflowers.
3. Homeopathic remedies include aconite and constitutional treatment.
4. B vitamins; avoidance of caffeine.
5. Aromatherapy: lavender, geranium, bergamot, sweet almond and peach kernel oils.
6. Flower essences include elm and aspen.

Influenza

1. Heated mustard oil compress, root ginger, honey and lime, bitter orange, sunflower, coriander, warmed apple juice, barley water, ginseng powder, hot lemon and honey in water, boneset, fenugreek, wormwood, sage, and licorice are among Ayurvedic, Chinese, traditional, and Western herbal remedies.
2. Homeopathic treatment includes gelsemium, rhus toxicodendron (rhus. tox.), bryonia, eupatorium perfoliatum, arsenicum, and baptisia.
3. Vitamin C, bioflavonoids, zinc, and royal jelly.
4. Aromatherapy: oils of eucalyptus, peppermint, tea tree, geranium, bergamot, chamomile, and melissa.

Pleurisy

1. Apple cider vinegar compress, comfrey root, leaf tea, plantain leaf, sage leaf, and corn silk are among herbal remedies.
2. Homeopathic remedies include aconite, cantharis, belladonna, bryonia, sulfur, and hepar sulfuris calcarcum, or calcium sulfide (hep. sulf.).

3. Aromatherapy includes oils of bergamot, calendula, chamomile, myrrh, and lavender.

Pneumonia

1. Heated mustard oil compress, root ginger, honey and lime, peach kernel, skullcap, fritillary bulb, raw garlic and onions, boneset, fenugreek, and ginseng are among Ayurvedic, Chinese, traditional, and Western herbal treatments.
2. Homeopathic treatment includes aconite, bryonia, sanguinaria, and phosphorus.
3. Vitamin C and zinc.
4. Aromatherapy: eucalyptus and tea tree oils, and niaouli or cajeput massage.

Tracheitis

1. Hollyhock, comfrey root or leaf tea, and plantain leaf compress are among Ayurvedic and herbal treatments.
2. Homeopathic remedies include rumex, stannum, bryonia, phosphorus, and kali bichronicum.
3. Vitamin C and zinc.
4. Aromatherapy: bergamot, calendula, chamomile, and myrrh.

Tuberculosis

1. Stramonium, licorice, garlic, Echinacea, and ginseng are included in Ayurvedic and herbal treatments.
2. Homeopathic remedies include baccillinium, arsenicum, and calcarea.
3. Aromatherapy: vaporized garlic, tea tree and lavender oils, and juniper, rosemary, bergamot or eucalyptus oils.

SOURCES

Shealy, C. Norman, M.D., Ph.D., *The Illustrated Encyclopedia of Natural Remedies,* Element Books Limited, Boston, 1998.

De Schepper, Luc, M.D., Ph.D., C.Hom, *The People's Pharmacy,* Full of Life Publishing, Santa Fe, NM, 1998.

APPENDIX XII
PROFESSIONAL AND LAY ORGANIZATIONS

Allergy and Asthma Network
Mothers of Asthmatics, Inc.
2751 Prosperity Avenue, Suite 150
Fairfax, VA 22031
(703) 641-9595
www.aanma.org

Allergy/Asthma Information Association
65 Tomley Drive, Suite 10
Etobicoke, Ontario, Canada M9B 5Y7

American Academy of Allergy, Asthma and Immunology (AAAAI)
611 East Wells Street
Milwaukee, WI 53202-3889
(800) 822-2762 or (800) 822-ASMA
http://www.aaaai.org

American Academy of Pediatrics
141 Northwest Point Boulevard
Elk Grove Village, IL 60007
(800) 433-9016 or (847) 228-5005
http://www.aap.org

American Association for Respiratory Care
11030 Ables Lane
Dallas, TX 75229-4593
(972) 243-2272
http://www.aarc.org

American College of Allergy, Asthma and Immunology (ACAAI)
85 West Algonquin Road, Suite 550
Arlington Heights, IL 60005
(800) 842-7777
http://allergy.mcg.educ

American Dietetic Association
216 West Jackson Boulevard
Chicago, IL 60606-6995
(312) 899-0040 or (800) 366-1655
www.eatright.org

American Lung Association (ALA)
1740 Broadway
New York, NY 10019
(800) LUNG-USA (800) 586-4872
www.lungusa.org

Asthma and Allergy Foundation of America (AAFA)
1233 20th Street NW, Suite 402
Washington, DC 20036
(202) 466-7643 or (800) 7-ASTHMA (800) 727-8462
www.aafa.org

U.S. CHAPTERS

AAFA Los Angeles Chapter
5225 Wilshire Boulevard, Suite 705
Los Angeles, CA 90036
(213) 937-7859

AAFA Florida State Chapter
c/o University Community Hospital
3100 East Fletcher Avenue
Tampa, FL 33613
(813) 972-7872

AAFA Greater Chicago Chapter
111 North Wabash, Suite 909
Chicago, IL 60602
(312) 346-0745

AAFA Maryland Chapter
5601 Loch Raven Boulevard
Baltimore, MD 21239
(301) 532-4135

AAFA Michigan State Chapter
6900 Orchard Lake Road, Suite 207
West Bloomfield, MI 48322
(313) 427-2202

AAFA Greater Kansas City Chapter
7905 East 134th Terrace
Grandview, MO 64030
(816) 966-8164

AAFA St. Louis Area Chapter
222 South Central, Suite 600
St. Louis, MO 63105
(314) 726-6866

AAFA
Community Health Place, Suite 209-D
7101 Newport Avenue
Omaha, NE 69152
(402) 572-3073

AAFA New England Chapter
220 Boylston Street, Suite 305A
Chestnut Hill, MA 02167
(617) 965-7771

AAFA S.E. Pennsylvania Chapter
P.O. Box 249
Plymouth Meeting, PA 19402
(215) 825-0583

**American Society of Health-System
  Pharmacists (ASHP)**
7272 Wisconsin Avenue
Bethesda, MD 20814
(301) 657-3000
http://www.ashp.org/public/news/breaking/asthma
  2000.html

breathnet
the breathing experts™
A Network of Respiratory Specialists
850 Third Avenue
New York, NY 10022
(646) 840-3901
www.breathnet.com

Center for Environmental Health
Centers for Disease Control and Prevention
Mail Stop F-29
4770 Buford Highway, NE
Atlanta, GA 20241-3724
(800) 311-3435
www.cdc.gov

The Food Allergy and Anaphylaxis Network
10400 Eaton Place, Suite 107
Fairfax, VA 22030-2208
(703) 691-3179 or (800) 929-4040
www.foodallergy.org

Food and Drug Administration
Office of Consumer Affairs/HFE-88
5600 Fishers Lane
Rockville, MD 20857

(888) INFO-FDA (888) 463-6332
www.fda.gov

Healthy Kids: The Key to Basics
Educational Planning for Students With Asthma
  and Other Chronic Health Conditions
79 Elmore Street
Newton, MA 02159-1137
(617) 965-9637

Immune Deficiency Foundation
P.O. Box 586
Columbia, MD 21045
(410) 461-3127

**Indoor Air Quality Information
  Clearinghouse**
(800) 438-4318
http://www.epa.gov/iaq

JAMA **Asthma Information Center**
American Medical Association
515 North State Street
Chicago, IL 60610
(312) 464-5374
www.ama.assn.org/special/asthma

**Joint Council of Allergy, Asthma and
  Immunology**
http://www.jcaai.org

**National Allergy and Asthma Network/
  Mothers of Asthmatics**
3554 Chain Bridge Road, Suite 200
Fairfax, VA 22030
(800) 878-4403

National Asthma Education Program
National Heart, Lung, and Blood Institute
  Information Center
P.O. Box 30105
Bethesda, MD 20824-0105
(301) 592-8573 or (301) 251-1222
http://www.nhlbi.nih.gov

**National Institute of Allergy and Infectious
  Diseases (NIAID)**
National Institutes of Health Office of
  Communications and Public Liaison
31 Center Drive MSC 2520
Building 31, Room 7A-50
Bethesda, MD 20892-2520
www.niaid.nih.gov

National Institute of Environmental Health Sciences
Office of Communications
P.O. Box 12233
Research Triangle Park, NC 27709
(919) 541-3345
www.niehs.nih.gov/airborne/prevent/intro.html

National Jewish Medical and Research Center (Lung Line)
1400 Jackson Street
Denver, CO 80206
(800) 222-5864
http://www.njc.org

U.S. Department of Education
Office of Civil Rights, Customer Service Team
Mary E. Switzer Building, 330 C Street, SW
Washington, DC 20202-1328
(800) 421-3481 or (202) 205-5413
http://www.ed.gov/offices/OCR

U.S. Environmental Protection Agency
Indoor Environments Division
401 M Street (66043)
Washington, DC 20460
(202) 233-9370

BIBLIOGRAPHY

Adams, Francis V., M.D. *The Asthma SourceBook: Everything You Need to Know.* Los Angeles: Lowell House, 1998.

———. *The Breathing Disorders SourceBook.* Los Angeles: Lowell House, 1998.

Allergy & Asthma Network/Mothers of Asthmatics. "AANMA Headquarters," Allergy & Asthma Network/Mothers of Asthmatics Website. Available online. URL: http://www.aanma.org/headquarters. Downloaded on May 29, 2002.

Altman, Lawrence K. "U.S. to Investigate Death in an Asthma Study." *New York Times,* June 16, 2001.

———. "Volunteer in Asthma Study Dies after Inhaling Drug." *New York Times,* June 15, 2001.

American College of Allergy, Asthma & Immunotherapy. "ACAAI Launches Asthma All-Stars," Allergy, Asthma & Immunology Online. Available online. URL: http://allergy.mcg.edu/news/allstars.html. Downloaded on June 4, 2000.

———. "International Evidence Shows Allergy Shots Improve Symptoms, Reduce Need for Drugs and Can Modify Disease Course," Allergy, Asthma & Immunology Online. Available online. URL: http://allergy.mcg.edu/news/inint.html. Posted on November 22, 1999.

———. "The Journal 'Annals of Allergy, Asthma & Immunology' Is Now Online," Allergy, Asthma & Immunology Online. Available online. URL: http://allergy.mcg.edu/news/annals.html. Downloaded on June 4, 2000.

———. "Kids' Asthma Check: For Ages 1–8," Allergy, Asthma & Immunology Online. Available online. URL: http://allergy.mcg.edu/lifeQuality/kac1.html. Posted on April 6, 2000.

———. "Nationwide Asthma Screening," Allergy, Asthma & Immunology Online. Available online. URL: http://allergy.mcg.edu/lifeQuality/nasp.html. Downloaded on May 29, 2002.

———. "1999 ACAAI Abstracts," Allergy, Asthma & Immunology Online. Available online. URL: http://allergy.mcg.edu/news/abstracts.html. Posted on November 12, 1999.

———. "Occupational Allergies and Asthma: Experts Say Occupational Allergies and Asthma Is a Growing Problem in the Industrialized World," Allergy, Asthma & Immunology Online. Available online. URL: http://allergy.mcg.edu/news/occall.html. Downloaded on June 4, 2000.

American Lung Association. "ALA State of the Air 2000," American Lung Association Website. Available online. URL: http://www.lungusa.org/air2000. Downloaded on June 4, 2000.

———. "Executive Summary: The American Lung Association Asthma Survey," American Lung Association Website. Available online. URL: http://www.lungusa.org/asthma.merck_summary.html. Downloaded on May 30, 2002.

———. "Progress Report 2000: The Asthma Research Centers," American Lung Association Website. Available online. URL: http://www.lungusa.org/arc/index_oo.html. Downloaded on May 30, 2002.

———. "Trends in Asthma Morbidity and Mortality, February 2000," American Lung Association Website. Available online. URL: http://www.lungusa.org/data/asthma/part1.pdf. Downloaded on May 30, 2002.

———. "Trends in Lung Cancer Morbidity and Mortality, December 2000," American Lung Association Website. Available online. URL: http://www.lungusa.org/data/lc/lcpart1.pdf. Downloaded on May 29, 2002.

"Asthma Ruled Cause of Death." *Asbury Park Press,* August 5, 2001.

Berkow, Robert, M.D.; Beers, Mark H., M.D.; Bogin, Robert M., M.D.; and Fletcher, Andrew J., M.B.,

B. Chir. *The Merck Manual of Medical Information.* Home ed. New York: Pocket Books, 1997.

Centers for Disease Control and Prevention. "Allergies/Hay Fever," National Center for Health Statistics Fast Stats. Available online. URL: http://www.cdc.gov/nchc/fastats/allergys.htm. Posted on May 15, 2000.

Chernick, Victor; Kendig, Edwin L.; and Boat, Thomas F. *Kendig's Disorders of the Respiratory Tract in Children.* Orlando, Fla.: W.B. Sanders, 1997.

Cook, Allan R., and Dresser, Peter D. *Respiratory Diseases and Disorders Sourcebook.* Vol. 6. Detroit, Mich.: Omnigraphics, Inc., 1995.

Cystic Fibrosis Foundation. "Cystic Fibrosis Foundation . . . Adding Tomorrows Every Day," Cystic Fibrosis Foundation Website. Available online. URL: http://www.cff.org. Downloaded on May 29, 2002.

De Schepper, Luc, M.D., Ph.D., C. Hom. *The People's Pharmacy.* Santa Fe, N.Mex.: Full of Life Publishing, 1998.

Edelman, Norman, M.D. *The American Lung Association's Family Guide to Asthma and Allergies.* Boston: Little, Brown, 1997.

Freudenheim, Milt. "Panel Says 3 Allergy Drugs Should Be Sold over the Counter." *New York Times,* May 12, 2001.

Gazoontite. "Allergy and Asthma Relief," Gazoontite Website. Available online. URL: http://www.gazoontite.com. Downloaded on May 18, 2000.

Gerdus, Marion K., B.S.N., R.N., CNOR. "Safer Sinus Surgery." *Advance for Nurses,* August 6, 2001.

Glanz, James. "Clues of Asthma Study Risks May Have Been Overlooked." *New York Times,* July 27, 2001.

GlaxoSmithKline. "Executive Summary," Asthma in America: A Landmark Survey Website. Available online. URL: http://www.asthmainamerica.com/execsum_over.htm. Downloaded on May 29, 2002.

Gosselin, Kim. *Taking Asthma to School.* Valley Park, Mo.: JayJo Books, LLC, 1998.

Greenhouse, Linda. "E.P.A.'s Right to Set Air Rules Wins Supreme Court Backing." *New York Times,* February 28, 2001.

Hale, Teresa. *Breathing Free: The Revolutionary 5-Day Program to Heal Asthma, Emphysema, Bronchitis, and Other Respiratory Ailments.* New York: Random House, 1999.

Harrington, Geri. *The Asthma Self-Care Book.* New York: HarperCollins, 1999.

Holgate, Stephen T. *An Atlas of Asthma.* London: Parthenon Publishers, 1999.

"Innovative Surgery Eases the Pain of Hearburn." *Health Link* (Long Branch, N.J.), spring 2001.

Instep International. "How to Grow out of Asthma," NQ Buteyko Asthma Relief Center Website. Available online. URL: http://nqnet.com/asma. Downloaded on May 28, 2000.

Ivker, Robert S., and Anderson, Robert A. *Sinus Survival: The Holistic Medical Treatment for Allergies, Asthma, Bronchitis, Colds, and Sinusitis.* New York: Jeremy P. Tarcher/Putnam, 1995.

Lipkowitz, Myron A., M.D., and Navarra, Tova, B.A., R.N. *The Encyclopedia of Allergies.* 2d ed. New York: Facts On File, 2001.

London, Jonathan. *The Lion Who Had Asthma.* Morton Grove, Ill.: Albert Whitman & Company, 1997.

Meltzer, Eli O., M.D. "The Pharmacological Basis for the Treatment of Perennial Allergic Rhinitis and Non-Allergic Rhinitis with Topical Corticosteroids." *Allergy* 52 (suppl. 36), 33–40.

Mikelberg, Felice. "Help Your Kids Breathe Easy." *Meridian HealthViews,* July/August 2000.

National Institutes of Health/National Heart, Lung, and Blood Institute. *Expert Panel Report 2: Guidelines for the Diagnosis and Management of Asthma.* NIH Publication No. 97-4051. Washington, D.C.: National Institutes of Health, 1997.

Navarra, Tova. *Your Body: Highlights of Human Anatomy.* Neptune, N.J.: Asbury Park Press, 1991.

OnHealth. "Asthma Inhalers Linked to Cataracts," OnHealth Website. Available online. URL: http://www.onhealth.com/conditions/in-depth/item. Downloaded on June 4, 2000.

———. "Inhalers Linked to Heart Attacks," OnHealth Website. Available online. URL: http://www.onhealth.com/conditions/briefs/item.39490.asp. Downloaded on May 28, 2000.

Perry, Angela R. *The American Medical Association Essential Guide to Asthma.* New York: Pocket Books, 1998.

Peterson, Melody. "A Push to Sell Top Allergy Drugs over the Counter." *New York Times,* May 11, 2001.

Pilbeam, Susan P. *Mechanical Ventilation: Physiological and Clinical Applications.* 3d ed. St. Louis, Mo.: Mosby-Year Book, Inc., 1992.

Placitella, Christopher, J. D. "Mesothelioma Alert." *StraightTalk,* summer 2000.

Prabhavananda, Swami, and Manchester, Frederick, trans. *The Upanishads: Breath of the Eternal.* New York: Mentor/Penguin Books, 1948.

PSL Group. "Scientists Identify Genetic Mutation That Makes People Allergic," PSL online. Available online. URL: http://www.pslgroup.com/dg/4D95A.htm. Downloaded on July 19, 2000.

Revkin, Andrew C. "New Pollution Tool: Toxic Avenger with Leaves." *New York Times,* March 6, 2001.

Sander, Nancy. *A Parentís Guide to Asthma: How You Can Help Your Child Control Asthma at Home, School, and Play.* New York: Penguin, 1994.

Schultz, Dodi. "Asthma: A Public Health Partnership Tackles a Neighborhood Terror." *Columbia University Alumni Magazine,* winter 2001.

Sciencewise. "FEDIX," Sciencewise Website. Available online. URL: http://content.sciencewise.com/fedix. Downloaded on May 31, 2000.

Shaver, Joan L. F., Ph.D., R.N., FAAN, and Rodgers, Ann E., Ph.D., R.N. "Screening for Sleep-Related Disorders: Sleep Apnea and Narcolepsy." *The American Nurse,* November/December 1994.

Shealy, C. Norman, M.D., Ph.D. *The Illustrated Encyclopedia of Natural Remedies.* Boston: Element Books Limited, 1998.

Simpson, Carolyn. *Everything You Need to Know about Asthma.* New York: Rosen Publishing Group, Inc., 1998.

Skidmore-Roth, Linda, R.N., M.S.N., N.P. *Mosby's 1999 Nursing Drug Reference.* St. Louis, Mo.: Mosby, Inc., 1999.

Spector, Nancy, R.N., DNSc; Klein, Diane, R.N., Ph.D.; and Rice-Wyllie, Laurie, R.N., M.S.N. "Terminally Ill Patients Breathe Easier with Nebulized Morphine." *Nursing Spectrum* 12, no. 25, December 11, 2000.

Sprott, Kendall, M.D. "Vaccine for Pneumococcal Infection Important at Early Age." *The Star Ledger,* August 15, 2000.

Stapleton, Stephanie. "Whiff of Danger: Sniffing Inhalants Continues to Be a Silent, Sometimes Deadly, Epidemic among Teens and Pre-Teens." *Asbury Park Press,* May 1, 2001.

Thomas, Clayton L., M.D., M.P.H. *Taber's Cyclopedic Medical Dictionary,* 17th ed. Philadelphia, Pa.: F.A. Davis Company, 1993.

"Tis the Season for the Flu." *Focus* (Horizon Blue Cross Blue Shield of New Jersey), fall 2000.

Vimy Park Pharmacy. "Zileutron (Leutrol) Drug for Asthma: Use, Side Effects, Interactions," Virtual Drugstore Website. Available online. URL: http://www.virtualdrugstore.com/asthma/zileutron.html. Downloaded on June 28, 2000.

Weinstein, Allan M. *Asthma.* Princeton, N.J.: McGraw-Hill, 1988.

Wilkens, Robert L., and Dexter, James R. *Respiratory Disease: A Case Study Approach to Patient Care.* 2d ed. Philadelphia, Pa.: F.A. Davis Company, 1997.

"Winter Coughs: What to Do and When to Worry." *Healthy Decisions,* winter 1997.

Woodman, Sue. "A Little Night Music: The Snoring Report." *My Generation,* March–April 2001.

Zurlinden, Jeffrey, R.N., M.S., ACRN. "Smoking Gun: Drug Regimens Can Pose Problem with Tobacco Cessation." *Nursing Spectrum* 13, no. 2, January 22, 2001, 22–23.

INDEX

Boldface page numbers indicate major treatment of a subject.

A

AAAAI. *See* American Academy of Allergy, Asthma and Immunology

AAFA. *See* Asthma and Allergy Foundation of America

AAMA. *See* American Academy of Medical Acupuncture

ABAI. *See* American Board of Allergy and Immunology

ABGs. *See* arterial blood gases

ABIM. *See* American Board of Internal Medicine

ABP. *See* American Board of Pediatrics

ABPA. *See* allergic bronchopulmonary aspergillosis

abscess, lung **120**

ACAAI. *See* American College of Allergy, Asthma and Immunology

acapnia **1**

accessory nasal sinuses **178**

Accolate **1**. *See also* Zafirlukast

Accreditation Council for Graduate Medical Education (ACGME) 14

Accurbron. *See* theophylline

acetaldehyde 148

acetaminophen, for bronchitis 49

acetanilide, and toxic-allergic syndrome 189

acetylsalicylic acid. *See* aspirin

ACGME. *See* Accreditation Council for Graduate Medical Education

Achromycin 187

acid-base balance 1, 26

acidity-alkalinity, and arterial blood gas tests 26

acidosis
　carbon dioxide 1
　hypercapnic 1
　respiratory 1

acquired immune deficiency syndrome (AIDS) **5–6,** 103

acrivistine 176

ACTH. *See* corticotropin

Actidil. *See* triprolidine

Actifed 198

actinomycetes, and air conditioning 6

active expiration 80

active immunity **1–2**

acupressure **2**

acupuncture **2,** 11

acute epiglottitis 29

Adam's apple 169

addiction **2**

adenocarcinoma 121

adenoid cystic carcinomas 121

adenoidectomy 3

adenoids **2–3,** 100

adenosine deaminase, and severe combined immunodeficiency disease 104

adenotonsillectomy **3**

adrenal glands, and corticosteroids 67

adrenaline. *See* epinephrine

Adrenaline Chloride. *See* epinephrine

adrenergic agonists, for allergies 10

adrenergic nervous system 170

adult-onset asthma 331

adult respiratory distress syndrome (ARDS) **3**

adverse drug reactions **3**

Advil. *See* ibuprofen

aeration **3**

aeroallergens **3–4**

aerobes 41

aerobic **4**

aerobic exercise 4

AeroBid **4**. *See also* flunisolide

Aerolate Slo-Phyllin. *See* theophylline

aeropathy **4**

aerophobia **4**

aerosol **4**

aerotherapy **4**

African Americans
　and asthma-related deaths 33
　lung cancer and 125

Afrin 147

Afrinol. *See* pseudoephedrine

agammaglobulinemias 103

agonist **4–5**

agranulocytes 118

ague, brass founder's **46**

AIDS. *See* acquired immune deficiency syndrome

AIDS-related complex 5

air **6**

air block **45**

airborne allergens 3–4

air bronchogram sign **6**

air cells, of lungs 12

air conditioning **6**

air curtain **6**

air-filtration systems 6

air flow, laminar **6**

air hunger **6,** 75, **95**

air pollution **7**

air pump **164**

grapeseed oil, and toxic-allergic syndrome 189

grass pollen allergy **86**

gravity principle, in postural drainage 161

green tobacco sickness **86**

grepafloxacin, for Legionnaire's disease 118

grindelia **86**

grinder's disease 177. *See also* silicosis

grippe. *See* influenza

growing out of allergies and asthma **86**

guaifenesin 80, **86,** 173

Guidelines for the Diagnosis and Management of Asthma 71

Guillain, Georges 86

Guillain-Barré syndrome (GBS) **86–87,** 110

gustatory rhinits **87**

H

H. *See* hemagglutinin

Habitrol. *See* nicotine patches

hacking cough 68, **88**

Haemophilus influenzae 69, 178

halitosis 46

hamartomas 121

Hamman, Louis 88

Hamman-Rich syndrome **88**

Hamman's disease **88**

Hansen's disease. *See* leprosy, tuberculoid

H$_1$ antihistamines 22
second-generation 23

H$_2$ antihistamines 22

haptens 16, 101, 152

Harrison, Edwin 88

Harrison's groove **88**

harsh cough 68

Harvard School of Public Health 180

hashish 88

hay fever **88–89,** 173. *See also* allergic rhinitis; pollinosis
seasonal **175–176**
trees that cause 190–197
weeds that cause 205–210

Hay Fever, a Key to the Allergic Disorders 83

headache
histamine **89**
sinus 178

Healthy Kids: The Key to Basics 375

heart 170

heartburn **89**

heart-lung bypass 89

heart-lung machine **89**

heart-lung preparation **162**

Heimlich, H. J. 89

Heimlich maneuver 60, **89**

Heimlich sign 89

Heiner's syndrome **89,** 97

helium 89

helper T cells 102

hemagglutinin (H) 109

hemithorax **89**

hemlock poisoning **90**

hemolytic anemia, and antihistamines 23

hemopleura **90**

hemopneumothorax **90,** 157

hemoptysis **90.** *See also* Goodpasture's syndrome

hemorrhage, lung **90, 129,** 157, 159

hemorrhagic bronchitis. *See* bronchospirochetosis

hemosiderosis 142, 177. *See also* Goodpasture's syndrome

hemothorax **90,** 155

hemp, and byssinosis 53

hemp plant 88. *See also* cannabis

hen cluck stertor 183

HEPA filters. *See* high-efficiency particulate air filters

heparin 76, 101

hepatopulmonary **90**

herbalism, for allergies 11

Hering, Heinrich Ewald 90

Hering-Breur reflex **90**

hernia
diaphragmatic **90**
of lung tissue 156
phrenic **90**
pulmonary 159

heroin toxicity **90**

hiccups/hiccough **90,** 177, 373

high-efficiency particulate air (HEPA) filters 6, 202

high frequency jet ventilation 203

high-molecular-weight allergens 141–142

hilitis **90**

Hippocrates **90–91**

hippus, respiratory **91**

Hirstia 93

Hismanal. *See* astemizole

histamine 15, 16, **91,** 101. *See also* antihistamines

histamine headache **89**

histamine H$_1$ receptor antagonist **91**

histamine H$_2$ receptor antagonist **91**

Histapan 133

Histoplasma capsulatum 91

histoplasmosis **91**

Histor-D 133

HIV. *See* human immunodeficiency virus

HIV-antibody test 5

hives. *See* urticaria

H1N1 virus 109

H3N2 virus 109

hoarseness **91–92**

holistic medicine **92**

home care, for asthma exacerbations 367

homeopathy 10, **92**

home remedies **92**

Hong Kong flu 109

Hopmann's papilloma **148**

hormonal changes, with corticosteroids 67

hormone **92**

horse-serum antitoxin, and anaphylaxis 15

hospital-based care, for asthma exacerbations 370

house-dust extract 107

house-dust mites **92–94,** 144

H$_1$ receptor antagonist **91**

H$_2$ receptor antagonist **91**